D1224129

Color Atlas and Text of
Pulmonary Pathology

Color Atlas and Text of Pulmonary Pathology

▶ Editor-in-Chief:

Philip T. Cagle, MD

Professor of Pathology
Director, Center for Pulmonary Pathology
Department of Pathology
Baylor College of Medicine
Attending Pathologist
The Methodist Hospital
Houston, Texas

▶ Associate Editors:

Timothy C. Allen, MD, JD
Chairman
Associate Professor
Department of Pathology
The University of Texas Health Center at Tyler
Tyler, Texas

Roberto Barrios, MD
Associate Professor
Department of Pathology
Baylor College of Medicine
Active Physician
Department of Pathology and Laboratory Medicine
The Methodist Hospital
Houston, Texas

Carlos Bedrossian, MD
Staff Member
Department of Pathology
Northwestern Memorial Hospital
Department of Pathology
Consulting Staff
Norwegian-American Hospital
Chicago, Illinois

Abida K. Haque, MD
Attending Surgical Pathologist
Professor
Department of Pathology
University of Texas Medical Branch
Galveston, Texas

Alvaro C. Laga, MD
Postdoctoral Research Fellow in Pulmonary Pathology
Department of Pathology
Baylor College of Medicine
Houston, Texas

Mary L. Ostrowski, MD
Associate Professor
Department of Pathology
Baylor College of Medicine
Staff Pathologist
Department of Pathology
The Methodist Hospital
Houston, Texas

Dani S. Zander, MD
Professor and Vice Chair
Director of Anatomic Pathology
Department of Pathology and Laboratory Medicine
University of Texas Health Science Center at Houston Medical School
Houston, Texas

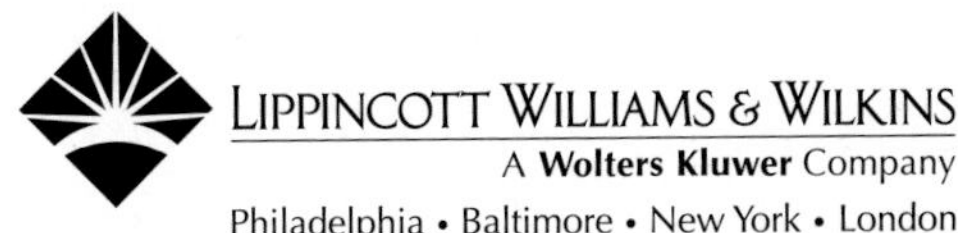

Acquisitions Editor: Jonathan Pine and Ruth W. Weinberg
Developmental Editors: Nicole T. Dernoski
Production Editor: Christiana Sahl
Manufacturing Manager: Benjamin Rivera
Compositor: Graphic World
Printer: Quebecor World

530 Walnut Street
Philadelphia, PA 19106 USA
LWW.com

Printed in the USA

Library of Congress Cataloging-in-Publication Data
Color atlas and text of pulmonary pathology / editor-in-chief, Philip C. Cagle ; associate editors, Timothy C. Allen . . . [et al.].
p. ; cm.
Includes bibliographical references and index.
ISBN 0-7817-3453-3
1. Lungs—Disease—Atlases. I. Cagle, Philip T. II. Allen, Timothy C.
[DNLM: 1. Lung Diseases—pathology—Atlases. WF 17 C719 2005]
RC756.C64 2005
616.2′4--dc22 2004048687

Care has been taken to confirm the accuracy of the information presented and to describe generally accepted practices. However, the authors, editors, and publisher are not responsible for errors or omissions or for any consequences from application of the information in this book and make no warranty, expressed or implied, with respect to the currency, completeness, or accuracy of the contents of the publication. Application of this information in a particular situation remains the professional responsibility of the practitioner.

The authors, editors, and publisher have exerted every effort to ensure that drug selection and dosage set forth in this text are in accordance with current recommendations and practice at the time of publication. However, in view of ongoing research, changes in government regulations, and the constant flow of information relating to drug therapy and drug reactions, the reader is urged to check the package insert for each drug for any change in indications and dosage and for added warnings and precautions. This is particularly important when the recommended agent is a new or infrequently employed drug.

Some drugs and medical devices presented in this publication have Food and Drug Administration (FDA) clearance for limited use in restricted research settings. It is the responsibility of the health care provider to ascertain the FDA status of each drug or device planned for use in their clinical practice.

10 9 8 7 6 5 4 3 2 1

This book is dedicated to the memory of S. Donald Greenberg, MD, one of the pioneers of modern lung pathology and academic father to many of us.

Contents

Section 1

Normal Cytology and Histology 1

Section 2

Artifacts and Age-Related Changes 19

Section 3

Malignant Neoplasms 33

Section 8

Granulomatous Diseases 249

Section 9

Diffuse Pulmonary Hemorrhage 275

Section 10

Pulmonary Hypertension and Emboli 295

Section 11

Large Airways 315

Section 12

Small Airways 327

Section 22

Metabolic Disorders/Storage Diseases 569

Section 23

Non-Neoplastic Lesions of the Pleura 577

Section 24

Pediatric Pulmonary Pathology 593

Contributing Authors

Ilkser Akpolat, MD
Associate Professor
Department of Pathology
Ondokuz Mayis Univeristy
Samsun, Turkey

Avissai Alcántara-Vázquez
Professor of Pathology
Department of Pathology
School of Medicine UNAM
Chairman
Pathology
General Hospital
Mexico City

Timothy Allen, MD, JD
Associate Professor
Department of Pathology
The University of Texas Health Center at Tyler
Chairman
Department of Pathology
The University of Texas Health Center at Tyler
Tyler, Texas

Mojghan Amrikachi, MD
Assistant Professor
Department of Pathology
Baylor College of Medicine
Assistant Professor
Department of Pathology
The Methodist Hospital
Houston, Texas

Judith Aronson, MD
Associate Professor
Director, Autopsy Service
Department of Pathology
University of Texas Medical Branch
Galveston, Texas

Roberto Barrios, MD
Associate Professor
Department of Pathology
Baylor College of Medicine
Active Physician
Pathology and Laboratory Medicine
The Methodist Hospital
Houston, Texas

Mary Beth Beasley, MD
Department of Pathology
Providence Portland Medical Center
Portland, Oregon

Carlos Bedrossian, MD
Staff member
Department of Pathology
Northwestern Memorial Hospital
Consulting Staff
Department of Pathology
Norwegian-American Hospital
Chicago, Illinois

Philip T. Cagle, MD
Professor of Pathology
Director, Center for Pulmonary Pathology
Department of Pathology
Baylor College of Medicine
Attending Pathologist
The Methodist Hospital
Houston, Texas

Hakan Cermik, MD
Visiting Fellow in Pulmonary Pathology
Department of Pathology
Baylor College of Medicine
Houston, Texas
Chief
Department of Pathology
Gulhane Military Medical Academy
Camlica Respiratory Disease Hospital
Istanbul, Turkey

Donna Coffey, MD
Assistant Professor
Department of Pathology
Baylor College of Medicine
Staff
Department of Pathology
The Methodist Hospital
Houston, Texas

Megan Dishop, MD
Assistant Professor
Department of Pathology
Baylor College of Medicine
Pathologist
Department of Pathology
Texas Children's Hospital
Houston, Texas

Florencio Dizon, MD
Research Institute for Tropical Medicine
Manila, Philippines

Armando Fraire, MD
Professor
Department of Pathology
University of Massachusetts Medical School
Pathologist
Department of Pathology
University of Massachusetts Health Care
Worcester, Massachusetts

Abida Haque, MD
Professor
Attending Surgical Pathologist
Department of Pathology
University of Texas Medical Branch
Galveston, Texas

Sajid A. Haque, MD
Fellow
Department of Internal Medicine
Division of Pulmonary, Critical Care, and Sleep Medicine
University of Texas Health Science Center at Houston
Houston, Texas

Jaishree Jagirdar, MD
Professor
Director of Anatomic Pathology
University Health Systems
Department of Pathology
The University of Texas Health Science Center at San Antonio
San Antonio, Texas

Jeffrey Jorgensen, MD, PhD
Assistant Professor
Department of Hematopathology
MD Anderson Cancer Center
Houston, Texas

Andras Khoor, MD
Assistant Professor
Department of Pathology
Mayo Medical School
Rochester, Minnesota
Consultant
Department of Pathology
Mayo Clinic
Jacksonville, Florida

Alvaro C. Laga, MD
Postdoctoral Research Fellow in Pulmonary Pathology
Department of Pathology
Baylor College of Medicine
Houston, Texas

Claire Langston, MD
Professor
Department of Pathology
Baylor College of Medicine
Pathologist
Department of Pathology
Texas Children's Hospital
Houston, Texas

Rodolfo Laucirica, MD
Associate Professor
Department of Pathology
Baylor College of Medicine
Director of Anatomic Pathology
Department of Pathology
Ben Taub General Hospital
Houston, Texas

Daniel Libraty, MD
Assistant Professor of Medicine
University of Massachusetts Medical School
Worcester, Massachusetts

Cesar Moran, MD
Professor of Pathology
Director of Thoracic Pathology
MD Anderson Cancer Center
Houston, Texas

Bruno Murer, MD
Chief
Clinical Laboratory and Anatomic Pathology
Umberto the 1st Hospital ASL N 12 Veneziana
Mestre—Venice, Italy

Juan P. Olano, MD
Assistant Professor
Department of Pathology
University of Texas Medical Branch
Galveston, Texas

Remigo M. Olveda, MD
Research Institute for Tropical Medicine
Manila, Philippines

Nelson Ordonez, MD
Professor of Pathology
Department of Pathology
MD Anderson Cancer Center
Director
Immunohistochemistry Section
MD Anderson Cancer Center
Houston, Texas

Mary Ostrowski, MD
Associate Professor
Department of Pathology
Baylor College of Medicine
Staff Pathologist
Department of Pathology
The Methodist Hospital
Houston, Texas

Helmut Popper, MD
Professor
Institute of Pathology, Laboratory Molecular Cytogenics, Environmental and Respiratory Pathology
University of Graz Medical School
Staff Member
University Hospital Graz
Graz, Austria

Vicki J. Schnadig, MD
Associate Professor
Department of Pathology
University of Texas Medical Branch
Associate Director of Cytopathology
Department of Pathology
University of Texas Medical Branch Hospital and Clinics
Galveston, Texas

Angela Shen, BS
Harvard University
Boston, Massachusetts
Post-Sophomore Fellow
Department of Pathology
Baylor College of Medicine and the Methodist Hospital
Houston, Texas

Charles Stager, PhD
Associate Professor
Department of Pathology
Baylor College of Medicine
Director of Microbiology
Ben Taub General Hospital
Houston, Texas

Bruce A. Woda, MD
Professor of Pathology
University of Massachusetts Medical School
Worcester, Massachusetts

Dani Zander, MD
Professor and Vice Chair
Director of Anatomic Pathology
Department of Pathology and Laboratory Medicine
University of Texas Health Science Center at Houston Medical School
Houston, Texas

Handan Zeren, MD
Professor
Department of Pathology
Cukurova University
Department of Pathology
Cukurova University Hospital
Adana, Turkey

Preface

We have attempted to compile a comprehensive atlas covering common, rare, and newly described lung diseases, both neoplastic and nonneoplastic, in one volume. Topics are organized into sections, chapters, parts, and subparts for ready accessibility. Although diseases are designated according to the most current classification schemes, topics are divided into chapters, parts, and subparts based on their histopathologic distinctiveness, a more intuitive approach for the practicing pathologist. Our objective is to provide a format of color figures and handy lists of diagnostic features that provide clear-cut essentials for diagnosis undiluted by other types of information that can be obtained from other sources when necessary. Our goal for the practicing pathologist is to expedite timely and accurate diagnosis when signing out cases. For students, residents, fellows, and specialty Board applicants, this same format facilitates rapid, comprehensible study of all topics in lung pathology. The use of gross pathology, cytopathology, and histopathology figures and tables in this book allows a multidimensional approach to pathologic diagnoses. We have attempted to illustrate common nonspecific findings, false positive features, and potential diagnostic traps that the practicing pathologist may encounter so that these can be distinguished from specific diseases.

This book was conceived as a tribute to our mentor, one of the outstanding pioneers of modern lung pathology in the 1960s, '70s, and '80s, Dr. S. Donald Greenberg. Dr. Greenberg spent most of his career at Baylor College of Medicine in the Texas Medical Center in Houston and worked closely with community and academic physicians throughout Texas. Above all else, Dr. Greenberg was highly respected as an inspiring teacher to students, housestaff, and practicing pathologists and clinicians, both in the community and in the university, and he received many teaching awards during his career. Therefore, a practical atlas of lung pathology that would be useful to students, housestaff, and practicing pathologists and clinicians, both community based and university based, was felt to be the best tribute to Dr. Greenberg's legacy.

Because of the logistics, it was not possible to include all of Dr. Greenberg's many protégés and students as contributors to this book, so an editorial staff composed of lung pathologists of the Houston-Galveston area plus one of Dr. Greenberg's first protégés, Dr. Carlos Bedrossian, was organized. In addition to the editors, other faculty from the Houston-Galveston area contributed to this book, as did those lung pathologists who came as Visiting Professors to the Texas Medical Center during the time when the book was in preparation.

Our hope is that this book represents a culmination of Dr. Greenberg's work through those who learned from him.

Philip T. Cagle, MD
2-17-2004

Acknowledgments

The editors gratefully acknowledge the following individuals for their generous assistance in the preparation of this book:

- **Francine Allen,** RRT, BSRT
  Research Assistant, Center for Pulmonary Pathology, Baylor College of Medicine, Houston, Texas

- **Richard Bedrossian**
  Information Technology Specialist, Biomedical Communications, Oak Park, Illinois

- **Subhendu Chakraborty,** MS, MSBS
  Instructor, Department of Pathology, Baylor College of Medicine, Houston, Texas

- **Kirsten A. Johnson,** MLIS
  Research Librarian, Center for Pulmonary Pathology, Baylor College of Medicine, Houston, Texas

- **Deanna E. Killen,** HTMLT
  Supervisor of Immunohistochemistry, Department of Pathology Histology Laboratory, Houston, Texas

Section 1

Normal Cytology and Histology

Bronchus

1

▸ Alvaro C. Laga
▸ Timothy Allen
▸ Philip T. Cagle

The airways of the lung are tubular or pipelike structures that conduct air through their lumens. The airways branch into tubes or pipes of increasingly smaller diameter, with larger bronchi dividing into smaller bronchi that branch into smaller bronchioles, which eventually lead into the air sacs or alveoli, where gas exchange occurs. The airways are accompanied by branches of the pulmonary artery that approximate their diameters in cross section.

Bronchi are conducting airways more than 1 mm in diameter. Multiple plates of cartilage in their walls prevent their collapse, permitting them to vary in caliber. In addition to their larger caliber, the histologic features that distinguish bronchi from bronchioles (see Chapter 2) are the presence of respiratory epithelium (pseudostratified ciliated columnar epithelium), bronchial seromucinous glands, cartilage plates, and smooth muscle. There are approximately 9 to 12 generations of bronchi. The left and right mainstem bronchi branch from the trachea at the carina and enter the left lung hilum and right lung hilum, respectively. The left mainstem bronchus is longer and narrower, and it has a greater angle than the right mainstem bronchus. The right upper lobe bronchus branches off the right mainstem bronchus before it enters the hilum. The mainstem bronchi branch into the lobar bronchi, which in turn branch into the segmental bronchi of the bronchopulmonary segments, which in turn branch into generations of smaller bronchi.

Histologic Features:

Histologically, the bronchus consists of a central lumen lined by a mucosa consisting of respiratory epithelium; a submucosa consisting of connective tissue containing bronchial seromucinous glands, capillaries, and lymphatics; a muscularis consisting of smooth muscle; and a connective tissue adventitia that contains lymphatics.

- Bronchial lumens are lined by pseudostratified ciliated columnar epithelium (respiratory epithelium) that rests on a basement membrane; the pseudostratified appearance consists of nuclei of cells arranged as if they are layered one upon another in different strata when actually the bases of all the cells are touching the basement membrane.
- Ciliated columnar epithelial cells make up the majority of the cells of the bronchial epithelium (mucosa); cilia arise from terminal bars in the apices of these cells and project into the bronchial lumen, where they participate in the mucociliary escalator by push-

ing the layer of mucin lying over the bronchial lumen surface cephalad; also present in lesser numbers are goblet cells (columnar cells containing apical mucin), basal cells, and neuroendocrine (Kulchitsky) cells.

- Beneath the surface epithelium is the submucosa, which contains loose connective tissue with longitudinally arranged elastic fibers; bronchial glands (mucous glands) are seromucinous glands with ducts opening into the bronchial lumen present within the submucosa.
- Cartilage plates and smooth muscle bundles lie beneath the mucosa and submucosa.
- Bronchus-associated lymphoid tissue (BALT) consists of lymphoid tissue aggregates in the bronchial submucosal tissue equivalent to the mucosa-associated lymphoid tissue (MALT) of the gastrointestinal tract.

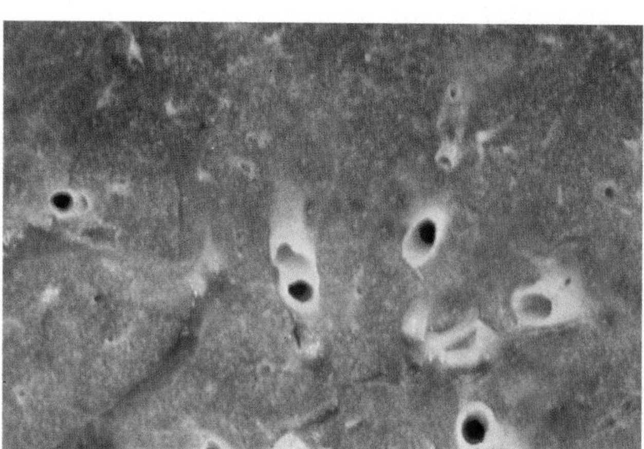

Figure 1.1 Gross figure of normal lung shows spongy tan lung parenchyma, interspersed bronchi, and pulmonary arteries forming bronchovascular bundles.

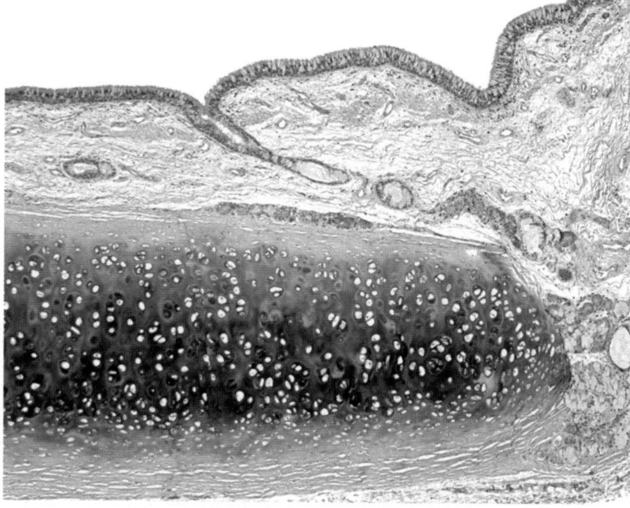

Figure 1.2 Bronchial wall with respiratory epithelium lining the lumen surface and underlying submucosal connective tissue containing a seromucinous gland with its duct connecting to the lumen surface and a cartilage plate.

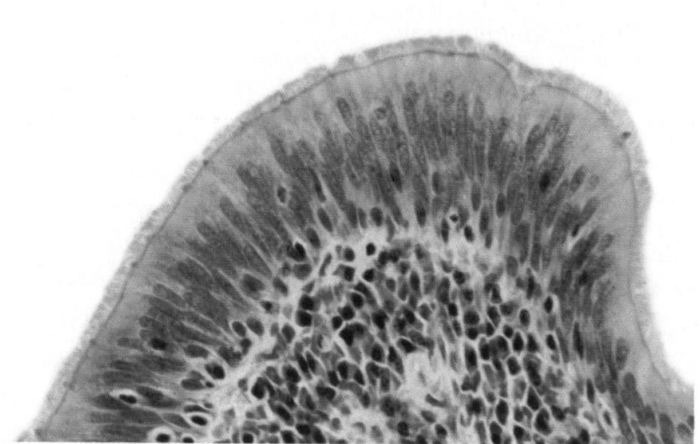

Figure 1.3 Ciliated pseudostratified columnar epithelium shows nuclei arranged as if they are lying in different layers or strata, giving a pseudostratified appearance, but in actuality the bases of all of the cells are touching the basement membrane; the surface of the columnar cells shows cilia arising from terminal bars, which form a dense line between the cell apical surfaces and the overlying cilia; there is an infiltrate of lymphocytes and plasma cells in the submucosa.

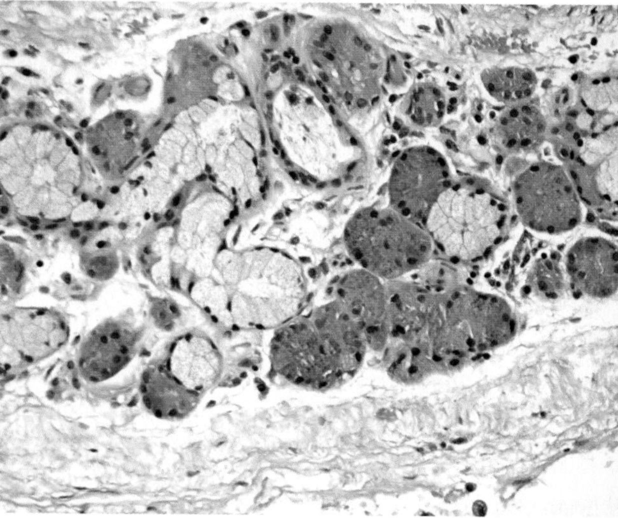

Figure 1.4 Bronchial glands are seromucinous glands in the submucosal connective tissue composed of both serous and mucinous acini.

Bronchioles and Alveolar Ducts

2

▶ Alvaro C. Laga
▶ Timothy Allen
▶ Philip T. Cagle

Bronchioles are defined as conducting airways less than 1 mm in diameter that lack cartilage in their walls. Bronchioles are divided into two groups. The larger (average diameter 0.5–1 mm) terminal (membranous) bronchioles branch from the smallest bronchi and give rise to the smaller (average diameter 0.15–0.2 mm) respiratory bronchioles. The terminal (membranous) bronchioles only conduct air, similar to bronchi, whereas the respiratory bronchioles both conduct air and participate in gas exchange via the alveoli in their walls. The respiratory bronchioles branch into about two more generations of respiratory bronchioles with increasing numbers of alveoli in their walls and give rise to the alveolar ducts.

Terminal bronchioles (membranous bronchioles) are the most distal generation of bronchioles that do not contain alveoli. Terminal bronchioles have a simple columnar epithelium (bronchiolar mucosa) composed of ciliated columnar cells and nonciliated Clara cells, a layer of smooth muscle, and a connective tissue adventitia. Terminal (membranous) bronchioles lack cartilage, and seromucinous glands and goblet cells are generally not observed or are minimal in the normal bronchiolar mucosa. The terminal bronchiole leads into the acinus (a functional unit composed of the structures distal to a single terminal bronchiole—its respiratory bronchioles, alveolar ducts, and alveoli). A lobule is an anatomic unit consisting of the acini of 3 to 10 terminal (membranous) bronchioles that are bounded together by the interlobular septum. As with the bronchi, the bronchioles are accompanied by branches of the pulmonary artery of approximately the same diameter.

Respiratory bronchioles have a bronchiolar wall with simple columnar to cuboidal bronchiolar epithelium and alveoli budding from their walls. The alveoli budding from the bronchiolar walls increase in numbers the higher the generation of the respiratory bronchiole. In two-dimensional longitudinal sections of glass slides, respiratory bronchioles often appear to have a bronchiolar mucosa and wall on one side of their lumen and alveolar spaces on the opposite side of their lumen. Respiratory bronchioles represent the first generation of airways in which exchange of gases occurs.

Alveolar ducts are straight tubular spaces bounded entirely by alveoli and lead to alveolar sacs. They contain numerous outpockets of alveoli protruding from their lumens and lack bronchiolar mucosa or wall.

Histologic Features:

- Membranous (terminal) bronchioles are lined by ciliated simple columnar epithelium.
- Respiratory bronchioles consist of both simple columnar epithelium and alveoli.
- Alveolar ducts are spaces lined by alveoli.

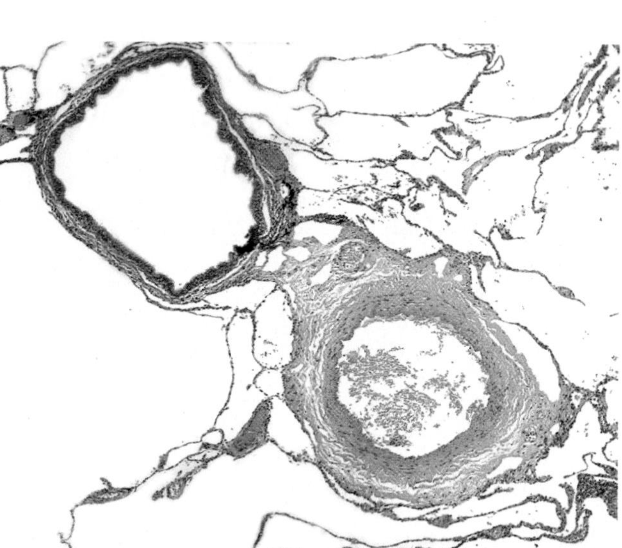

Figure 2.1 Cross section of a terminal (membranous) bronchiole with its lumen lined by simple ciliated columnar epithelium and an accompanying small muscular pulmonary artery.

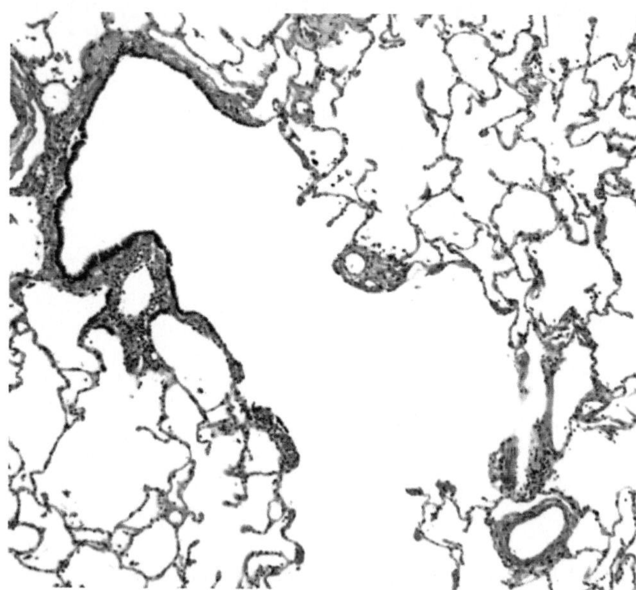

Figure 2.2 Longitudinal section of a terminal (membranous) bronchiole opening into a respiratory bronchiole; the latter consists of a bronchiole with alveoli budding from its wall, displaying simple columnar epithelium on one side of the lumen and alveoli on the other side.

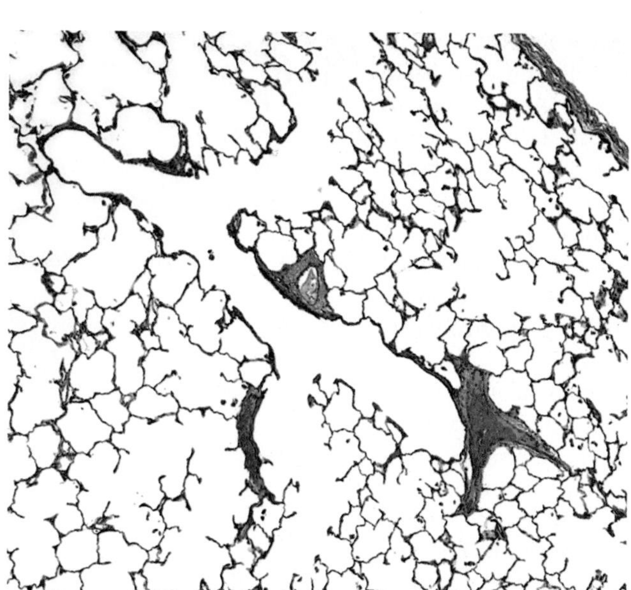

Figure 2.3 Longitudinal section of respiratory bronchiole (lumen lined by bronchiolar epithelium and alveoli) branching into alveolar ducts (lumens lined by alveoli only).

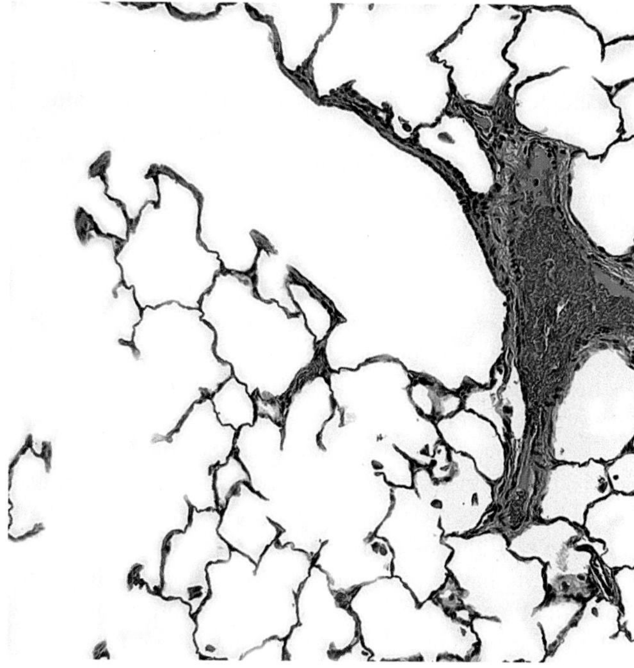

Figure 2.4 Higher power shows respiratory bronchiole lined on one side by simple columnar epithelium and alveoli on the other side; it is accompanied by a small arterial vessel.

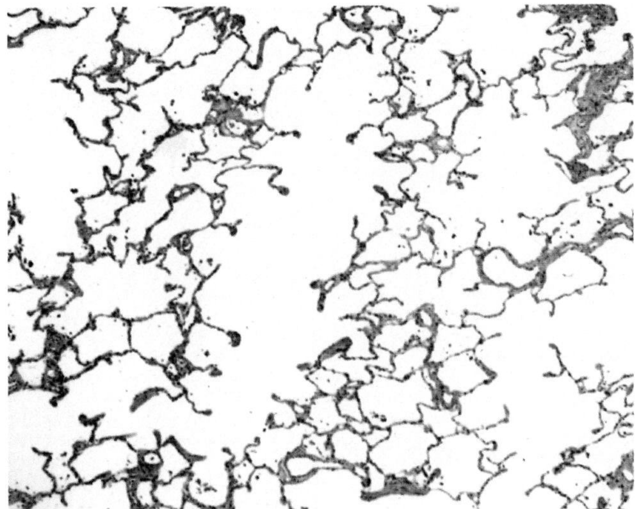

Figure 2.5 Alveolar duct consists of tubular space lined by alveoli and terminates in alveolar sacs.

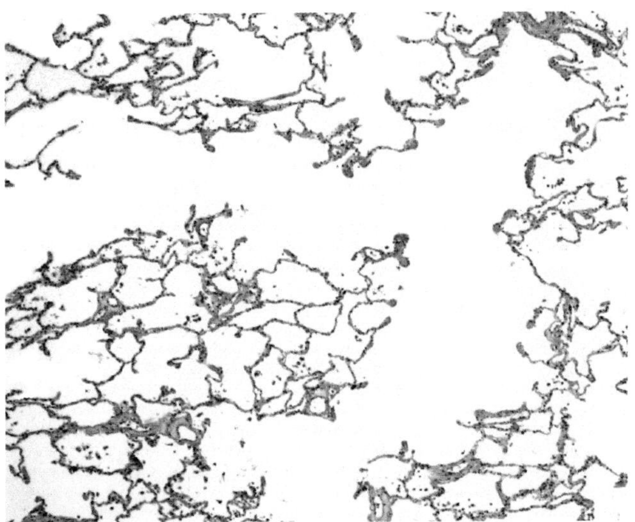

Figure 2.6 Alveolar ducts have walls composed of alveoli.

Blood Vessels and Lymphatics

3

▶ Alvaro C. Laga
▶ Timothy Allen
▶ Philip T. Cagle

The pulmonary vasculature involved in gas exchange includes pulmonary arteries and arterioles that bring blood relatively low in oxygen and high in carbon dioxide from the heart to the gas exchange areas, alveolar capillaries where the gas exchange occurs, and pulmonary venules and veins that return oxygenated blood to the heart. Bronchial arteries and veins are part of the systemic circulation and provide oxygen and nutrients to the bronchi.

Pulmonary arteries branch into increasingly smaller vessels accompanying the bronchi and bronchioles, often with a common connective tissue sheath (bronchovascular bundle), and have a cross-section diameter approximately equal to that of the accompanying airway. Gas exchange occurs in capillaries in the alveolar septa, and venules merge into increasingly larger veins that return oxygenated blood to the heart. Veins are found in the interlobular septa and pleura.

The large branches of the pulmonary artery are elastic arteries, although the elastic fibers are more fragmented than in the aorta. The elastic pulmonary arteries give rise to the muscular pulmonary arteries that accompany the bronchioles. Arteries have two elastic lamina, but smaller arterioles often have only one elastic lamina. Veins also have only one elastic lamina. Histologic differentiation of venules from arterioles may be very difficult.

Lymphatic channels are found in the bronchovascular bundles, in the interlobular septa, along pulmonary veins, and in the pleura. Lymphatics are generally histologically inconspicuous. Certain diseases, such as sarcoidosis, tend to be distributed along lymphatics (lymphangitic distribution).

Histologic Features:

- Muscular pulmonary arteries have a tunica media of circularly oriented smooth muscle lying between internal and external elastic lamina.
- Pulmonary arteries have a thin tunica media compared to systemic arteries.
- Pulmonary veins have a single elastic lamina and gradually acquire a muscular media downstream.
- The tunica media of pulmonary veins consists of circularly oriented smooth muscle with interspersed elastic fibers.

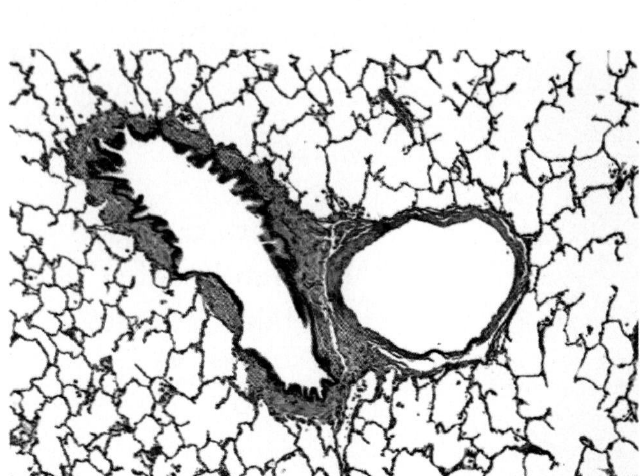

Figure 3.1 Bronchovascular bundle containing cross sections of a small muscular pulmonary artery and an accompanying terminal (membranous) bronchiole of equivalent diameter.

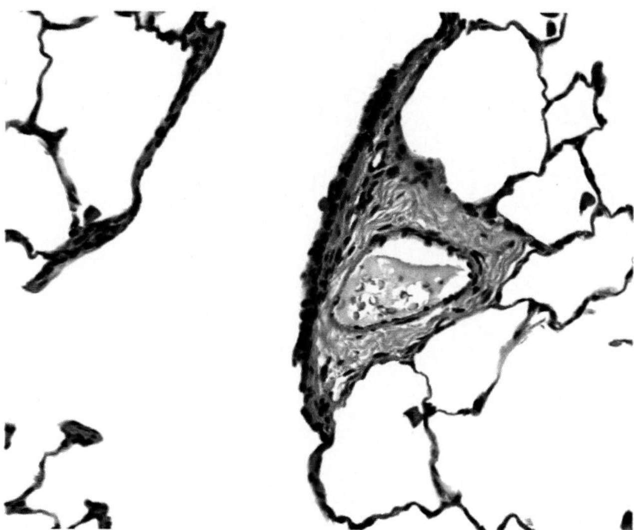

Figure 3.2 Small vessel associated with respiratory bronchiole.

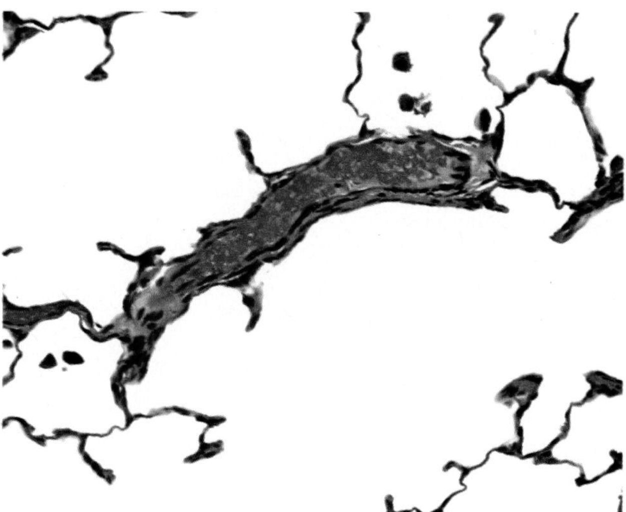

Figure 3.3 Small vessel lying between alveolar ducts.

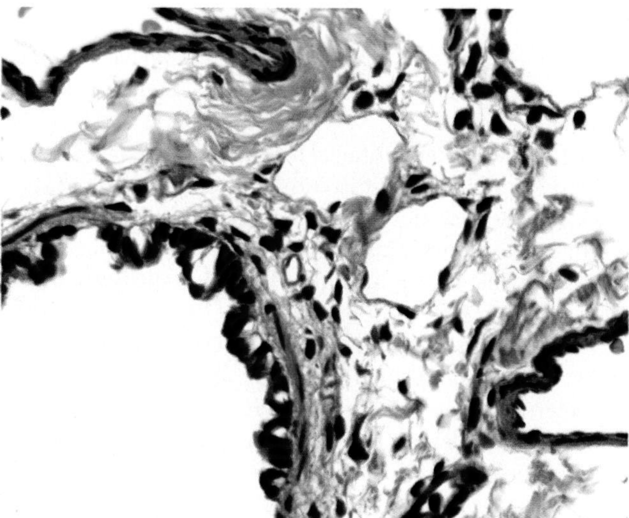

Figure 3.4 Cross section of lumens of two lymphatic vessels lined by inconspicuous flat endothelial cells within the connective tissue of a bronchovascular bundle.

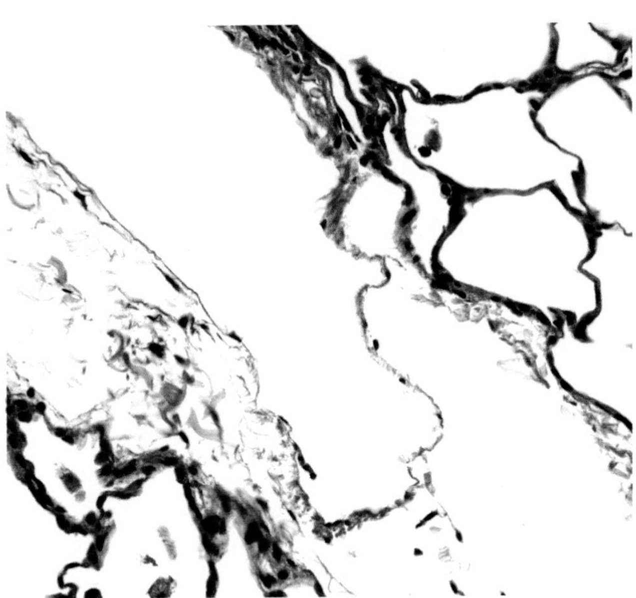

Figure 3.5 High power of a lymphatic vessel within an interlobular septum.

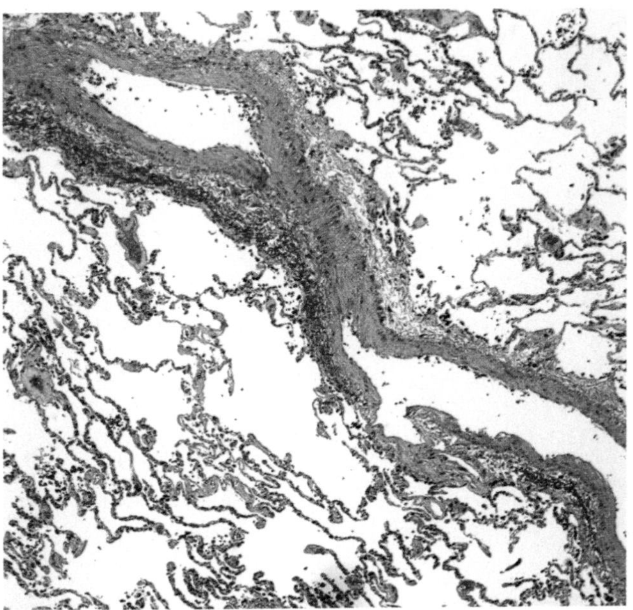

Figure 3.6 Longitudinal section of a pulmonary vein within an interlobular septum.

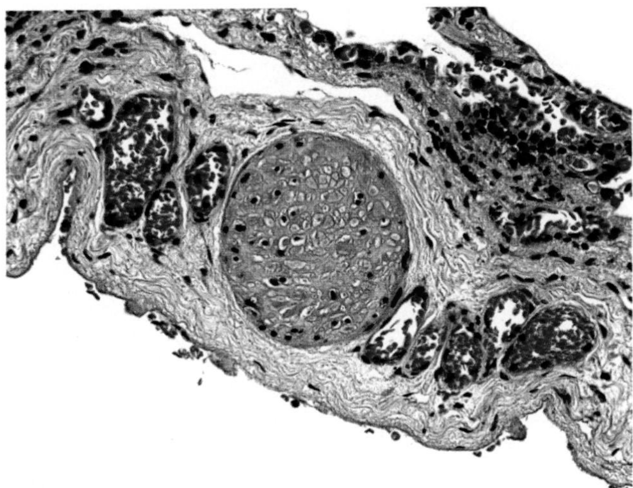

Figure 3.7 Pleura showing a cross section of the media of a vessel (which should not be mistaken for nerve or granuloma) and adjacent small blood vessels and lymphatics.

4

Alveoli

▶ Alvaro C. Laga
▶ Timothy Allen
▶ Philip T. Cagle

Alveoli are saclike evaginations of the respiratory bronchioles, alveolar ducts, and alveolar sacs where the exchange of gases between the inhaled air and the blood in the alveolar capillaries occurs. The numerous tiny alveoli produce a tremendous surface area for gas exchange that is compactly arranged in the lungs. The wall or septum of each alveolus is normally very thin in order to permit gas exchange. It consists of epithelial cells on the surface of the lumen (pneumocytes), the endothelial cells of the capillaries, and basement membranes of the pneumocytes and endothelial cells that are typically fused. The pneumocytes are divided into two types. (i) Type 1 pneumocytes are thin flat cells that make up 90% of the surface of the alveolar lumen. They have a very thin cytoplasm across which gas exchange occurs. (ii) Type 2 pneumocytes are cuboidal cells that produce and secrete surfactant, give rise to type 1 pneumocytes, and are involved in alveolar repair. An occasional myofibroblast may be encountered in the alveolar septum. The orifices of alveoli along the alveolar ducts and alveolar sacs are composed of elastic and collagen bundles that are a continuation of the bronchial and bronchiolar elastic bundles. All of the elastic fibers, including the alveolar meshwork, are interconnected in all directions, forming an integrated elastic network essential to the uniform expansion and contraction of the lung during respiration.

Histologic Features:

- The interalveolar septum consists of two thin epithelial layers, between which lie capillaries, occasional myofibroblasts, and elastic and reticular fibers; macrophages may be present on the surface or within the septum.
- There are two types of alveolar lining cells: type 1 and type 2 pneumocytes.
- Type 1 alveolar pneumocytes are large flat cells lining the lumen surface; they cover approximately 90% of the alveolar surface and are believed to be incapable of division.
- Type 2 alveolar pneumocytes are cuboidal cells characterized by a large basal nucleus with a prominent nucleolus and abundant ultrastructural lamellar inclusions (surfactant); they are capable of division and therefore may become hyperplasic in response to alveolar damage.

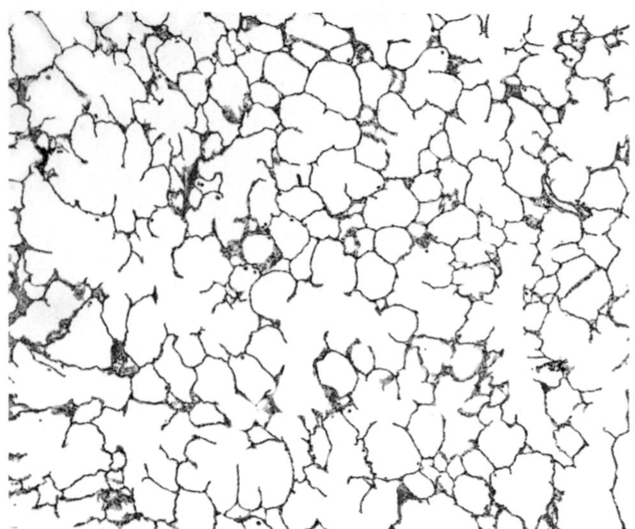

Figure 4.1 Low power shows normal lung parenchyma with numerous alveoli cut in cross section, many of them arising from alveolar sacs and alveolar ducts, creating a tremendous surface area for gas exchange between the air in the alveolar lumens and the capillaries within their very thin walls or septa.

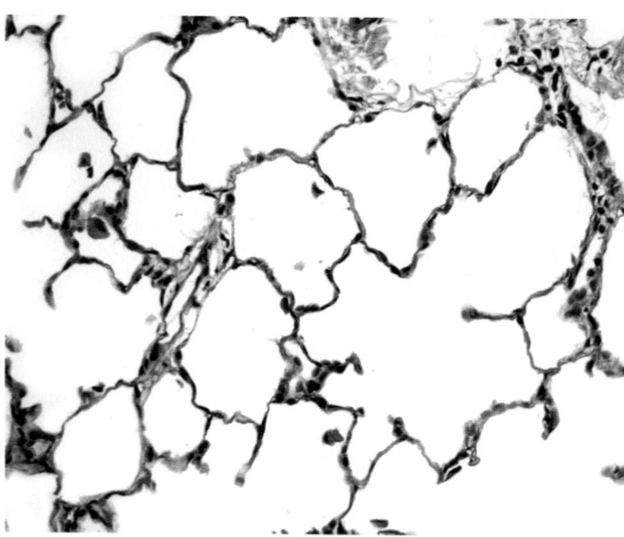

Figure 4.2 Higher power shows the alveoli's thin delicate walls or septa containing inconspicuous capillaries; nuclei of several types of cells, which are not always distinguishable by light microscopy, represent nuclei of flat, simple, lining epithelial cells (type 1 pneumocytes), nuclei of occasional cuboidal epithelial cells (type 2 pneumocytes), capillary endothelial cell nuclei, and scattered lymphocytes, mesenchymal cells, and macrophages.

5

Pleura

▶ Alvaro C. Laga
▶ Timothy Allen
▶ Philip T. Cagle

The pleura is the serous membrane that covers the lung and thoracic pleural cavity. The lung sits within the thoracic cavity. The visceral pleura covers the outer surface of the lung parenchyma, and the parietal pleura covers the inner surface of the thoracic cavity, creating a pleural cavity between them. Under normal conditions, the pleural cavity contains only a thin film of liquid that acts as a lubricant, facilitating the sliding of the two surfaces against each other during respiratory movements.

Both outer pleural surfaces are covered by a single layer of flattened mesothelial cells. The connective tissue of the visceral pleura contains arteries and veins that are mostly thought to be part of the bronchial (systemic) circulation, but this is controversial and probably does not account for all of the visceral pleural circulation. Shunts between the systemic and pulmonary arteries and veins occur increasingly with age and chronic disease. In older patients, bronchial arteries in the visceral pleura may be sclerotic and obliterated. In inflammatory conditions, systemic blood vessels may invade the visceral pleura in adhesions between the visceral pleura and chest wall. The visceral pleura has branches of the vagus nerve and sympathetic trunk but does not contain pain nerve fibers. Pleuritic chest pain always originates in the parietal pleura.

Histologic Features:

- The pleural membranes are composed of a single layer of simple flat surface cells known as mesothelial cells resting on a connective tissue layer that contains collagen and elastic fibers.
- The mesothelium is composed of a single layer of flat polygonal cells with central nuclei.
- Ultrastructurally, the mesothelium possesses long sinuous microvilli covered by a thick glycocalyx.
- Both the visceral and parietal pleurae carry lymphatics and blood vessels.

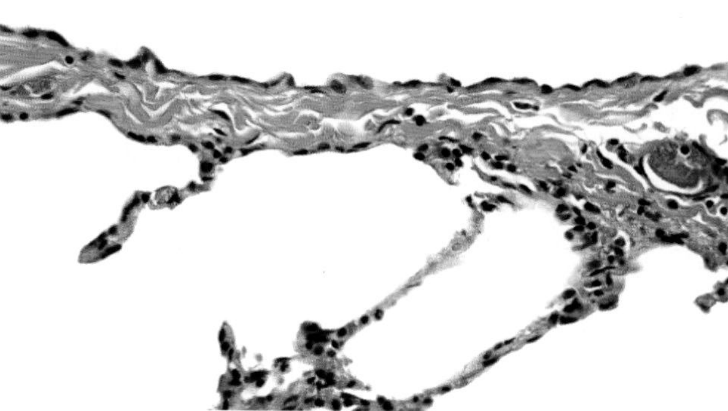

Figure 5.1 Visceral pleura shows a connective tissue layer overlying alveolar parenchyma and is lined on the outer pleural surface by a single layer of simple flat mesothelial cells.

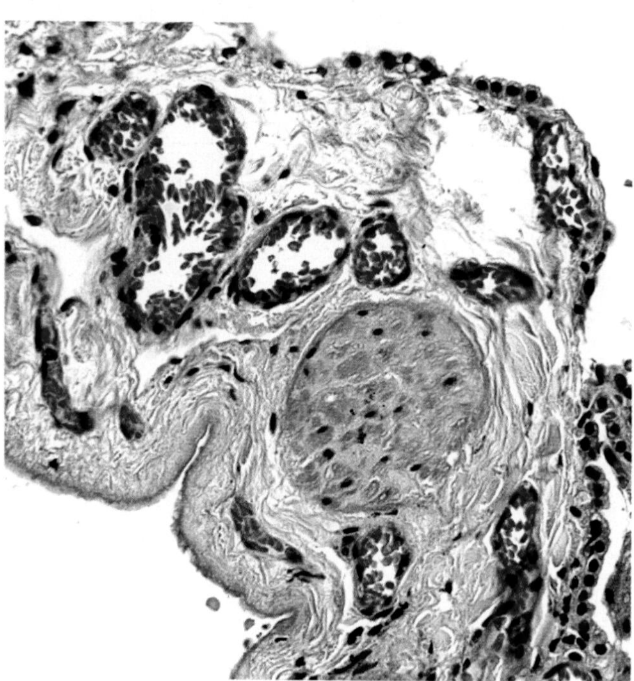

Figure 5.2 Pleura shows the thickened media of a vessel cut in cross section (which should not be confused with nerve or granuloma) and smaller blood vessels and lymphatics.

Normal Cytology of the Lung and Pleura

6

- Alvaro C. Laga
- Timothy Allen
- Mary Ostrowski
- Philip T. Cagle

Normal cells lining the airways and alveolar spaces are encountered in exfoliative cytology specimens from the lung. The normal cell population in exfoliative cytology specimens includes ciliated columnar cells, mucous goblet cells, basal reserve cells, macrophages, and inflammatory cells. There is some variation in the cells encountered, depending on the procedure used. An essential assessment for all exfoliative pulmonary cytology specimens is whether there has been an adequate sampling. The criterion used in sputum cytology is the presence of alveolar macrophages. For bronchial brush and wash specimens, ciliated columnar cells, in addition to alveolar macrophages, should be identified for the specimen to be considered satisfactory. These same cells, including macrophages, are encountered in bronchoalveolar lavage.

Mesothelial cells are frequently encountered in exfoliative cytology specimens of pleural fluid. Generally, mesothelial cells shed into pleural effusions are considered to be reactive. The cytologic reactive changes of exfoliated mesothelial cells may be minimal, or they may be so severe as to mimic malignancy (see Chapter 130). In addition, acute and chronic inflammatory cells and red blood cells frequently appear in cytologic specimens.

Histologic Features:

Lung

- Ciliated columnar cells have a columnar or flask shape, cilia, and a terminal bar.
- Goblet cells possess basal nuclei and a clear cytoplasm.
- Basal reserve cells are usually seen attached to a strip of ciliated columnar cells or as a honeycomb arrangement of small cells with scant cytoplasm.
- Alveolar macrophages characteristically show a single nucleus and abundant cytoplasm; anthracotic pigment can often be seen in their cytoplasm.
- Type 2 alveolar pneumocytes can be recognized in bronchial washings and lavages as round cells with foamy cytoplasm, medium-sized nuclei, and prominent nucleoli.
- Squamous cells are often seen in sputum specimens and occasionally in bronchial specimens; if single superficial or intermediate cells are present in a bronchial specimen, they generally represent oral contamination.

Pleura

- So-called "normal" mesothelial cells that are shed into pleural fluid are generally reactive.
- Mesothelial cells have round or oval nuclei, thin nuclear membranes, single or multiple nucleoli, and vesicular or finely granular chromatin.
- Mesothelial cells possess dark cyanophilic cytoplasm and microvilli on the cell surface, giving the cells a fuzzy outer border.
- Vacuolization within the cytoplasm may occur.
- Multinucleation and mitotic figures may occur.
- Small aggregates with intercellular spaces ("windows") may be seen.

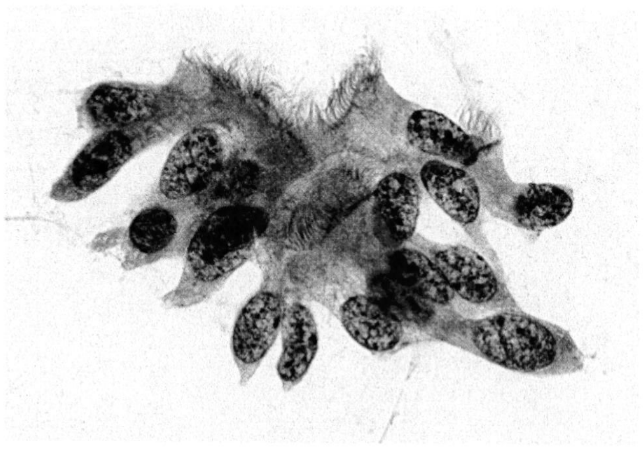

Figure 6.1 Bronchial epithelial cells in an exfoliative cytology specimen consist of flask-shaped columnar cells with prominent apical cilia and terminal bars, and smooth-contoured basal nuclei with finely granular chromatin and small nucleoli.

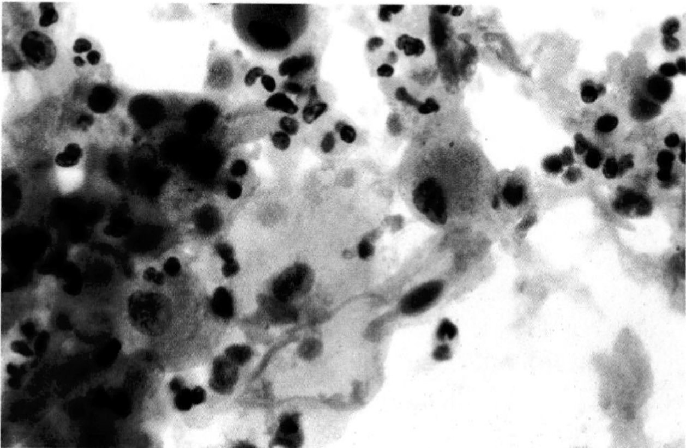

Figure 6.2 Sputum cytology with benign squamous cells, alveolar macrophages, some of which are pigmented, and neutrophils.

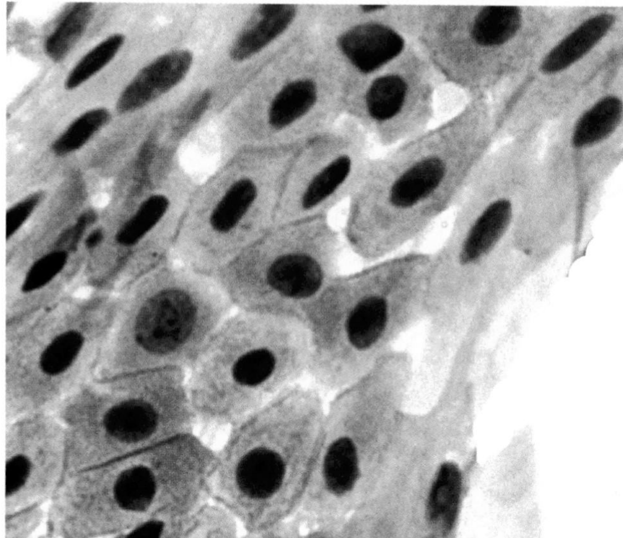

Figure 6.3 Sheet of mildly reactive mesothelial cells in a pleural fluid shows uniform polygonal cells with round to oval nuclei, sharp cell borders, and spaces or "windows" between some of the cells.

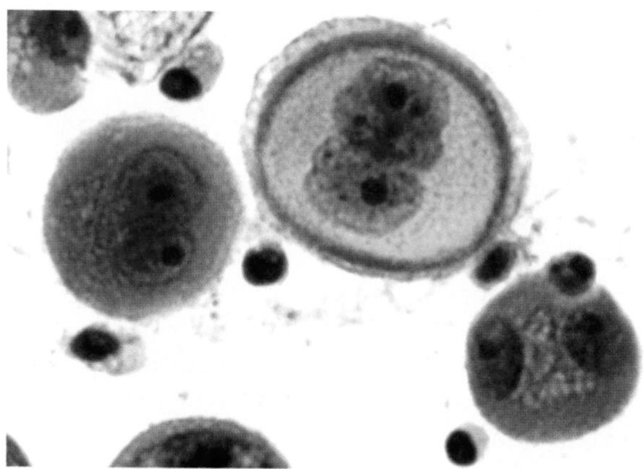

Figure 6.4 High power shows multinucleated reactive mesothelial cells; the distinct cell membrane and fuzzy outer border of the larger cell are prominent in this exfoliative cytology specimen.

Section 2

Artifacts and Age-Related Changes

Procedural and Laboratory Artifacts

7

▶ Alvaro C. Laga
▶ Timothy Allen
▶ Philip T. Cagle

The biopsy procedure itself, both transbronchial biopsies performed with biopsy forceps and surgical procedures to obtain wedge biopsies, and subsequent events related to the handling of the biopsy can result in artifacts that should not be misinterpreted as pathologic processes. Several of the commonly encountered artifacts in lung biopsies are listed and illustrated here.

Histologic Features:

- Crush artifact from forceps including (i) compression of alveolar parenchyma that gives a false impression of interstitial fibrosis or cellular infiltrates, (ii) compression of alveolar parenchyma creating rounded spaces that may be confused with fungus or lipid vacuoles, (iii) compression of bronchial lymphocytes or other cells that may be misinterpreted as small cell carcinoma, and (iv) compression of large bronchial vessels or other components of the bronchial wall that may give a false impression of interstitial fibrosis.
- Intraalveolar hemorrhage caused by the biopsy procedure may give a false impression of intraalveolar hemorrhage from disease.
- Materials from surgical gloves (starch or talc), cotton fibers from pads, or sutures may mimic organisms or exposures to exogenous dusts or other materials; these may be highlighted on special stains or polarized light (cotton fibers are "Gomori methenamine-silver [GMS] positive").
- Ordinary dust, dirt, and fibers that may settle on a slide in the laboratory will often be birefringent on polarized light and should not be mistaken for foreign material present in the patient's lungs.
- Drying or improper fixation of the specimen may make tissue difficult to interpret.
- Overinflation of specimens may mimic emphysema, whereas lack of inflation may give a false impression of fibrosis or cellular infiltrates in the alveolar parenchyma.
- Clamping of specimen may cause lymphatic dilation and edema.
- Neutrophils may marginate during surgery and give a false impression of acute inflammation or acute capillaritis.

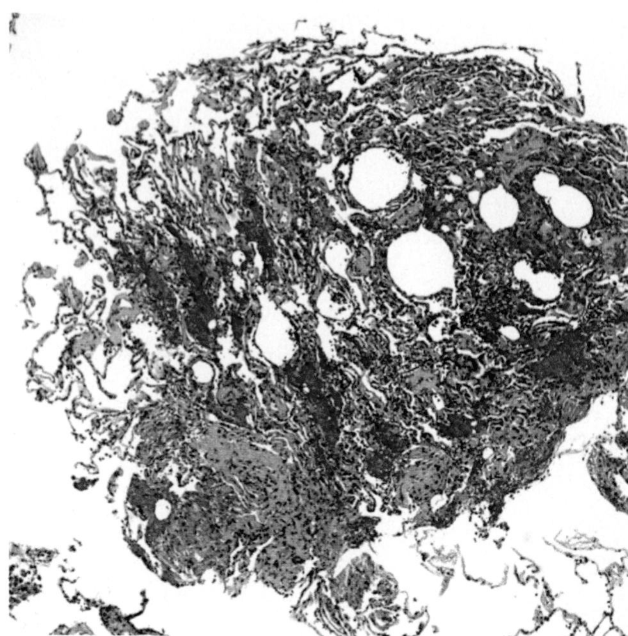

Figure 7.1 Low power of a transbronchial biopsy shows compression of the specimen, creating a false impression of increased interstitial cellularity and fibrosis and artifactual rounded holes that might be mistaken for fungal organisms or lipid.

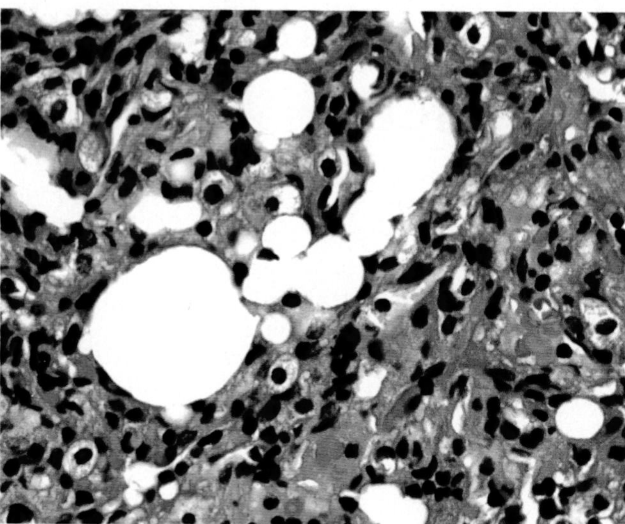

Figure 7.2 Higher power of transbronchial biopsy with compression of the specimen causing a false appearance of increased interstitial cellularity and fibrosis and artifactual rounded holes that might be mistaken for fungal organisms or lipid.

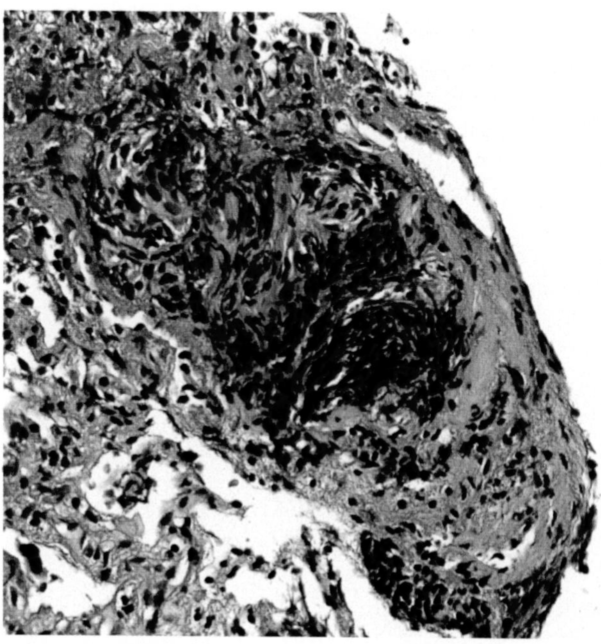

Figure 7.3 High power of transbronchial biopsy with crush artifact of lymphocytes, suggesting the possibility of small cell carcinoma.

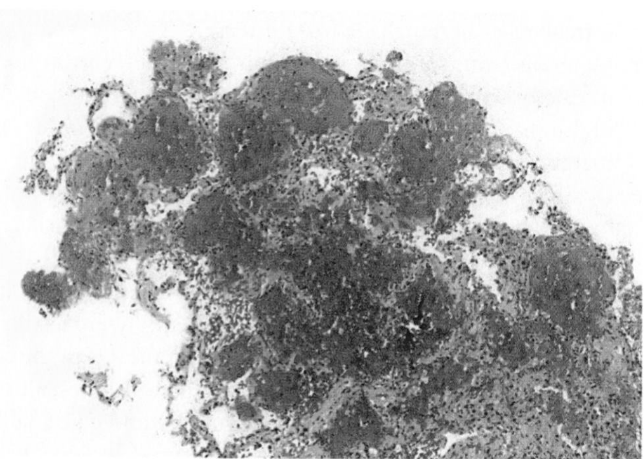

Figure 7.4 Low power of transbronchial biopsy with fresh intraalveolar hemorrhage secondary to the biopsy procedure.

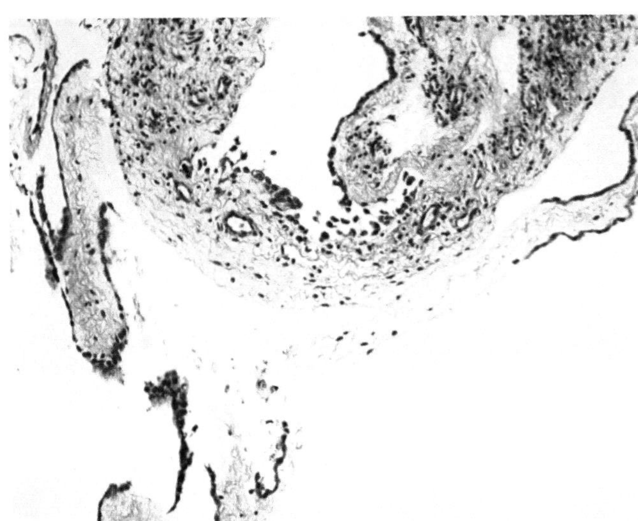

Figure 7.5 This transbronchial biopsy has penetrated and sampled pleura with mesothelial cells, resulting in an unexpected finding that may be confusing.

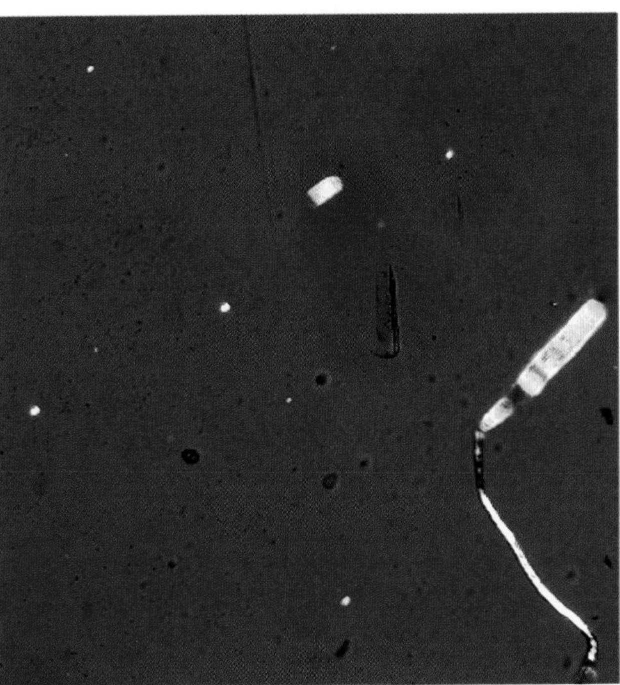

Figure 7.6 Examination of this transbronchial biopsy with polarized light shows birefringent ordinary dust, dirt, and fibers that have accumulated on the slide in the laboratory and should not be mistaken for foreign materials from the patient's lung.

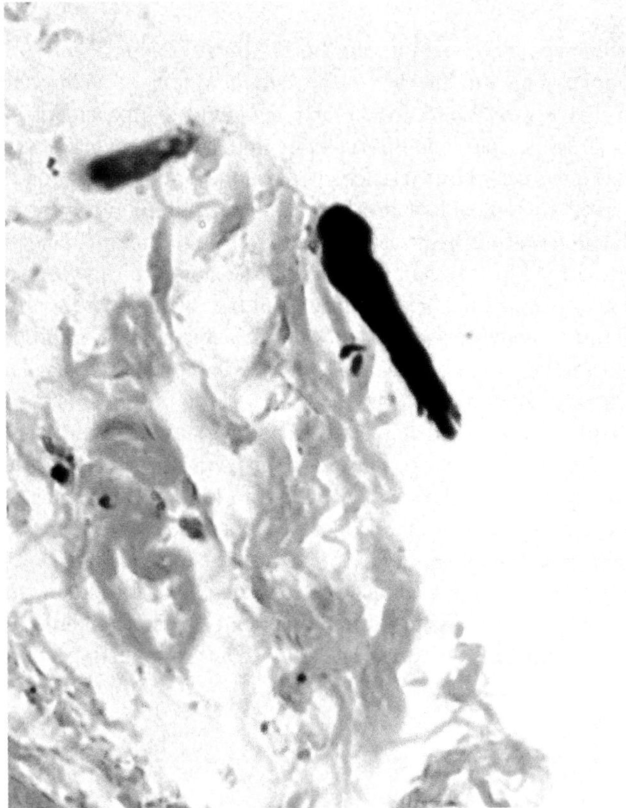

Figure 7.7 GMS stain of a cotton fiber may give a false impression of a fungal organism.

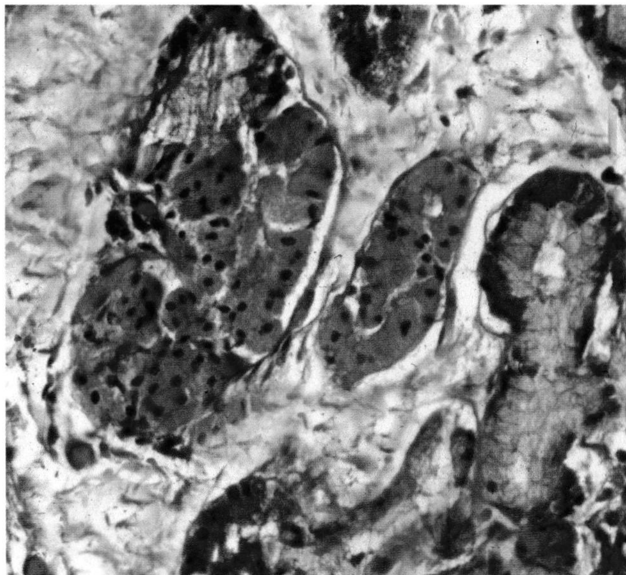

Figure 8.1 Bronchial seromucinous glands may show oncocytic change of glandular epithelium (cells with abundant granular eosinophilic cytoplasm) with age.

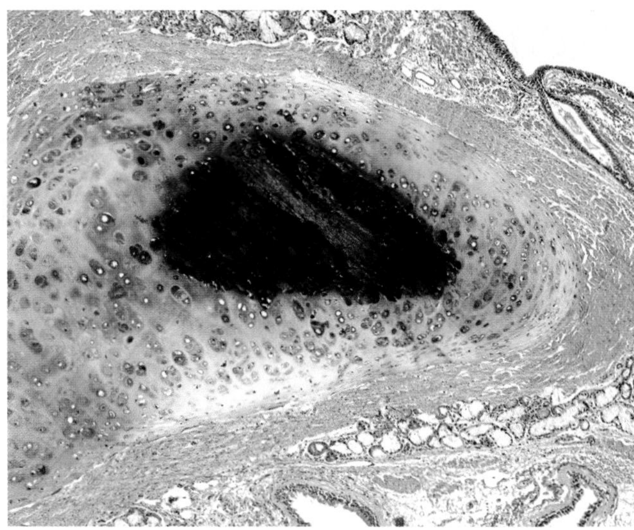

Figure 8.2 Bronchial cartilage may show calcification and/or ossification as patients age.

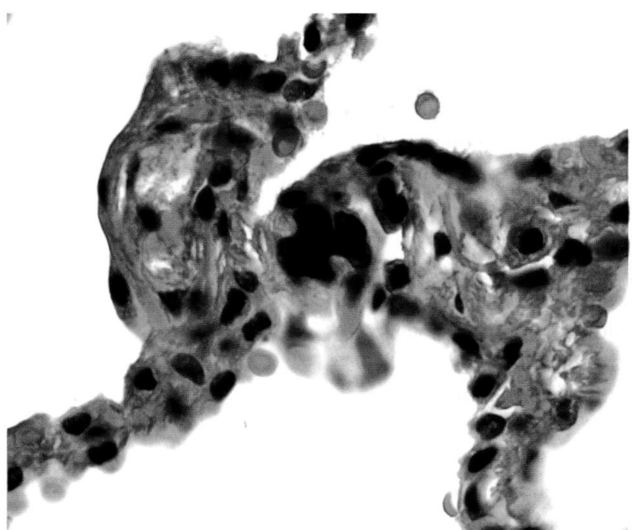

Figure 8.3 Megakaryocytes are normally found in the pulmonary circulation and may increase in certain conditions; the large, dark, multilobed appearance of these cells may suggest viral inclusions or malignant cells.

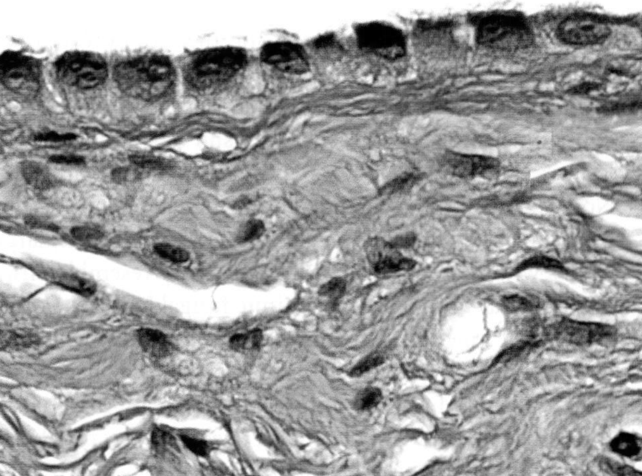

Figure 8.4 A row of reactive cuboidal mesothelial cells on the pleural surface stands out compared to normally flat inconspicuous mesothelial cells.

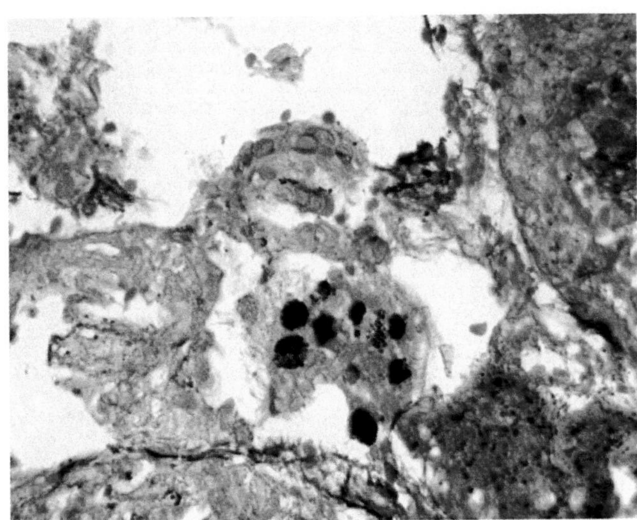

Figure 8.5 Mucin stains positive with GMS and may suggest fungus when round mucin droplets in goblet cells (shown here) or seromucinous glands are stained.

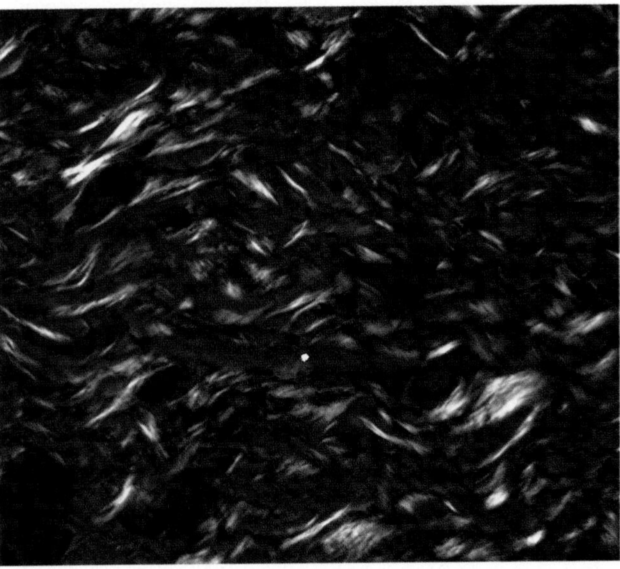

Figure 8.6 Collagen often is birefringent under polarized light and should not be mistaken for foreign material.

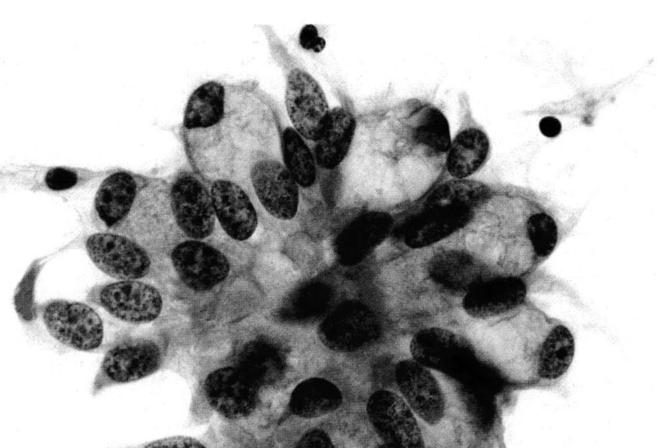

Figure 8.7 Goblet cells from the bronchial epithelium in this exfoliative cytology specimen are distended by cytoplasmic mucin.

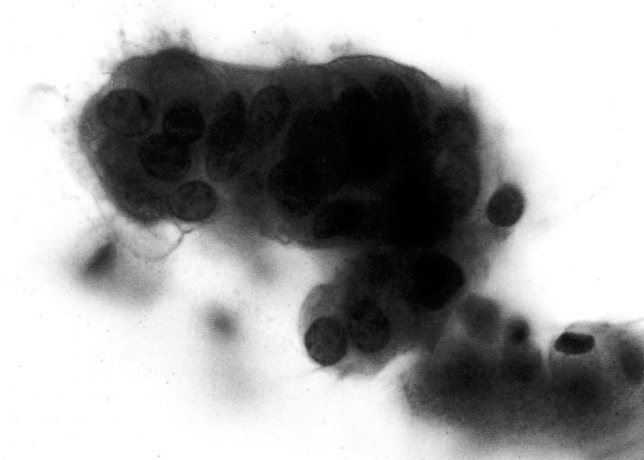

Figure 8.8 Creola body consists of densely cellular, tightly cohesive papillary fragments of bronchial epithelium with cilia visible along the border.

Noncellular Structures

9

- Alvaro C. Laga
- Timothy Allen
- Carlos Bedrossian
- Mary Ostrowski
- Philip T. Cagle

A variety of noncellular structures may be incidentally observed in lung tissue samples. They may be produced endogenously in both pathologic and nonpathologic conditions or may be exogenous materials inhaled into the lungs. The exogenous and endogenous materials associated with specific disease conditions are discussed elsewhere, including Chapters 35, 55, 59, 64, 78, 79, 80, 85, 125, 126, and 127.

Histologic Features:

- Corpora amylacea (30–200 μm) are round to oval endogenous concretions arranged in concentric layers; radiating lines may cross the more prominent concentric laminations; they may have a black or birefringent central core; typically pale pink on hematoxylin and eosin (H&E) stain: found in alveoli and alveolar walls; may be surrounded by a rim of macrophages; periodic acid-Schiff (PAS) positive (stain bright magenta); composed of glycoproteins and lack iron and calcium; no known clinical significance but may form around irritating inhaled particles or secretions.
- Psammoma bodies are round calcified basophilic endogenous concretions arranged in concentric layers; PAS-positive center; may be birefringent with a Maltese cross pattern; occur in papillary malignancies.
- Blue bodies, Schaumann bodies, asteroid bodies, and calcium oxalate crystals are formed by histiocytes and multinucleated giant cells; they may be found either within these cells or in the interstitium or alveolar spaces after extrusion from the cells or death of the cells; more than one type of these structures may be found in the same specimen; these structures are often seen in sarcoidosis granulomas but are found in many other types of granuloma.
- Blue bodies (15–40 μm) are round to oval, basophilic calcified concretions arranged in concentric layers; formed in histiocytes and macrophages but found in interstitium and alveolar spaces; positive for PAS, Alcian blue, and iron stain; birefringent; they should not be mistaken for exogenous foreign material.
- Schaumann bodies (25–200 μm) are irregularly shaped, basophilic calcified concretions arranged in concentric layers; formed in multinucleated giant cells in granulomatous

diseases but may be seen in interstitium; composed of calcium, iron, and mucopolysaccharides; positive for iron stain; may be birefringent; they should not be mistaken for exogenous foreign material.

- Asteroid bodies (5–30 μm) consist of eosinophilic needle-shaped structures arranged in a stellate pattern within a cleared space in the cytoplasm of multinucleated giant cells in granulomatous diseases; they are composed of cell organelles; they should not be mistaken for organisms, such as fungus, or exogenous foreign material.
- Calcium oxalate crystals (1–20 μm) are translucent, irregular sheet crystals that are brightly birefringent on polarized light; they are found in the cytoplasm of multinucleated giant cells in granulomatous inflammation; large numbers of calcium oxalate crystals may be produced by *Aspergillus niger;* they should not be mistaken for exogenous foreign material.
- Other endogenous structures include rhomboid to needle-shaped Charcot-Leyden crystals, which are formed from eosinophil granules and associated with asthma and other eosinophilic conditions (see Chapter 59, part 2); needle-shaped cleared spaces or cholesterol clefts within multinucleated giant cells (see Chapter 82); and foam cells consisting of macrophages with numerous bubbly cytoplasmic vacuoles containing lipid (see Chapter 73).
- Inhaled or aspirated materials or structures including pollen, vegetable matter, anthracotic pigment, smoker's pigment, and inorganic dusts and fibers can be seen in pulmonary histology and cytology specimens.
- Curschmann spirals are spiral-shaped mucinous casts of bronchioles seen in exfoliative cytology specimens from patients with asthma or chronic bronchitis.

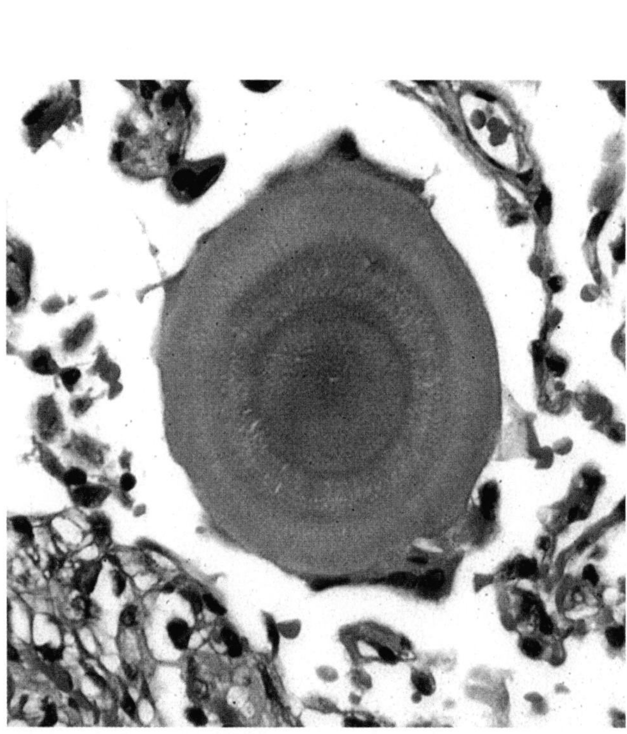

Figure 9.1 Corpora amylacea "free floating" in an alveolar space shows oval pink body with concentric rings, fine radiating lines, and macrophages along the outer rim.

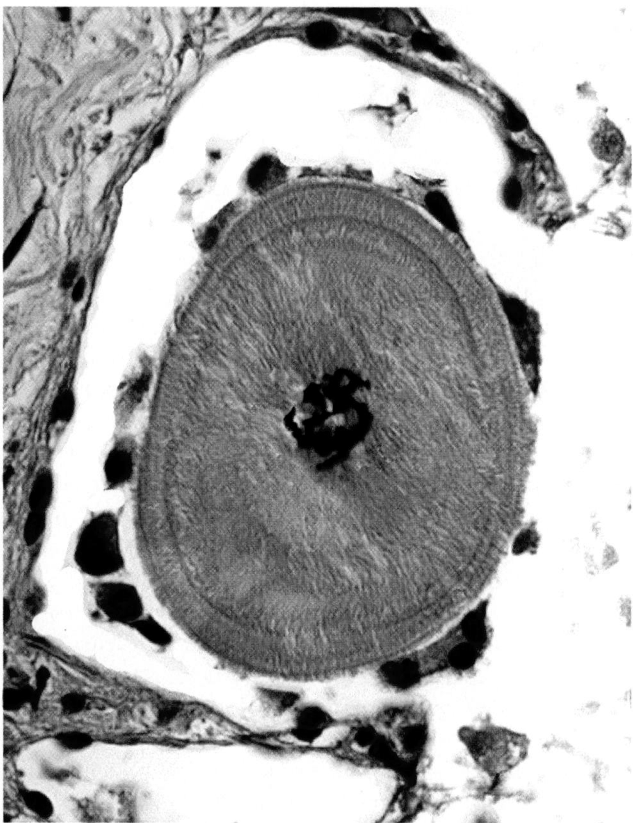

Figure 9.2 Corpora amylacea in an alveolar space with black filaments as a central core surrounded by oval bluish-pink body with concentric rings, finely fibrillar radiating lines, and macrophages on the outer periphery.

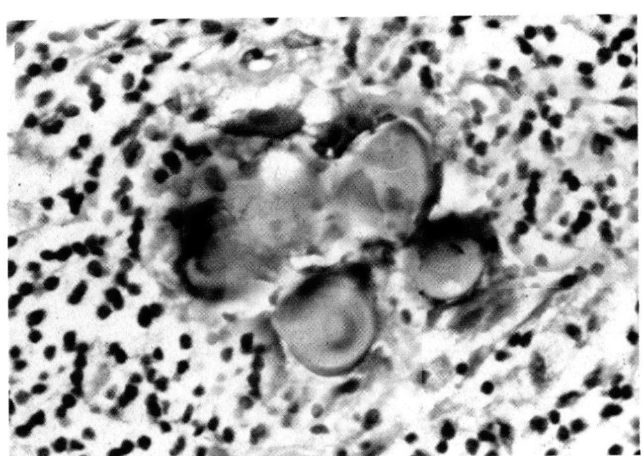

Figure 9.3 Blue bodies consist of an interstitial cluster of oval basophilic calcified structures with focal concentric rings.

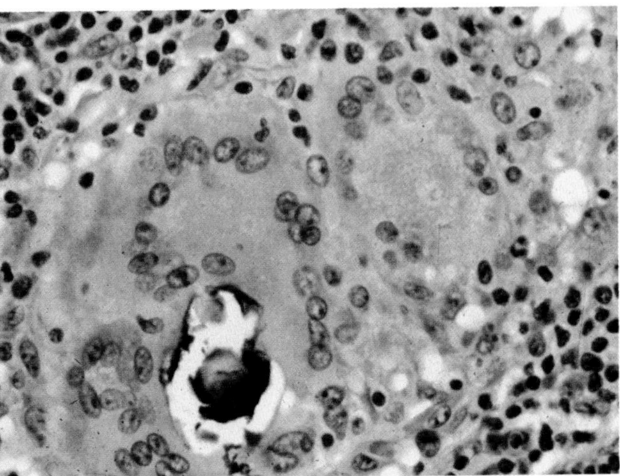

Figure 9.4 Schaumann body consists of fragmented irregular calcified basophilic refractile structure in the cytoplasm of a multinucleated giant cell in a sarcoidosis granuloma.

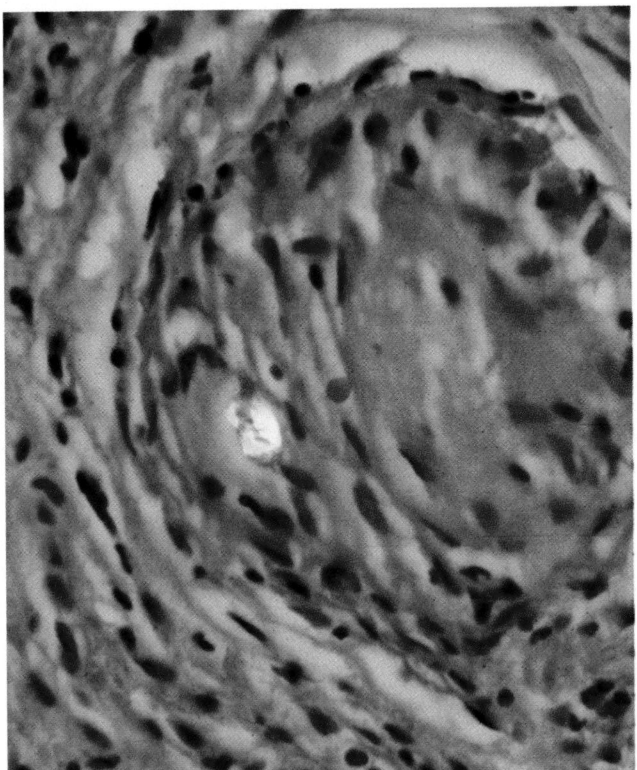

Figure 9.5 Calcium oxalate crystal in the cytoplasm of a multinucleated giant cell in a sarcoidosis granuloma is highly birefringent on polarized light.

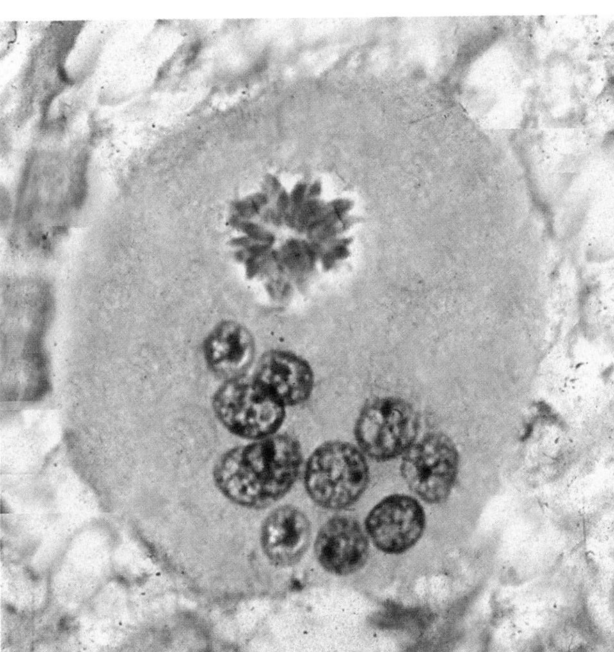

Figure 9.6 Asteroid body consists of a stellate arrangement of needle-shaped eosinophilic structures within a space in the cytoplasm of a multinucleated giant cell in a sarcoidosis granuloma.

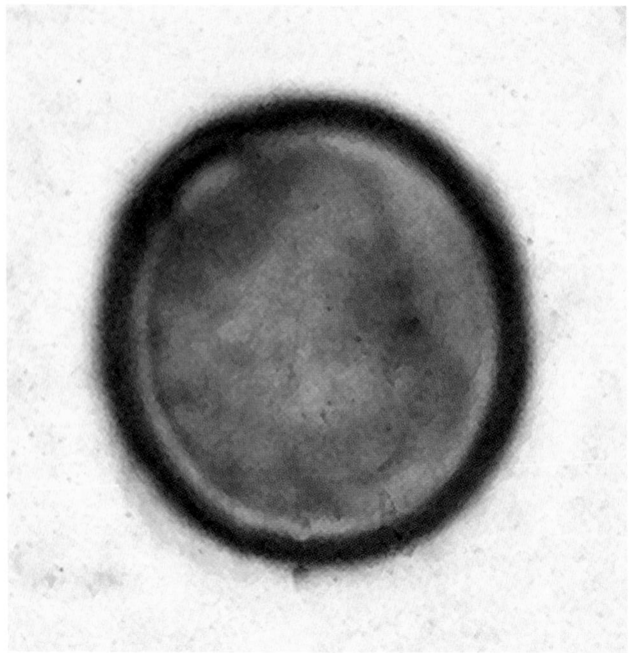

Figure 9.7 Inhaled pollen granule in an exfoliative cytology specimen consists of a round structure with a thick wall.

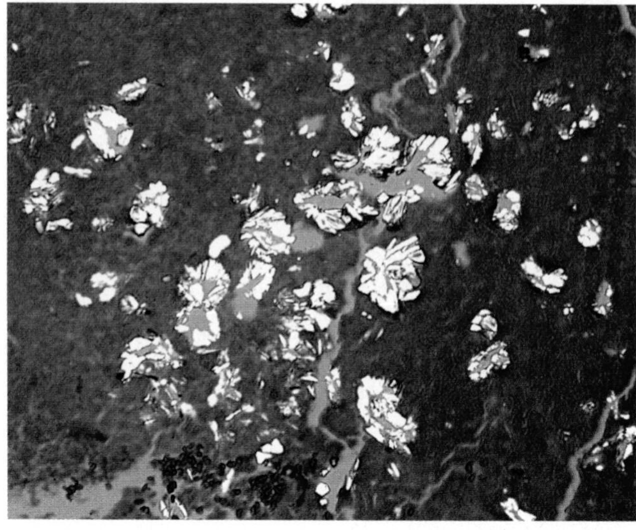

Figure 9.8 Large numbers of brightly birefringent calcium oxalate crystals are seen on polarized light in an exfoliative cytology specimen from a patient with *Aspergillus*.

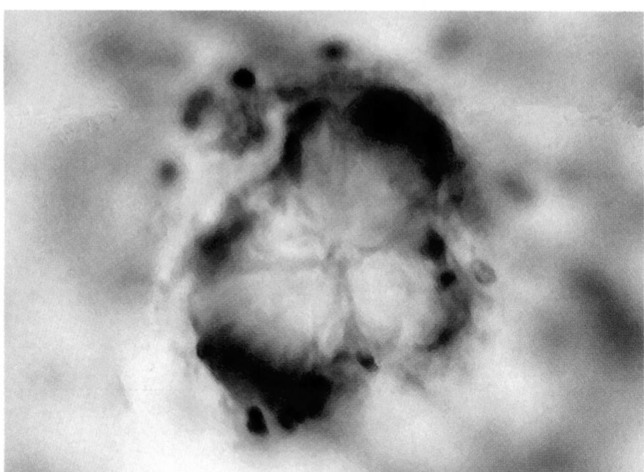

Figure 9.9 Higher power of calcium oxalate crystals from exfoliative cytology specimen.

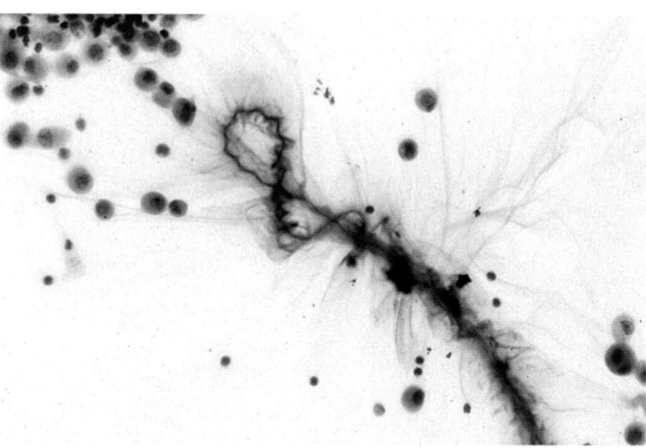

Figure 9.10 Curschmann spiral shows corkscrew-shaped mucinous cast with radiating filaments in an exfoliative cytology specimen from a patient with asthma.

Section 3

Malignant Neoplasms

Carcinomas

10

Primary lung carcinomas account for the highest number of cancer deaths in the United States each year. Carcinomas are tumors of the lung epithelium, including the bronchial mucosa. The four primary histopathologic cell types of lung carcinoma are adenocarcinoma, squamous cell carcinoma and large cell carcinoma (collectively referred to as *non–small cell carcinomas*), and small cell carcinoma. Subtypes of the four major cell types and other, often rare, histopathologic types of primary pulmonary carcinoma occur and are included in this chapter. Several tumors that have been categorized together in some of the classification schemes are illustrated separately here according to the distinctiveness of their histopathology to emphasize pattern recognition for the practicing pathologist. For a classification scheme of lung carcinomas, please refer to the 2004 World Health Organization Classification of Tumours: Pathology and Genetics of Tumours of the Lung, Pleura, Thymus and Heart.

Part 1

Adenocarcinoma

▶ Alvaro C. Laga, Timothy Allen, Mary Ostrowski, and Philip T. Cagle

Adenocarcinomas are glandular epithelial cancers and are the most common cell type of lung cancer, accounting for slightly more than 30% of all lung cancers in many series. Adenocarcinomas are frequently histologically heterogeneous. Major histologic subtypes include acinar (gland-forming), papillary, bronchioloalveolar carcinoma, solid adenocarcinoma with mucin, and adenocarcinoma with mixed subtypes. Most adenocarcinomas consist of two or more of the subtypes and therefore fall into the mixed subtype. It is common to see central scarring in pulmonary adenocarcinomas and a focal bronchioloalveolar-like pattern at the periphery of the tumor. Due to distinctive clinicopathologic features, bronchioloalveolar carcinomas are discussed in Part 2 of this chapter.

Cytologic Features:

- Tissue fragments, cell clusters, single cells.
- Eccentric nuclei with finely granular chromatin.
- Central macronucleoli, acinar type.
- Foamy or vacuolated, usually cyanophilic, cytoplasm.
- Occasional large cytoplasmic vacuoles.

Histologic Features:

- Gray-white, grossly lobulated lesions often with central scarring and anthracotic pigment.
- Histopathologically, adenocarcinomas form acinar structures like glands and tubules and often produce mucin.
- Microscopic subtypes include acinar, papillary, bronchioloalveolar, and solid with mucin production.
- More poorly differentiated tumors tend to loose gland formation and tend toward solid pattern.
- Most adenocarcinomas are histologically heterogeneous and therefore have mixed subtypes.
- Variant patterns include fetal adenocarcinoma (well-differentiated fetal adenocarcinoma), mucinous ("colloid") adenocarcinoma, mucinous cystadenocarcinoma, signet ring adenocarcinoma, clear cell adenocarcinoma, and sarcomatoid (sarcomatous or spindle-cell) adenocarcinoma.
- True bronchioloalveolar carcinoma currently can be diagnosed only in the setting of an adenocarcinoma growing in a lepidic fashion without stromal invasion and is discussed separately.
- True papillary adenocarcinoma can be distinguished from bronchioloalveolar carcinoma by the following criteria: papillary morphology with complex secondary and tertiary branching in greater than 75% of the tumor, stromal invasion and destruction of normal lung architecture, and marked nuclear atypia with occasional "dirty necrosis".
- Micropapillary pattern can be distinguished from papillary pattern by the absence of fibrovascular cores in the projections and is discussed in Subpart 1.1.
- Positive immunoreactivity usually with CK7 and AE1/AE3, CEA, TTF-1, EMA, and HMFG-2, often with LeuM1 (CD-15), BerEP4, and B72.3, and occasionally with vimentin.
- Negative immunoreactivity with CK5/CK6 and CK20 in the vast majority of cases.

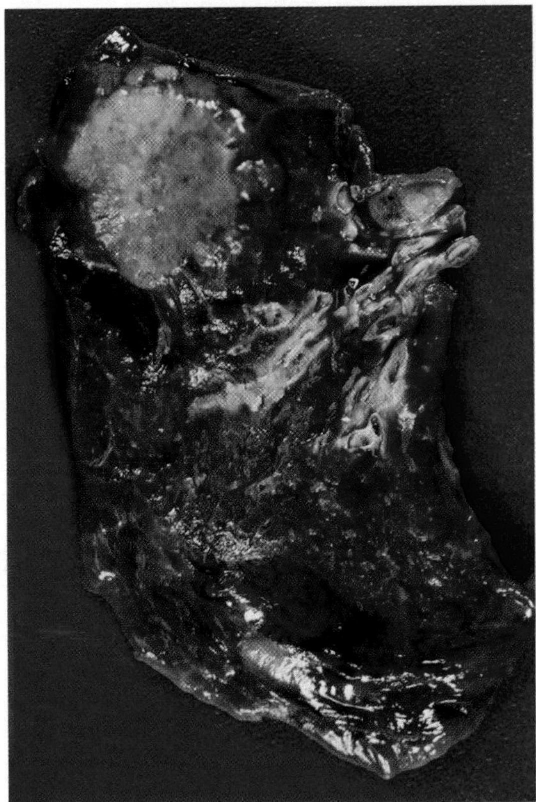

Figure 10.1 Gross figure showing a peripheral tumor mass; adenocarcinoma.

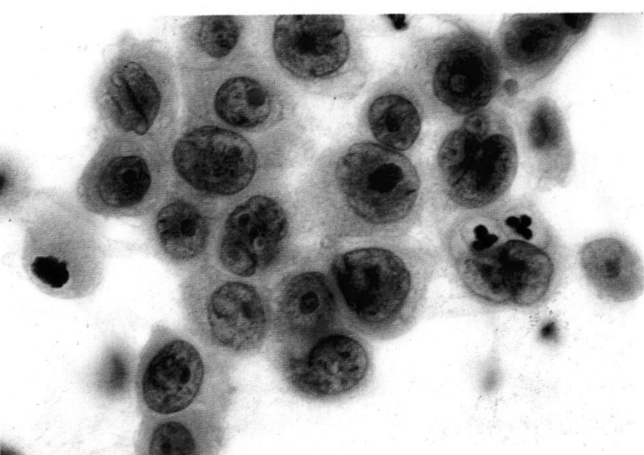

Figure 10.2 Cytology figure showing abundant cytoplasm with enlarged nuclei with finely granular chromatin.

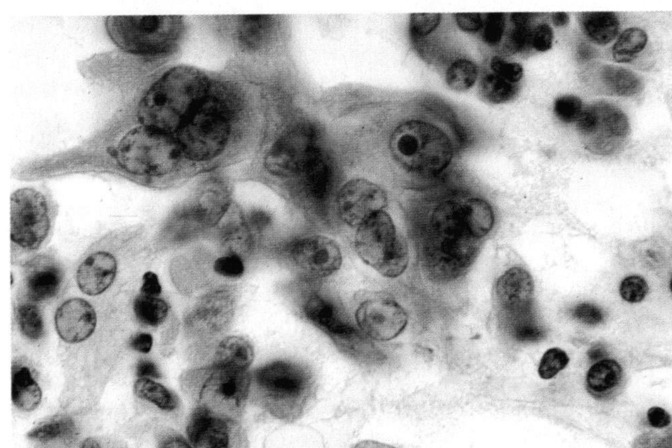

Figure 10.3 Cytology figure showing enlarged nuclei, some of which have macronucleoli.

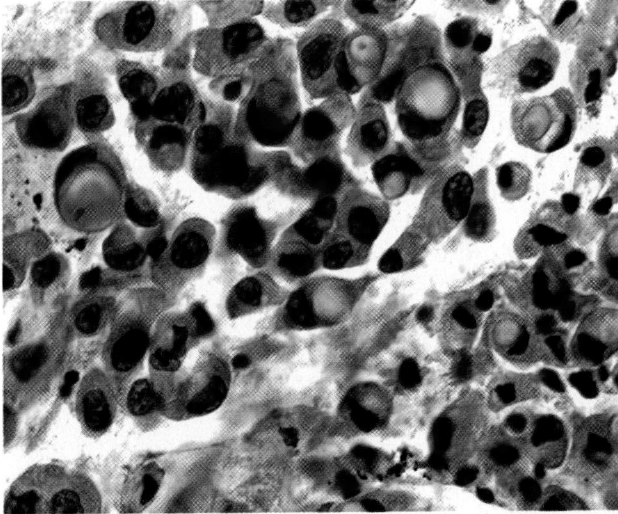

Figure 10.4 Cytology figure showing mucinous adenocarcinoma with large cytoplasmic vacuoles and eccentric nuclei.

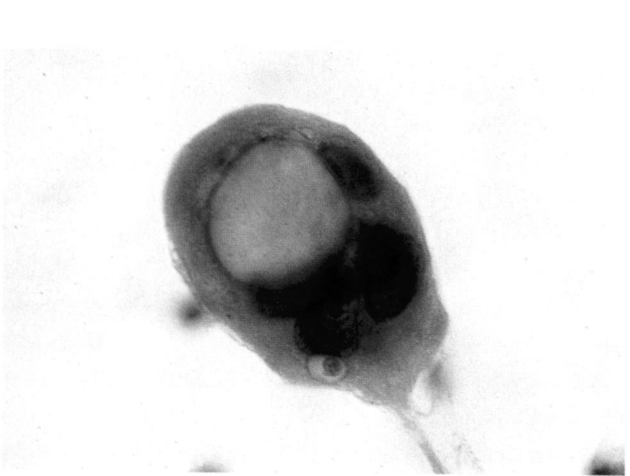

Figure 10.5 Cytology figure showing cytoplasmic vacuolization and multinucleation.

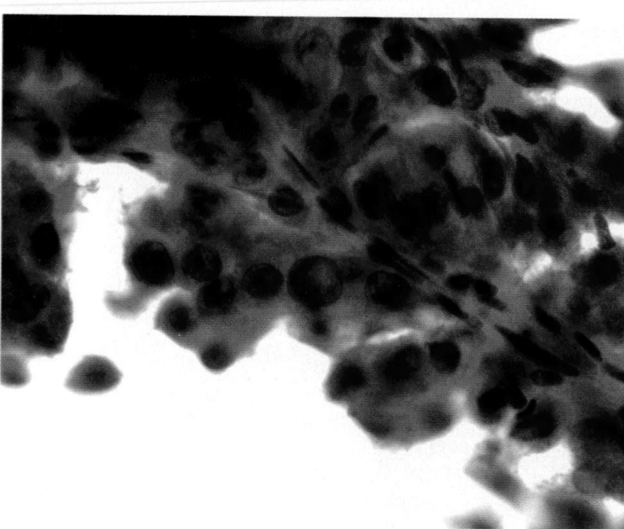

Figure 10.6 Cytology figure showing papillary adenocarcinoma with central fibrovascular core.

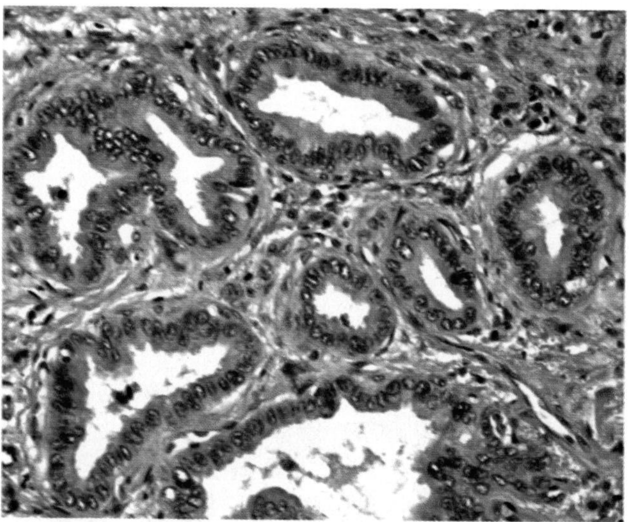

Figure 10.7 Acinar pattern of adenocarcinoma composed of glands lined by malignant cells.

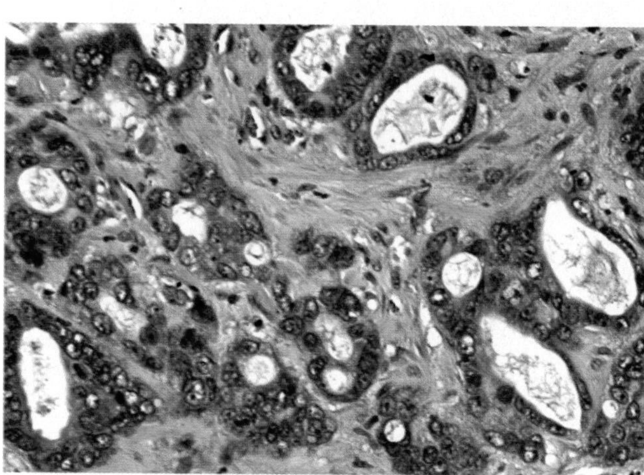

Figure 10.8 Acinar pattern of adenocarcinoma with desmoplastic stroma containing glands with malignant cells exhibiting pleomorphic nuclei.

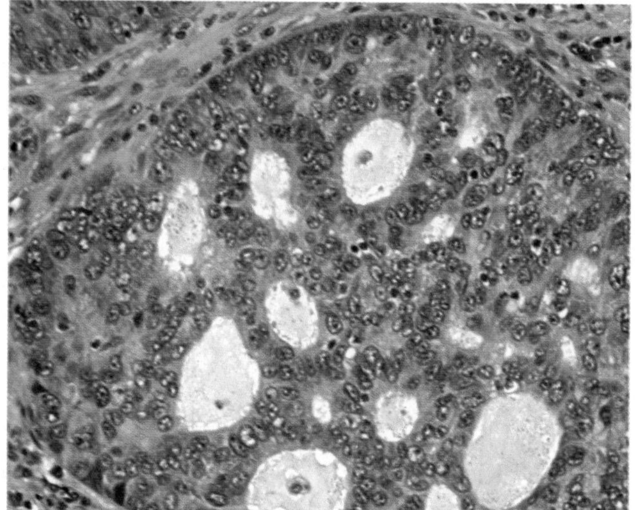

Figure 10.9 Cribriform pattern of adenocarcinoma showing small regular round back-to-back glands.

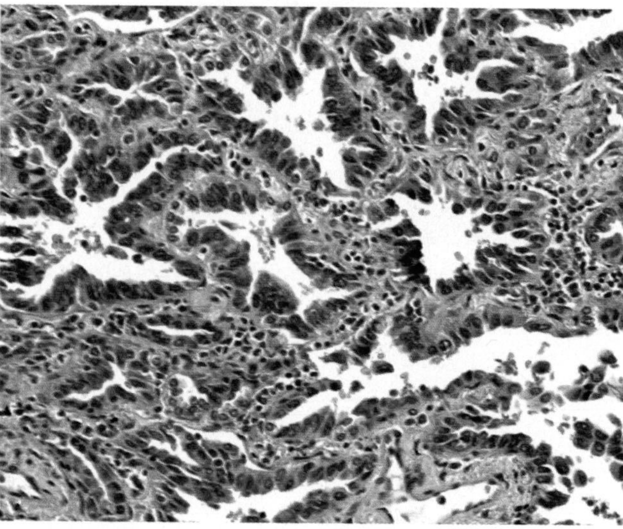

Figure 10.10 Irregularly shaped invasive glands of adenocarcinoma at periphery of so-called central scar.

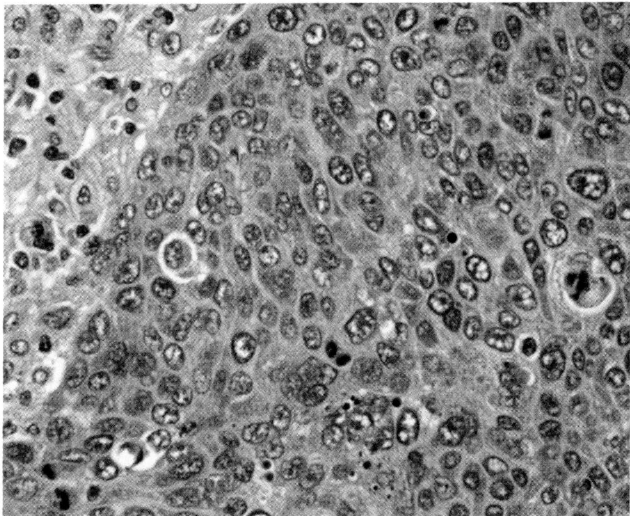

Figure 10.11 Solid pattern of adenocarcinoma with a sheet of malignant cells with abundant cytoplasm and scattered mitotic figures lacking gland formation.

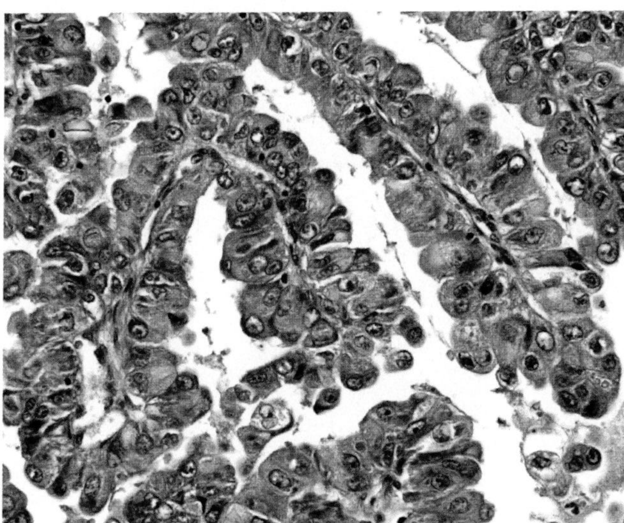

Figure 10.12 Papillary adenocarcinoma with fibrovascular cores surrounded by malignant cells.

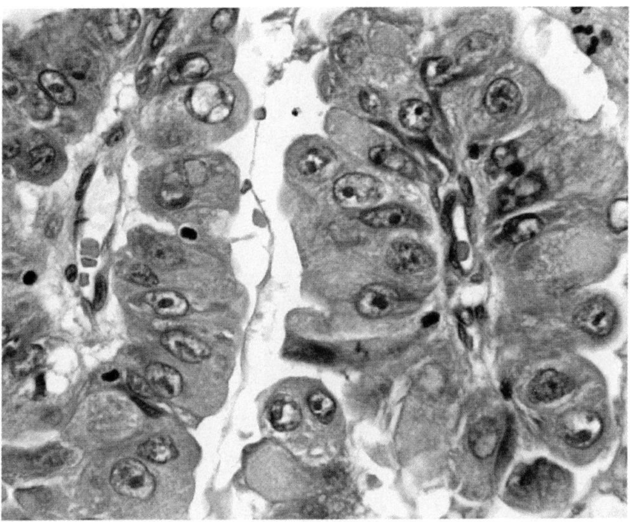

Figure 10.13 Higher power of papillary adenocarcinoma showing matypical vesicular nuclei and prominent nucleoli.

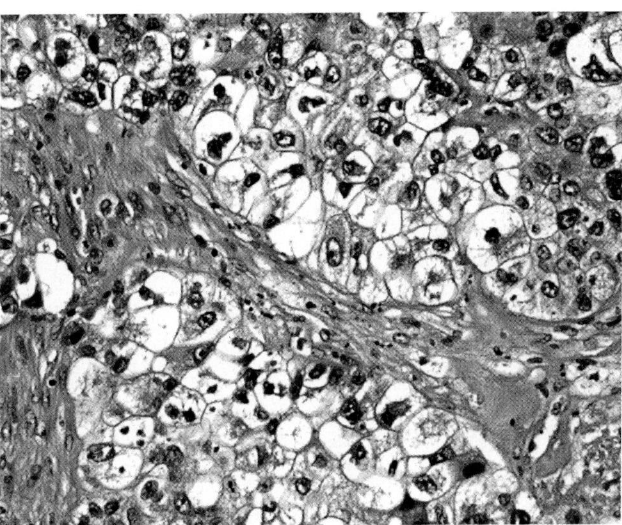

Figure 10.14 Clear cell pattern of adenocarcinoma composed of malignant cells with clear cytoplasm.

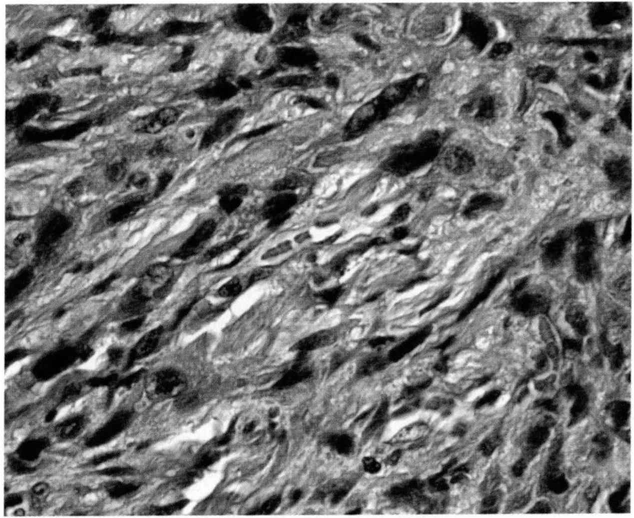

Figure 10.15 Sarcomatoid (sarcomatous) pattern of adenocarcinoma composed of spindled cells with elongated pleomorphic nuclei.

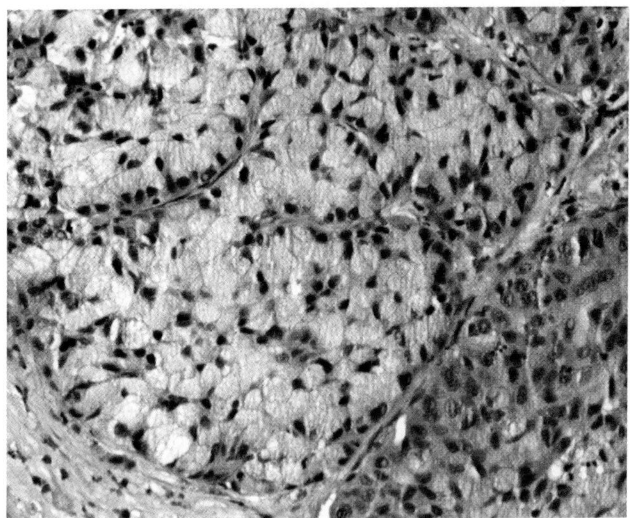

Figure 10.16 Signet ring pattern of adenocarcinoma with cells containing vacuolated mucin-filled cytoplasm and eccentric nuclei resembling signet rings.

Subpart 1.1

Adenocarcinoma with Micropapillary Component

▶ Andras Khoor

Adenocarcinomas of the lung may possess a micropapillary component. This component can range from focal to prominent and may be associated with any conventional histologic subtype. Adenocarcinomas with a micropapillary component are more likely to metastasize and have a poorer prognosis..

Histologic Features:

- The micropapillary component displays small papillary tufts, which lack a central fibrovascular core.

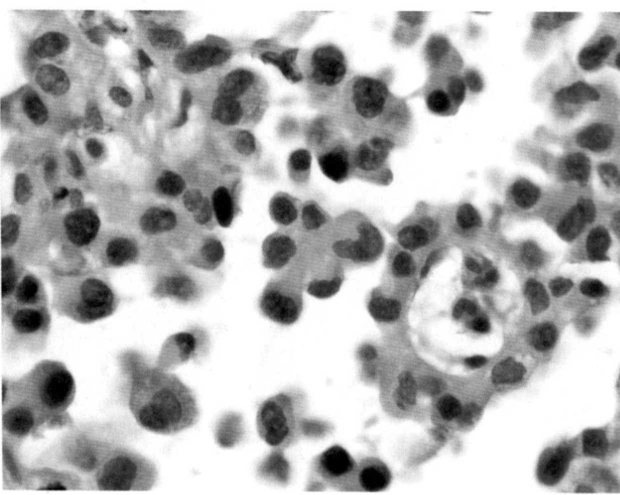

Figure 10.17 Small papillary tufts are seen focally in an adenocarcinoma.

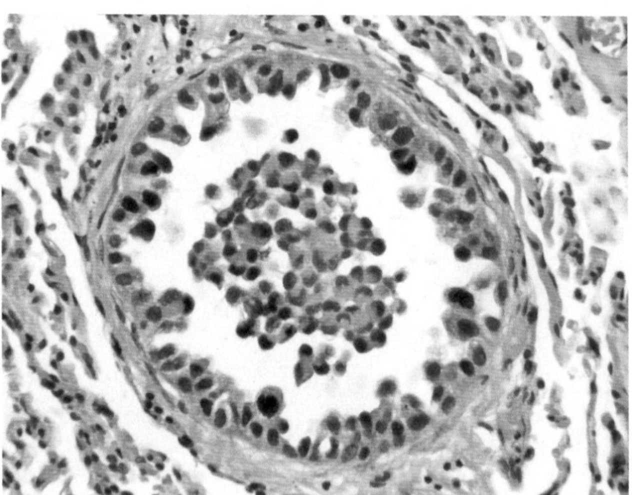

Figure 10.18 A micropapillary pattern can also be observed in the lymphangitic spread of the same tumor.

Subpart 1.2

Fetal Adenocarcinoma

▶ Dani Zander and Philip T. Cagle

Fetal adenocarcinoma is usually a well-differentiated malignancy accounting for less than 1% of all pulmonary neoplasms. A poorly differentiated or high-grade variant of fetal adenocarcinoma is now recognized. The peak incidence of fetal adenocarcinoma is in the fourth decade, and both sexes are equally affected. Despite histologic similarities between fetal adenocarcinoma and the epithelial component of pulmonary blastoma, these tumors have distinct clinical features. Fetal adenocarcinoma typically presents as an asymptomatic solitary pulmonary mass that may be located centrally or peripherally. It is rarely associated with pleural effusion. Well-differentiated fetal adenocarcinoma has a better prognosis than more common types of adenocarcinoma or biphasic pulmonary blastoma.

Histologic Features:

- Fetal adenocarcinoma is composed of glands and tubules lined by glycogen-rich columnar cells resembling a fetal lung at 10 to 15 weeks of gestation.
- The histopathology of the neoplastic glands is said to resemble that of endometrial glands with supranuclear and subnuclear vacuolization.
- The glycogen-rich cytoplasm of the columnar cells is diastase sensitive and periodic acid-Schiff (PAS) positive, and is negative for mucin stains.
- Rounded morules of polygonal cells with abundant eosinophilic and finely granular cytoplasm are frequently seen at the margin of tumor glands.
- The adjacent stroma is benign and consists of inconspicuous spindle-shaped cells in a sparse myxomatous connective tissue background.
- Immunoreactivity is typically positive for AE1/EA3, CAM5.2, TTF-1, CEA, GATA-6, β-catenin, and EMA.
- Immunoreactivity is negative for ER, PR, NSE, chromogranin, synaptophysin, desmin, α-fetoprotein, p53, and S-100.
- Histopathologic features of high-grade fetal adenocarcinoma include disorganized glands, large vesicular nuclei, prominent nucleoli, variation in nuclear size (anisonucleosis), absence of morules, transition to conventional adenocarcinoma, broad areas of necrosis, and desmoplastic stroma.

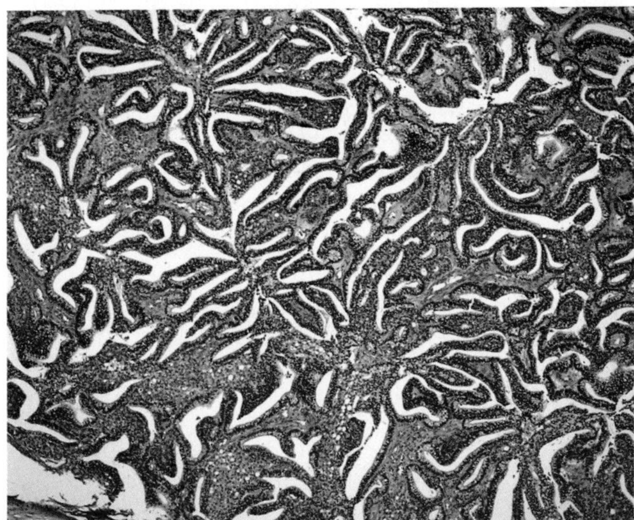

Figure 10.19 Fetal adenocarcinoma with a villiform glandular pattern resembling endometrial glands or fetal lung, low-grade or well-differentiated variant.

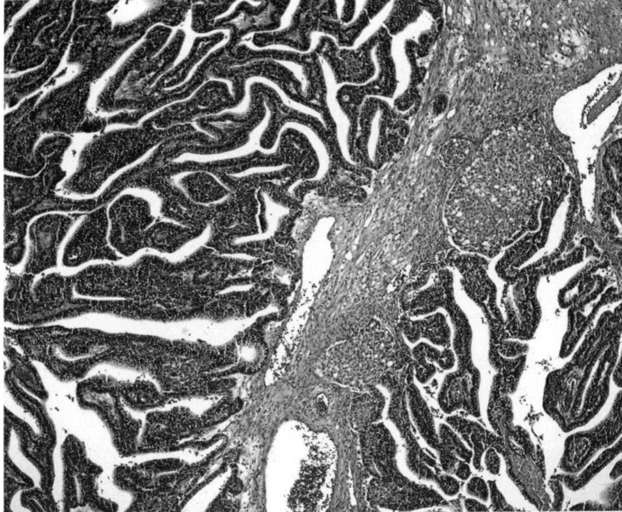

Figure 10.20 Two squamoid morules are found at the margin of the glandular component of a well-differentiated or low-grade fetal adenocarcinoma.

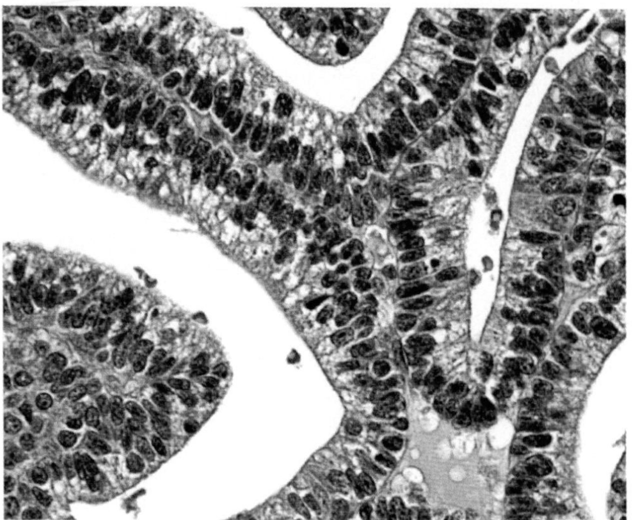

Figure 10.21 Higher power of the glandular component shows columnar cells with glycogen-rich cytoplasm and basally arranged uniform nuclei in well-differentiated fetal adenocarcinoma.

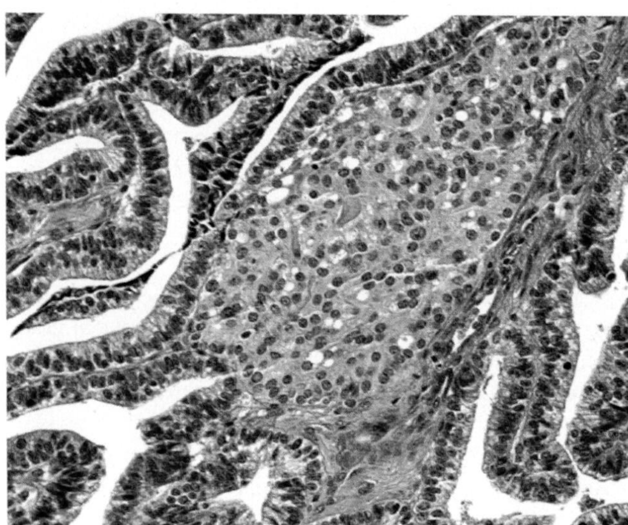

Figure 10.22 Rounded squamoid morule is composed of polygonal cells with abundant eosinophilic cytoplasm in well-differentiated fetal adenocarcinoma.

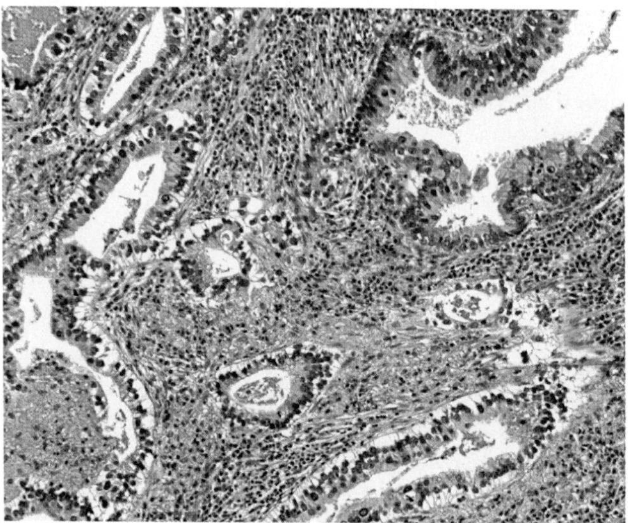

Figure 10.23 High-grade fetal adenocarcinoma shows irregular glands in a desmoplastic stroma.

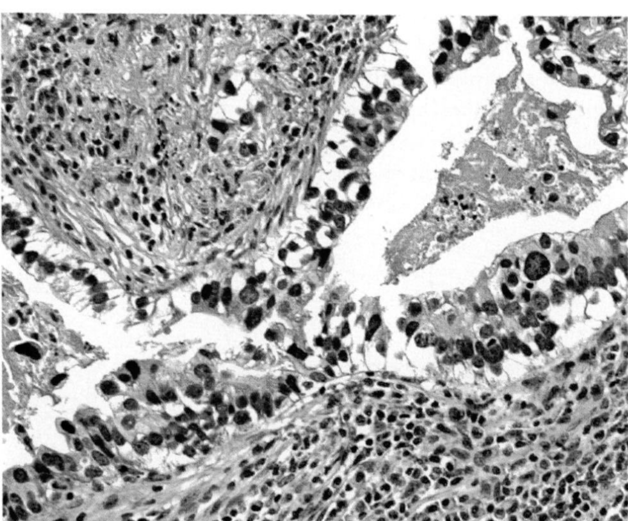

Figure 10.24 High-grade fetal adenocarcinoma with glycogen-rich columnar cells exhibiting anisonucleosis and necrotic debris in gland lumen.

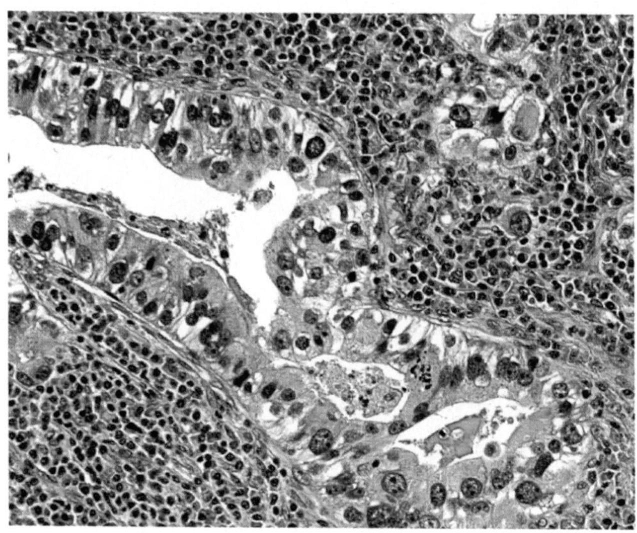

Figure 10.25 High-grade fetal adenocarcinoma with stratification of glycogen-containing columnar cells, anisonucleosis, and several nuclei with prominent nucleoli.

Part 2

Bronchioloalveolar Carcinomas

▶ Alvaro C. Laga, Timothy Allen, Mary Ostrowski, and Philip T. Cagle

Bronchioloalveolar carcinoma (BAC) is defined as adenocarcinoma of the lung that grows in a lepidic fashion along intact alveolar septa without invasion. BAC can be nonmucinous, mucinous, or a mixture of these two subtypes. BACs, particularly the nonmucinous subtype, may be associated with areas of subpleural alveolar collapse, fibrosis, and pleural puckering apparently without stromal invasion, referred to in the past as a *scar.* Some BACs, particularly the mucinous subtype, grow in a pneumonic pattern spreading through the air spaces. BAC-like growth around the edge of an invasive adenocarcinoma is very common but is only a component of an adenocarcinoma of mixed cell type in that setting. A final diagnosis of BAC can be achieved only on a surgical resection specimen because bronchoscopic or needle biopsies are insufficient to exclude the presence of invasive growth. Metastatic adenocarcinomas to the lung may grow in a lepidic pattern on intact alveolar septa mimicking BAC, including metastatic adenocarcinomas of the colon, pancreas, and breast.

Cytologic Features:

- Ball-like clusters (three dimensional), papillary fronds, florets.
- Single cells.
- Round to oval nuclei, bland chromatin.
- Nucleoli (sometimes small).
- Occasional secretory vacuoles, intranuclear cytoplasmic inclusions, psammoma bodies.

Histologic Features:

- Mucinous BACs tend to be multicentric and characteristically have mucin production evident by gross and microscopic examination; they can cause lobar consolidation resembling pneumonia.
- Mucinous BACs consist of tall columnar cells with abundant apical cytoplasmic mucin and small basally oriented nuclei growing along intact alveolar septa; the alveolar septa are usually thin and delicate.
- Mucinous BACs may form discontinuous tufts of cells on the alveolar septal surfaces, may project into the alveolar spaces as pseudopapillae, or may shed into mucin-filled alveolar spaces.
- Nonmucinous BACs are more likely to be solitary tumors and may be associated with subpleural alveolar collapse, fibrosis, and pleural puckering without apparent invasion previously referred to as a *scar.*
- Nonmucinous BACs are composed of cuboidal-to-columnar cells proliferating along intact alveolar septa; the cells may have a hobnail or sawtooth appearance and may project into the alveolar spaces as tufts or pseudopapillae; the alveolar septa may be thickened.

- Nuclear inclusions may be found in the nonmucinous variant and may be PAS and surfactant apoprotein positive.
- Generally, BACs are immunopositive for CEA and B72.3.
- Nonmucinous BACs are typically immunopositive for TTF-1 and CK7.
- Mucinous BACs are typically immunonegative for TTF-1 and may be immunopositive for CK20.

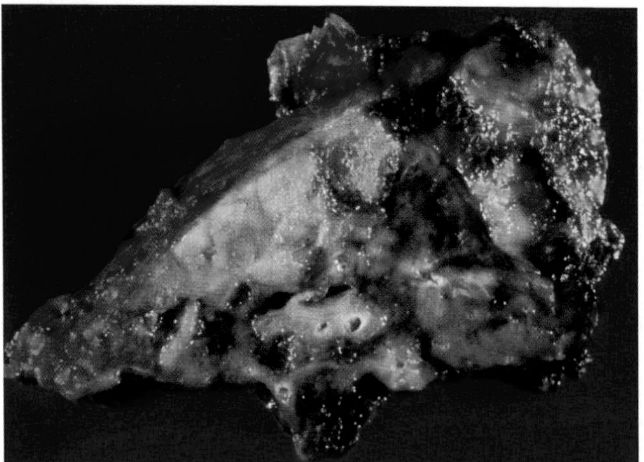

Figure 10.26 Wedge resection of nonmucinous BAC showing subpleural tumor with associated subpleural consolidation or so-called *scar.*

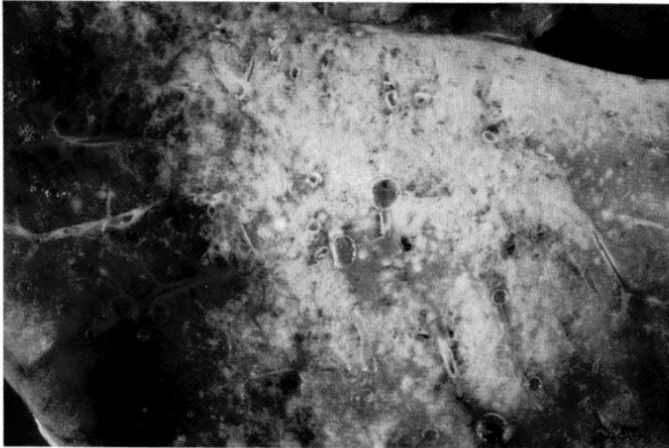

Figure 10.27 Gross figure of mucinous BAC showing pneumonic tumor spread.

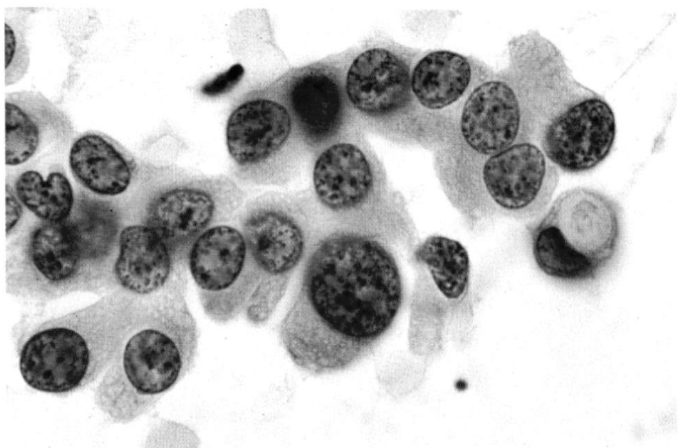

Figure 10.28 Cytology figure showing round to oval nuclei with occasional small nucleoli and a secretory vacuole.

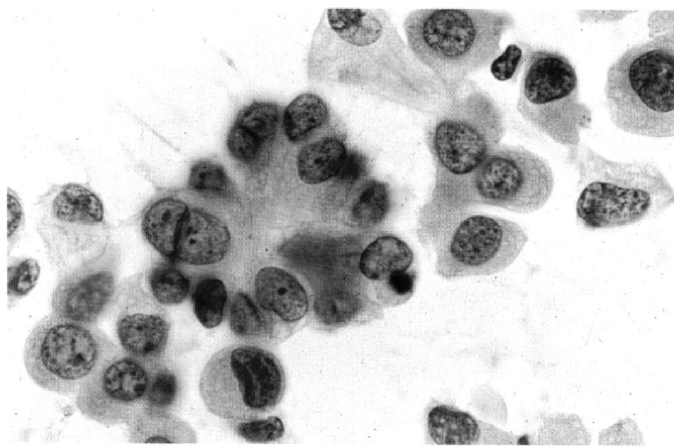

Figure 10.29 Cytology figure showing a floret of BAC cells and scattered single cells.

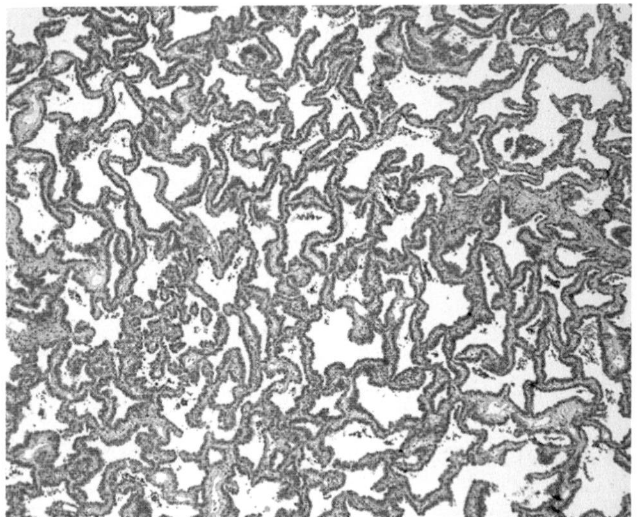

Figure 10.30 Lepidic growth of nonmucinous BAC along intact alveolar septa.

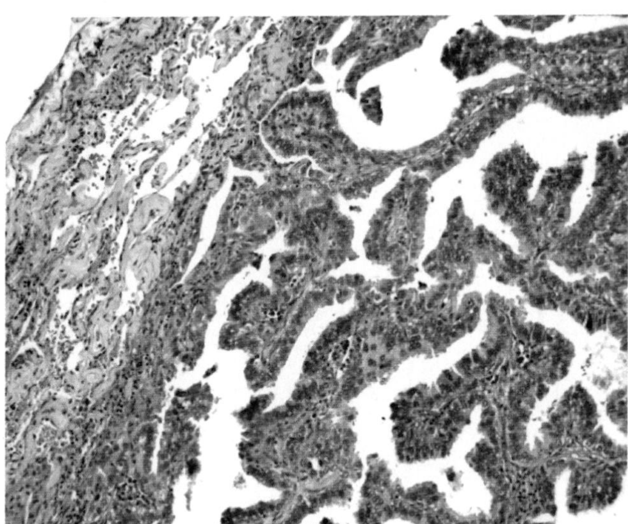

Figure 10.31 Subpleural nonmucinous BAC showing circumscription and mildly thickened alveolar septa.

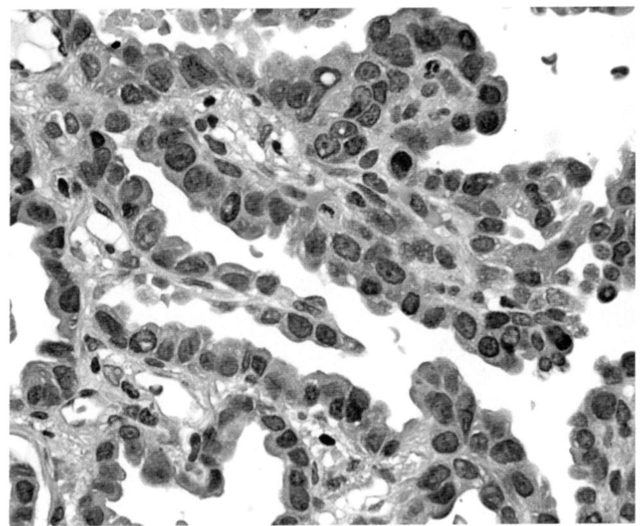

Figure 10.32 Nonmucinous BAC showing cuboidal to columnar cells with focal intranuclear cytoplasmic inclusions.

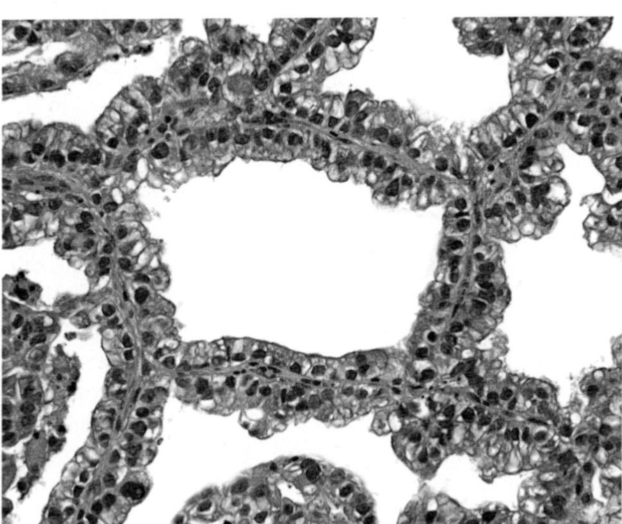

Figure 10.33 BAC with cuboidal to columnar cells with basally oriented nuclei and eosinophilic or vacuolated cytoplasm proliferating along intact alveolar septa.

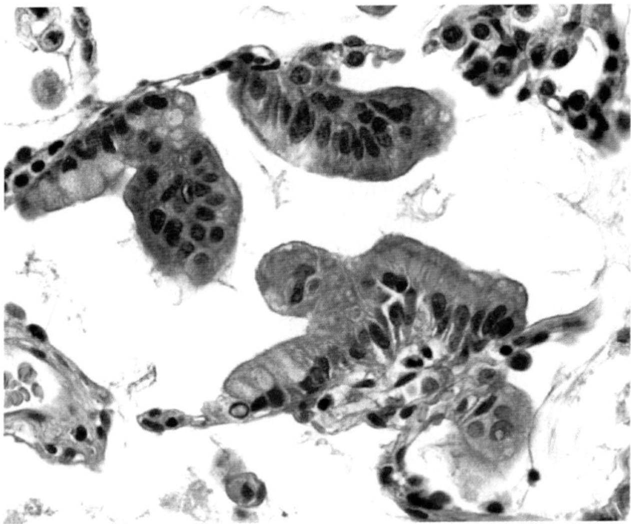

Figure 10.34 Mucinous BAC cells with abundant apical mucin and small basal nuclei lining thin, delicate alveolar septa and projecting into the alveolar spaces as tufts or pseudopapillae.

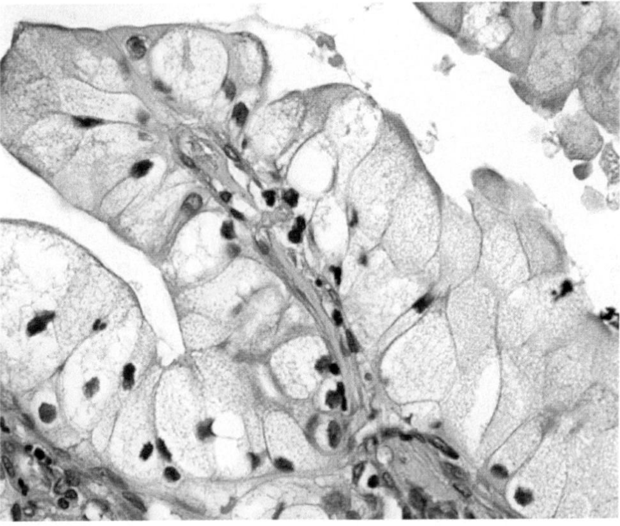

Figure 10.35 Mucinous BAC with abundant mucin-rich apical cytoplasm and basally oriented small nuclei growing along thin, delicate alveolar septa.

Part 3

Squamous Cell Carcinoma

▶ Handan Zeren, Alvaro C. Laga, Timothy Allen, Carlos Bedrossian, Mary Ostrowski, and Philip T. Cagle

Squamous cell carcinoma is a cancer with keratinization and/or intercellular bridges. It accounts for about 30% of all lung cancers in many series. Two thirds present as central lung tumors. Squamous cell carcinomas of the lung may have clear cell, small cell, papillary, and basaloid subtypes. Papillary squamous cell carcinomas often show a pattern of exophytic endobronchial growth and are discussed in Subpart 3.1 of this chapter. Basaloid carcinomas are discussed in Part 10.

Cytologic Features:

- Single cells and small clusters in sputum.
- Sheets of cells ("fish in a stream"), bronchial brushings, and fine needle aspiration.
- Marked cellular pleomorphism due to bizarre cytoplasmic shapes (tadpole or caudate cells, spindle or fiber cells).
- Hyperchromatic, "ink blot" nuclei.
- In poorly differentiated cases, nucleoli may be prominent.
- Cytoplasm ranges from dense and orangeophilic to deeply cyanophilic (Papanicolaou stain) due to keratin, and may be abundant with prominent cell borders.
- Herxheimer spirals composed of keratin in the cytoplasm, endoectoplasm, and intercellular bridges are present in well-differentiated cases.

Histologic Features:

- Squamous cell carcinomas arise most often in bronchi, particularly segmental bronchi.
- Squamous differentiation is identified by intercellular bridges, squamous pearl formation, and individual cell keratinization.
- These features are apparent in well-differentiated tumors but are difficult or impossible to find in poorly differentiated tumors.
- The small cell variant is a poorly differentiated squamous cell carcinoma with small tumor cells with nuclear and cytoplasmic features of squamous cell carcinoma.
- Positive immunoreactivity usually with AE1/AE3, CK5/CK6, 34BE12, EMA, and HMFG-2, often with polyclonal CEA, and occasionally with vimentin.
- Negative immunoreactivity with TTF-1 in the great majority of squamous cell carcinomas.

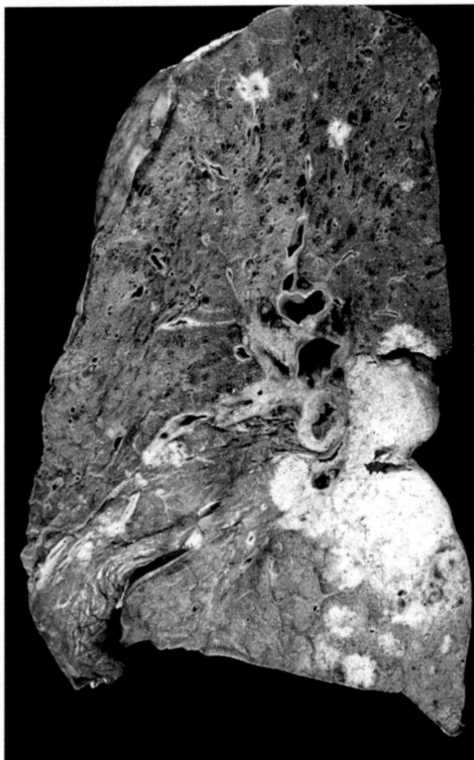

Figure 10.36 Gross figure of squamous cell carcinoma showing a central tumor mass with bronchial and hilar lymph node involvement, and peripheral satellite lesions.

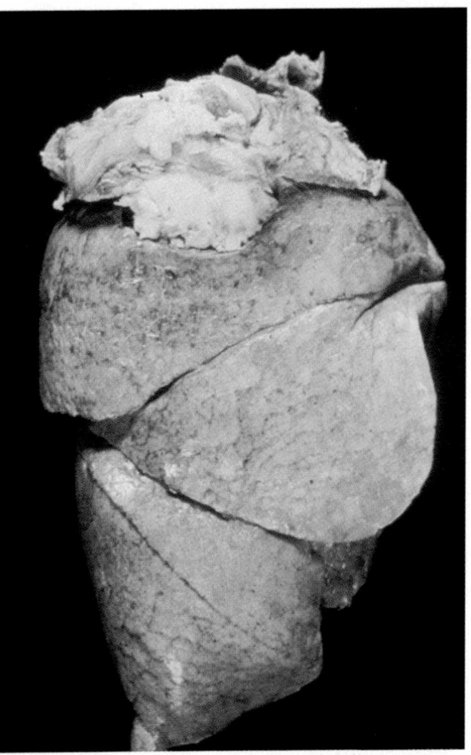

Figure 10.37 Gross figure of a squamous cell carcinoma showing a superior sulcus tumor (Pancoast tumor) arising from apex of the right lung.

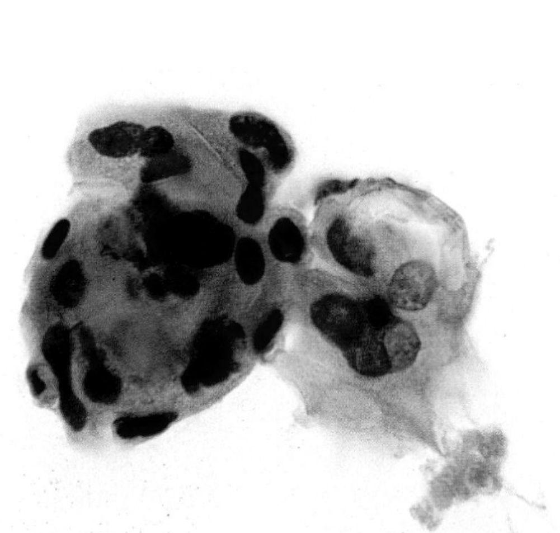

Figure 10.38 Cytology figure showing small clusters of squamous cells exhibiting nuclear pleomorphism and hyperchromatic "ink blot" nuclei.

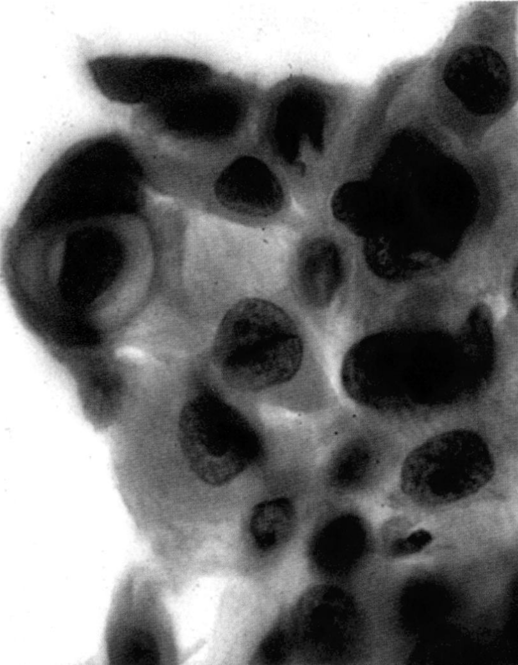

Figure 10.39 Cytology figure showing a cell with prominent endoectoplasm.

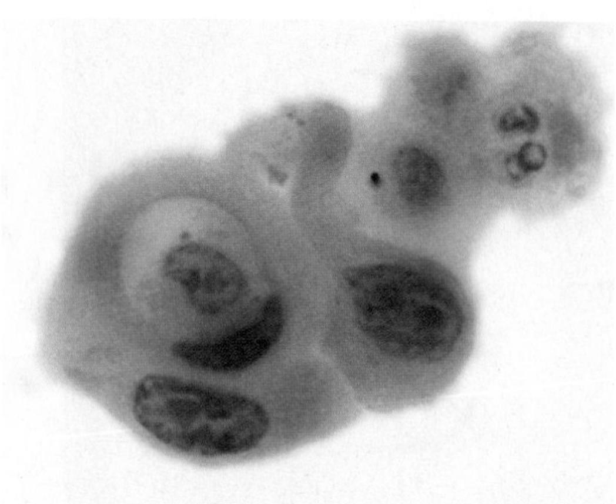

Figure 10.40 Cytology figure showing Herxheimer spiral and pleomorphic nuclei, some containing prominent nucleoli.

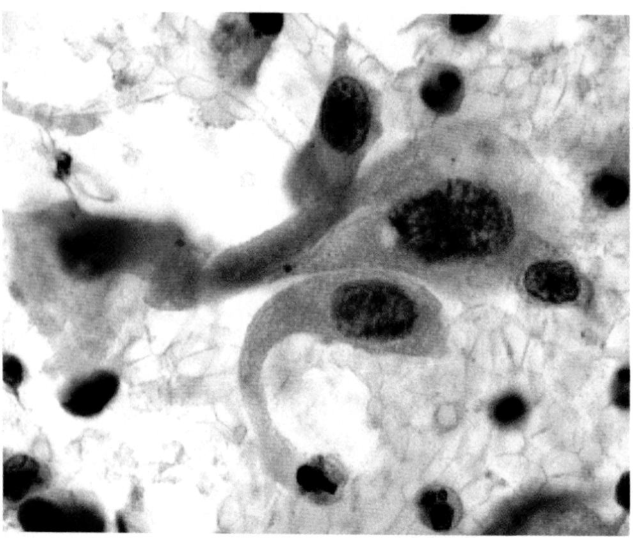

Figure 10.41 Cytology figure showing a tadpole cell.

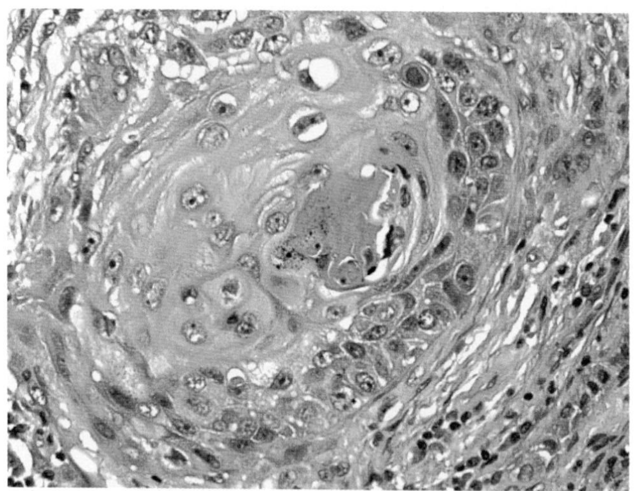

Figure 10.42 Well-differentiated squamous cell carcinoma with focal keratin pearl formation.

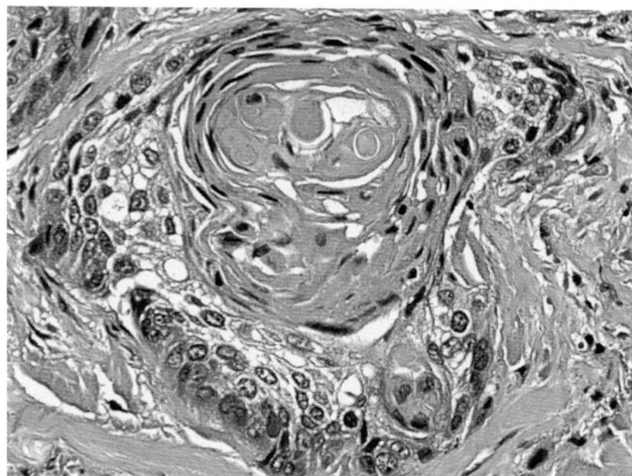

Figure 10.43 Well-differentiated squamous cell carcinoma with prominent keratinization and keratin pearl formation.

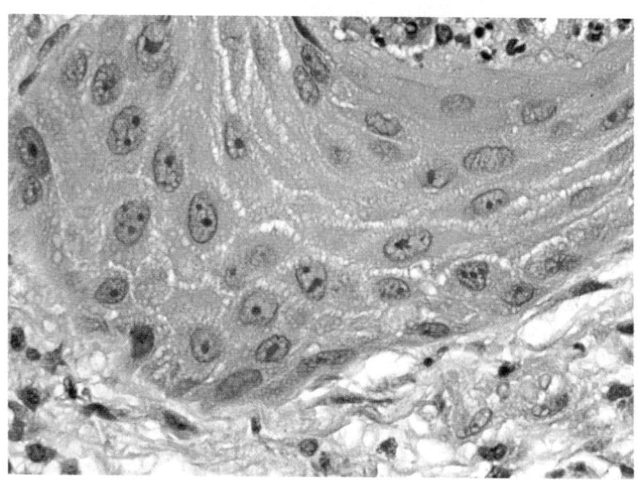

Figure 10.44 Squamous cell carcinoma with distinct intercellular bridges.

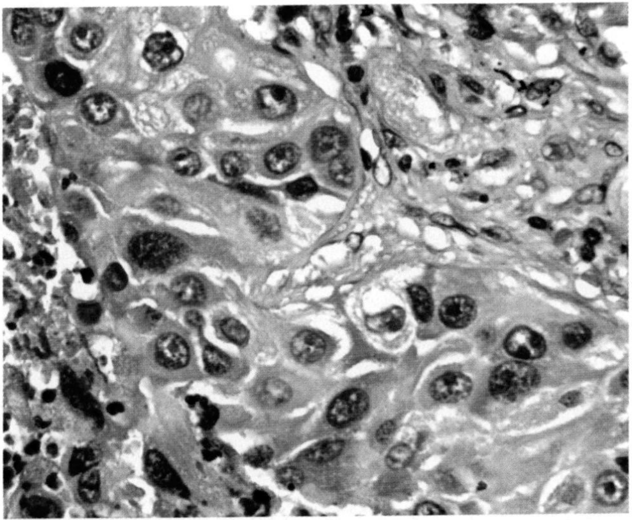

Figure 10.45 Moderately differentiated squamous cell carcinoma.

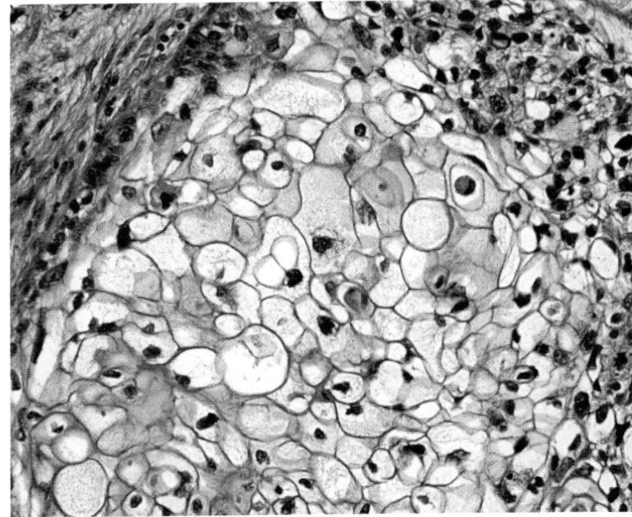

Figure 10.46 Clear cell pattern of squamous cell carcinoma showing cells with clear cytoplasm.

Subpart 3.1

Papillary Squamous Cell Carcinoma

▶ Alvaro C. Laga, Timothy Allen, and Philip T. Cagle

Papillary squamous cell carcinoma is a rare subtype of squamous cell carcinoma with a unique growth pattern. These tumors grow as exophytic, papillary endobronchial tumors but may invade the underlying bronchus and lung tissue. Papillary squamous cell carcinoma typically is a solitary neoplasm in middle-aged to older smokers but may arise in the setting of squamous papillomatosis. Squamous papillomas and papillomatosis are discussed in Chapter 14, Part 2. It may be very difficult to differentiate papillary squamous cell carcinoma from squamous papilloma in the absence of invasion. The squamous epithelium of a squamous papilloma may extend into the bronchial glands and should not be confused with invasion. Rare verrucous carcinomas of the lung are also classified with papillary squamous cell carcinomas.

Histologic Features:

- Papillary fibrovascular cores protruding into the bronchial lumen are lined by squamous cell carcinoma.
- Invasion into underlying bronchus and lung parenchyma may be present.

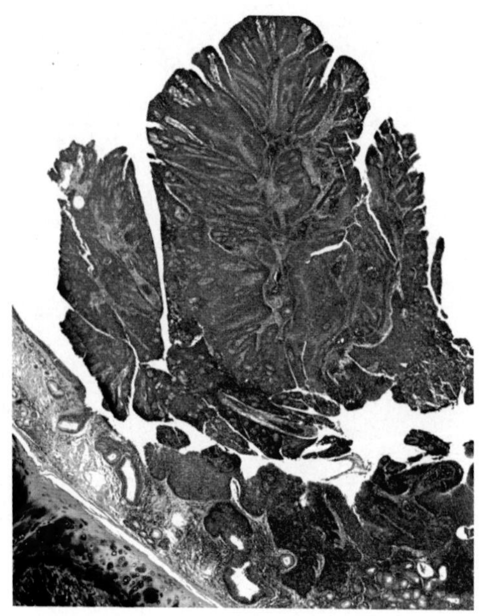

Figure 10.47 Papillary squamous cell carcinoma with underlying invasion.

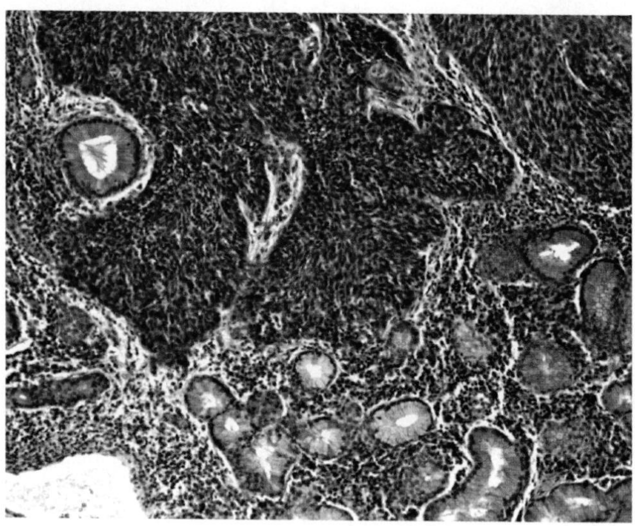

Figure 10.48 Higher power of malignant squamous cells invading underlying bronchial wall.

Part 4

Large Cell Carcinoma

▶ Alvaro C. Laga, Timothy Allen, Carlos Bedrossian, Mary Ostrowski, and Philip T. Cagle

Large cell carcinoma is defined as a poorly differentiated malignant epithelial tumor that lacks glandular, squamous, or small cell differentiation by light microscopy. It accounts for approximately 10% of all lung carcinomas in many series and often presents as a peripheral tumor. There are several variants of large cell carcinoma, including large cell neuroendocrine carcinoma, basaloid carcinoma, clear cell carcinoma, lymphoepithelioma-like carcinoma and large cell carcinoma with rhabdoid phenotype. Large cell neuroendocrine carcinoma is discussed in Part 8 of this chapter and basaloid carcinoma is discussed in Part 10. Large cell carcinomas frequently appear as large, necrotic tumors.

Cytologic Features:

- Syncytial groups and single cells.
- Large, round to oval nuclei, sometimes lobulated, with irregular borders, 60% of cell volume.
- Markedly irregular nuclear chromatin.
- Large, irregular, often multiple, nucleoli.
- Indistinct, variably stained cytoplasm.

Histologic Features:

- Large cell carcinomas usually consist of sheets and nests of large polygonal cells with vesicular nuclei and prominent nucleoli.
- These tumors do not show squamous or glandular differentiation by light microscopy; however, by electron microscopy, features of adenocarcinoma or squamous cell carcinoma may be found.
- It has been proposed that large cell carcinomas may have rare mucin droplets; if abundant mucin-producing cells (a minimum of five mucin droplets per two high-power fields has been proposed) can be demonstrated by mucin stains such as mucicarmine or PAS with diastase digestion, the tumor is classified as solid adenocarcinoma with mucin formation.

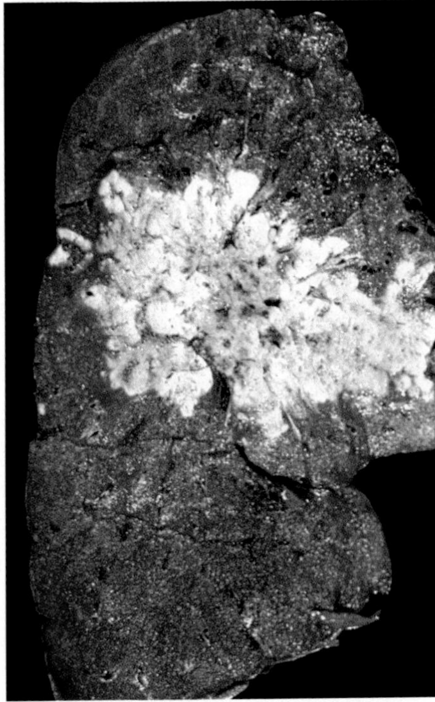

Figure 10.49 Gross figure of large cell carcinoma showing an extensive tumor mass.

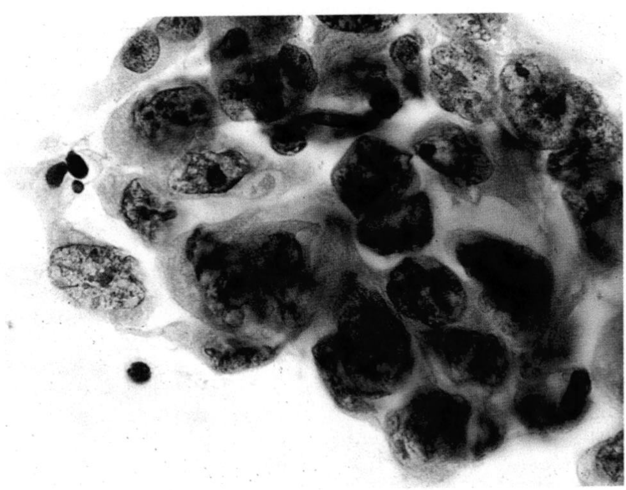

Figure 10.50 Cytology figure showing a syncytial cluster of cells with large nuclei having irregular nuclear chromatin and scattered nucleoli.

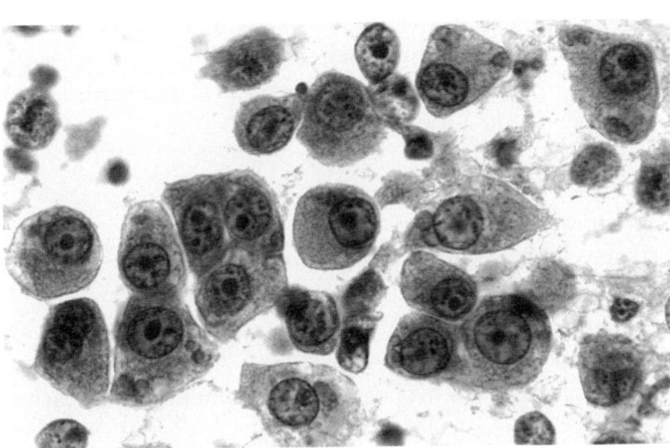

Figure 10.51 Cytology figure showing plasmacytoid cells with prominent nucleoli within round to oval nuclei and abundant cytoplasm.

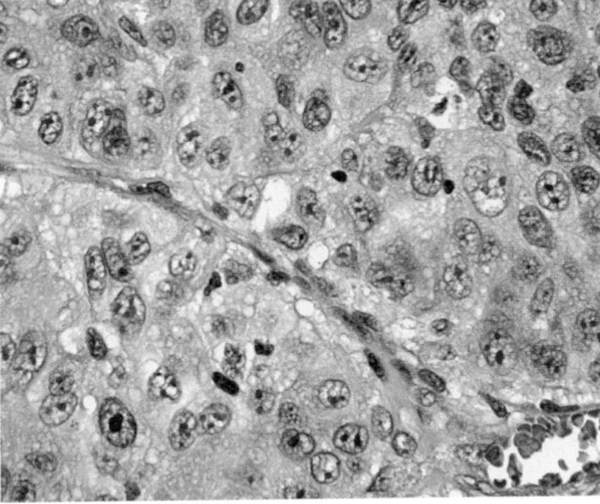

Figure 10.52 Nests of large polygonal cells with vesicular nuclei and prominent nucleoli.

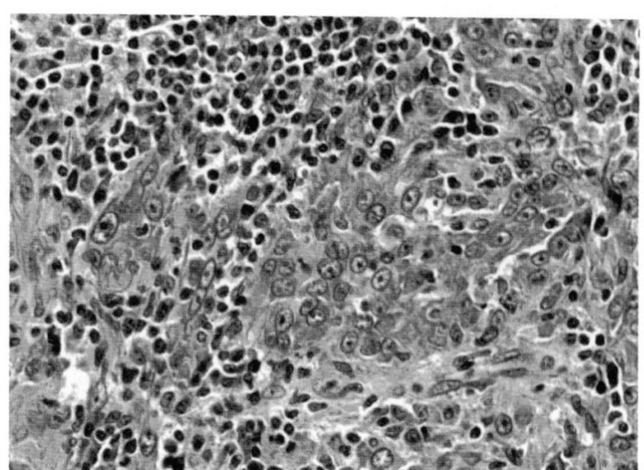

Figure 10.53 Lymphoepithelioma-like variant of large cell carcinoma with abundant lymphocytes infiltrating clusters of polygonal large cell carcinoma cells.

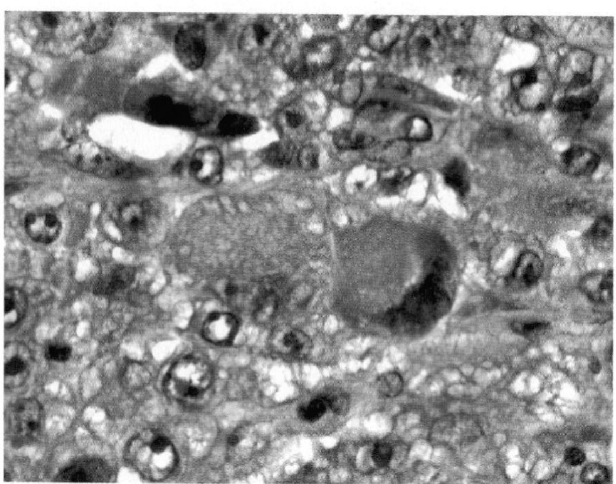

Figure 10.54 Large cell carcinoma with rhabdoid differentiation showing cells with abundant eosinophilic cytoplasm reminiscent of muscle cell differentiation.

Part 5

Small Cell Carcinoma

▶ Mary Beth Beasley and Mary Ostrowski

Small cell carcinoma is a high-grade neuroendocrine carcinoma with a mitotic rate greater than 10 per 10 high-power fields and characteristic small cell morphology as described in the following.

Cytologic Features:

- Small cell carcinomas show cells in loose clusters, clumps (vs. lymphoma), single cells with necrosis, mitotic figures, cell compression with molding, and cells along mucus strands in sputum and bronchial samples.
- Cells are 1.5 to 3 times the size of a normal lymphocyte and have extremely scant cytoplasm.
- Chromatin is present in a finely granular pattern but is extremely dense, yielding marked hyperchromasia or "salt and pepper" stippled pattern.
- Small nucleoli may be present in fine needle aspiration and bronchial specimens.

Histologic Features:

- Small cell carcinomas have small cell size, approximately 3 to 4 times the size of a resting lymphocyte.
- Cells have scant cytoplasm, granular chromatin, oval to spindle cell shape, absent or inconspicuous nucleoli, and typically prominent necrosis.
- In larger biopsies or resection specimens, cells may appear better preserved and larger, with more discernible cytoplasm.
- Transbronchial biopsies typically show sheets of cells with prominent crush artifact.
- Larger specimens may show a more obvious neuroendocrine growth pattern, including organoid pattern with peripheral palisading, rosettes, and pseudopapillary pattern.

- Small cell carcinomas are generally immunopositive for pancytokeratin, CAM5.2, CK7, NCAM (CD56), and TTF-1, and immunonegative for CK20 and CK34βe12; keratin tends to immunostain in a punctate or stippled pattern in the cytoplasm.
- Neuroendocrine markers synaptophysin and chromogranin are positive in approximately 70%.
- Immunohistochemistry does not discriminate between large cell neuroendocrine carcinoma and small cell carcinoma.

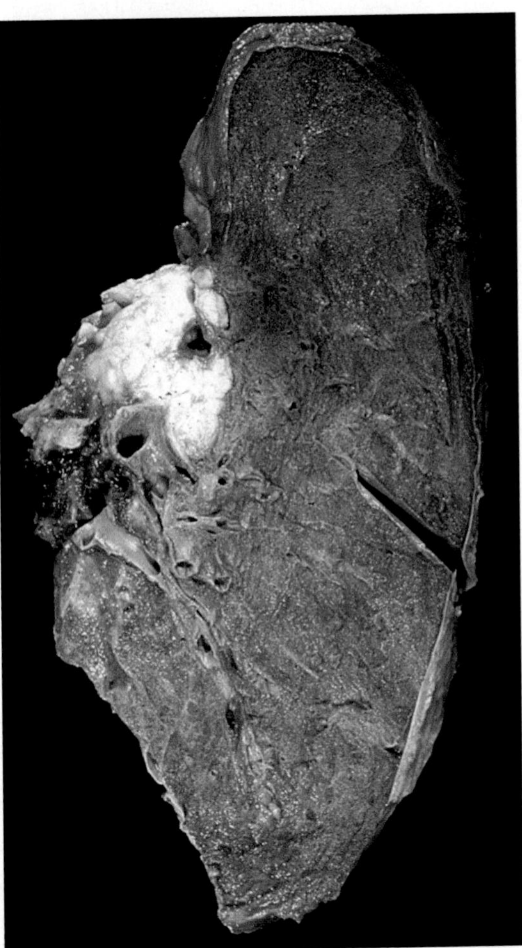

Figure 10.55 Gross figure of small cell carcinoma showing a central tumor mass not involving bronchial lumen but involving hilar lymph nodes.

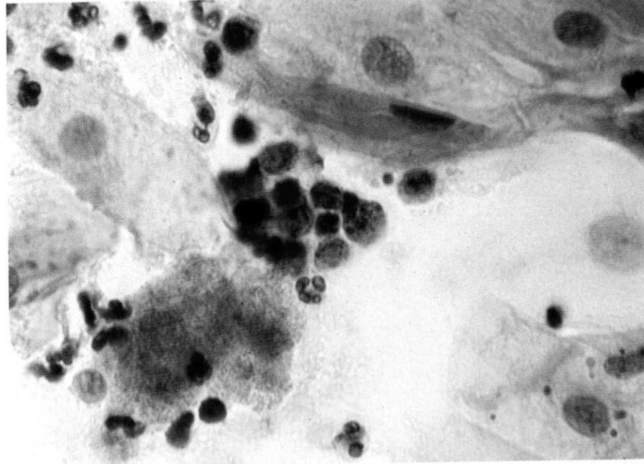

Figure 10.56 Sputum cytology figure showing a cluster of hyperchromatic small cells with indistinct cytoplasm and surrounding benign squamous cells.

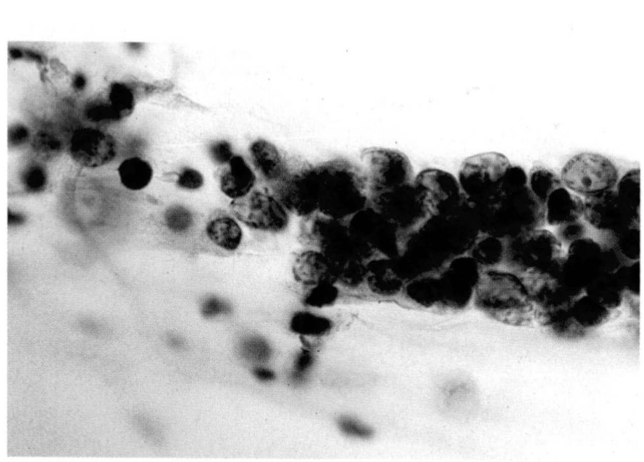

Figure 10.57 Cytology figure showing a mucus strand containing a three-dimensional cluster of small hyperchromatic cells with focal molding.

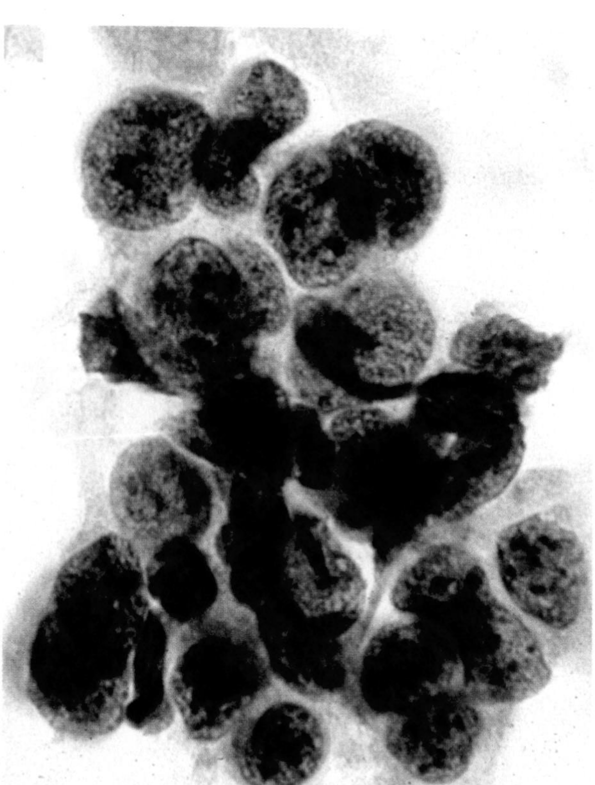

Figure 10.58 Cytology figure showing typical cytologic features of small cell carcinoma, including finely granular ("salt and pepper") chromatin pattern, inconspicuous nucleoli, molding, and scant cytoplasm.

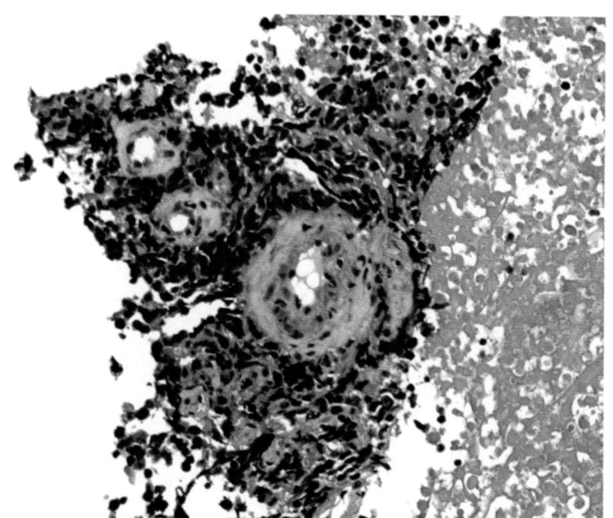

Figure 10.59 Transbronchial biopsy of small cell carcinoma with abundant crush artifact and tumor necrosis.

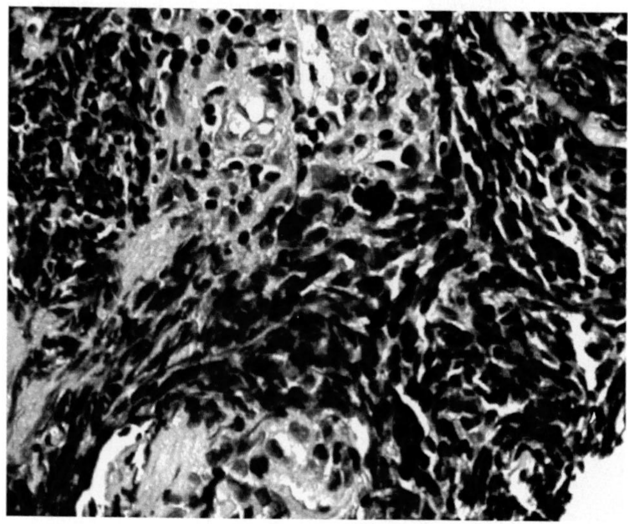

Figure 10.60 Higher power of transbronchial biopsy of small cell carcinoma showing prominent crush artifact.

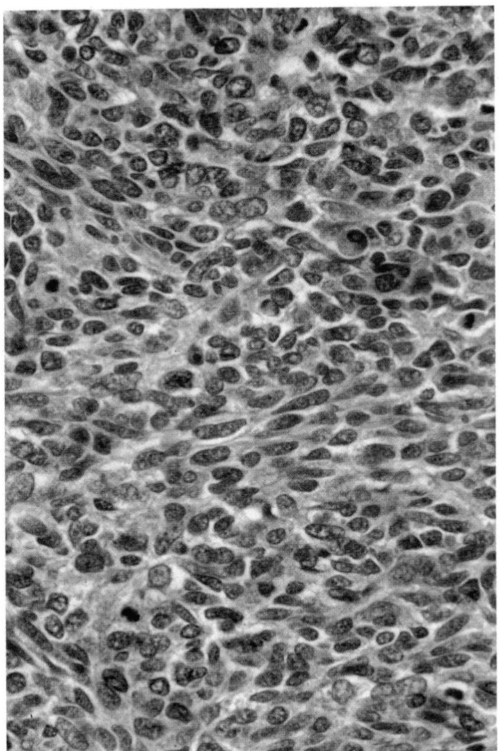

Figure 10.61 Classic appearance of small cell carcinoma, with sheets of small cells, slightly spindled shape, finely granular chromatin, and very scant cytoplasm.

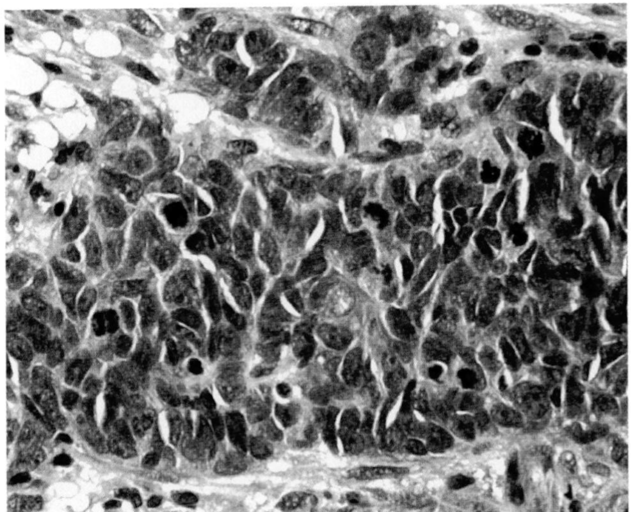

Figure 10.62 Higher power of the classic appearance of small cell carcinoma with numerous mitotic figures, scant cytoplasm, "salt and pepper" chromatin, and nuclear molding.

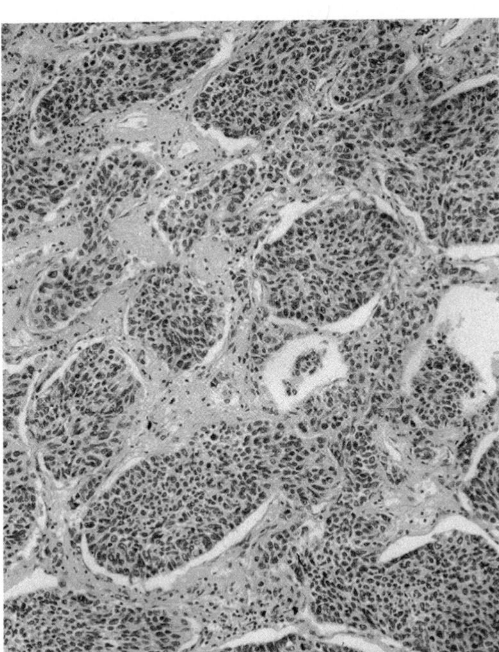

Figure 10.63 Resected small cell carcinoma with overt organoid growth pattern.

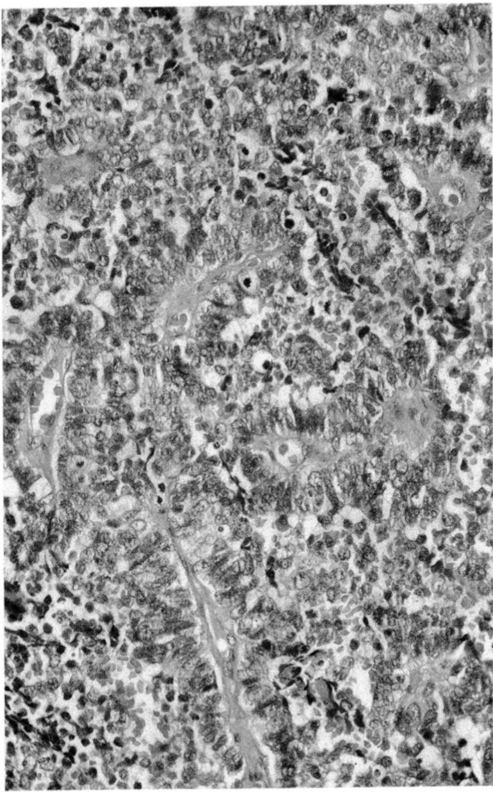

Figure 10.64 Resected small cell carcinoma with pseudopapillary pattern.

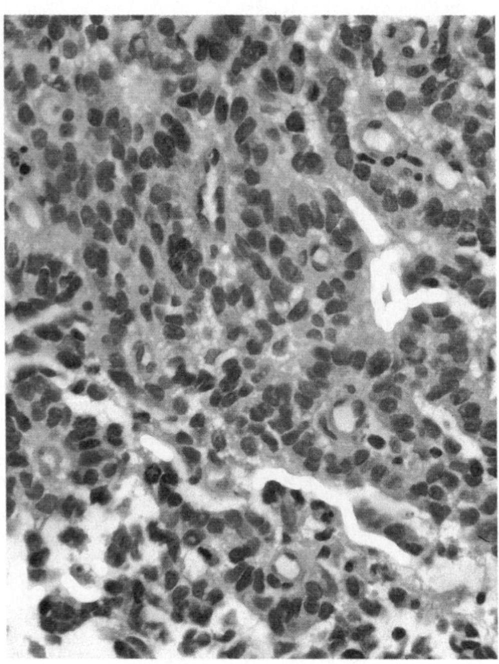

Figure 10.65 Small cell carcinoma with prominent pseudorosettes and rosettes.

Subpart 5.1

Combined Small Cell and Non–Small Cell Carcinoma

▶ Mary Beth Beasley, Alvaro C. Laga, Timothy Allen, and Philip T. Cagle

Some lung cancers may show combined small cell carcinoma and non–small cell carcinoma histopathology. A minority of small cell carcinomas show combination with squamous cell carcinoma, adenocarcinoma, or large cell carcinoma (10% or more of tumor cells) and less often with spindle cell or giant cell components. Non–small cell carcinoma components may be recognized within a treated small cell carcinoma subsequent to chemotherapy.

Histologic Features:

- Features of a small cell carcinoma component combined with features of a non–small cell carcinoma component in the same tumor.

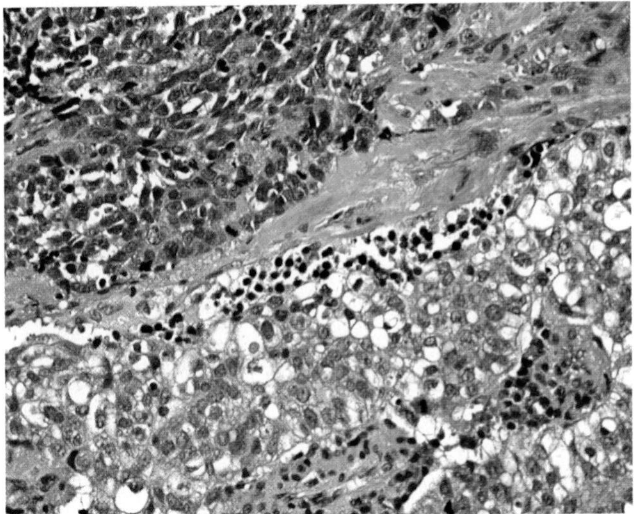

Figure 10.66 Lung cancer composed of combined small cell carcinoma in the *upper portion* of the figure and large cell carcinoma in the *lower portion* of the figure.

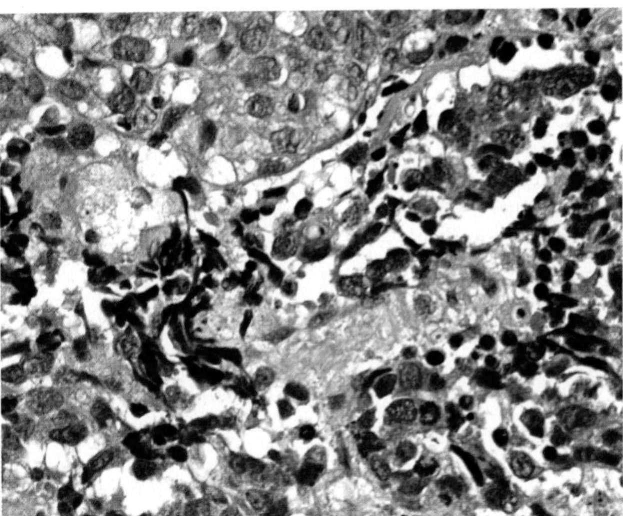

Figure 10.67 Higher power of combined small cell and non–small cell carcinoma showing large cell carcinoma with round to oval nuclei and abundant cytoplasm, and small cell carcinoma with hyperchromatic nuclei and scant cytoplasm.

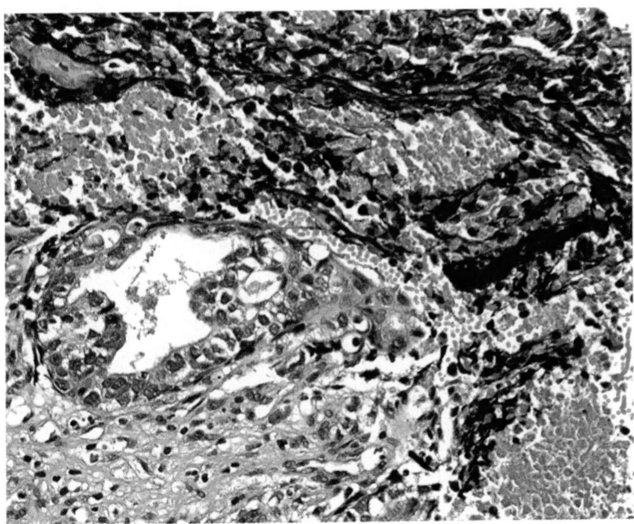

Figure 10.68 Combined tumor with adenocarcinoma in the center of the figure and small cell carcinoma showing prominent crush artifact and necrosis in the *upper* and *right-hand portions* of the figure.

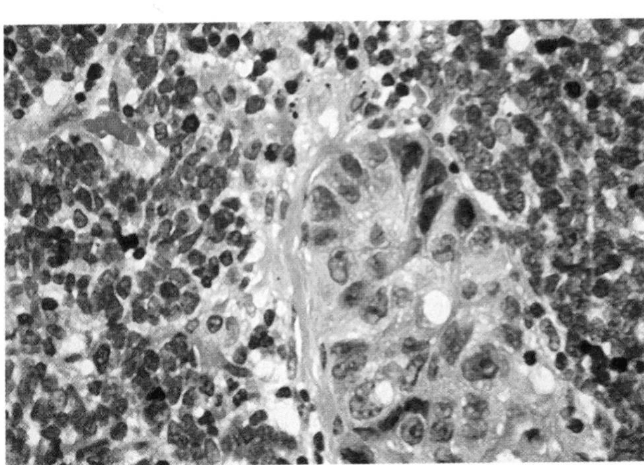

Figure 10.69 Higher power of combined small cell and adenocarcinoma showing glands and surrounding small cells with scattered mitotic figures.

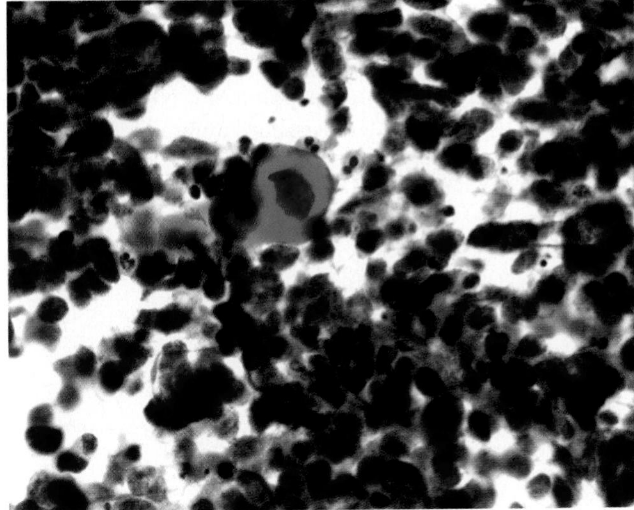

Figure 10.70 Cytology figure from a combined carcinoma showing a malignant squamous cell surrounded by small cell carcinoma cells.

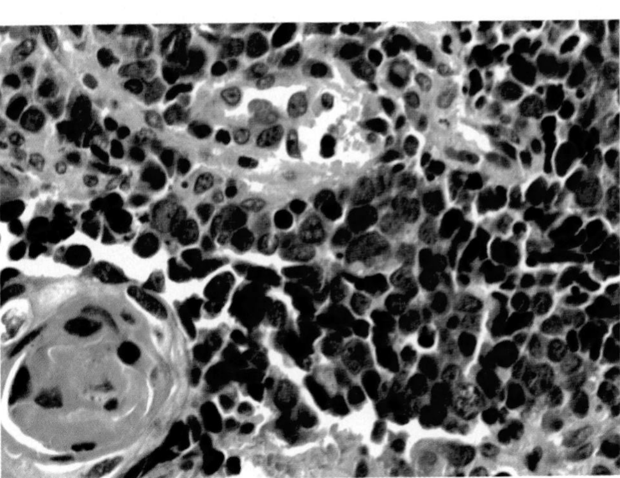

Figure 10.71 Malignant squamous cells forming a keratin pearl, with adjacent small cell carcinoma cells in a combined tumor.

Part 6

Carcinoid Tumor

▶ Mary Beth Beasley and Mary Ostrowski

Carcinoid tumors are neuroendocrine tumors that are divided in the lung into typical and atypical varieties according to strictly defined World Health Organization criteria. A typical carcinoid is defined as a carcinoid tumor that lacks necrosis and has fewer than two mitoses per 10 high-power fields. Although they are carcinomas, typical carcinoids are generally indolent cancers that only occasionally metastasize and are rarely fatal.

Cytologic Features:

- Carcinoid cells show monotonously round and regular nuclei and relatively abundant cytoplasm that is basophilic on Papanicolaou stain.
- Carcinoid cells may have a plasmacytoid appearance.

Histologic Features:

- Classic growth patterns of carcinoid tumor include organoid and trabecular patterns.
- Unusual growth patterns include papillary, pseudoglandular, follicular, prominent rosettes, and spindle cell.
- More than one growth pattern is often present in the same tumor.
- Carcinoid cells generally have uniform, round nuclei with finely granular chromatin, inconspicuous nucleoli, and scant to moderately abundant eosinophilic cytoplasm.
- Prominent nucleoli may occasionally occur.
- Carcinoid cells may occasionally show clear cytoplasm, oncocytic cytoplasm, granular basophilic "acinic" cytoplasm, and intracytoplasmic melanin pigment.
- Cellular pleomorphism may be marked, even in typical carcinoid, and is not a criterion for distinguishing typical carcinoid from atypical carcinoid.
- Stroma is typically delicate and highly vascular; however, dense hyaline collagen, amyloid-like stroma, metaplastic cartilage, or bone may occasionally occur.
- Typical carcinoids are generally immunopositive with cytokeratins (AE1/AE3, CAM5.2, CK7) and neuroendocrine markers (chromogranin, synaptophysin, NCAM [CD56], Leu-7), occasionally immunopositive with TTF-1, and usually immunonegative with CK20.

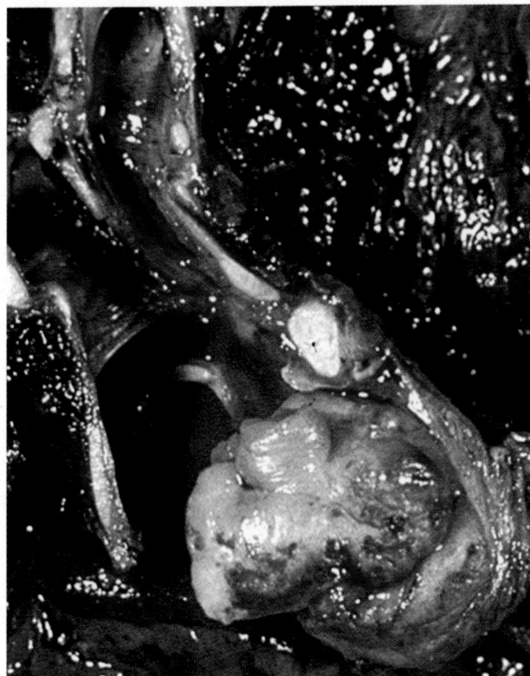

Figure 10.72 Gross figure of carcinoid tumor protruding into bronchial lumen.

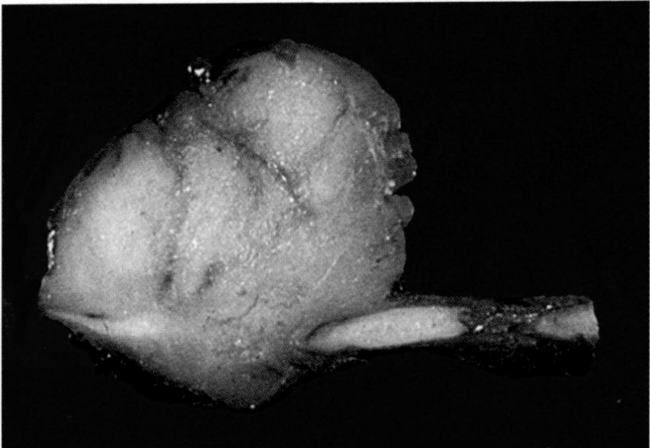

Figure 10.73 Gross figure of resected carcinoid tumor cut in cross section to show invasion through bronchial cartilage.

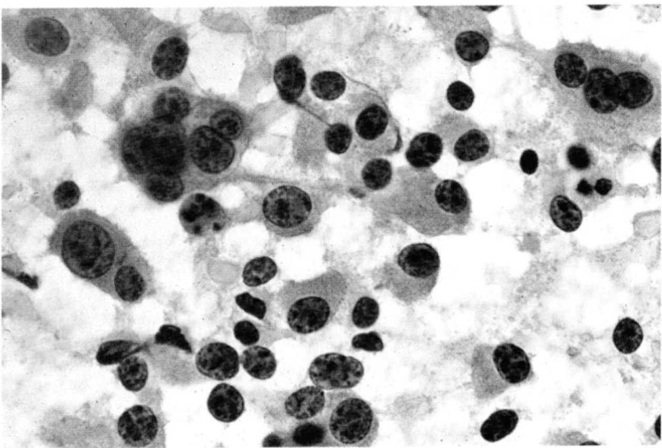

Figure 10.74 Cytology figure showing carcinoid tumor cells with plasmacytoid features including round, regular eccentric nuclei and abundant cytoplasm.

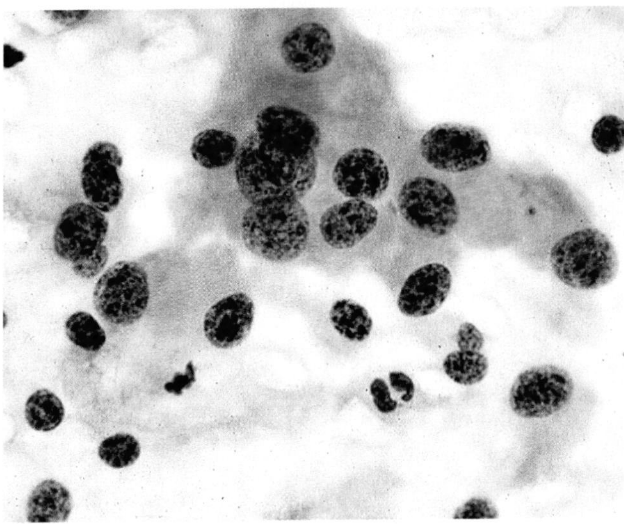

Figure 10.75 Cytology figure showing carcinoid tumor cells with round, regular nuclei with relatively abundant cytoplasm.

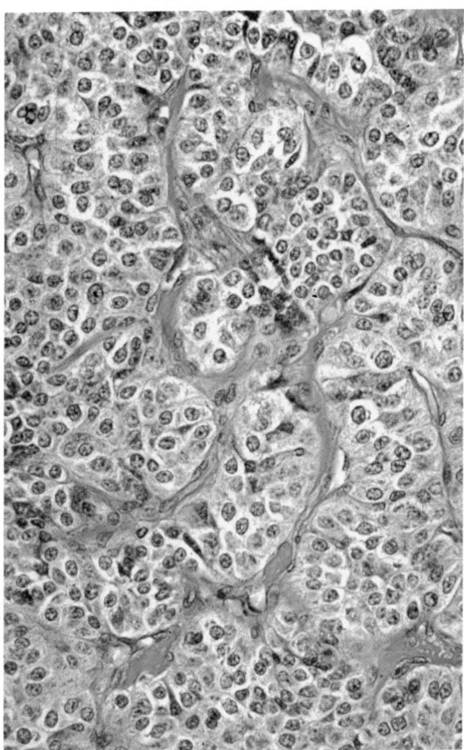

Figure 10.76 Carcinoid tumor with nests of tumor cells in classic organoid pattern.

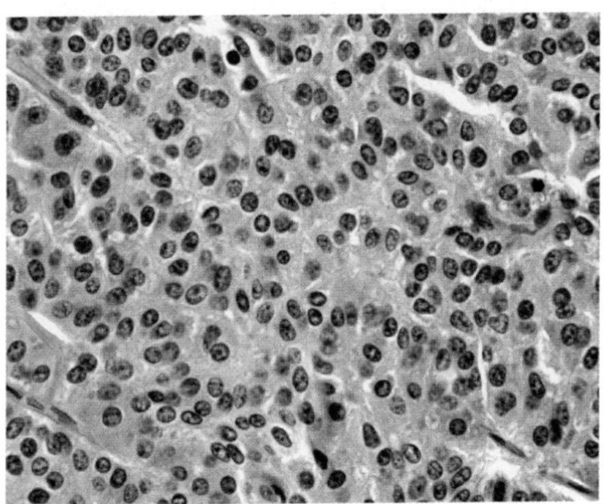

Figure 10.77 Higher power of organoid pattern with uniform nuclei and no mitoses.

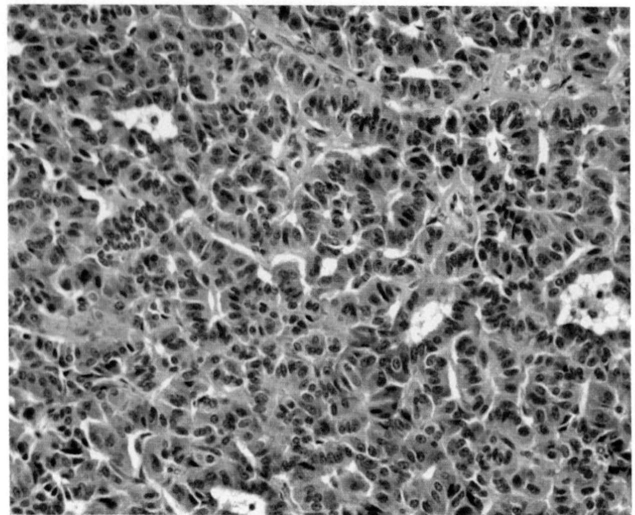

Figure 10.78 Carcinoid tumor with trabecular pattern.

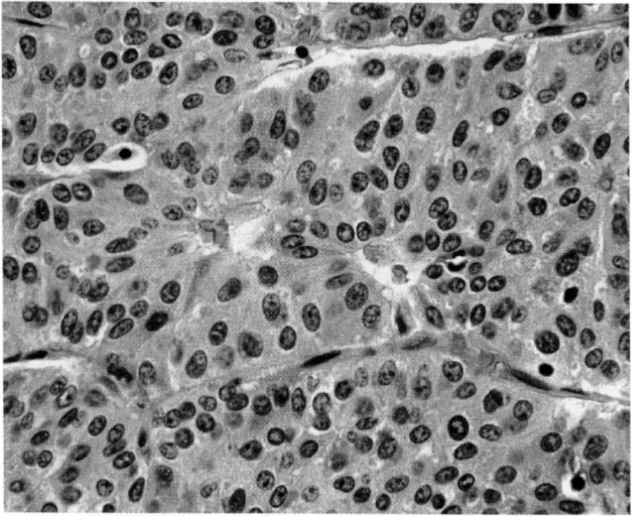

Figure 10.79 Higher power showing nests of carcinoid tumor cells with delicate intervening vascular stroma.

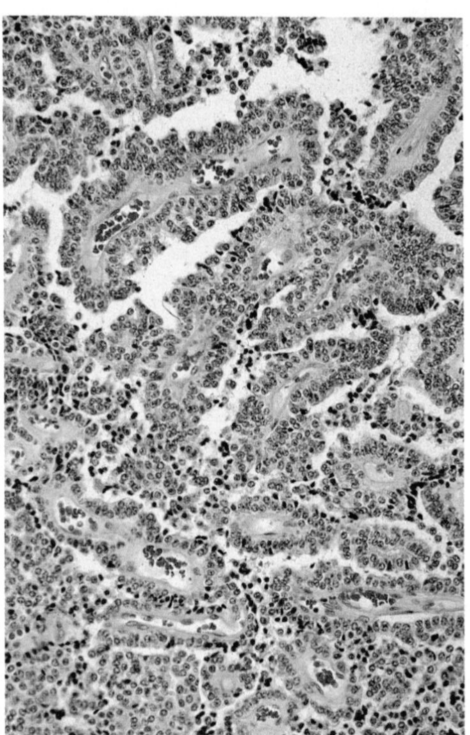

Figure 10.80 Carcinoid tumor with papillary growth pattern.

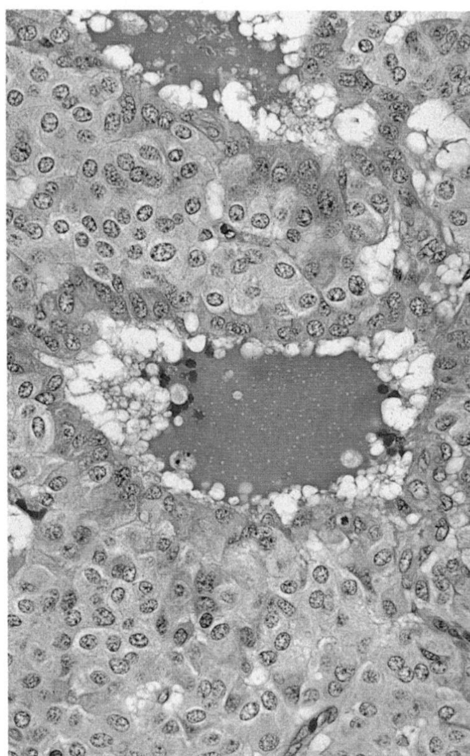

Figure 10.81 Carcinoid tumor with follicular growth pattern.

Part 7

Atypical Carcinoid

▶ Mary Beth Beasley

An atypical carcinoid is defined as a carcinoid tumor that has 2 to 10 mitoses per 10 high-power fields (2 mm^2) and/or necrosis. Carcinoid tumors with necrosis and fewer than 2 mitoses per 10 high-power fields should be classified as atypical carcinoids, as studies have supported their more aggressive behavior. The vast majority of atypical carcinoids fulfill both criteria. Atypical carcinoids have a higher metastatic rate and worse prognosis than typical carcinoids.

Cytologic Features:

- Atypical carcinoids have cytologic features similar to typical carcinoids but with additional findings of necrosis and increased mitoses.

Histologic Features:

- Atypical carcinoids show histologic features similar to typical carcinoids but with additional findings of necrosis and more than 2 mitoses per high-power field.
- Necrosis is typically present centrally within organoid nests and may be punctate; zones of "infarctlike" necrosis may occur.
- Mitotic activity should be assessed in the most active areas; ideally, three sets of 10 high-power fields should be counted and averaged.
- Atypical carcinoids, like typical carcinoids, are typically immunopositive for cytokeratins (AE1/AE3, CAM5.2, CK7) and neuroendocrine markers (chromogranin, synaptophysin, Leu-7, NCAM [CD56]) and typically immunonegative for CK20.
- In contrast to typical carcinoids, most atypical carcinoids are immunopositive for TTF-1.

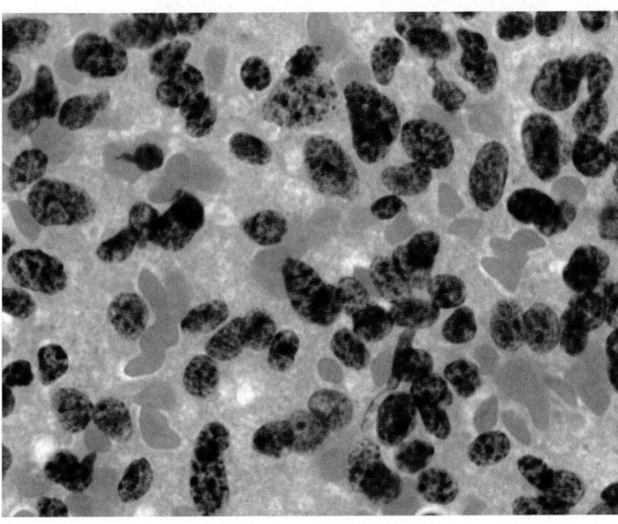

Figure 10.82 Cytology figure of an atypical carcinoid showing relatively uniform cells similar to those of a typical carcinoid.

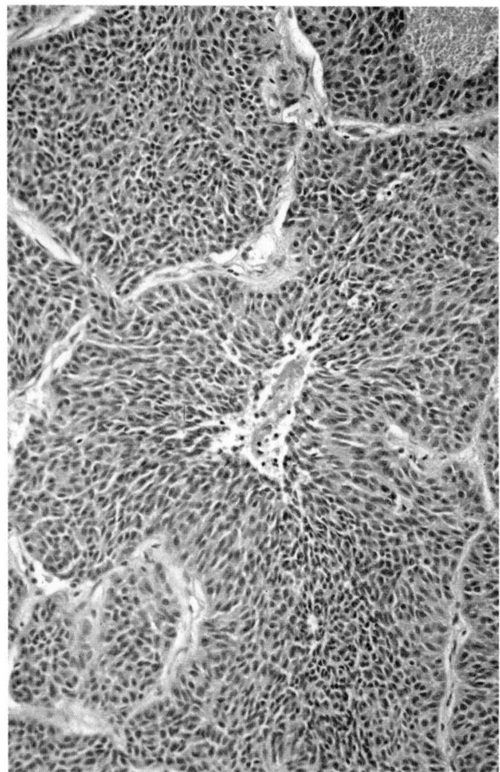

Figure 10.83 Atypical carcinoid with classic pattern of necrosis within organoid nest in upper right.

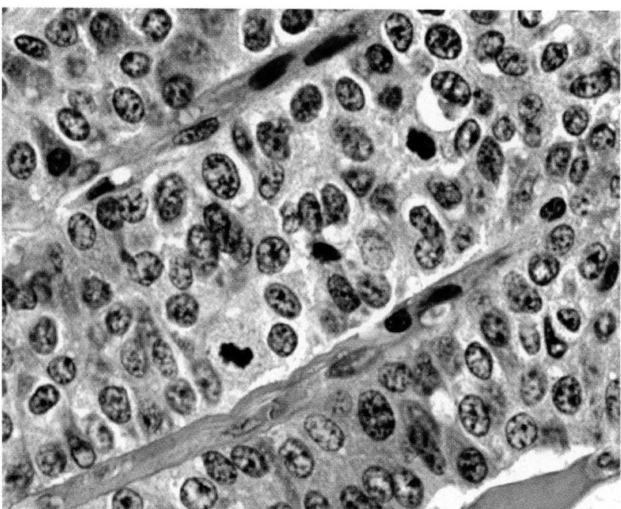

Figure 10.84 Higher power of atypical carcinoid showing scattered mitotic figures.

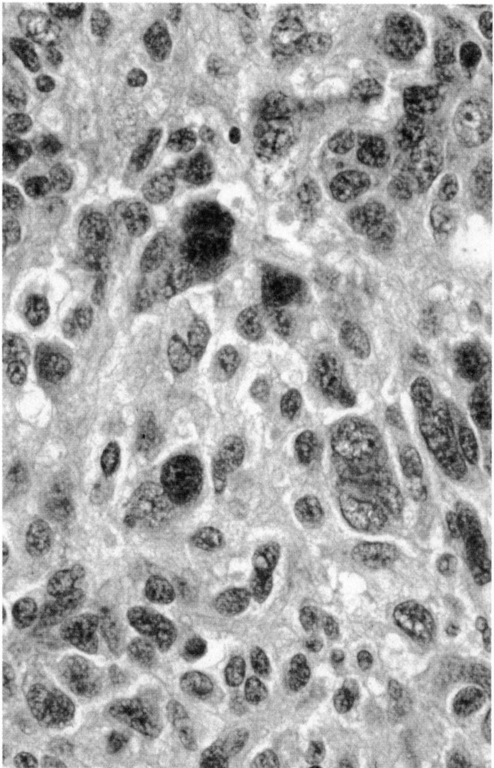

Figure 10.85 Cellular pleomorphism (may be marked in either typical carcinoid or atypical carcinoid).

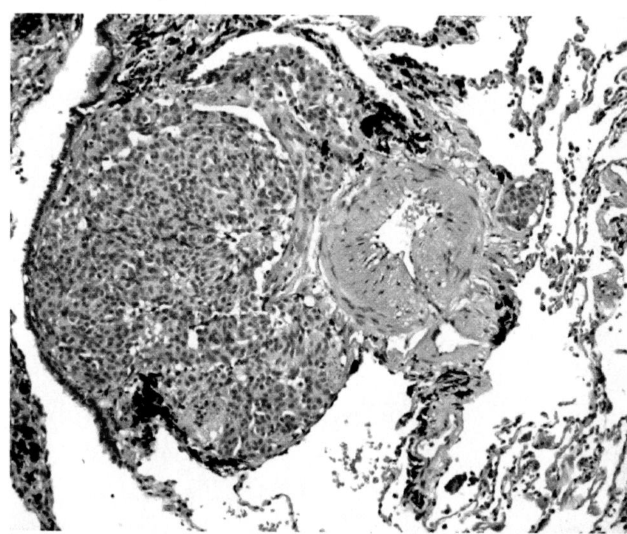

Figure 10.86 Metastatic atypical carcinoid within a perivascular lymphatic.

Part 8

Large Cell Neuroendocrine Carcinoma

▶ Mary Beth Beasley

Large cell neuroendocrine carcinoma (LCNEC) is a high-grade carcinoma with neuroendocrine morphology, cytologic features of large cell carcinoma, and a mitotic rate of greater than 10 per 10 high-power fields. Neuroendocrine differentiation by immunohistochemistry must be demonstrated to fulfill the World Health Organization criteria.

Histologic Features:

- Neuroendocrine morphology, typically consisting of an organoid or nested pattern, must be present.
- Peripheral palisading around tumor nests is common, and rosette formation may be prominent.
- Necrosis may occur centrally within nests.
- LCNECs have a mitotic rate greater than 10 per 10 high-power fields, typically averaging 70 per 10 high-power fields.
- Features differentiating LCNEC from small cell carcinoma include large cell size; polygonal shape; moderately abundant cytoplasm; course or vesicular, rather than finely granular, chromatin; frequent nucleoli; and lack of prominent spindle morphology.
- LCNEC may occur combined with conventional adenocarcinoma, squamous carcinoma, or carcinoma with spindle cell features.
- LCNECs are generally immunopositive for TTF-1, pan-keratin, and CK7, and immunonegative for CK34βe12 (distinguishing LCNEC from basaloid carcinoma).
- World Health Organization criteria require that at least one neuroendocrine marker such as chromogranin or synaptophysin be immunopositive.

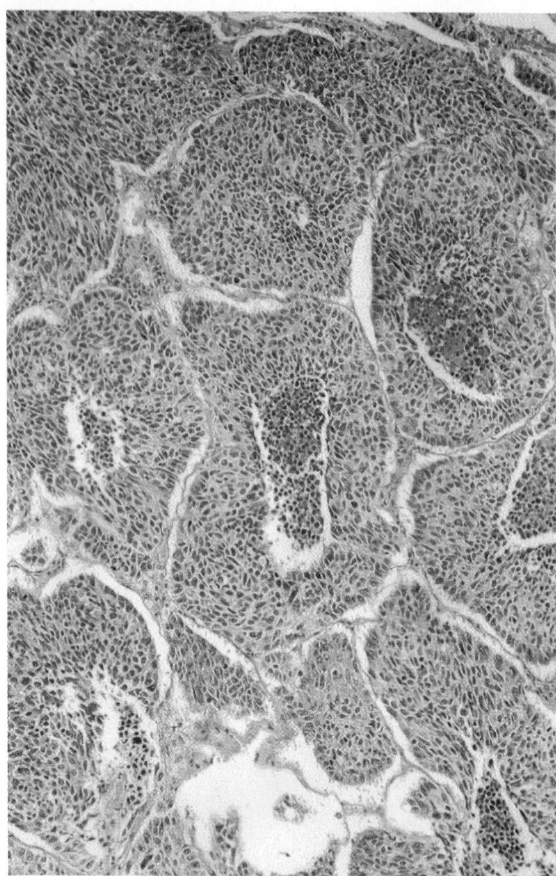

Figure 10.87 Typical organoid growth pattern; LCNEC may resemble atypical carcinoid at low power but they are easily distinguished by the increased mitotic activity in LCNEC.

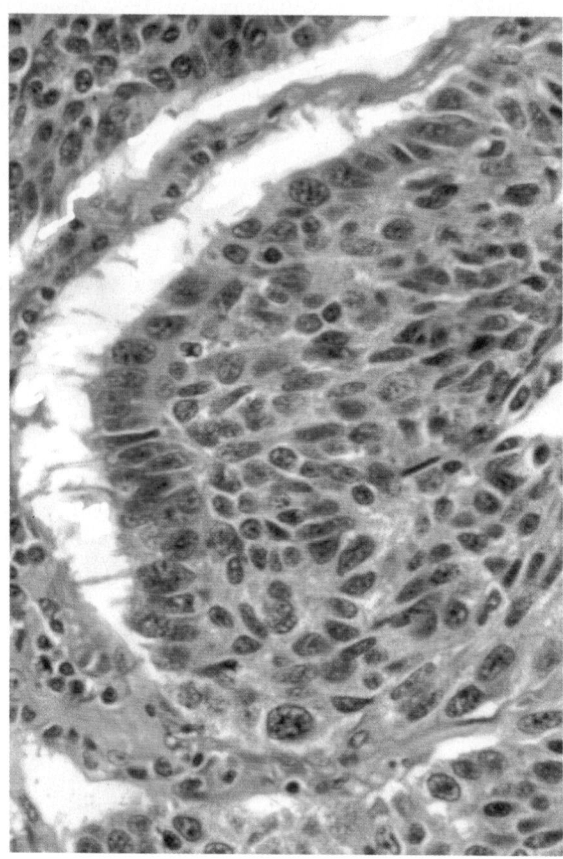

Figure 10.88 Peripheral palisading around organoid nests.

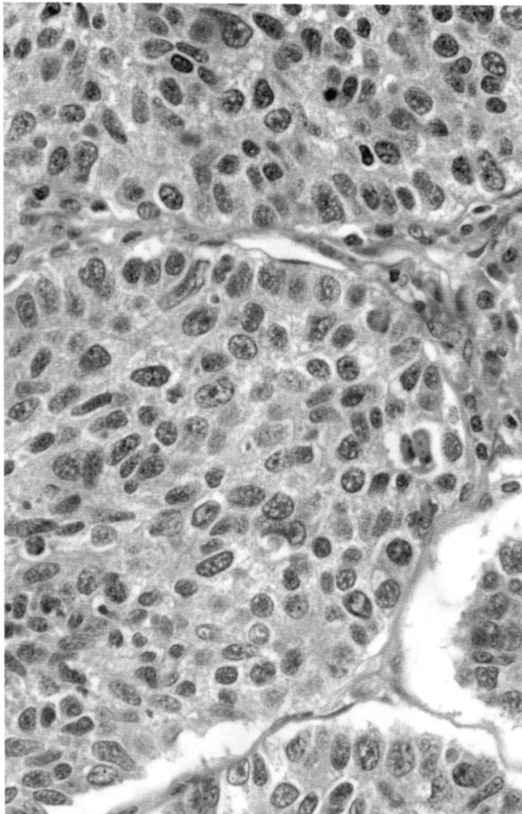

Figure 10.89 Large cell features include moderately abundant cytoplasm, vesicular nuclei, and prominent nucleoli.

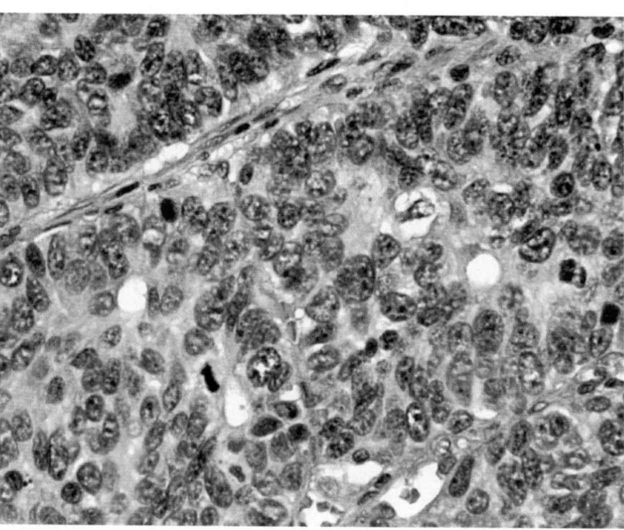

Figure 10.90 Higher power of LCNEC showing organoid nests with scattered mitotic figures.

Part 9

Adenosquamous Carcinoma

▶ Alvaro C. Laga, Timothy Allen, and Philip T. Cagle

Adenosquamous carcinoma is a rare subtype of lung cancer containing components of both adenocarcinoma and squamous carcinoma. A definitive diagnosis requires the presence of unequivocal squamous differentiation in the form of keratin or intercellular bridges and unequivocal glandular differentiation in the form of acini, tubules, or papillary structures, and requires a minimum of 10% of each component in the whole tumor. Some studies have shown a poorer prognosis for lung adenosquamous carcinoma than for adenocarcinoma or squamous carcinoma.

Cytologic Features:

- Cytologic features of both squamous cell carcinoma and adenocarcinoma may be present.

Histologic Features:

- Minimum of 10% of squamous component and minimum of 10% of adenocarcinoma component.
- Unequivocal squamous differentiation consists of keratin or intercellular bridges.
- Unequivocal glandular differentiation consists of acini, tubules, or papillary structures.

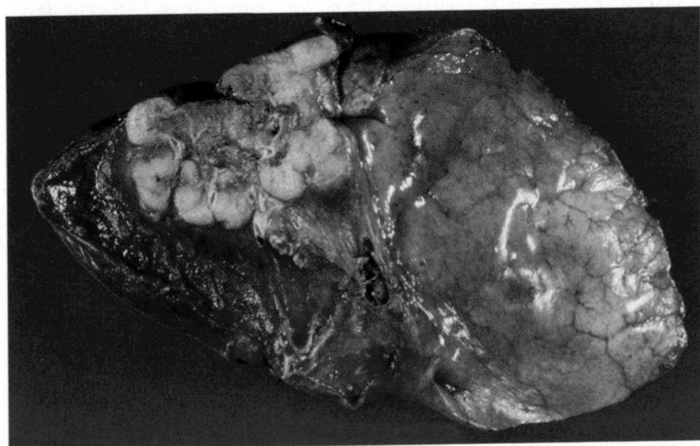

Figure 10.91 Gross figure of adenosquamous carcinoma showing large peripheral mass.

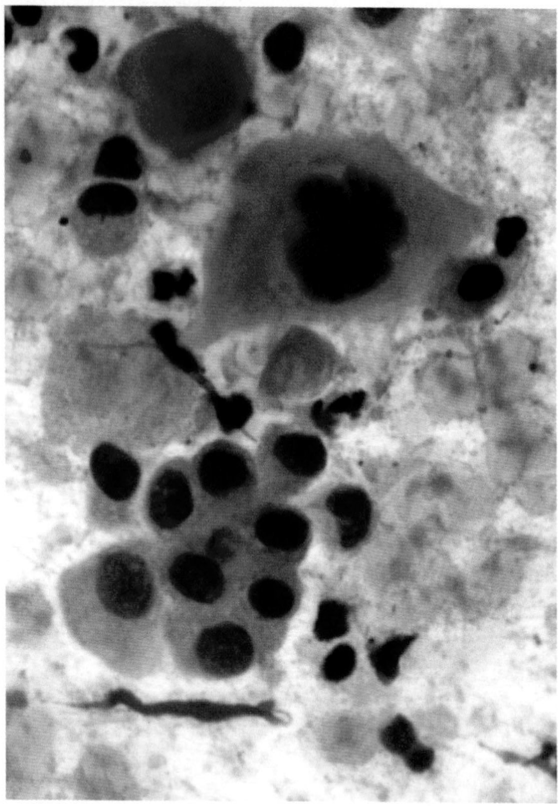

Figure 10.92 Cytology figure showing a malignant squamous cell *(upper)* adjacent to adenocarcinoma cells *(lower)*.

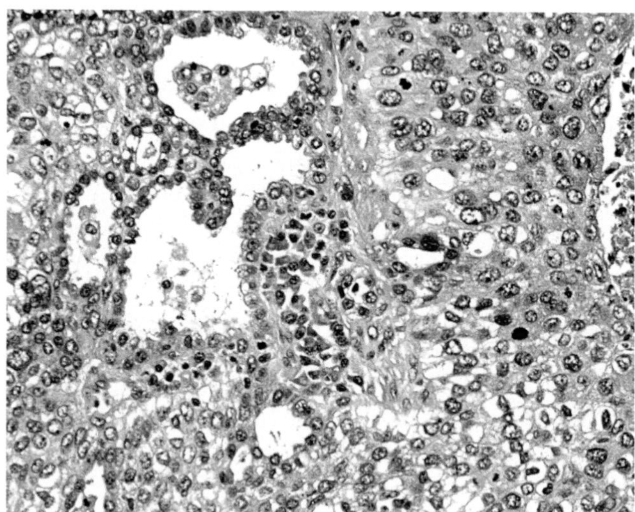

Figure 10.93 Glands of adenocarcinoma on the *left*, adjacent to moderately differentiated squamous cell carcinoma on the *right*.

Part **10**

Basaloid Carcinoma

▶ Alvaro C. Laga, Timothy Allen, Mary Ostrowski, and Philip T. Cagle

Basaloid carcinoma is a rare form of non–small cell lung carcinoma that is classified as a variant of large cell carcinoma when histologically pure and as a variant of squamous cell carcinoma when a squamous cell carcinoma component is also present. Basaloid carcinoma has a solid lobular or trabecular pattern of small cuboidal to fusiform cells with moderately hyperchromatic nuclei, finely granular chromatin, inconspicuous nucleoli, a high nuclear-to-cytoplasm ratio, peripheral palisading, and prominent mitotic figures. Comedo-type necrosis may be present. Approximately one third contain rosettes. Only about 10% of basaloid carcinomas express a neuroendocrine marker and, in these cases, in only 5% to 20% of cells. Basaloid carcinoma is immunonegative for TTF-1.

Cytologic Features:

- Small cuboidal to spindle cells with scant cytoplasm.

Histologic Features:

- Small cuboidal to fusiform cells with moderately hyperchromatic nuclei containing finely granular chromatin and inconspicuous nucleoli.
- High nuclear-to-cytoplasm ratio.
- Peripheral palisading.
- Prominent mitotic figures.
- Focally positive for neuroendocrine markers in 10% of cases and immunonegative for TTF-1.

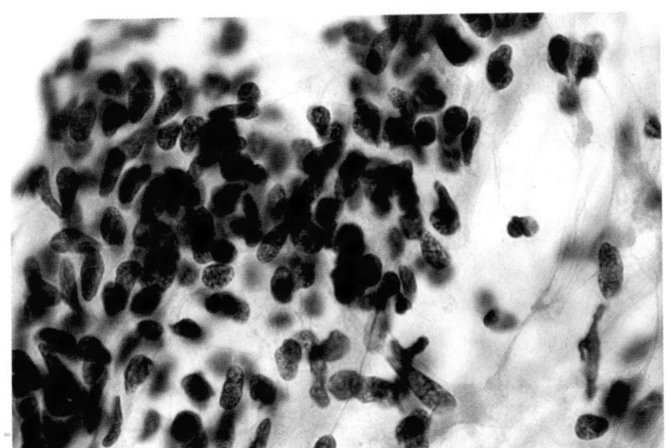

Figure 10.94 Cytology figure showing small cuboidal to spindle cells with scant cytoplasm.

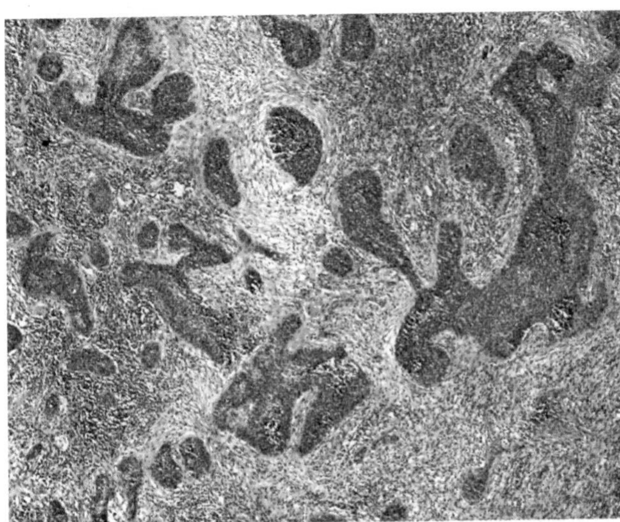

Figure 10.95 Low power of basaloid carcinoma showing nests of cells within a desmoplastic stroma with aggregates of inflammatory cells.

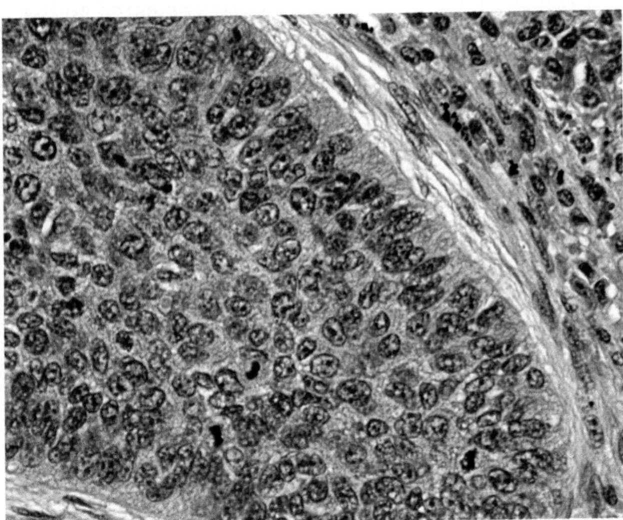

Figure 10.96 High power showing small cuboidal to fusiform cells and peripheral palisading.

Part 11

Sarcomatoid (Sarcomatous) Carcinoma

▶ Alvaro C. Laga, Timothy Allen, Mary Ostrowski, and Philip T. Cagle

Rarely poorly differentiated non–small cell carcinomas may have a spindle cell or sarcomatoid component or may be entirely spindle cell or sarcomatoid. Carcinomas with these histopathologic features have been given many different designations and classifications over the years. This group includes pleomorphic carcinoma, spindle cell carcinoma, giant cell carcinoma, carcinosarcoma, and pulmonary blastoma. Due to their distinctive histopathology, giant cell carcinoma and pulmonary blastoma are discussed in Parts 12 and 13 of this chapter, respectively.

Cytologic Features:

- Cytologic features include sarcomatoid (spindle cell) elements with or without carcinoma (epithelial) components, giant cells, and/or heterologous elements (malignant bone, cartilage, or muscle).

Histologic Features:

- Sarcomatoid carcinomas consist of carcinomas with sarcoma or sarcomalike features, including malignant spindle cells, giant cells, and/or heterologous elements.
- Pleomorphic carcinomas consist of non–small cell carcinomas with spindle cell and/or giant cell components (at least 10%) or consist purely of spindle cell and/or giant cell components.
- Spindle cell carcinomas are non–small cell carcinomas composed purely of malignant spindle cells.
- Carcinosarcomas are mixtures of carcinoma and sarcoma with heterologous (differentiated) elements, including malignant cartilage, bone, or skeletal muscle.
- Malignant spindle cells in sarcomatoid carcinomas are typically vimentin positive. Immunopositivity for cytokeratin in the malignant spindle cells supports a diagnosis of sarcomatoid carcinoma. However, a negative cytokeratin immunostain does not rule out this diagnosis.
- Due to their poor differentiation, sarcomatoid carcinomas are typically immunonegative for carcinoma markers such as CEA.
- Small cell carcinoma with a sarcomatoid component is classified as combined small cell carcinoma with sarcomatoid component (see Part 5, Subpart 5.1).

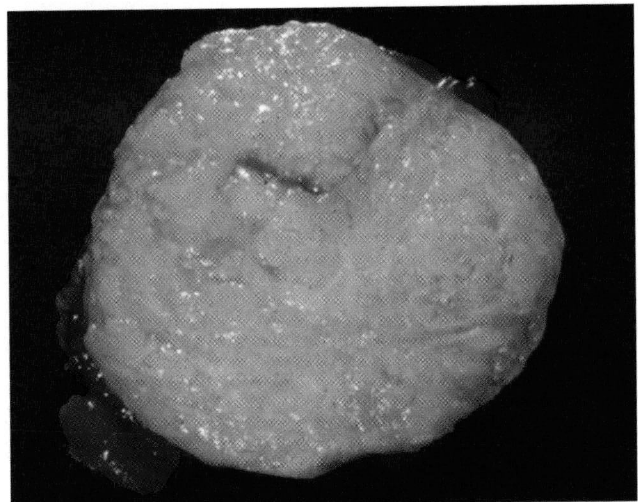

Figure 10.97 Gross of peripheral carcinosarcoma shows well-circumscribed mass with heterogeneous cut surface.

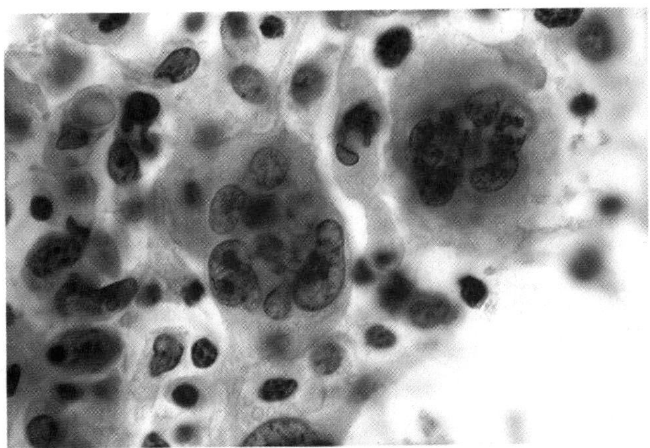

Figure 10.98 Cytology of pleomorphic carcinoma with multinucleated giant cells.

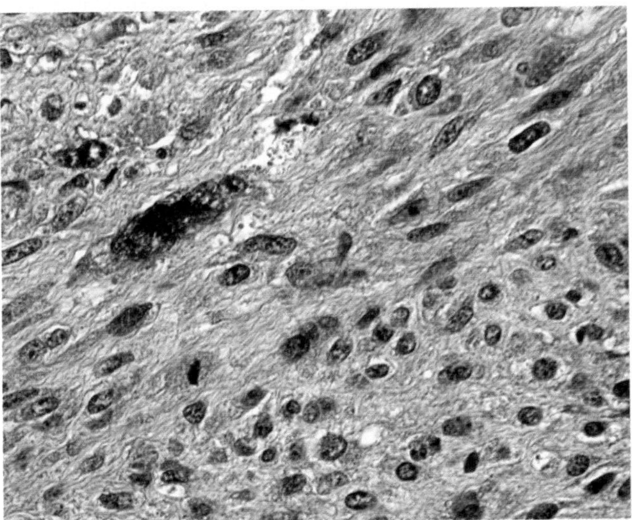

Figure 10.99 Histology of spindle cell carcinoma shows malignant spindle cells.

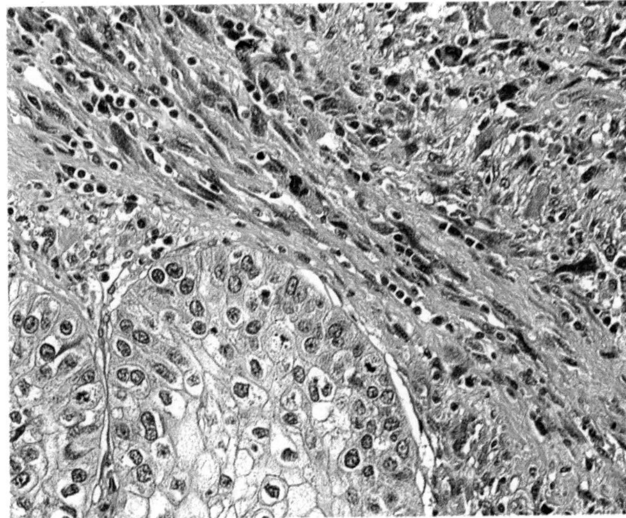

Figure 10.100 Sarcomatoid (pleomorphic) carcinoma with combined squamous cell carcinoma *(lower left)* and malignant spindle cell component.

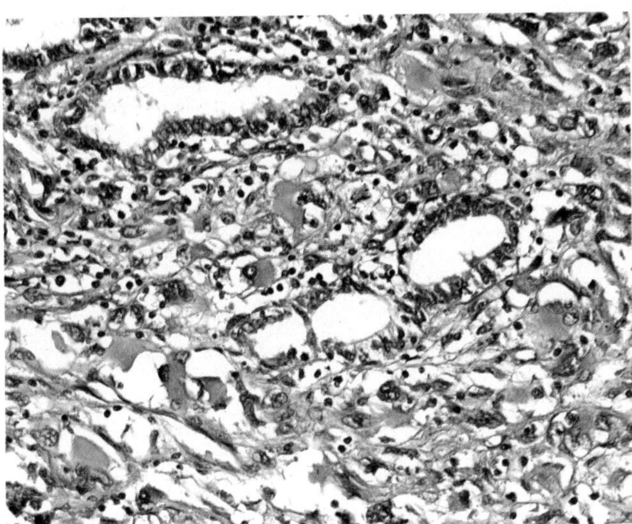

Figure 10.101 Sarcomatoid (pleomorphic) carcinoma with glands of adenocarcinoma combined with malignant spindle cell component.

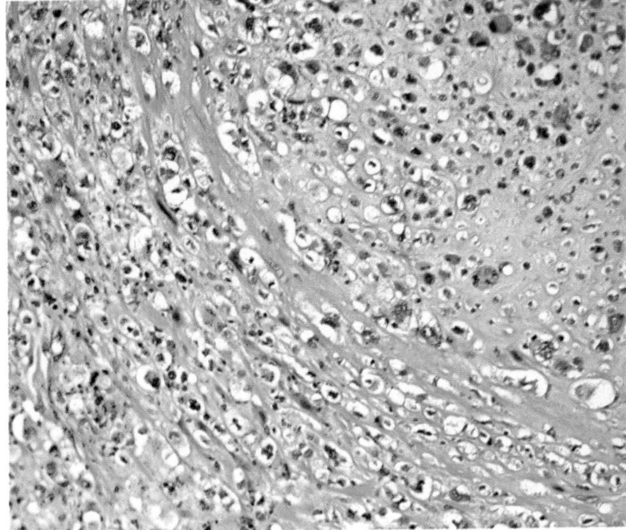

Figure 10.102 Carcinosarcoma with malignant cartilage *(upper right)*.

Part 12

Giant Cell Carcinoma

▶ Alvaro C. Laga, Timothy Allen, and Philip T. Cagle

Giant cell carcinoma is a rare tumor composed of highly pleomorphic tumor giant cells currently classified with the sarcomatoid carcinomas. Tumor cells are discohesive pleomorphic tumor giant cells that may be bizarre and multinucleated or have multilobed nuclei. There is an associated inflammatory infiltrate that includes many neutrophils and neutrophils typically penetrating the cytoplasm of the giant cells (emperipolesis). Although other types of lung cancer may occasionally contain giant cells, especially after radiation therapy, they lack the diagnostic features of giant cell carcinoma.

Histologic Features:

- Discohesive pleomorphic giant cells, typically very large, often bizarre, with multinucleated or multilobed nuclei.
- Inflammatory infiltrates including numerous neutrophils.
- Neutrophils often penetrate the cytoplasm of the giant tumor cells (emperipolesis).

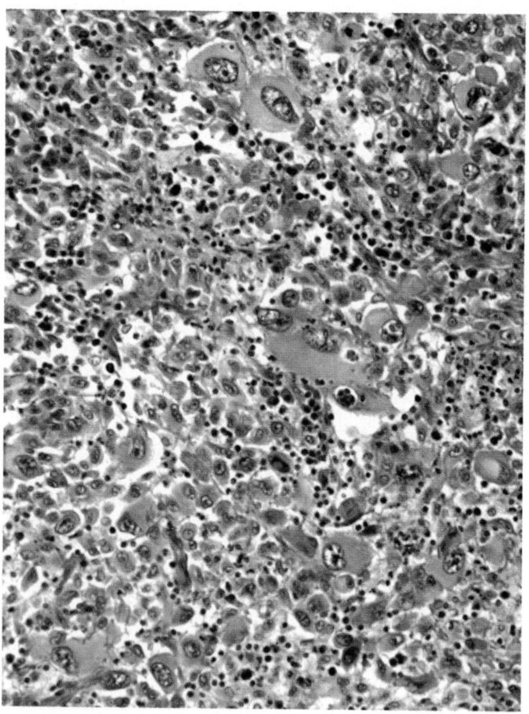

Figure 10.103 Giant cell carcinoma with discohesive pleomorphic giant cells with a neutrophilic infiltrate and focal emperipolesis (penetration of giant cell cytoplasm by neutrophils).

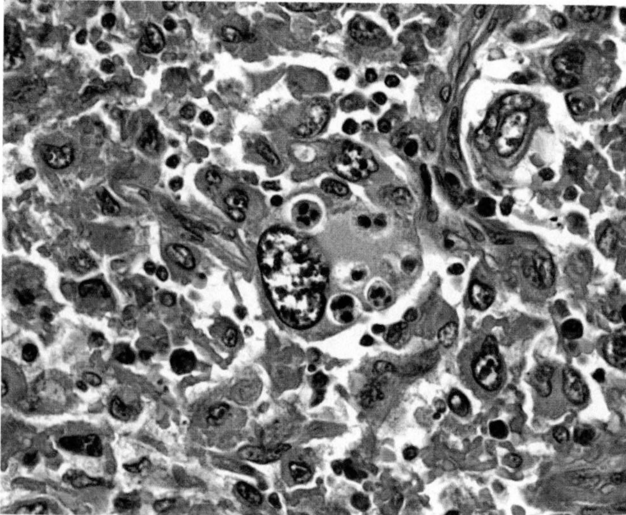

Figure 10.104 Higher power showing a pleomorphic giant cell with infiltration of its cytoplasm by neutrophils (emperipolesis).

Part 13

Pulmonary Blastoma

▶ Alvaro C. Laga, Timothy Allen, Carlos Bedrossian, and Philip T. Cagle

Pulmonary blastoma is a rare biphasic tumor consisting of immature or primitive epithelial and mesenchymal components, resembling embryonic lung. These tumors commonly present as large masses with satellite lesions and are associated with pleural effusion in about 50% of the cases. Both the epithelial and mesenchymal components are malignant. The epithelial component consists of glands lined by columnar cells with glycogen-filled vacuoles similar to fetal adenocarcinoma (see Part 1, Subpart 1.2). The mesenchymal component consists of blasteme-like primitive spindle to oval cells in a myxoid stroma. Foci of adult-type sarcoma with or without heterologous (differentiated) elements such as malignant osteoid, cartilage, or skeletal muscle may be present. The histologic distinction between pulmonary blastoma and fetal adenocarcinoma has prognostic significance because the prognosis of pulmonary blastoma usually is much worse than that of fetal adenocarcinoma.

Histologic Features:

- Pulmonary blastomas are biphasic with malignant epithelial and mesenchymal components.
- The epithelial component of pulmonary blastoma consists of glands lined by columnar cells with glycogen-filled vacuoles, often resembling fetal adenocarcinoma.
- Squamoid morules may be seen in the epithelial component of pulmonary blastomas.
- The mesenchyme in pulmonary blastoma is histologically primitive, consisting of spindle to oval cells in a myxoid stroma, occasionally with foci of adult-type sarcoma, sometimes including osteosarcoma, chondrosarcoma, or rhabdomyosarcoma.

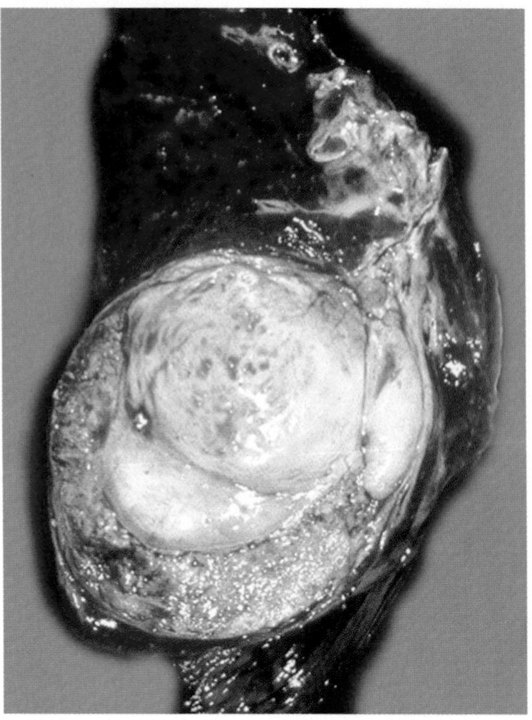

Figure 10.105 Gross figure of pulmonary blastoma consisting of a large, solid, fleshy mass.

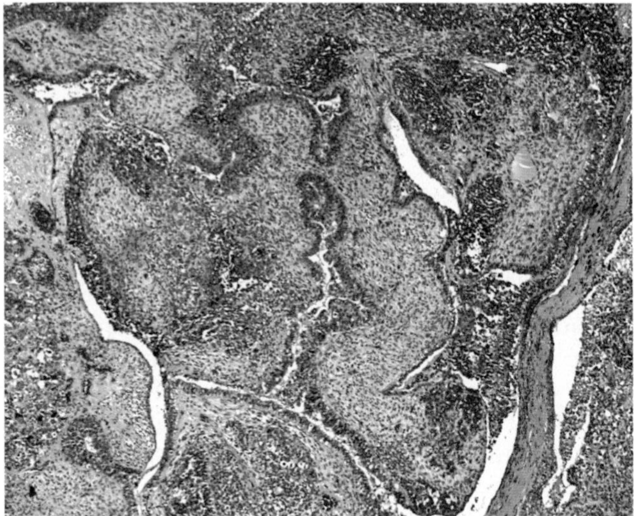

Figure 10.106 Pulmonary blastoma consisting of a primitive spindle cell mesenchymal component with myxoid stroma and a malignant glandular component.

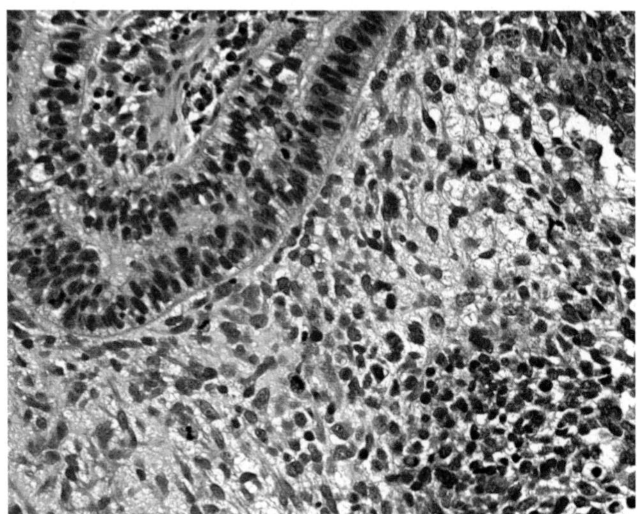

Figure 10.107 Glandular component of pulmonary blastoma resembles the columnar cells of fetal adenocarcinoma; mesenchymal component consists of primitive malignant spindle cells in a myxoid stroma.

Part 14

Mucoepidermoid Carcinoma

▶ Alvaro C. Laga, Timothy Allen, Handan Zeren, and Philip T. Cagle

Morphologically similar to mucoepidermoid carcinoma of salivary gland origin, mucoepidermoid carcinoma of the lung is uncommon, accounting for less than 1% of primary lung cancers, and arises from the submucosal bronchial glands. Mucoepidermoid carcinoma is composed of varying mixtures of mucinous glandular cells, squamoid cells, and intermediate cells. It is classified as either high-grade or low-grade mucoepidermoid carcinoma based on its histologic appearance.

Low-grade mucoepidermoid carcinomas typically have prominent cystic areas. Solid areas are composed of glands and small cysts lined by mucinous cells and columnar cells. In low-grade tumors, the mucinous cells have mild cytologic atypia and rare mitoses. Typically intermixed with the mucinous cells are sheets of nonkeratinizing squamoid cells and oval intermediate cells with eosinophilic cytoplasm. The stroma tends to be myxoid with focal hyalinization.

High-grade mucoepidermoid carcinoma generally shows areas of solid growth composed mostly of squamoid and intermediate cells with a lesser glandular component. The cells show increased cytologic atypia and mitotic figures, and tumor necrosis is more prominent. Despite some resemblance to adenosquamous carcinoma, keratinization and squamous pearl formation are not expected in high-grade mucoepidermoid carcinomas.

Cytologic Features:

- Low-grade mucoepidermoid carcinoma shows predominantly bland glandular cells, with other cells such as mucous goblet cells, intermediate cells, and squamoid cells.
- High-grade mucoepidermoid carcinoma shows features similar to low-grade tumors but with increased pleomorphism, a larger component of squamoid differentiation, and a solid growth pattern.

Histologic Features:

- Exophytic, with smooth or papillary contours, soft, cystic, solid, and mucoid, approximately 0.5 to 6 cm.
- Low-grade mucoepidermoid carcinomas have abundant mucinous cysts and predominantly bland glandular components with sheets of squamoid cells, rare mitoses, and mild cytologic atypia.
- High-grade mucoepidermoid carcinomas have sheets of squamoid and intermediate cells with fewer glandular components, frequent mitotic figures, moderate cytologic atypia, and necrosis.

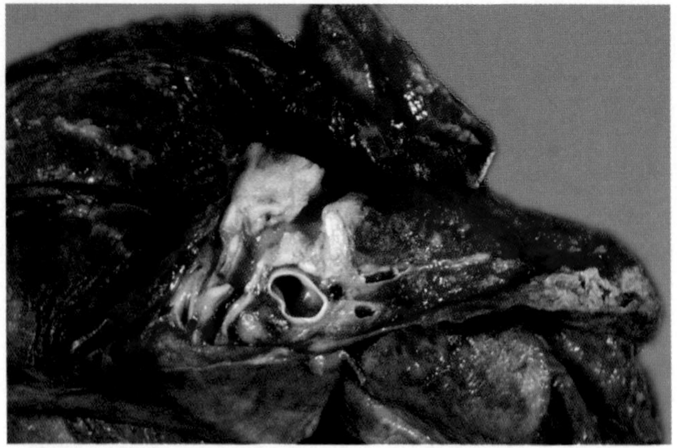

Figure 10.108 Gross figure of a centrally located mucoepidermoid carcinoma.

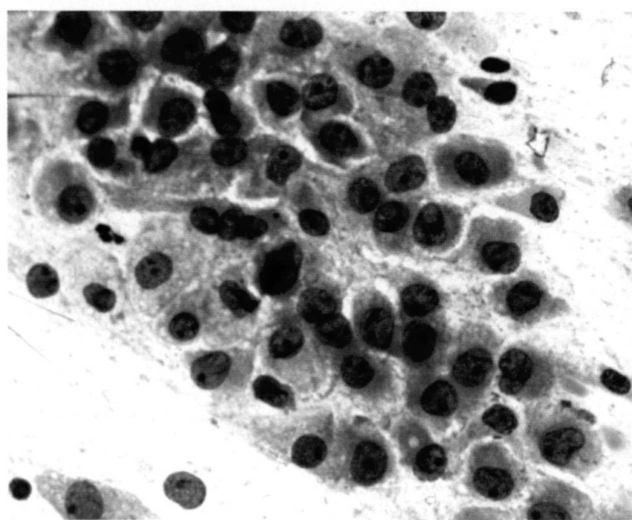

Figure 10.109 Cytology figure showing bland glandular epithelial cells with distinct nucleoli.

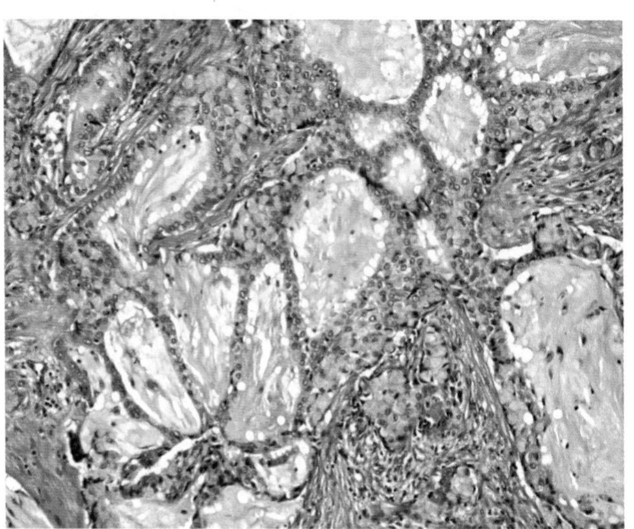

Figure 10.110 Mucoepidermoid carcinoma with mucin-filled glands lined by bland glandular cells and goblet cells, with mild atypia.

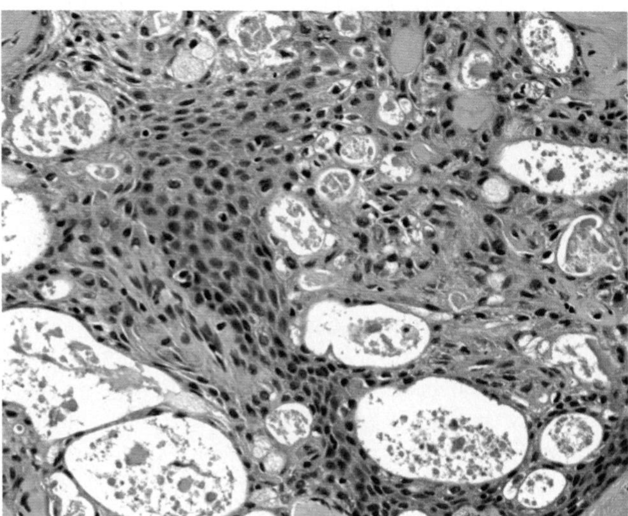

Figure 10.111 Mucoepidermoid carcinoma with a combination of well-differentiated glands and squamous cells.

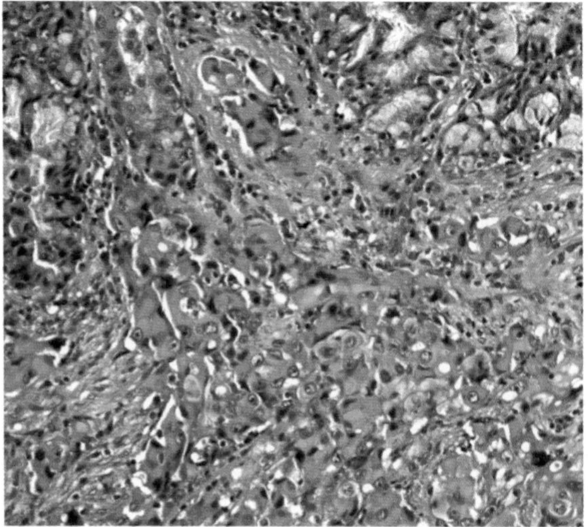

Figure 10.112 High-grade mucoepidermoid carcinoma consists primarily of solid squamoid areas without keratinization *(lower portion)* with glands lined by more cytologically atypical cells *(upper portion)*.

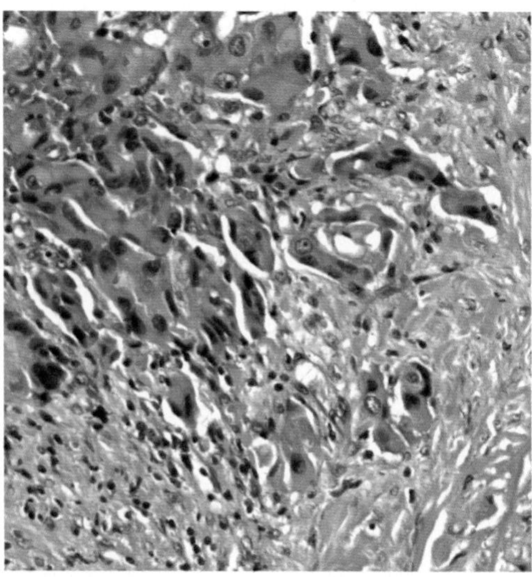

Figure 10.113 Solid squamoid area of high-grade mucoepidermoid carcinoma infiltrates fibrous tissue and lacks individual cell keratinization or keratin pearls.

Part 15

Adenoid Cystic Carcinoma

▶ Handan Zeren and Carlos Bedrossian

Primary pulmonary adenoid cystic carcinoma (ACC) is a rare, endobronchial, exophytic (polypoid or intraluminal) or endophytic, epithelial tumor that is histologically similar to adenoid cystic carcinoma of the salivary glands. ACC is generally a well-circumscribed endobronchial mass that histologically demonstrates most commonly cribriform, but also tubular and solid, growth patterns. A slow-growing tumor, ACC often contains no necrosis, mitotic figures, or angiolymphatic invasion. ACC generally infiltrates along the tracheobronchial wall and shows perineural invasion. ACC is characteristically immunopositive for S-100, actin, calponin, and CAM5.2.

Cytologic Features:

- Adenoid cystic carcinoma contains epithelial cells, generally uniform small cells with a high nuclear-to-cytoplasm ratio, oval regular nuclei, and characteristic hyaline eosinophilic or myxoid stroma.

Histologic Features:

- Exophytic (polypoid or intraluminal) or endophytic, soft, tan well-circumscribed mass, typically approximately 1 to 4 cm.
- Cribriform, tubular, and solid growth patterns.
- Hyalinized, sclerotic, or myxoid basement membranelike material is deposited in the lumens of cribriform cylinders or tubules.
- Often infiltrates tracheobronchial wall and shows perineural invasion.
- Generally immunopositive for S-100, actin, calponin, and CAM5.2.

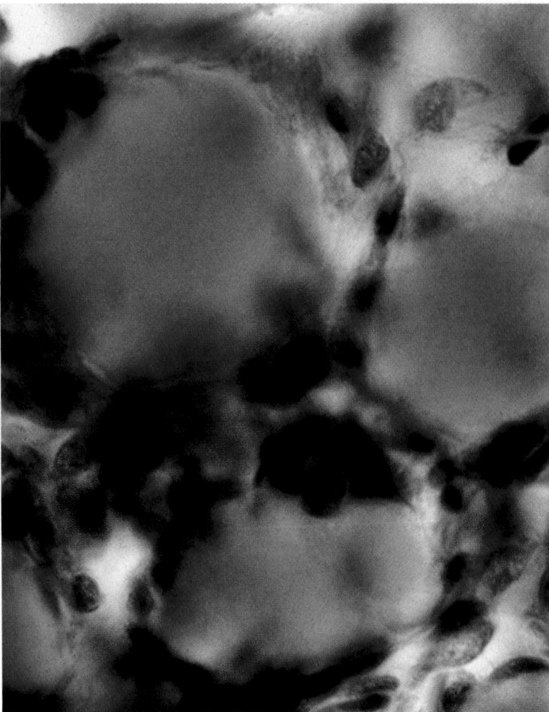

Figure 10.114 Cytology figure showing acinar structures containing central amorphous hyaline material ringed by small hyperchromatic oval cells with scant cytoplasm.

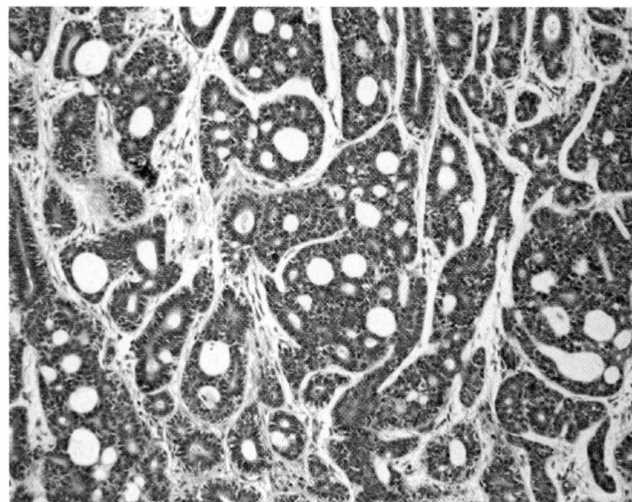

Figure 10.115 Low power of adenoid cystic carcinoma with predominantly cribriform and tubular pattern, and loose myxoid stroma.

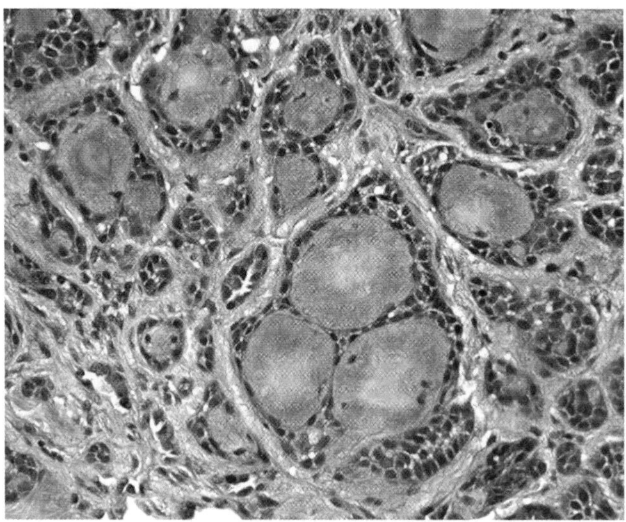

Figure 10.116 Adenoid cystic carcinoma with cylindrical mucinous matrix surrounded by small hyperchromatic oval cells with scant cytoplasm.

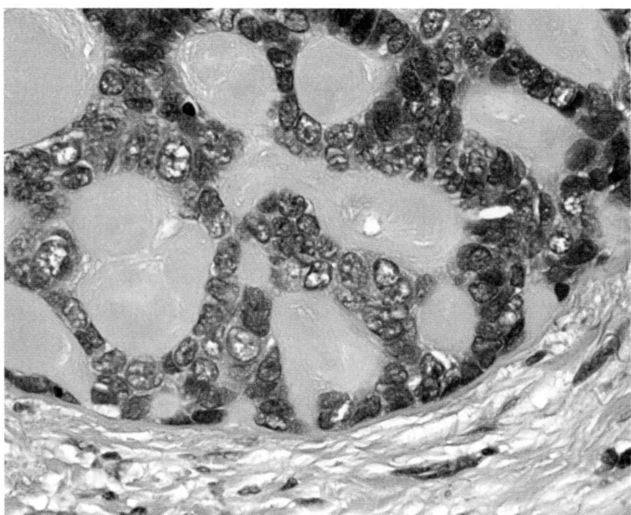

Figure 10.117 High power of adenoid cystic carcinoma showing cylindrical hyalinized matrix surrounded by small oval cells with scant cytoplasm.

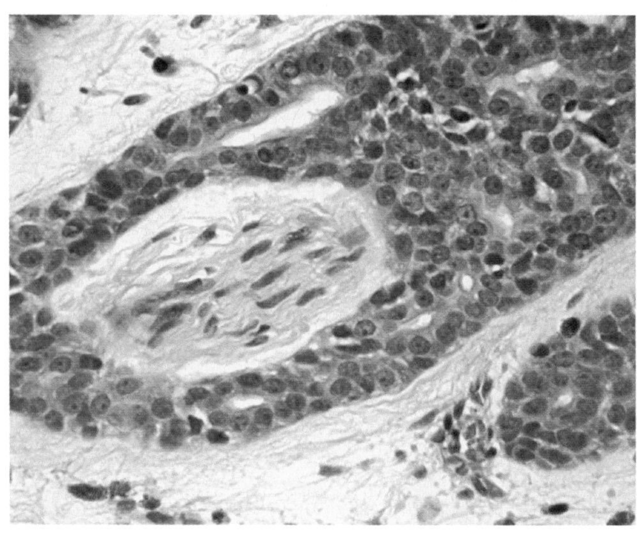

Figure 10.118 Perineural invasion with adenoid cystic carcinoma surrounding a nerve.

Part 16

Metastatic Carcinoma

▶ Alvaro C. Laga, Timothy Allen, Carlos Bedrossian, Mary Ostrowski, and Philip T. Cagle

The most common neoplasm in the lungs is metastatic carcinoma. When a primary lung cancer cannot be excluded, carcinomas metastatic to the lung may be biopsied. Tumors known to be metastatic may occasionally be resected. Metastases may occur by lymphangitic spread, hematogenous spread, or direct invasion from adjacent organs. The most common metastatic carcinomas in the lung are from lung, breast, and gastrointestinal primary sites. Lymphangitic spread is seen most often with metastatic carcinomas of the breast, stomach, prostate, ovary, and lung. Hematogenous spread is seen most often with metastatic carcinoma of the breast, colon, kidney, and testes.

Cytologic Features:

- Cytologic features of metastatic carcinomas are the same as those of the respective primary carcinomas.

Histologic Features:

- Metastatic carcinomas may be observed as nodules in the lung parenchyma, as nodules beneath bronchial mucosa, and as clusters of cells within lymphatic and/or blood vessels.
- Metastatic carcinomas may occasionally be observed as tumor thromboemboli.
- Metastatic carcinomas may occasionally grow in a lepidic pattern on intact alveolar septa mimicking bronchioloalveolar carcinoma.
- Metastatic carcinomas generally show the same histologic and immunohistochemical phenotype as the respective primary carcinomas.

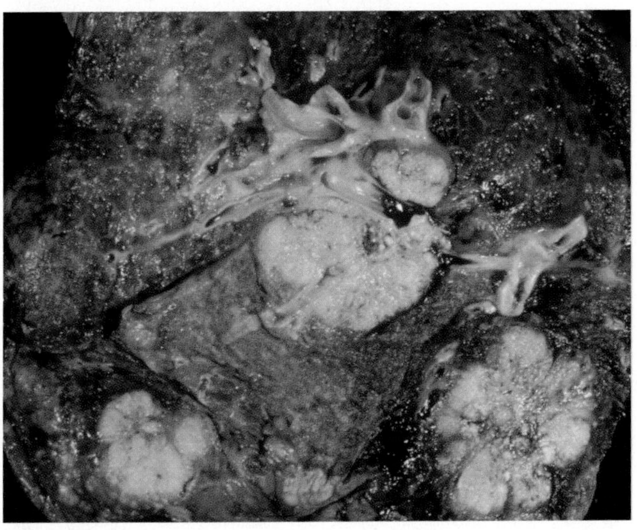

Figure 10.119 Gross figure of lung with multiple tumor masses of metastatic carcinoma.

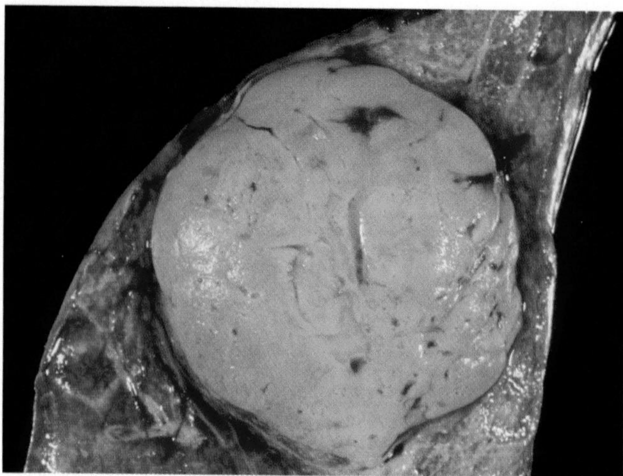

Figure 10.120 Gross figure of lung with metastatic renal cell carcinoma with typical yellow coloration.

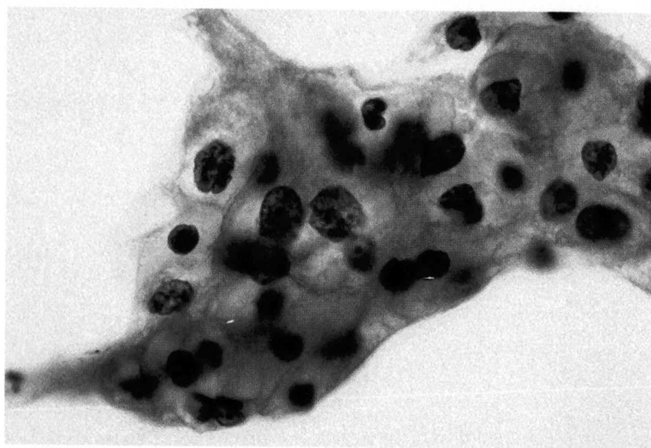

Figure 10.121 Cytology figure of metastatic renal cell carcinoma showing pleomorphic nuclei and abundant cytoplasm.

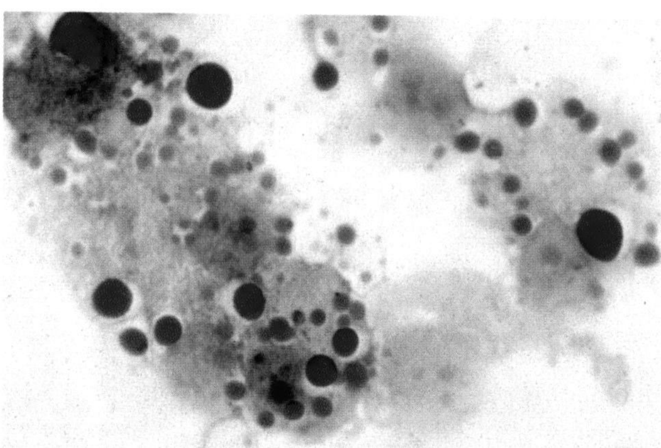

Figure 10.122 Cytology of oil red O stain of metastatic renal cell carcinoma showing positive oil red O staining of lipid within the carcinoma cells typical of renal cell carcinoma.

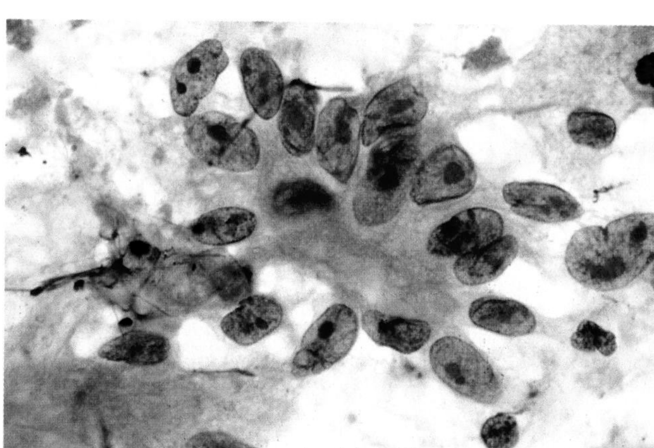

Figure 10.123 Cytology figure of metastatic colon adenocarcinoma, with enlarged nuclei and prominent nucleoli.

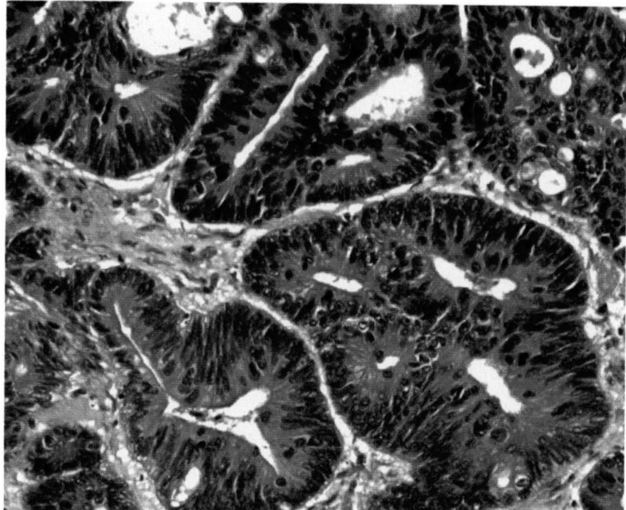

Figure 10.124 Metastatic colon carcinoma with complex glands lined by malignant columnar cells with pleomorphic nuclei.

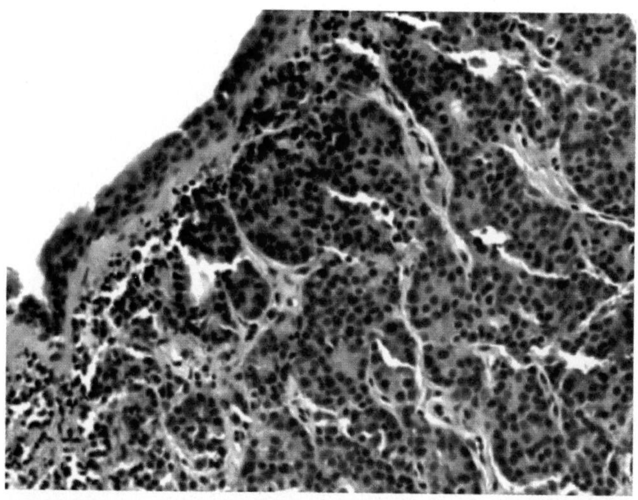

Figure 10.125 Metastatic prostate carcinoma in bronchial submucosa forming nests and small glands of relatively bland carcinoma cells suggestive of primary carcinoid tumor of the lung.

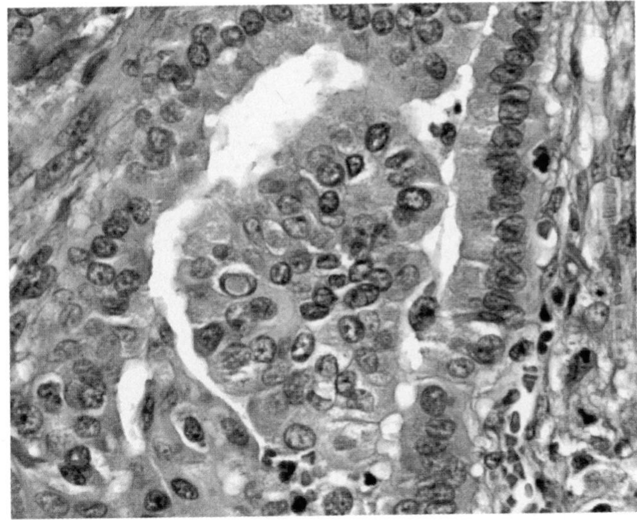

Figure 10.126 Metastatic papillary carcinoma of the thyroid with focal intranuclear inclusions. Similar to most primary adenocarcinomas of the lung, this metastatic thyroid carcinoma is likely to be TTF-1 immunopositive.

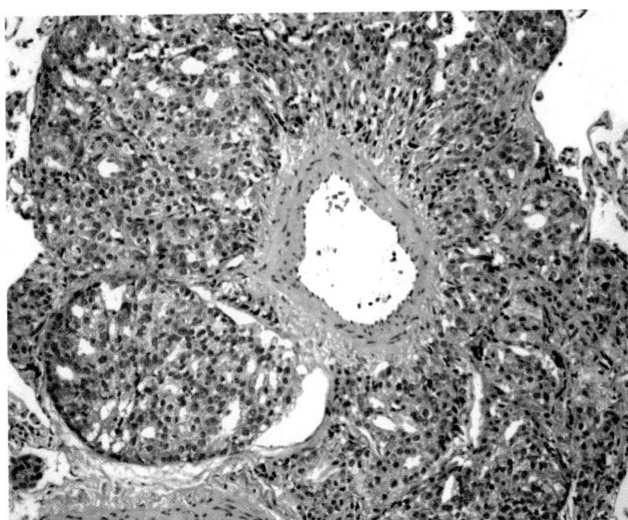

Figure 10.127 Perivascular lymphatic spread of metastatic prostate carcinoma.

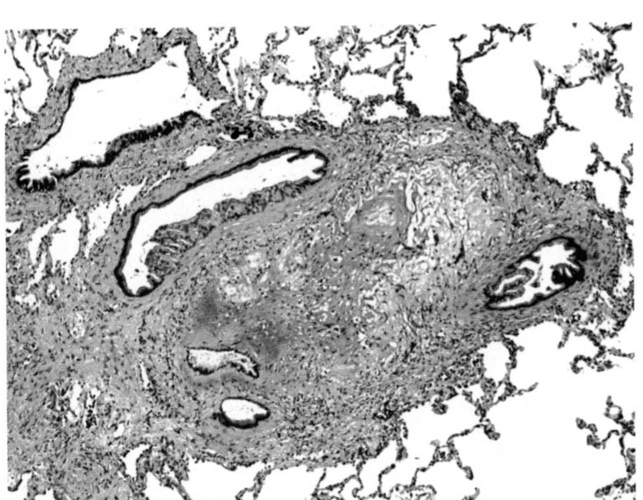

Figure 10.128 Hematogenous spread of metastatic adenocarcinoma obliterating arterial lumen with tumor thrombus.

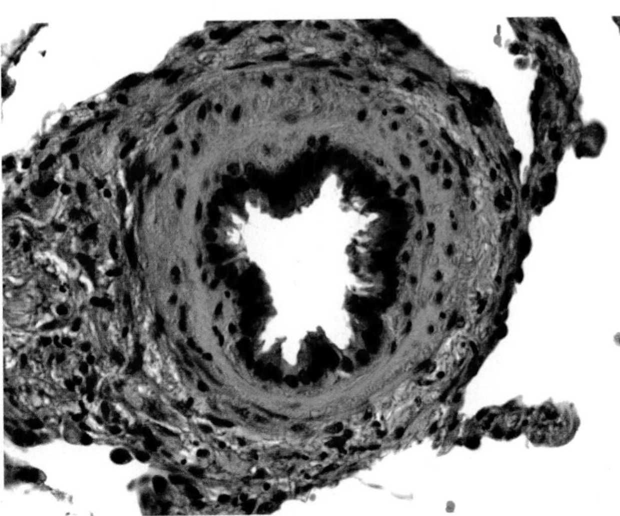

Figure 10.129 Higher power of hematogenous spread of metastatic adenocarcinoma showing adenocarcinoma gland within center of thrombus in vessel lumen.

Sarcomas

11

Primary sarcomas of the lung are very rare. Most sarcomas in the lung are metastases from other primary sites. The histopathologic features of sarcomas in the lung are generally the same whether they are rare primary tumors or metastases from other sites.

Part 1

Sarcoma of the Pulmonary Artery and Vein

▶ Mojghan Amrikachi and Timothy Allen

Sarcomas of the pulmonary artery and vein are rare primary pulmonary sarcomas, generally occurring in adults in the fourth to sixth decades. Grossly, sarcomas of the pulmonary artery and vein form fleshy, occasionally polypoid, masses, distending the pulmonary trunk or pulmonary artery by gray tumor mixed with thrombus. The tumor may extend tó pulmonary valve and right ventricle. Extravascular extension of tumor from the vessel lumen or wall may occur. Metastases, especially to distal lung, may occur.

Histologic Features:

- Hemorrhagic lesion with a uniform spindle cell proliferation within the vessel lumen and tumor cells infiltrating vascular intima and media.
- Some tumors may demonstrate marked pleomorphism with occasional giant cells (undifferentiated intimal sarcoma).

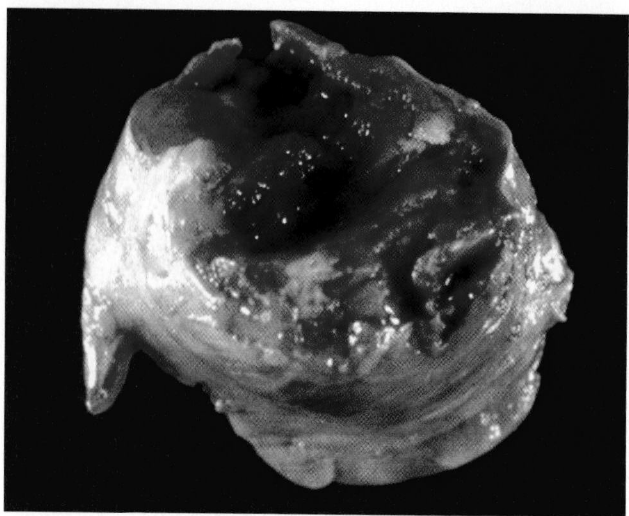

Figure 11.1 Gross figure of pulmonary artery sarcoma, with fleshy tumor within the vessel.

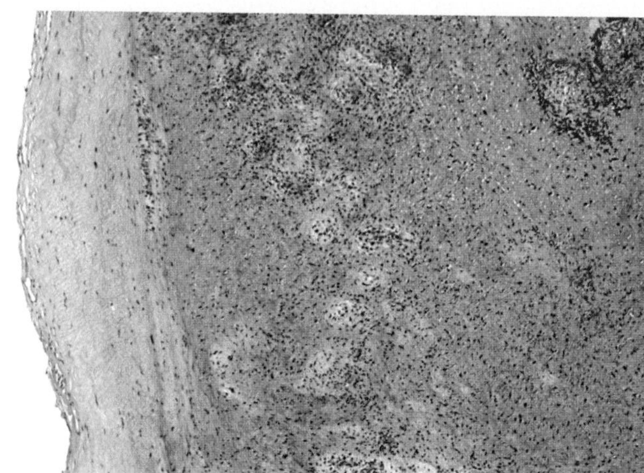

Figure 11.2 Artery with a spindle cell proliferation filling the lumen and infiltrating the vessel wall.

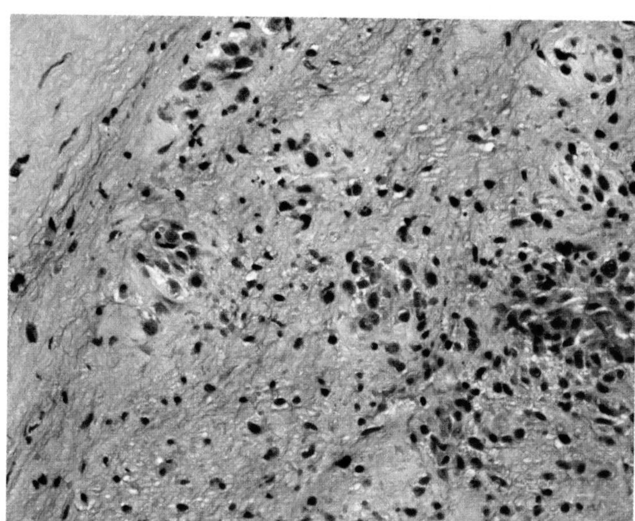

Figure 11.3 Higher power showing spindle cells and round to oval cells with myxoid stroma and admixed scattered blood vessels. Malignant cells infiltrate the vessel wall.

Part 2

Angiosarcoma

▶ Mojghan Amrikachi and Timothy Allen

Angiosarcomas generally occur in older adults. Angiosarcomas in the lung are generally metastatic tumors; however, primary pulmonary angiosarcomas may very rarely occur. Angiosarcomas in the lung often present with hemoptysis and commonly appear grossly as ill-defined hemorrhagic areas. The histologic features of primary pulmonary angiosarcomas are similar to angiosarcomas arising from other sites.

Histologic Features:

- Malignant tumors with endothelial differentiation.
- Well to moderately differentiated angiosarcomas show irregular anastomosing vascular spaces lined by large endothelial cells, hyperchromatic nuclei, and papillary tufting along the lumina.
- Poorly differentiated angiosarcomas show high-grade pleomorphic spindle cells with rudimentary lumen formation in some areas and prominent mitotic activity.
- Ultrastructurally show tight junction between cells, pinocytic vesicles, and Weibel-Palade bodies (in small number of angiosarcomas).
- Generally immunopositive for CD34, CD31, and von Willebrand factor (less sensitive in high-grade tumors).

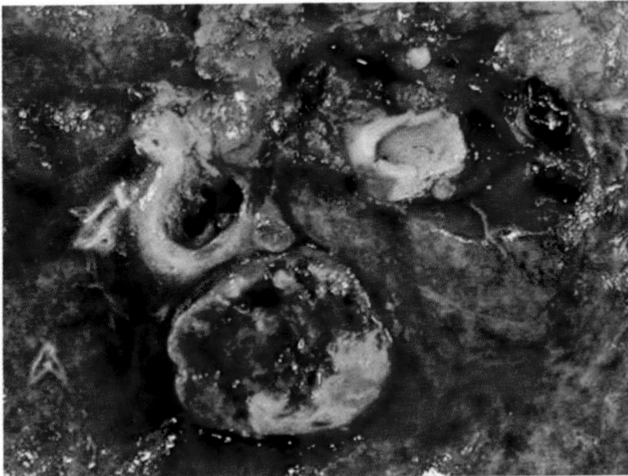

Figure 11.4 Gross figure of angiosarcoma, fleshy tumor containing necrosis, and hemorrhage lying near a large bronchus.

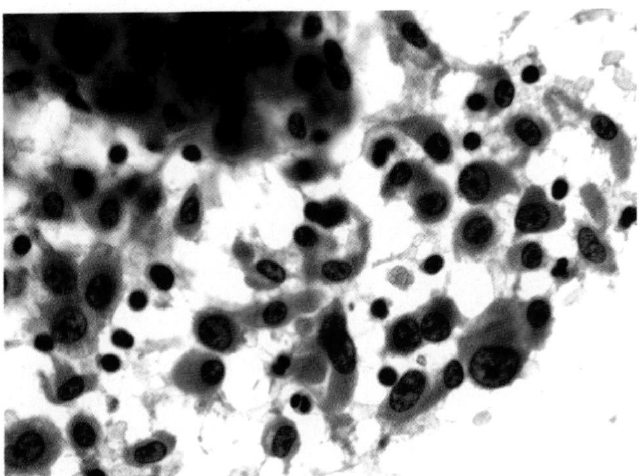

Figure 11.5 Cytology figure showing spindle to oval cells with hyperchromatic nuclei.

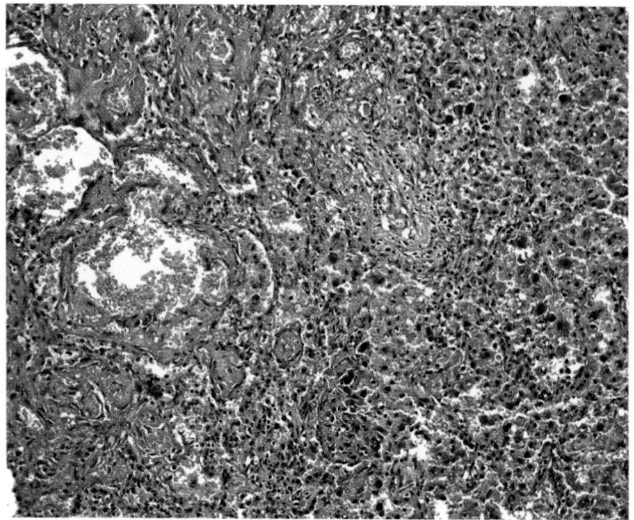

Figure 11.6 Angiosarcoma with irregular anastomosing vascular spaces and blood in airspaces peripheral to the tumor.

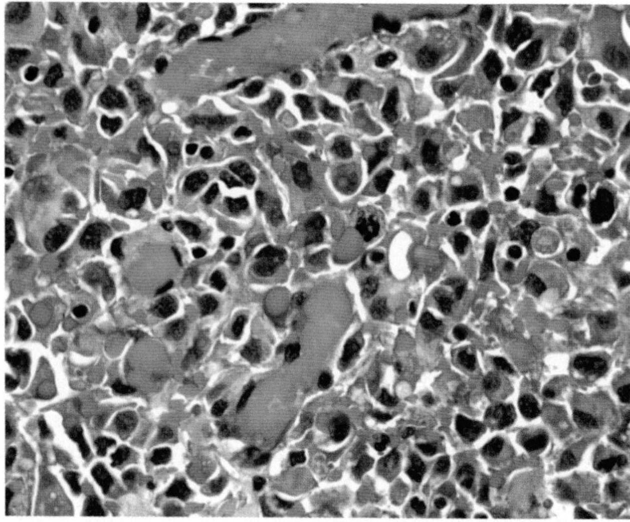

Figure 11.7 Higher power of angiosarcoma showing malignant spindle cells and round to oval cells with hyperchromatic nuclei and mitotic figures.

Part 3

Epithelioid Hemangioendothelioma

▶ Mojghan Amrikachi, Mary Ostrowski, and Alvaro C. Laga

Epithelioid hemangioendothelioma is a vascular tumor typically occurring around medium-sized and large veins in the soft tissue of adults. Although epithelioid hemangioendotheliomas occurring in the lung are most often metastases, rare primary pulmonary epithelioid hemangioendotheliomas occur. Differential diagnosis includes epithelioid angiosarcoma.

Cytologic Features:

- Large, polygonal eosinophilic cells, often vacuolated, with periodic acid–Schiff (PAS)-positive stroma.

Histologic Features:

- Usually a low-grade sarcoma with little mitotic activity.
- Cords, strands, and nests of cells infiltrating a myxoid or hyalinized stroma.
- Round to spindled cells with pale eosinophilic cytoplasm, vesicular nuclei, and inconspicuous nucleoli.
- Intracytoplasmic vacuoles with occasional intraluminal erythrocytes occur.
- High-grade tumors contain solid sheets of cells with marked nuclear atypia and increased mitotic activity.
- Generally immunopositive for CD31 and von Willebrand factor; approximately one third can be focally immunopositive for cytokeratin.

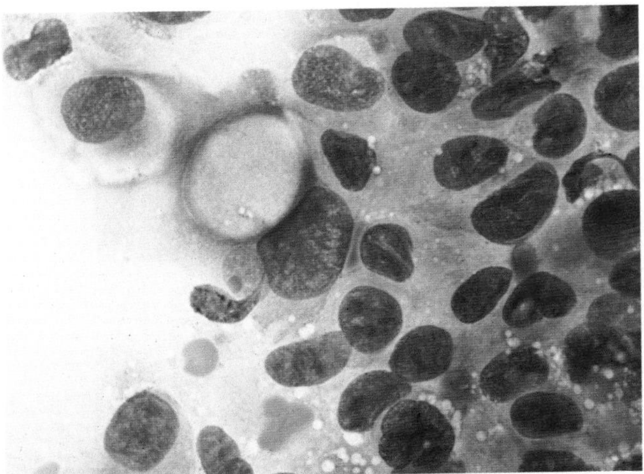

Figure 11.8 Cytology figure showing round and polygonal cells with a prominent cytoplasmic vacuole.

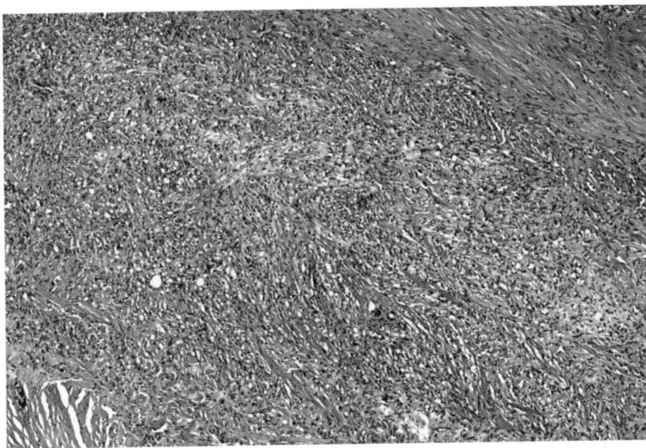

Figure 11.9 Nests, cords, and clusters of round to spindled cells within a myxoid and hyalinized stroma.

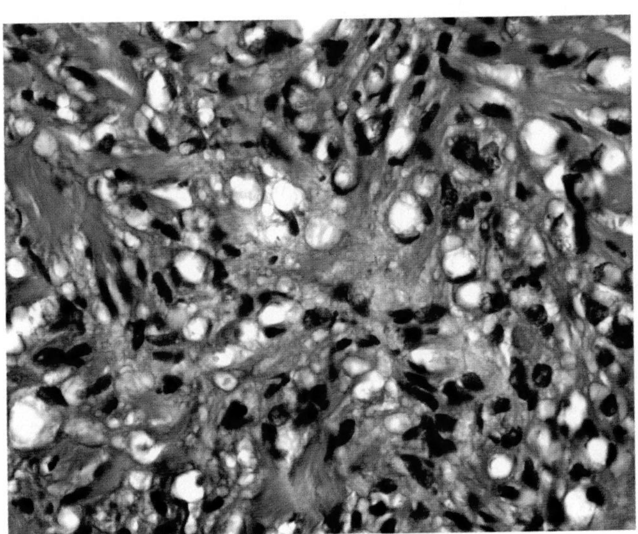

Figure 11.10 Higher power of myxoid stroma showing round to spindled cells with prominent cytoplasmic vacuoles.

Part 4

Kaposi Sarcoma

▶ Mojghan Amrikachi, Carlos Bedrossian, and Timothy Allen

Kaposi sarcoma is commonly associated with acquired immunodeficiency syndrome (AIDS) and may arise as a primary pulmonary neoplasm. Grossly, lung lesions generally occur as multiple hemorrhagic lesions. Differential diagnosis includes angiosarcoma, fibrosarcoma, arteriovenous malformation, spindle cell hemangioendothelioma, inflammatory granulation tissue, and bacillary angiomatosis.

Cytologic Features:

- Bland to mildly atypical oval to spindled cells with a background of red blood cells.

Histologic Features:

- Diffuse infiltrative lesion along lymphatic pathways, interlobular septa, and pleura.
- Bland monomorphic spindle cells separated by slitlike vascular spaces.
- Spindle cells resemble fibroblasts and form network of irregular vascular channels, with erythrocytes scattered between spindle cells.
- Sparse to abundant plasma cells and lymphocytes may occur.
- PAS-positive, diastase-resistant intracellular and extracellular hyaline globules may occur
- Generally immunopositive for CD34, CD31, and HHV-8.

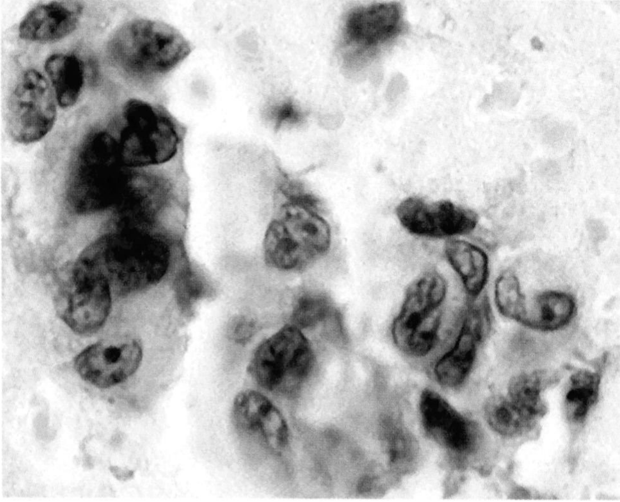

Figure 11.11 Cytology figure showing mildly atypical oval to spindled cells with a background of red blood cells.

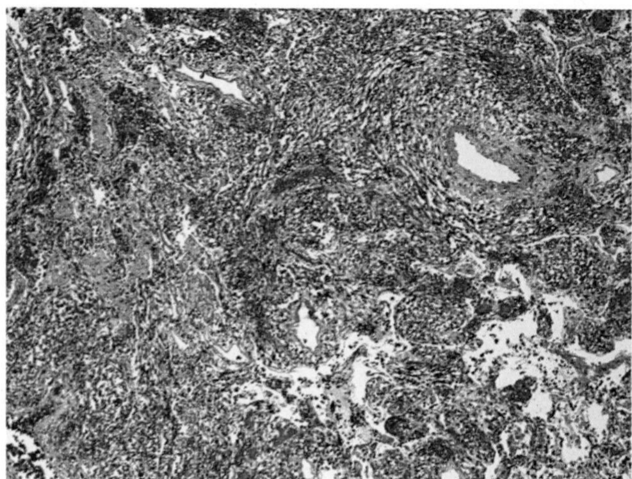

Figure 11.12 Kaposi sarcoma showing nests of spindled cells and surrounding lung parenchyma containing hemorrhage and hemosiderin-laden macrophages.

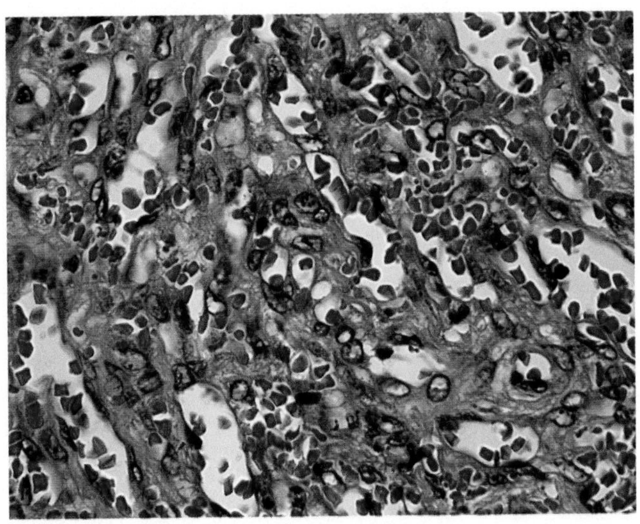

Figure 11.13 Higher power of Kaposi sarcoma showing monomorphic spindle cells separated by slitlike vascular spaces.

Part 5

Hemangiopericytoma

▶ Mojghan Amrikachi, Alvaro C. Laga, Timothy Allen, and Philip T. Cagle

Most, if not all, neoplasms previously designated as hemangiopericytoma are now considered solitary fibrous tumors. Tumors designated hemangiopericytomas have been described in the lungs as rare primary and metastatic tumors. Tumors diagnosed as hemangiopericytomas in the lung typically appear grossly as well-circumscribed masses with grey-white cut surfaces and areas of cystic degeneration.

Histologic Features:

- Dilated branching blood vessels with staghorn configuration surrounded by tightly packed round to fusiform small cells.
- Faint cytoplasm with indistinct cytoplasmic borders, round to oval nuclei, and rare to absent mitotic figures.
- Foci of spindle cell changes and myxoid changes can occur.
- Generally immunopositive for CD34, and immunonegative for CD31, actin, desmin and CD99.

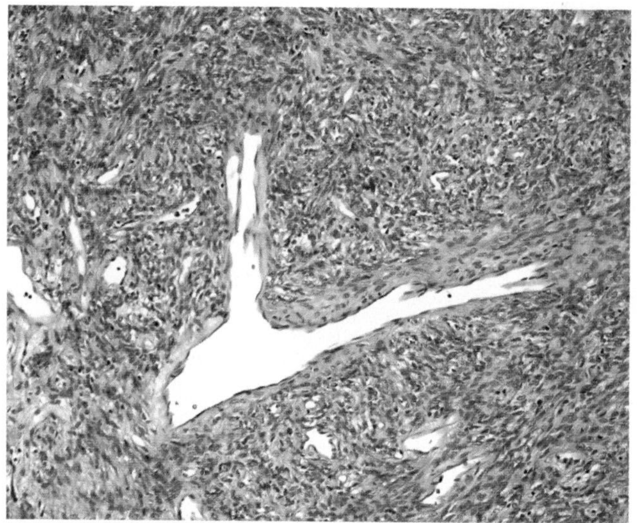

Figure 11.14 Branching blood vessel surrounded by tightly packed round to fusiform cells.

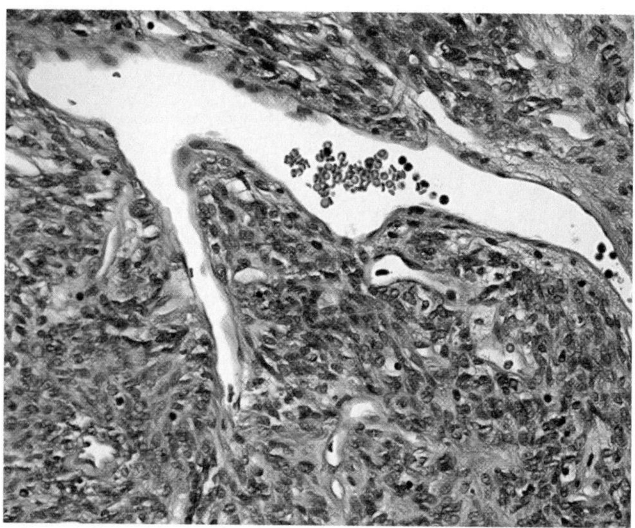

Figure 11.15 Higher power showing a vessel with staghorn configuration with surrounding cells containing faint cytoplasm with round to oval nuclei.

Part 6

Undifferentiated Sarcomas

Mojghan Amrikachi, Carlos Bedrossian, Alvaro C. Laga, and Philip T. Cagle

Sarcomas without differentiating features, including those formerly referred to as "malignant fibrous histiocytomas," are generally metastatic in the lung and very rarely occur as primary lung tumors. Generally sarcomas in the lung form gray-white masses, commonly with areas of necrosis.

Cytologic Features:

- Mixture of malignant spindle cells, and occasional giant cells, with areas of myxoid stromal tissue.

Histologic Features:

- Spindle cells in short fascicles or storiform pattern, with bizarre pleomorphic spindled cells including multinucleated cells.
- Some may have myxoid stroma.
- Abnormal mitotic activity is common.
- Differentiated elements such as malignant osteoid, cartilage or muscle are not observed.

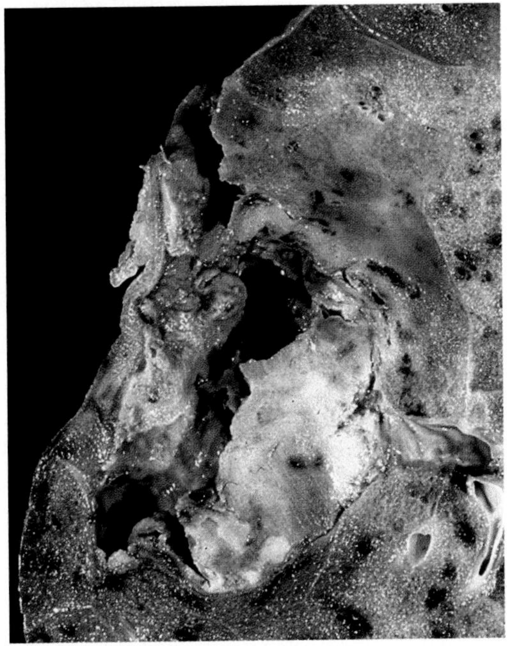

Figure 11.16 Gross figure of undifferentiated sarcoma with central cystic necrosis.

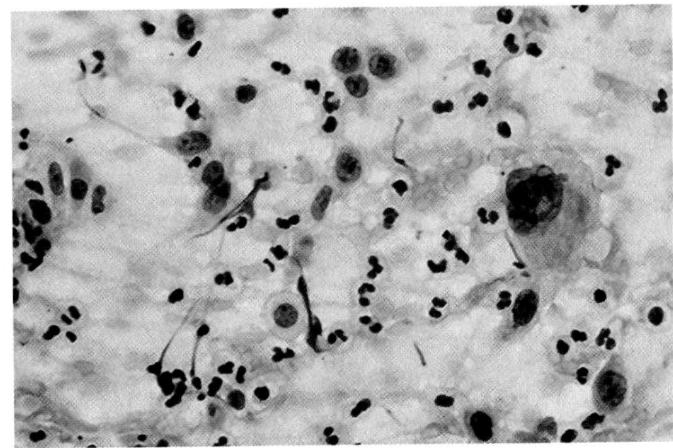

Figure 11.17 Cytologic figure showing malignant giant cells.

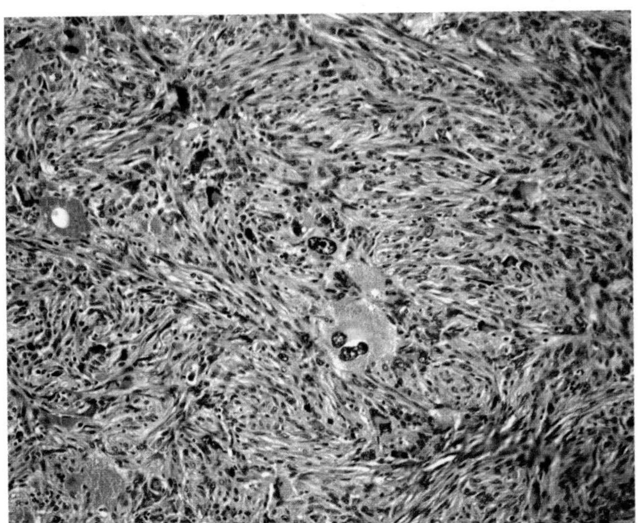

Figure 11.18 Storiform pattern of spindled cells with scattered multinucleated cells.

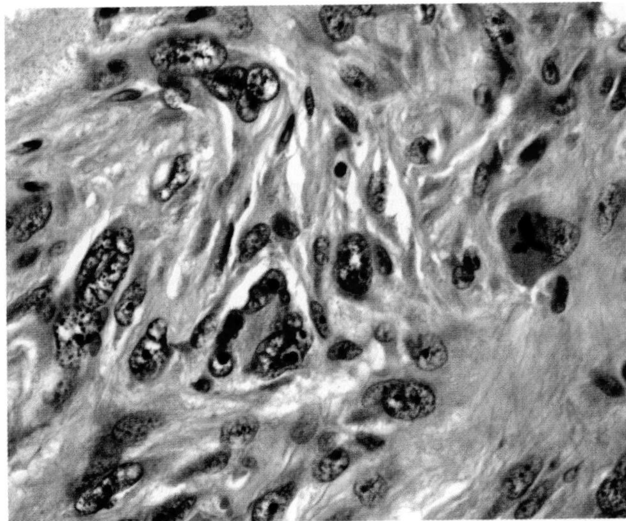

Figure 11.19 Higher power showing bizarre multinucleated cells and an atypical mitotic figure.

Part 7

Fibrosarcoma

▶ Mojghan Amrikachi and Timothy Allen

Most fibrosarcomas in the lung are metastatic tumors, but rare primary pulmonary fibrosarcomas may occur.

Cytologic Features:

- Atypical spindled cells, occasionally arranged in dense fascicles.
- The malignant cells may be elongated with tapered, irregular, hyperchromatic nuclei, and cytoplasm is generally indistinct.

Histologic Features:

- Elongated uniform spindled cells arranged in fascicles in a herringbone pattern, with variable amounts of stromal collagen present.
- Numerous mitotic figures including some abnormal forms.
- Immunonegative for desmin and CD34; some are immunopositive for actin.

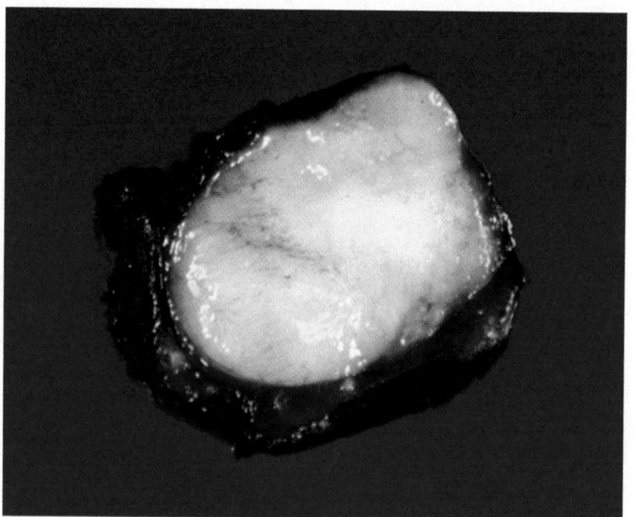

Figure 11.20 Gross figure of fibrosarcoma showing firm tan nodular mass.

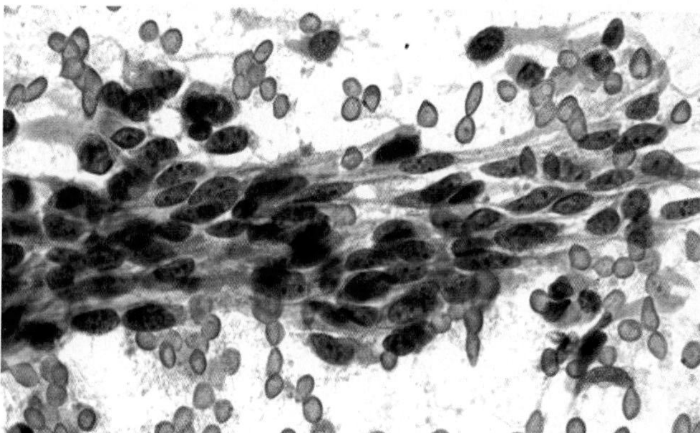

Figure 11.21 Cytology figure showing a fascicle of atypical spindled cells.

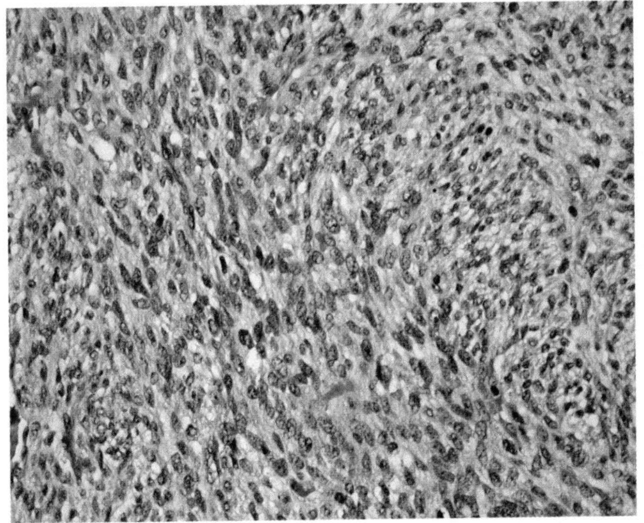

Figure 11.22 Fibrosarcoma with fascicles of elongated spindle cells.

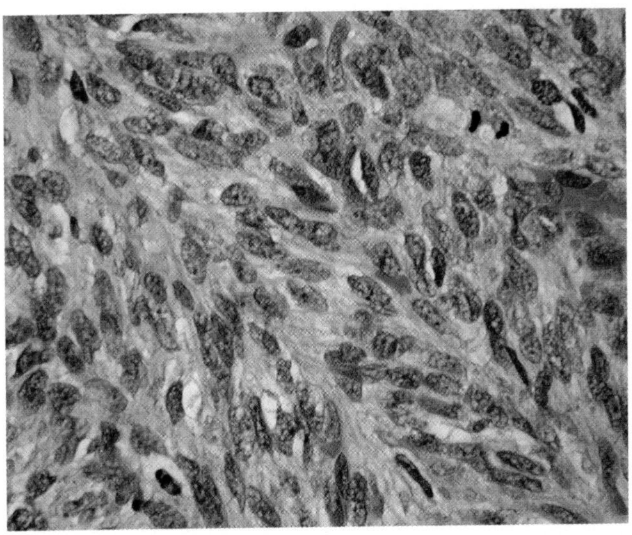

Figure 11.23 Malignant spindle cells with a mitotic figure present in the upper right.

Part 8

Malignant Peripheral Nerve Sheath Tumor

▶ Mojghan Amrikachi and Timothy Allen

Malignant peripheral nerve sheath tumors (malignant schwannoma) arise *de novo* or from transformation of a plexiform neurofibroma in patients with von Recklinghausen disease. They arise commonly in the neck, forearm, lower leg, and buttocks. Malignant peripheral nerve sheath tumors in the lung are predominantly metastatic tumors, but pulmonary primaries can occur. Differential diagnosis includes fibrosarcoma, monophasic synovial sarcoma, and leiomyosarcoma.

Histologic Features:

- Densely cellular and hypodense fascicles alternating in a marblelike pattern.
- Asymmetrically tapered spindled cells with wavy or comma-shaped nuclei and pale indistinct cytoplasm.
- Malignant peripheral nerve sheath tumors are generally immunopositive for S-100, Leu-7, and myelin basic protein.

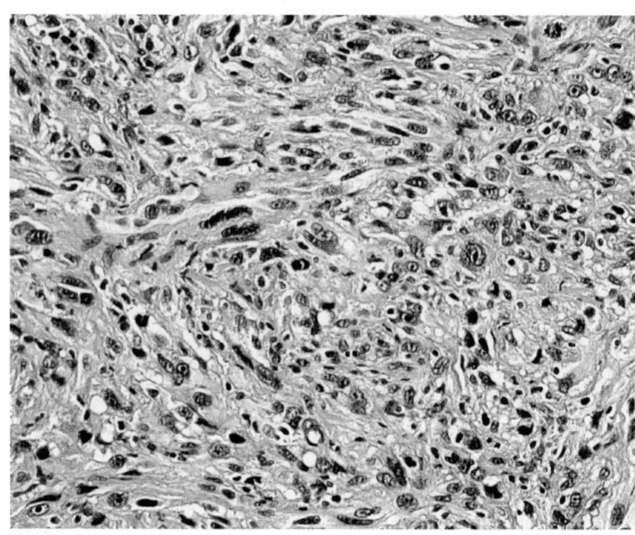

Figure 11.24 Medium power of malignant peripheral nerve sheath tumor showing malignant spindle cells.

Part 9

Osteosarcoma

▶ Mojghan Amrikachi, Carlos Bedrossian, and Timothy Allen

Most osteosarcomas arise in the medullary cavity of the metaphyses of long bones of the extremities. Osteosarcoma in the lung is most often metastatic tumor; however, primary pulmonary osteosarcomas very rarely occur. Osteosarcoma in the lung typically presents grossly as a gray-white mass with hemorrhage, necrosis, and cystic change.

Cytologic Features:

- Sarcoma cells and osteoid.

Histologic Features:

- High-grade sarcoma composed of pleomorphic and anaplastic cells.
- Sarcoma cells may be spindled, epithelioid, plasmacytoid, fusiform, ovoid, small and round, clear, or multinucleated.
- Osteoid formation with a trabecular and lacelike pattern.
- Abnormal mitotic figures.
- Sarcoma cells may also form cartilage.

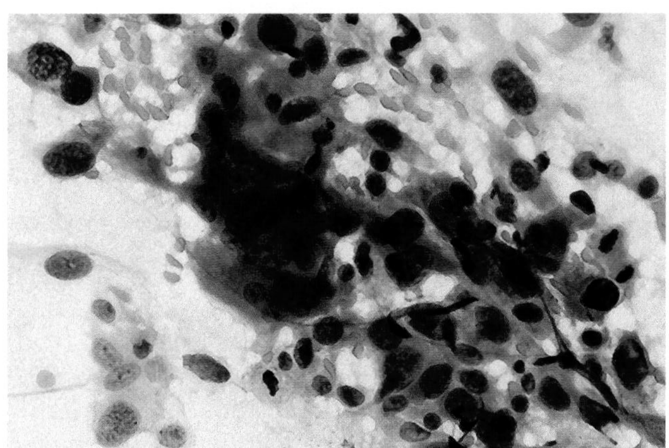

Figure 11.25 Cytology figure of osteosarcoma showing tumor cells including a multinucleated cell.

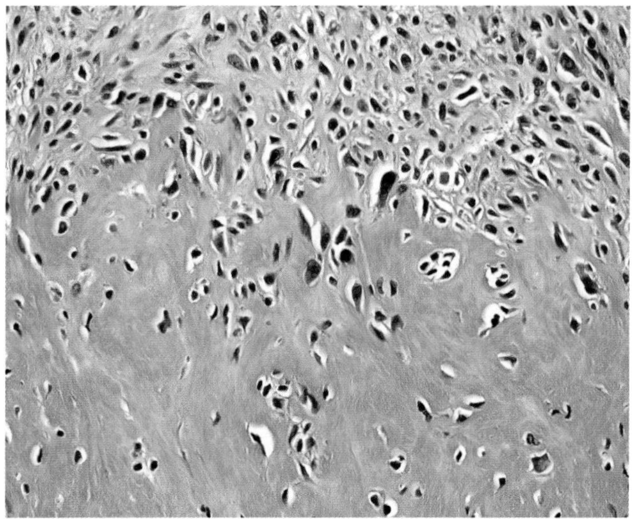

Figure 11.26 Osteosarcoma showing osteoid formation with cytologically malignant cells.

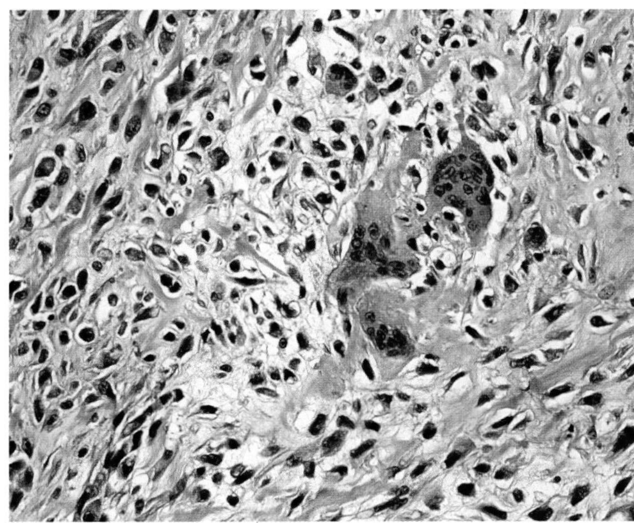

Figure 11.27 Higher power of osteosarcoma showing pleomorphic spindle cells and multinucleated cells with osteoid formation.

Part 10

Chondrosarcoma

▶ Mojghan Amrikachi, Carlos Bedrossian, and Timothy Allen

Chondrosarcomas generally arise in the pelvis, ribs, and shoulders in middle-aged and older adults. They arise either *de novo* or secondarily in preexisting benign cartilaginous tumors. Variants include clear cell, mesenchymal, myxoid, and dedifferentiated chondrosarcomas. Chondrosarcomas primarily occur in the lung as metastatic tumors, but primary pulmonary chondrosarcoma may rarely occur. Grossly, chondrosarcomas typically appear as lobulated masses with a gelatinous cut surface and with areas of necrosis and hemorrhage.

Cytologic Features:

- Malignant chondrocytes with large irregular nuclei and small to prominent nucleoli.

Histologic Features:

- Lobules of variable cellularity surrounded by fibrous tissue with a myxoid matrix.
- Uniform round to stellate cells with eosinophilic cytoplasm and dark chromatin, arranged in rows and in a chainlike pattern.
- Generally immunopositive for S-100 and Leu-7 and occasionally immunopositive for EMA.

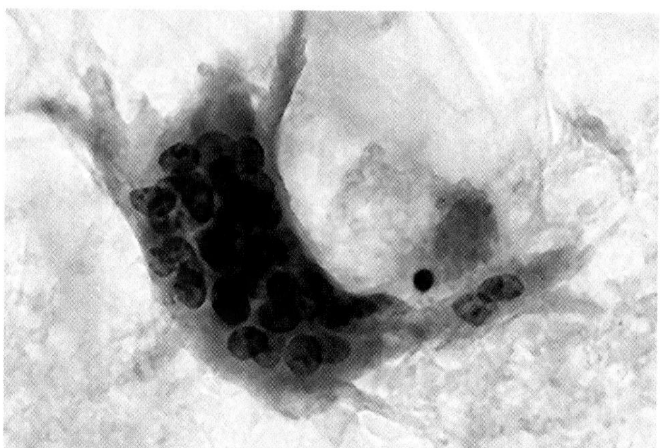

Figure 11.28 Cytology figure showing a malignant chondrocyte with hyperchromatic nuclei and small nucleoli.

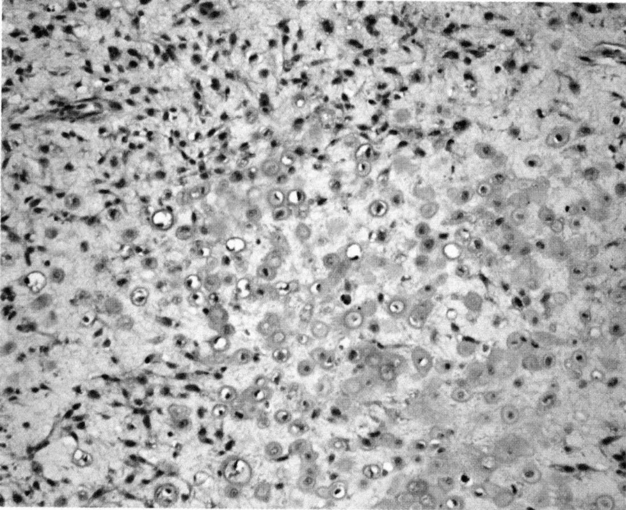

Figure 11.29 Chondrosarcoma with myxoid matrix containing malignant chondrocytes.

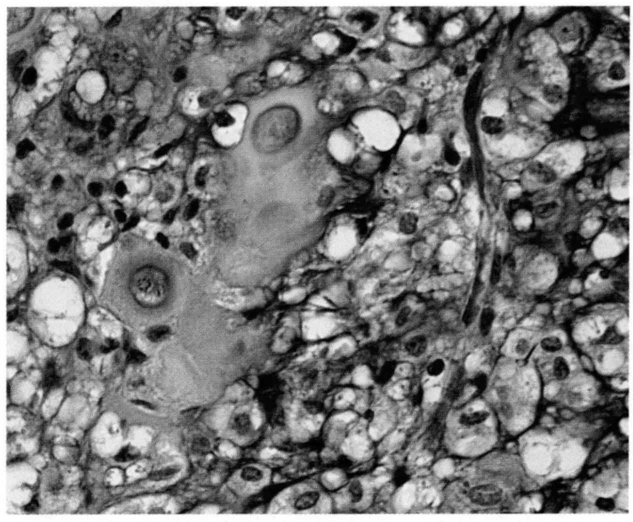

Figure 11.30 Higher power of chondrosarcoma showing malignant chondrocytes within a myxoid matrix.

Part 11

Synovial Sarcoma

▶ Mojghan Amrikachi, Bruno Murer, Carlos Bedrossian, and Timothy Allen

Most synovial sarcomas in the lung are metastatic tumors; however, primary pulmonary synovial sarcomas very rarely occur. Typical synovial sarcomas arise in the lower limbs, predominantly around the knee and ankle in patients aged 10 to 35. They may be monophasic or biphasic. The great majority of studied synovial sarcomas are reported to have a tumor-specific chromosome t(X;18)(p11.2;q11.2) translocation resulting in the production of fusion genes, and identification of these may be used to assist in diagnosis.

Cytologic Features:

- Monophasic spindled cell pattern, with occasional acinar structures in some biphasic synovial sarcomas.

Histologic Features:

- Most often monophasic sarcomas composed of spindle cells when they are primary in the lung.
- Biphasic tumors composed of both epithelial and spindle cells also occur in lung.
- The epithelial component consists of large, pale cells with distinct cell borders forming solid nests of glandular or tubular structures, with round vesicular nuclei.

- The spindle cell component consists of closely packed small monomorphic spindle cells with indistinct cell margins, hemangiopericytoma-like vascular structures, stroma with thick collagen bundles and calcifications, and mast cells.
- Generally immunopositive in the epithelial component for cytokeratin, EMA, CD56, and Bcl-2, often immunopositive for calretinin and CD99, and immunonegative for CD34.

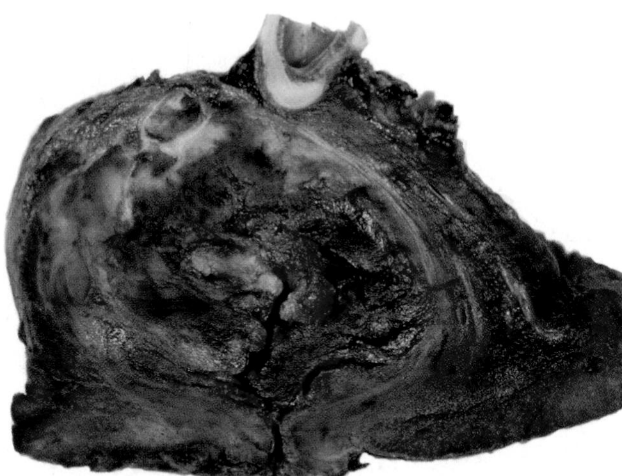

Figure 11.31 Gross specimen of large synovial sarcoma tumor mass with heterogeneous cut surface in the lung; note bronchial cartilage at *top* of figure.

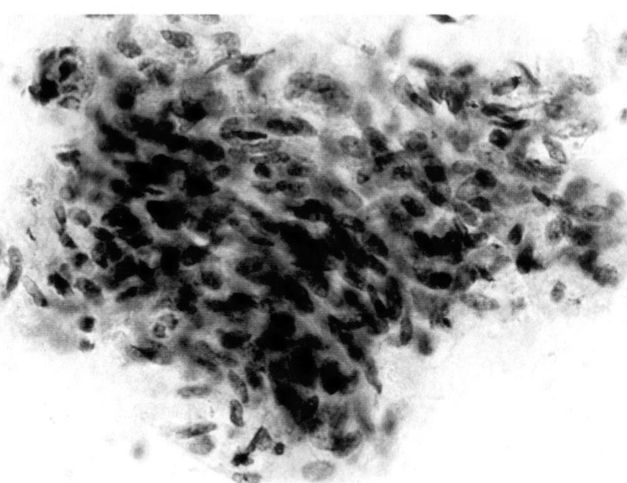

Figure 11.32 Cytology figure of synovial sarcoma showing a cluster of spindled cells with irregular coarse nuclei and moderate cytoplasm.

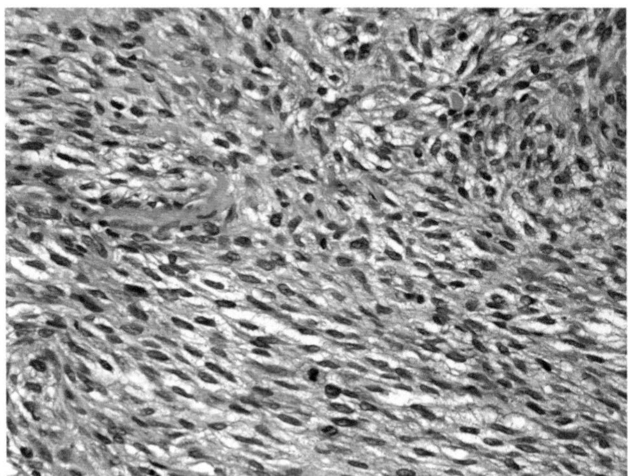

Figure 11.33 Synovial sarcoma showing spindled cells with scattered blood vessels.

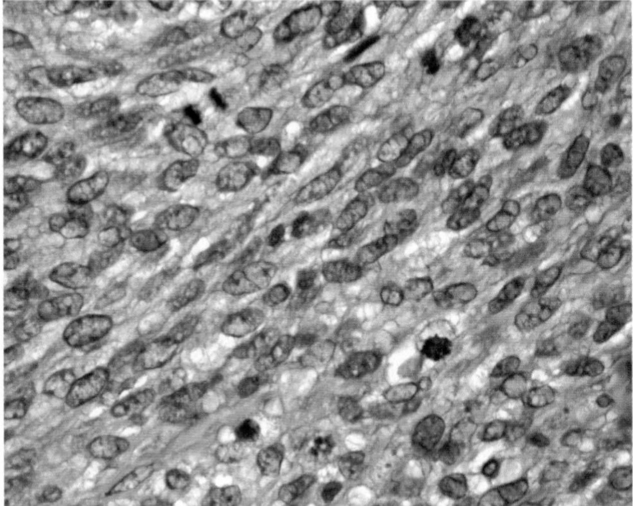

Figure 11.34 Higher power of synovial sarcoma showing spindle cells with round to oval vesicular nuclei and multiple mitotic figures.

Part 12

Leiomyosarcoma

▶ Mojghan Amrikachi, Carlos Bedrossian, and Timothy Allen

Leiomyosarcomas are malignant neoplasms with smooth muscle differentiation, generally arising from soft tissue in the extremities. In immunocompromised individuals such as AIDS patients and organ transplant patients, cases are often associated with Epstein-Barr virus. Most leiomyosarcomas in the lung are metastatic tumors, but rare primary pulmonary leiomyosarcomas occur. They generally present grossly in the lung as gray-white masses with foci of hemorrhage, necrosis, and cystic degeneration.

Cytologic Features:

- Highly cellular fascicular arrangements of oval to spindled cells.

Histologic Features:

- Well-differentiated leiomyosarcomas show elongated spindle cells, eosinophilic cytoplasm, elongated nuclei with rounded ends, occasional hyalinized or myxoid stroma, necrosis, and hemorrhage.
- Poorly differentiated leiomyosarcomas show marked pleomorphism with abnormal mitotic figures.
- Generally immunopositive for desmin and/or actin.

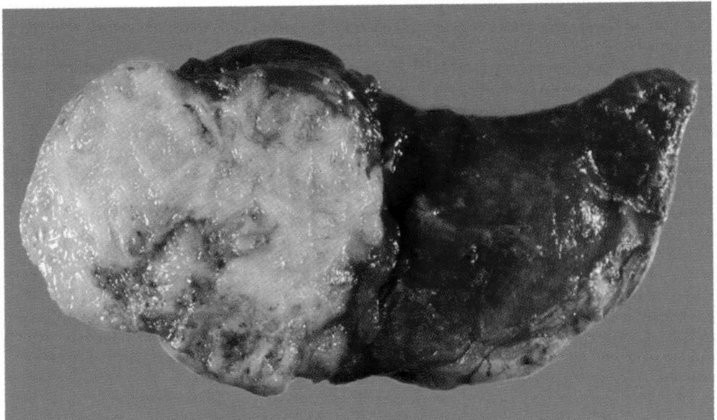

Figure 11.35 Gross figure of leiomyosarcoma showing a fleshy well-circumscribed mass with focal hemorrhage.

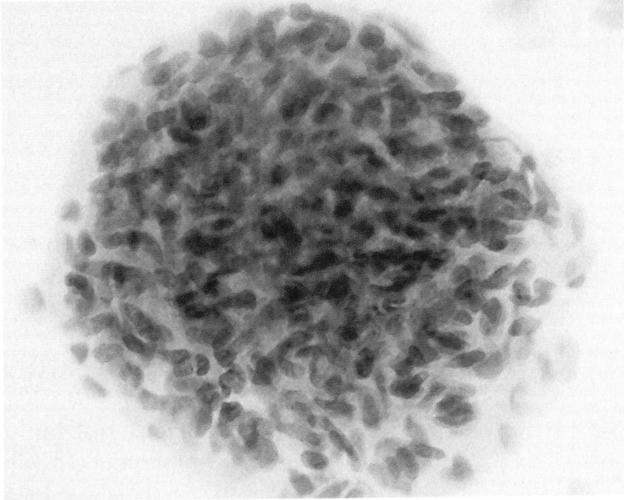

Figure 11.36 Cytology figure showing a cellular fragment of intermingled oval to spindled cells.

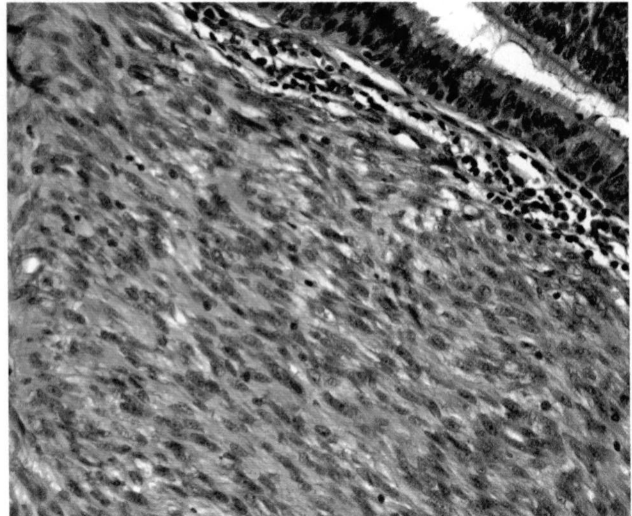

Figure 11.37 Leiomyosarcoma compressing ciliated bronchial epithelium, with spindle cells containing eosinophilic cytoplasm and elongated nuclei.

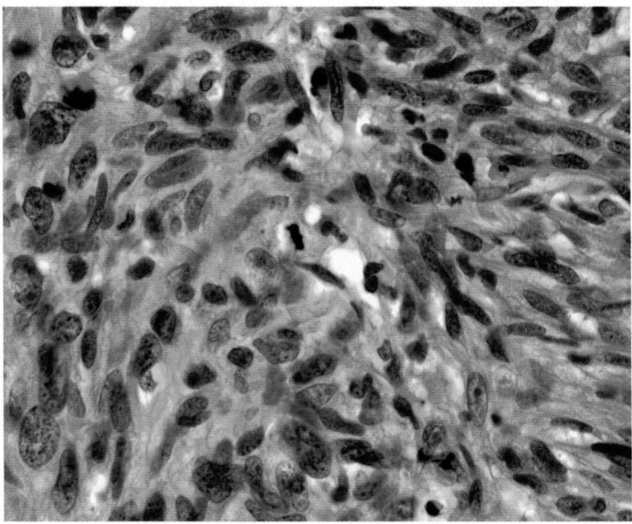

Figure 11.38 Higher power of leiomyosarcoma showing spindled and oval nuclei and mitotic figures.

Part 13

Rhabdomyosarcoma

▶ Mojghan Amrikachi, Carlos Bedrossian, and Timothy Allen

Rhabdomyosarcomas are sarcomas of skeletal muscle differentiation and occur in the lung as metastases. Rhabdomyosarcoma is a common soft tissue sarcoma in children, often arising in the head and neck area and urogenital area in children. Variants include embryonal, botryoid, alveolar, and pleomorphic. Differential diagnosis includes Ewing sarcoma, lymphoma, rhabdoid tumor, and other small blue cell tumors.

Cytologic Features:

- Embryonal rhabdomyosarcoma contains small- or medium-sized spindle and round cells, with hyperchromatic nuclei and scant or inconspicuous cytoplasm, occasional spindle rhabdomyoblasts, and rare multinucleation.
- Alveolar rhabdomyosarcoma contains pleomorphic cells including giant cells, tadpole cells with cytoplasmic tails and single large eccentric nuclei, and multinucleated strap cells.

Histologic Features:

- Embryonal rhabdomyosarcoma generally is a small blue cell tumor containing a nondescript sheet of cells with nuclei having fine chromatin and small nucleoli, round to oval to spindle cells, some with cross striations, and fibrotic or myxoid stroma.
- Alveolar rhabdomyosarcoma generally is a high-grade sarcoma containing nests of cells separated by fibrous septa, with discohesive cells toward the center of the nests resulting in an alveolar pattern, and polygonal or elongated cells with eosinophilic cytoplasm and some with cross striations at the periphery of the nests.

- The discohesive cells at the center of the alveolar spaces in alveolar rhabdomyosarcoma are round and small with sparse cytoplasm and with multinucleated cells.
- Rhabdomyoblasts and necrosis are common in alveolar rhabdomyosarcoma.
- Cytogenetic alterations include t(2;13) or t(1;13).
- Rhabdomyosarcomas are generally immunopositive for desmin, actin, and MyoD1.

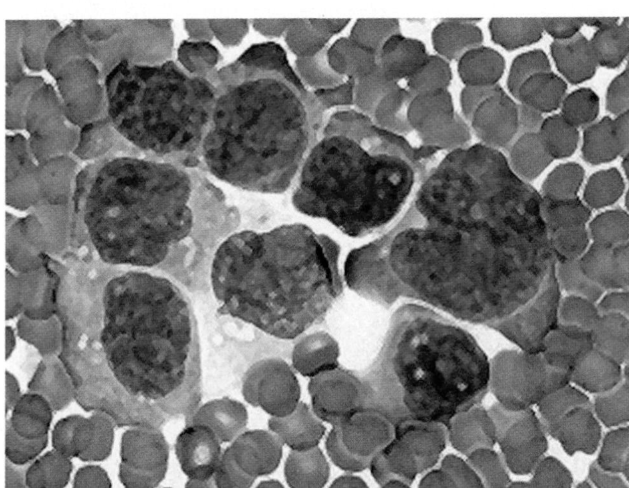

Figure 11.39 Cytology figure showing pleomorphic rhabdomyoblasts.

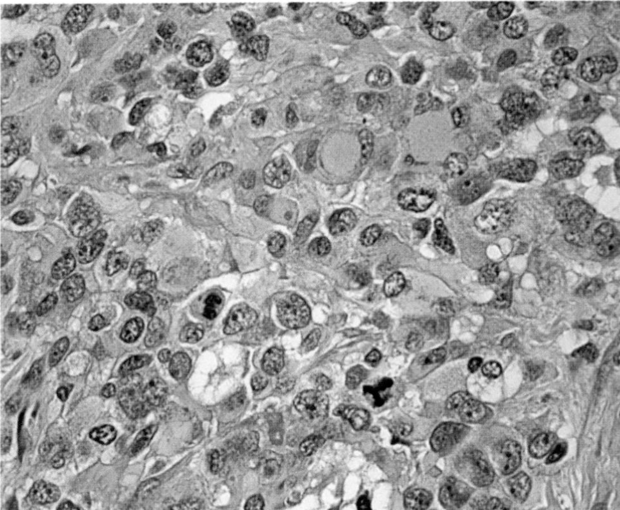

Figure 11.40 Rhabdomyosarcoma with atypical mitotic figure.

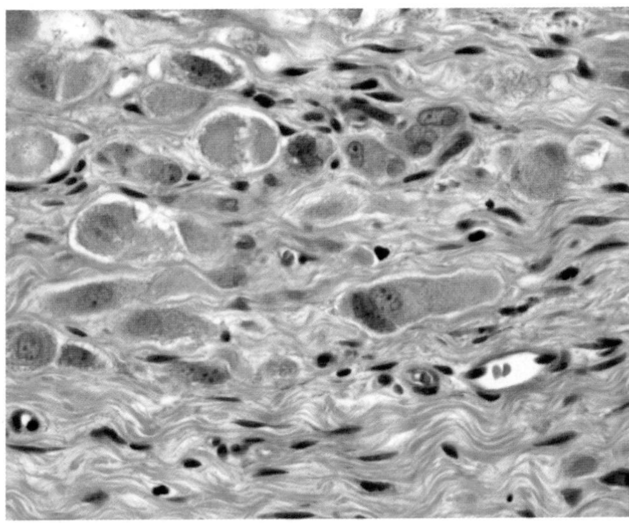

Figure 11.41 Rhabdomyoblasts within a fibrous stroma.

Part 14

Liposarcoma

▶ Mojghan Amrikachi, Carlos Bedrossian, and Timothy Allen

Liposarcomas are sarcomas of adipose tissue differentiation. Liposarcomas in the lung are generally metastatic tumors, but rare primary pulmonary liposarcomas occur. Liposarcomas are one of the most common sarcomas in adults and generally occur in deep soft tissues such as thigh, retroperitoneum, omentum, breast, mediastinum, and axilla, generally in the fifth to seventh decade. Liposarcomas may occur as well-differentiated, myxoid, pleomorphic, or dedifferentiated forms. Grossly, liposarcomas in the lung are typically gray-white, frequently containing areas of cystic change, hemorrhage, or necrosis.

Cytologic Features:

- Spindled cells with nuclear pleomorphism, hyperchromasia, and mitotic figures.
- Three general features of liposarcoma include a delicate capillary network, foamy extracellular matrix, and the presence of lipoblasts.

Histologic Features:

- Myxoid liposarcomas contain small uniform cells with cytoplasmic vacuoles (signet ring lipoblasts) and small uniform nonlipogenic cells with scant cytoplasm, a myxoid matrix, and numerous arborizing vascular structures.
- Differential diagnosis of myxoid liposarcoma includes myxoid malignant fibrous histiocytoma and myxoid chondrosarcoma.
- Pleomorphic liposarcoma contains cellular pleomorphic sarcomatous cells and multinucleated giant cells, with some cells differentiated as lipoblasts.
- Dedifferentiated liposarcoma contains both an atypical lipomatous component and a nonlipogenic high-grade sarcoma component.

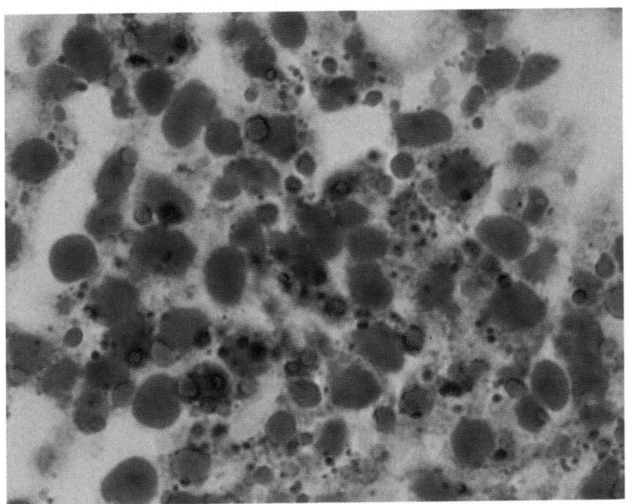

Figure 11.42 Cytology figure of lipoblasts on oil red O stain.

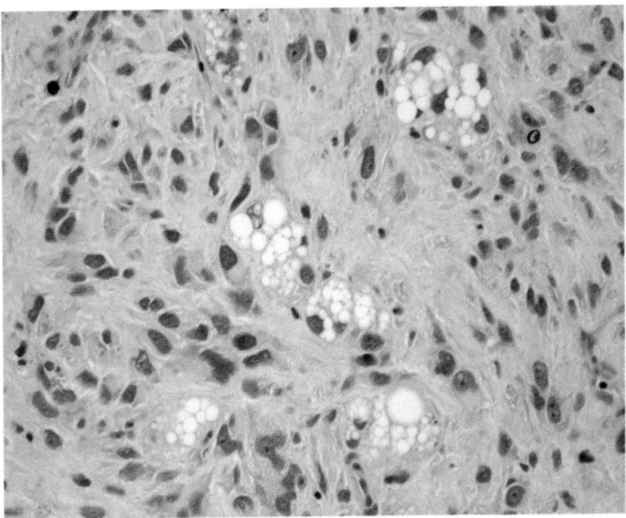

Figure 11.43 Pleomorphic liposarcoma with sarcomatous pleomorphic cells and lipoblasts.

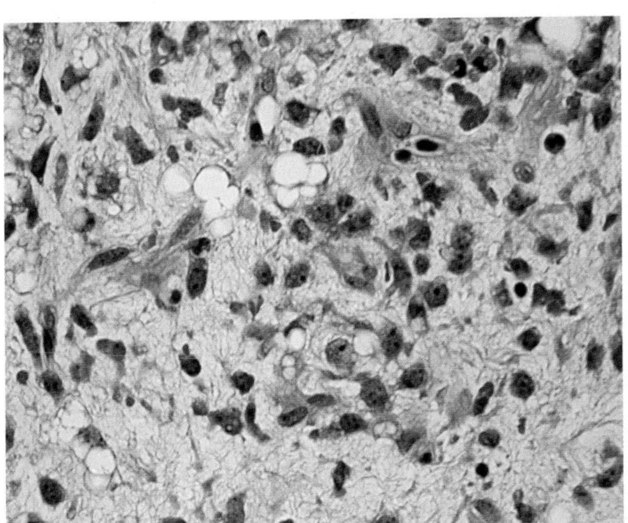

Figure 11.44 Myxoid liposarcoma with lipoblasts within a myxoid background.

Part 15

Alveolar Soft Part Sarcoma

▶ Mojghan Amrikachi and Timothy Allen

Alveolar soft part sarcoma (ASPS) is a rare malignant tumor, commonly occurring in deep soft tissues such as thigh and leg, in young adults generally between 15 and 35 years old. ASPS most often occurs in the lung as metastatic disease, but it may very rarely occur as a primary lung malignancy. Differential diagnosis of ASPS includes metastatic renal cell carcinoma, paraganglioma, and granular cell tumor.

Histologic Features:

- Sharply defined nodules of tumor cells with central degeneration and necrosis resulting in pseudoalveolar pattern.
- Nodules separated by thin-walled vascular channels.
- Uniform large round to polygonal cells with distinct cell borders and abundant eosinophilic granular or vacuolated cytoplasm.
- Vesicular nuclei and prominent nucleoli.
- PAS-positive, diastase-resistant rhomboid or rod-shaped crystals (intracellular glycogen).
- Immunonegative for cytokeratins, EMA, GFAP, and neurofilament.
- Ultrastructurally, cells contain rhomboid or rod-shaped crystals.

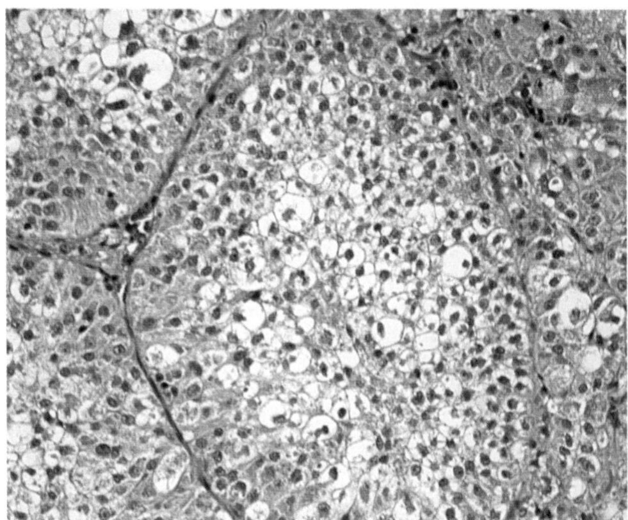

Figure 11.45 Sharply defined nodule of tumor exhibiting pseudoalveolar pattern.

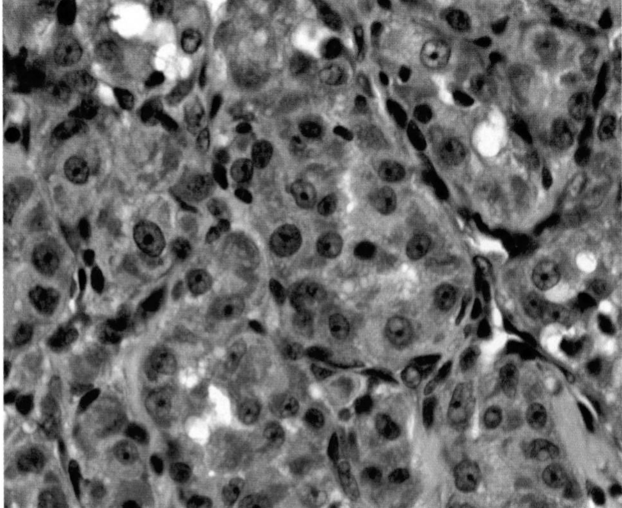

Figure 11.46 Higher power showing uniform large round to polygonal cells with abundant eosinophilic granular cytoplasm.

Part 16

Glomangiosarcoma (Malignant Glomus Tumor)

▶ Donna Coffey

Glomangiosarcomas (malignant glomus tumors) are rare tumors that are subdivided histologically in two categories: glomangiosarcoma arising within a glomus tumor and *de novo* glomangiosarcoma. Glomangiosarcomas arising within a glomus tumor display histopathologic features of benign glomus tumors but with features of malignancy described in the following. Glomangiosarcomas arising *de novo* may be more difficult to diagnose due to the absence of the more characteristic benign component. Glomangiosarcomas are commonly indolent, with an increased risk of local recurrence. Metastases may occur. Differential diagnosis includes carcinoid tumor, hemangiopericytoma, primitive neuroectodermal tumors, paraganglioma, and epithelioid leiomyoma. Generally, gross features include a large poorly circumscribed mass with necrosis and hemorrhage.

Cytologic Features:

- Clusters of uniform, round to oval cells admixed with intercellular myxoid material may be seen.
- Cytologic atypia, necrosis, and increased mitotic figures.

Histologic Features:

- Glomangiosarcomas arising within a glomus tumor display features of benign glomus tumor and malignant features including cytologic atypia, necrosis, increased mitotic figures, and cystic degeneration.
- Combination of blood vessels, polygonal cells with well-defined cell borders, and varying stroma.
- Uniform epithelioid cells with distinct cell borders, scant clear to eosinophilic cytoplasm, and central round nuclei.
- Solid, fascicular, or vaguely nested growth pattern.
- Occasional mast cells can be appreciated.
- Generally immunopositive for actin and collagen IV.
- May be immunopositive for desmin and CD34.
- Generally immunonegative for cytokeratins, chromogranin, NSE, S-100, and CD99.

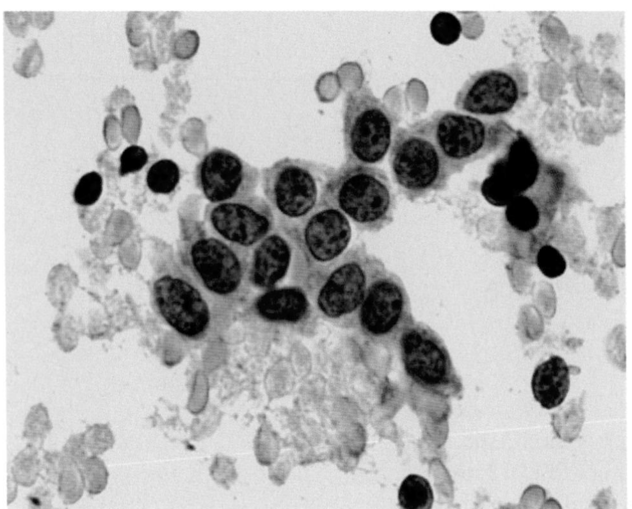

Figure 11.47 Cytology figure of glomangiosarcoma shows a cluster of uniform oval cells with scant cytoplasm and distinct cell borders.

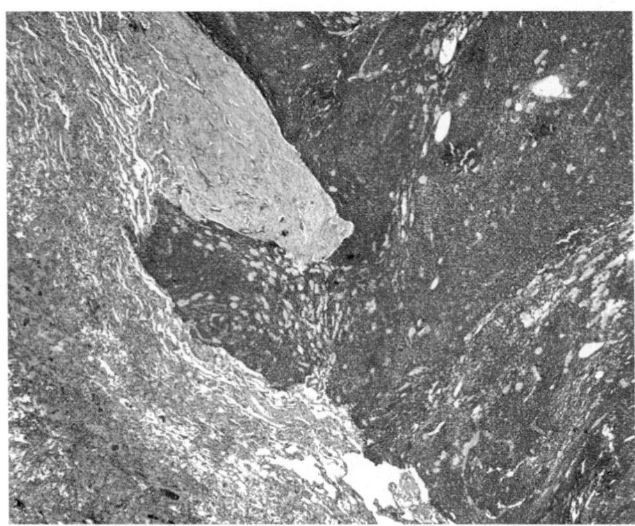

Figure 11.48 Low power of glomangiosarcoma shows a very cellular tumor infiltrating lung parenchyma.

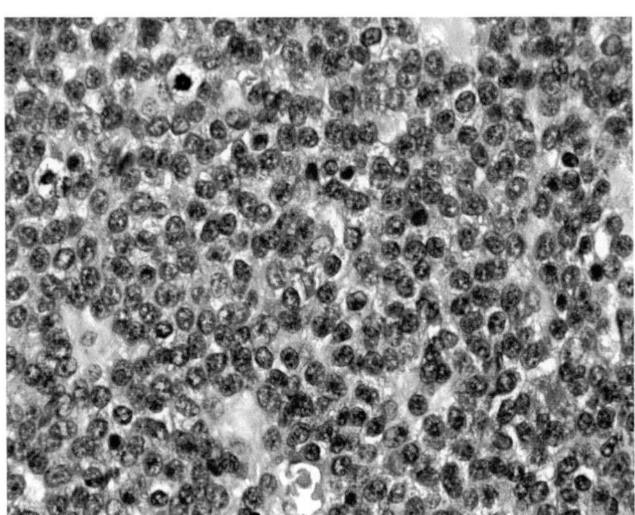

Figure 11.49 Higher power of glomangiosarcoma showing uniform oval to round epithelioid cells with distinct cell borders and mitotic figures.

12 Hematologic Malignancies

Primary non-Hodgkin lymphomas (NHLs) of the lung are relatively rare, composing less than 1% of primary pulmonary neoplasms and less than 10% of extranodal lymphomas. The most common entity is extranodal marginal zone B-cell lymphoma of mucosa-associated lymphoid tissue (MALT lymphoma). Large B-cell lymphomas, including the distinctive entity lymphomatoid granulomatosis, make up most of the remaining primary NHLs. Hodgkin lymphoma and other subtypes of NHLs may rarely present as pulmonary primaries.

On the other hand, the lungs are frequently involved by systemic lymphomas, leukemias, and plasma cell dyscrasias. Many of the features of these lesions are similar to those seen in the primary nodal or extranodal sites.

The malignant cells in MALT lymphomas usually show a range of morphologic features, and lymphomatoid granulomatosis, T-cell lymphomas, and Hodgkin lymphoma all are notable for their association with a polymorphous inflammatory background. Given these factors, primary diagnosis may be difficult on small biopsies, and open or thoracoscopic biopsy may be required.

Many cases may be diagnosed using immunoperoxidase studies on paraffin sections. B- and T-cell clonality may often be confirmed using polymerase reaction studies, also using paraffin-embedded material. If fresh material is available, flow cytometric analysis may confirm B-cell clonality or T-cell marker aberrancies in most cases. *In situ* hybridization is the most sensitive technique for detection of Epstein-Barr virus (EBV) infection. Cytogenetic studies are rarely required, although *in situ* hybridization for the t(11;18) translocation seen in some MALT lymphomas may play a diagnostic role in the near future.

Part 1

Extranodal Marginal Zone B-Cell Lymphoma

▸ Jeffrey Jorgensen

MALT lymphoma is the most common primary lymphoma involving the lung. This is a low-grade B-cell lymphoma that occurs primarily in older individuals (average age about 60). Only about half of patients are symptomatic at presentation. This lymphoma usually presents as solitary or multiple nodules, or less commonly as patchy or diffuse infiltrates. Grossly, most cases show an ill-defined fleshy mass with preservation of the lung architecture. Hilar lymph nodes are involved in a minority of cases, and most cases do not show bone marrow involvement. Multiple extranodal sites are involved in a few cases. These lymphomas are generally indolent and may respond well to localized therapy. Large cell transformation occurs in a minority of cases.

Differential diagnosis includes benign and borderline lymphoid proliferations such as nodular lymphoid hyperplasia and lymphocytic interstitial pneumonia, and other low-grade NHLs such as chronic lymphocytic leukemia/small lymphocytic lymphoma, follicular lymphoma, and mantle cell lymphoma.

Histologic Features:

- Dense lymphoid infiltrate with a lymphatic distribution along septa and bronchovascular bundles.
- Pleural involvement or erosion of bronchial cartilage may be seen; if present, either of these features favor a malignant process.
- Composed of varying proportions of small lymphocytes, intermediate-sized lymphocytes with moderately abundant pale cytoplasm (monocytoid, marginal zone lymphocytes), plasma cells and plasmacytoid lymphocytes, and scattered large cells with vesicular chromatin and distinct nucleoli.
- Dutcher bodies (nuclear pseudoinclusions) may be present in plasma cells or plasmacytoid lymphocytes; these are much more common in malignant lymphomas than in benign reactive conditions.
- Lymphocytic infiltration of bronchial or bronchiolar epithelium, forming lymphoepithelial lesions, is seen in nearly all cases; however, this feature may also be seen in reactive conditions.
- Most cases are associated with benign reactive germinal centers; some cases show "colonization" (infiltration) of germinal centers by lymphoma cells.
- Plasma cells are most often reactive, with polyclonal staining for κ and λ light chains.
- Some cases will show extensive plasmacytic differentiation, with monoclonal light-chain staining of plasma cells.
- Many cases are associated with multinucleated giant cells and/or epithelioid granulomas
- Immunopositive for B-cell markers (CD20; also CD22, CD79a, Pax-5).
- Aberrant coexpression of CD43 on B cells in some cases (note that T cells, histiocytes, and plasma cells are usually positive for CD43).

- Negative for CD5, CD10, BCL-6, and cyclin D1.
- Staining of lung epithelium with pan-keratin may highlight lymphoepithelial lesions.
- Diagnosis may hinge on demonstration of clonality by either flow cytometry of a fresh specimen (if necessary by repeat biopsy, possibly by fine needle aspiration) or analysis of immunoglobulin heavy chain genes by polymerase chain reaction (PCR).
- Some cases carry the characteristic translocation t(11;18), involving the API2 and MLT loci; this translocation can be identified by fluorescence *in situ* hybridization (FISH) or potentially by reverse transcription and polymerase chain reaction (RT-PCR).

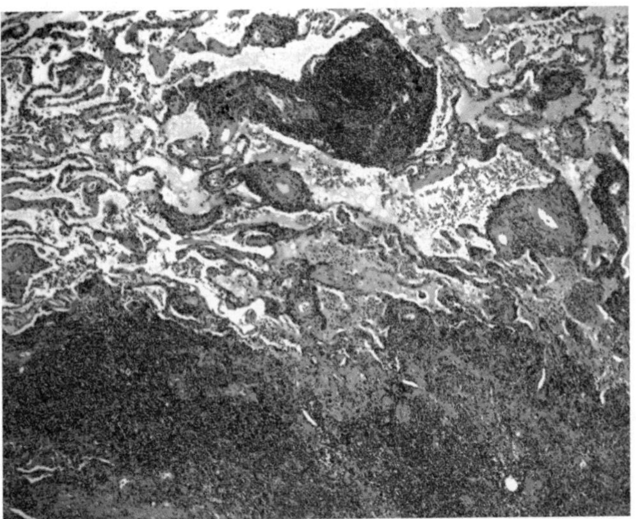

Figure 12.1 Sheets of small lymphocytes form a confluent mass in the center of the lesion (lower part of figure); lymphoid infiltrates at the periphery of the lesion show a lymphatic distribution around blood vessels.

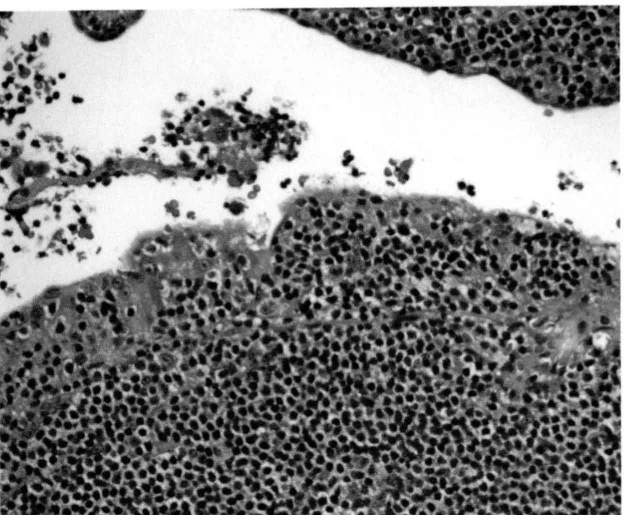

Figure 12.2 Small lymphocytes infiltrate bronchial epithelium, forming lymphoepithelial lesions.

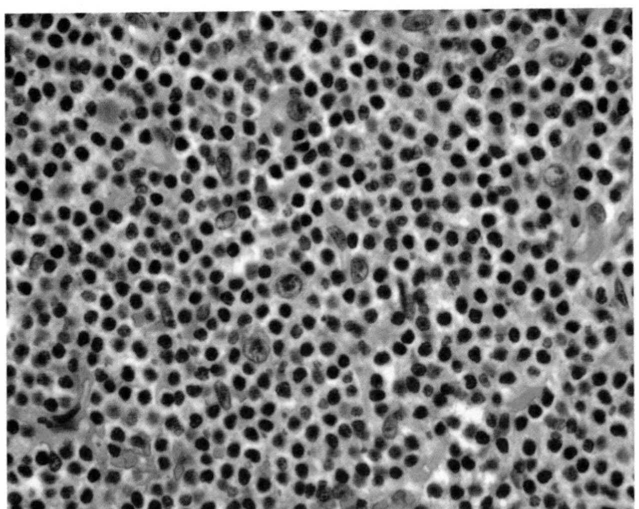

Figure 12.3 Scattered large cells are present in a background of small lymphocytes, some of which have increased pale cytoplasm (monocytoid lymphocytes).

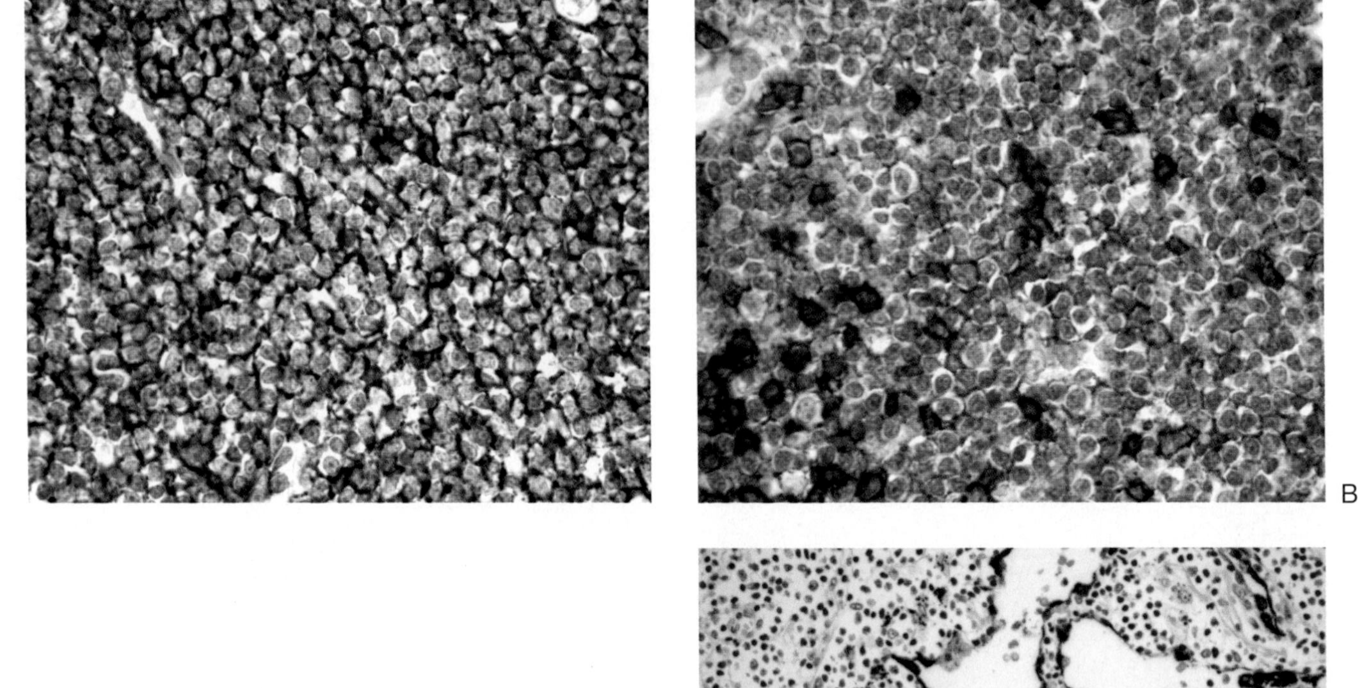

Figure 12.4 **A:** CD20 immunostain: Sheets of lymphocytes are immunopositive for this B-cell marker; this finding alone is highly worrisome for lymphoma. **B:** CD43 immunostain: B lymphocytes show weak-to-moderate aberrant staining (as seen in a minority of cases), whereas scattered reactive T lymphocytes show stronger staining. **C:** Pan-keratin immunostain: Lymphoepithelial lesion.

Part 2

Primary Large B-Cell Lymphoma

▶ Jeffrey Jorgensen

Large B-cell lymphoma is the second most common primary NHL in the lung after MALT lymphoma. There is a wide age range, from children to adults. Patients are often symptomatic (dyspnea, chest pain, and/or hemoptysis). Differential diagnosis primarily includes poorly differentiated carcinoma. Other primary large cell lymphomas of the lung are much less common; they include peripheral T-cell lymphoma (PTCL), Hodgkin lymphoma, and anaplastic large cell lymphoma.

Histologic Features:

- Sheets of discohesive large cells with oval to irregular nuclei, vesicular chromatin, and distinct nucleoli.
- Pulmonary architecture is usually effaced, often with associated necrosis, with vascular invasion in some cases.
- Tumor cells and fibrin may fill airspaces ("tumoral pneumonia").
- Diffuse areas or edges of a mass lesion often show infiltration in a lymphatic distribution.
- Usually immunopositive for CD45 (LCA) and B-cell markers such as CD20.
- Flow cytometric analysis may yield a false-negative result because of necrosis and/or cell fragility.

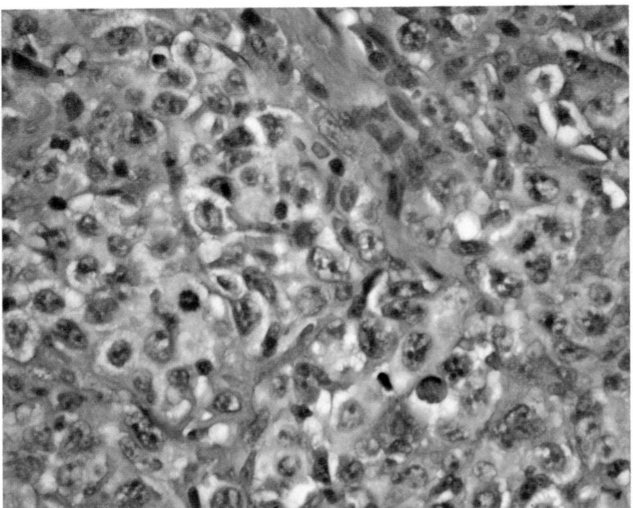

Figure 12.5 Large atypical lymphoid cells effacing the pulmonary architecture.

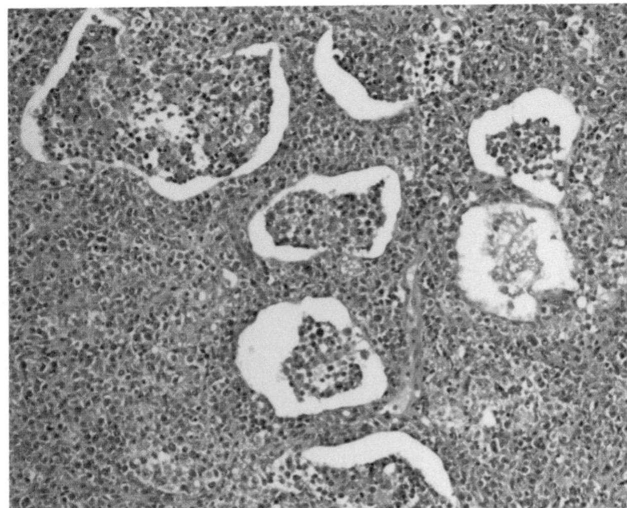

Figure 12.6 Tumor cells may be present in alveolar spaces ("tumoral pneumonia").

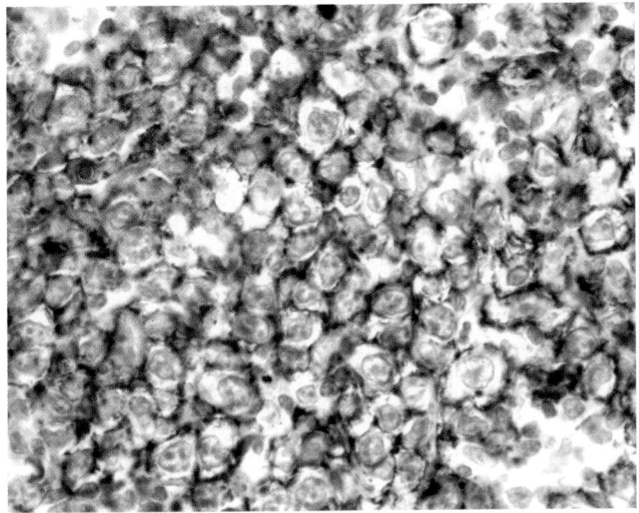

Figure 12.7 CD20 immunostain highlights malignant B cells.

Part 3

Lymphomatoid Granulomatosis

▶ Jeffrey Jorgensen

Lymphomatoid granulomatosis (LYG) is now regarded as a T-cell-rich, large B-cell lymphoma in which the malignant B cells are positive for EBV. It usually presents in adults and is more common in males. Immunodeficiency is a risk factor (human immunodeficiency virus [HIV], congenital or iatrogenic), and LYG may occur in immunodeficient children. Most patients have pulmonary disease and often have respiratory symptoms. Other common sites of involvement are skin, central nervous system, kidney, and liver. Systemic symptoms are frequent. In the lung, LYG most often shows multiple, bilateral nodules, with possible cavitation in larger nodules. The disease is aggressive in the majority of patients, although occasional cases may be more indolent.

Differential diagnosis of low-grade lesions includes infectious and inflammatory conditions (Wegener's granulomatosis, necrotizing sarcoid, bronchocentric granulomatosis). Granulomatous inflammation is actually uncommon in LYG, and the presence of granulomas or neutrophils favors an alternate diagnosis. Differential diagnosis of high-grade lesions includes carcinoma, melanoma, large cell lymphoma, and Hodgkin lymphoma.

Histologic Features:

- Polymorphous angiocentric lymphoid infiltrate.
- Lymphocytic vasculitis often leads to vascular compromise and central necrosis.
- Large atypical lymphocytes are usually in the minority and are occasionally pleomorphic or multinucleated.
- Most cells are small- to intermediate-sized reactive lymphocytes that may show some nuclear irregularity.
- Plasma cells and histiocytes may also be present, but granulomas, neutrophils, and eosinophils usually are not seen.
- Diagnostic areas including large cells may be focal, and thorough sampling is warranted
- Large atypical cells are immunopositive for the B-cell marker CD20, and many of these are also immunopositive for EBV latent membrane protein 1 (LMP1).
- Large cells are variably immunopositive for CD30 but negative for CD15.
- Most small background lymphocytes are immunopositive for the T-cell marker CD3.
- *In situ* hybridization studies on paraffin sections for EBV-expressed RNAs (EBER) may be a more sensitive detection technique for diagnosis and grading.
- Grading is based on the number of EBV-positive B cells: grade I with <5 EBV-positive cells per high-power field and rare or absent large cells; grade II with 5 to 20 EBV-positive cells and scattered large cells; and grade III with numerous EBV-positive large cells.

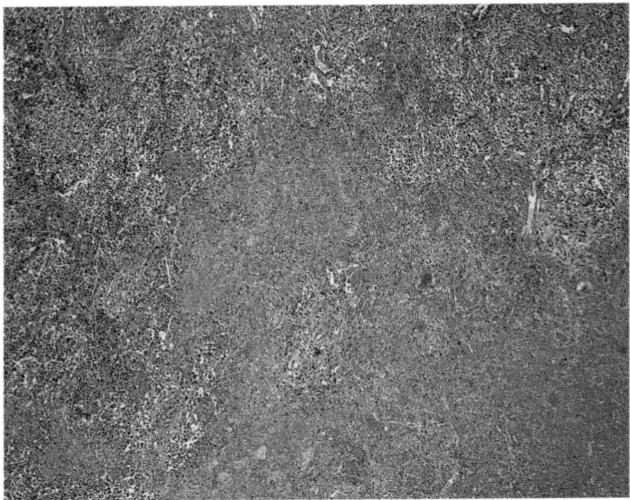

Figure 12.8 Large nodule containing a polymorphous lymphoid infiltrate, with central necrosis.

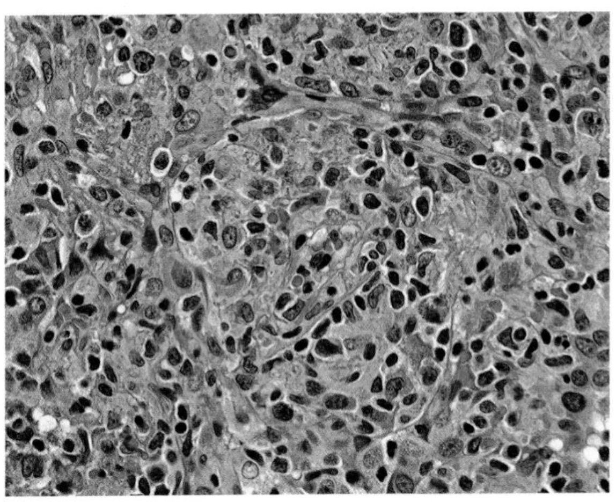

Figure 12.9 Scattered large atypical neoplastic lymphocytes are present in a background of small- and intermediate-sized reactive lymphocytes, some with irregular or "twisted" nuclei.

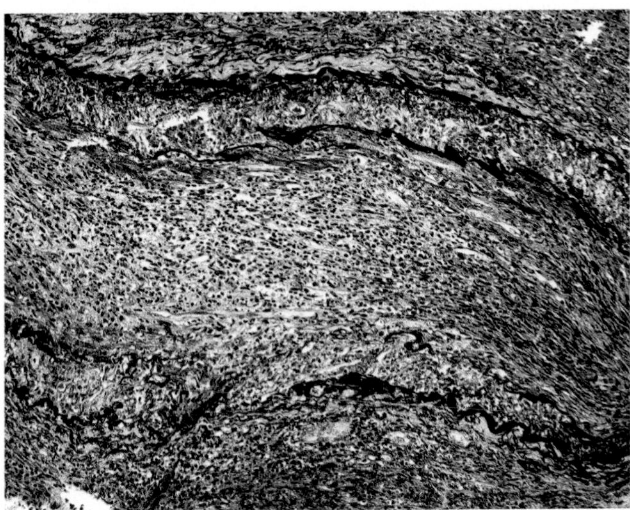

Figure 12.10 Elastin stain demonstrating lymphoid infiltration and destruction of vessel walls.

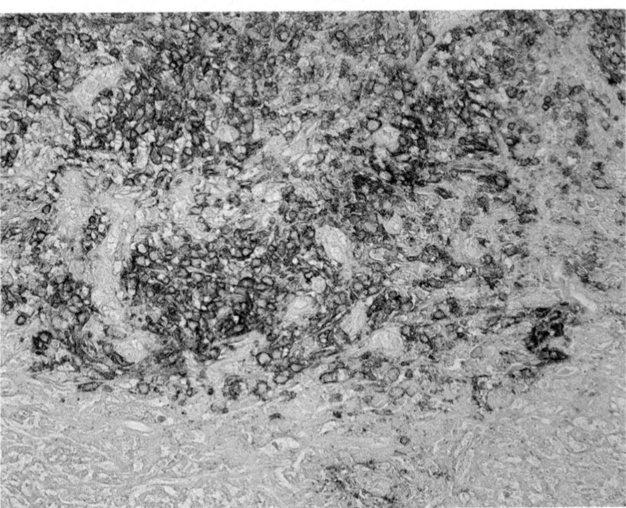

A B

Figure 12.11 A: CD20 immunostain highlights large cells in clusters in this focus. B: EBV LMP1 immunostain highlights a subset of large cells.

Part 4

Primary Hodgkin Lymphoma

▶ Jeffrey Jorgensen

Primary Hodgkin lymphoma of the lung, with no demonstrated extrapulmonary involvement, is rare. Patients often present with pulmonary symptoms, and systemic B symptoms are common. Multiple lesions are usually present, although solitary nodules or localized infiltrates may also be seen. There may be extensive granulomatous inflammation; thus, differential diagnosis includes inflammatory and infectious processes, as well as large-cell NHLs and poorly differentiated carcinomas. Reed-Sternberg-like cells may occur in occasional lymphomas and even carcinomas, and the presence of an appropriate inflammatory background is essential for the diagnosis of Hodgkin lymphoma.

Histologic Features:

- Large pleomorphic cells in a polymorphous inflammatory background.
- Diagnostic Reed-Sternberg cells have bilobated or multilobated nuclei with prominent eosinophilic nucleoli.
- Mononuclear (Hodgkin) cells may include pyknotic mummified cells and lacunar variants with cytoplasmic retraction artifact.
- Some cases contain Hodgkin and Reed-Sternberg (HRS) cells in large clusters or sheets
- Background reactive cells include histiocytes, small lymphocytes, eosinophils, plasma cells, and neutrophils.
- Tumor nodules may show central necrosis and/or neutrophilic microabscesses.
- Nodular sclerosis subtype shows dense collagen bands.
- HRS cells are immunopositive for CD30 in nearly all cases.
- Immunostaining for CD15 is seen in the majority of cases but sometimes in only a few cells, with only cytoplasmic or paranuclear Golgi staining.
- HRS cells are weakly to moderately immunopositive for the B-lineage marker PAX-5 in most cases and variably immunopositive for CD20 in some cases.
- HRS cells are negative for CD45, CD79a, and CD43.

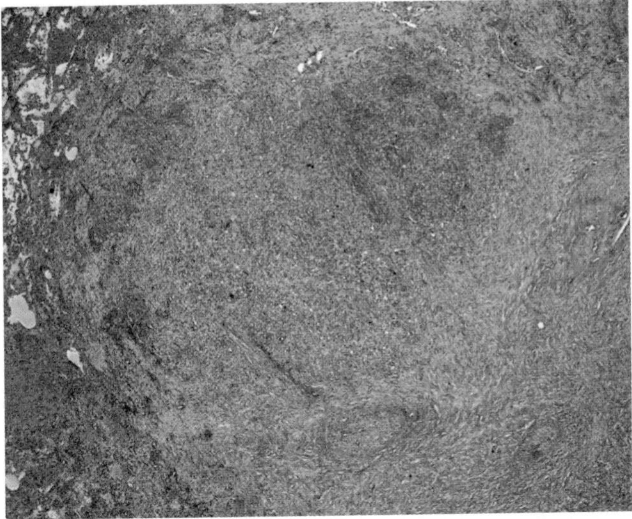

Figure 12.12 Large nodule containing a polymorphous inflammatory infiltrate, with associated dense sclerosis.

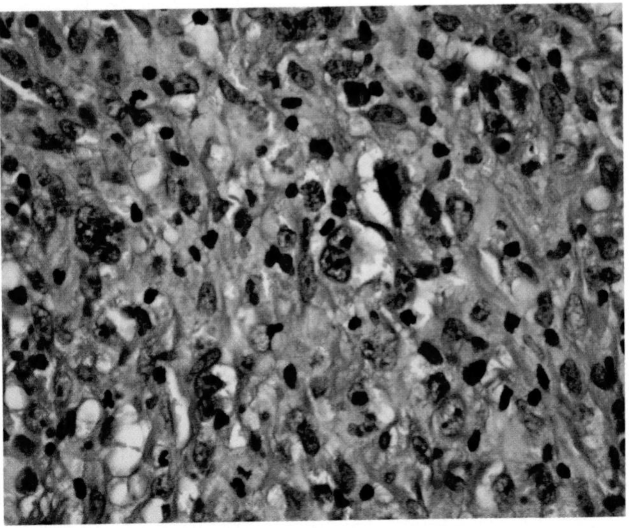

Figure 12.13 Several multinucleated Reed-Sternberg cells are present in an inflammatory background including histiocytes, lymphocytes, and a few plasma cells and eosinophils.

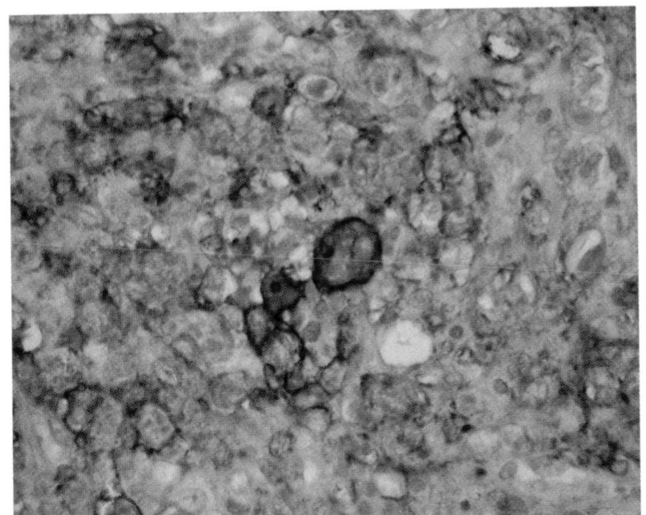

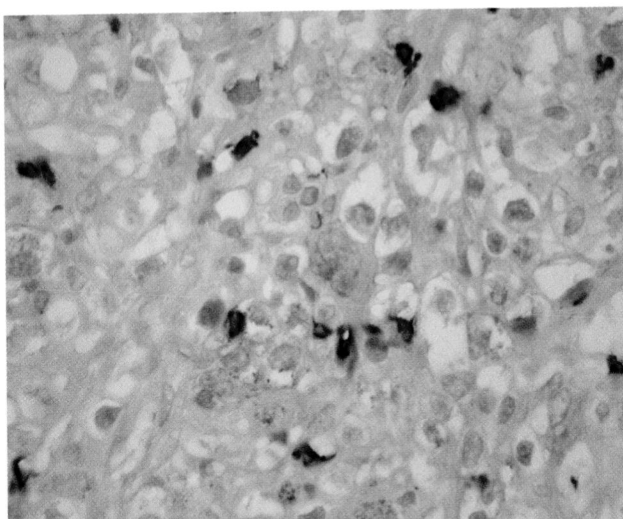

Figure 12.14 **A:** CD30 immunostain, with a Reed-Sternberg cell showing a predominantly membrane and paranuclear Golgi staining pattern. **B:** CD15 immunostain, with focal weak cytoplasmic staining of a Reed-Sternberg cell. Neutrophils and eosinophils show strong cytoplasmic staining, a normal finding.

Part 5

Systemic Lymphomas and Leukemias Involving the Lung and Pleura

Secondary involvement of the lungs and pleura by systemic lymphomas and leukemias is much more common than involvement by primary hematologic malignancies. The former are discussed in the following subparts.

Subpart 5.1

Acute Myeloid Leukemia

▶ Dani S. Zander

At autopsy, pulmonary infiltration by leukemic cells is a common finding in patients with acute myeloid leukemia. Symptomatic involvement during life is much less common, however, and occurs primarily in patients with high peripheral blast counts. Radiographic manifestations include thickening of bronchovascular bundles, patchy consolidation, prominence of peripheral pulmonary arteries, ground glass opacities, and nodules. Uncommon pulmonary complications associated with very high peripheral blast counts ($>100{,}000/mm^3$) include leukostasis with thrombosis of capillaries and diffuse alveolar damage secondary to chemotherapy-induced leukemic cell lysis. Opportunistic infections and complications of chemotherapy and radiation therapy represent other more common causes of pulmonary infiltrates in these patients.

Histologic Features:

- Perilymphatic and perivascular infiltrates in bronchovascular bundles, interlobular septa, and pleura.
- Nodular parenchymal or airway infiltrates less common.
- Large cells with large nuclei and open chromatin; may have prominent nucleoli.
- Cytoplasm may be granular.
- Chloroacetate esterase stain may highlight cytoplasmic granules.
- Immunohistochemistry for myeloperoxidase demonstrates granular cytoplasmic positivity; CD15 also may be expressed.

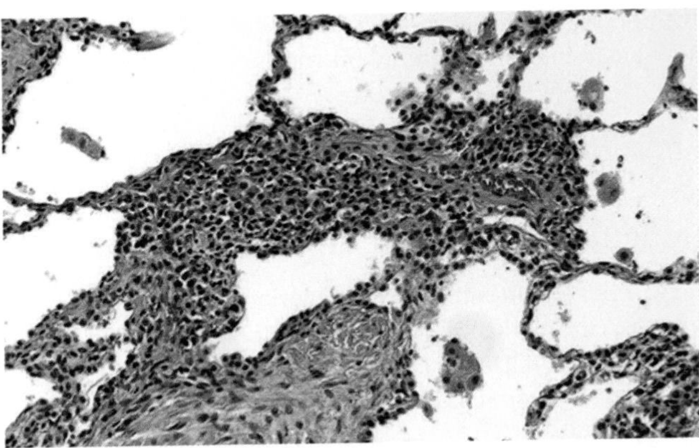

Figure 12.15 Perivascular myeloblasts with an adjacent focus of parenchymal fibrosis.

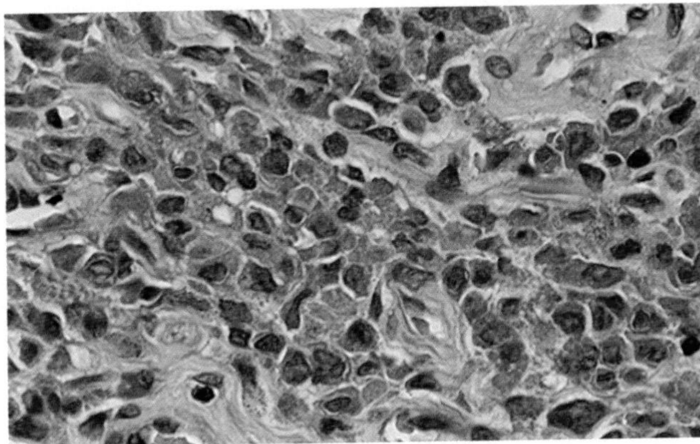

Figure 12.16 Myeloblasts with irregular nuclei and granular cytoplasm.

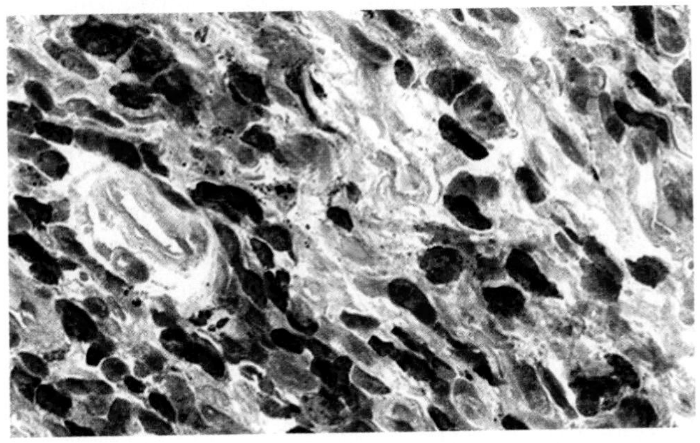

Figure 12.17 Chloroacetate esterase stain showing cytoplasmic granules staining red, confirming myeloid differentiation.

Subpart 5.2

B-Cell Lymphoproliferative Disorders

▶ Jeffrey Jorgensen

Neoplastic small B-cell infiltrates may be distinguished in most cases by careful immunophenotyping, flow cytometry of fresh material, or immunohistochemical staining. In patients with a known history of systemic lymphoma, fine needle aspiration of a pulmonary mass may yield sufficient material for flow cytometric immunophenotyping. Occasionally the lung is involved by large-cell transformation of a low-grade lymphoma, so both morphologic and immunophenotypic findings must be assessed.

A relatively comprehensive immunohistochemical marker panel for differentiating low-grade B-cell malignancies would include CD20, CD3, CD5, CD10, CD23, CD43, BCL-2, BCL-6, and cyclin D1. Some of these may be omitted in a given case, depending on the morphologic differential diagnosis. Note that CD43 may more reliably stain chronic lymphocytic leukemia and mantle cell lymphoma than CD5 (which may be expressed at a lower level and may be more technically challenging to perform).

Intravascular large B-cell lymphoma is a rare, aggressive tumor usually occurring in adults. Patients often present with widespread disease involving the central nervous system, skin, lung, and other organs, with occasional initial pulmonary presentation. Unfortunately, a significant proportion of cases remain undiagnosed until postmortem examination.

Histologic Features:

Chronic lymphocytic leukemia/small lymphocytic leukemia

- Usually interstitial infiltrate, without significant nodule formation.
- Small lymphocytes with clumped chromatin and scant cytoplasm.
- Immunopositive for CD20, CD5, CD23, CD43, and BCL-2.
- Immunonegative for cyclin D1, CD10, and BCL-6.

Follicular Lymphoma

- Nodular proliferation in a lymphatic distribution.
- Small- to intermediate-sized cells with angulated or cleaved nuclei, admixed with large cells with vesicular chromatin and distinct nucleoli.
- Most cases show a relative paucity of mitotic figures and macrophages with nuclear debris in comparison with reactive follicles.
- Immunopositive for CD20, CD10, and BCL-6.
- Most cases immunopositive for BCL-2, in contrast to reactive follicles, which are always BCL-2 negative (note, however, that most other subtypes of low-grade B-cell lymphoma are also BCL-2 positive).
- Immunonegative for CD5, CD43, and cyclin D1.

Mantle Cell Lymphoma

- Small- to intermediate-sized cells with round to irregular, often notched nuclei.
- Immunopositive for CD20, CD5, CD43, and cyclin D1.
- Immunonegative for CD10, CD23, and BCL-6.
- Prognosis is significantly worse than for other B-cell lymphomas with predominantly small cells.

Intravascular Large B-Cell Lymphoma

- Interstitial infiltrate, often subtle.
- Large atypical cells with open chromatin and distinct nucleoli.
- Tumor cells are largely confined to small vessels, sometimes associated with fibrin thrombi.
- Immunopositive for B-cell markers such as CD20.

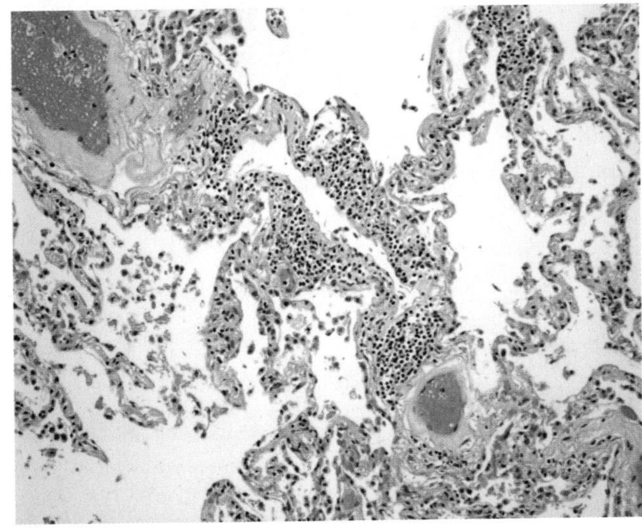

Figure 12.18 Chronic lymphocytic leukemia (autopsy specimen), with focal expansion of interstitial lymphatics by small lymphocytes.

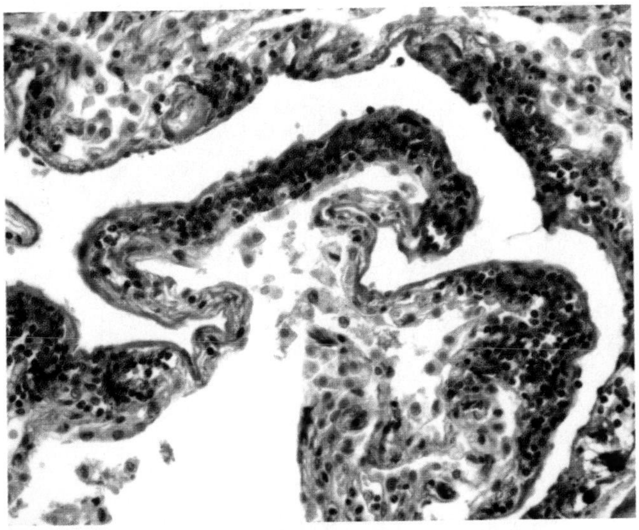

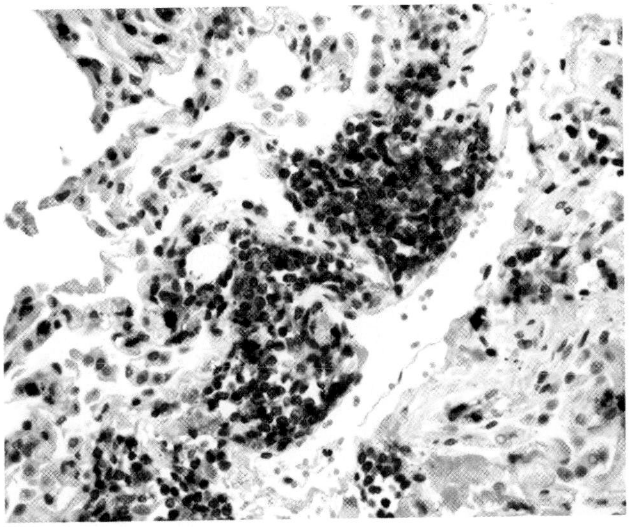

Figure 12.19 Chronic lymphocytic leukemia. **A:** CD20 immunostain; **B:** CD5 immunostain; **C:** CD43 immunostain. Neoplastic B cells show aberrant coexpression of the T-lineage-associated molecules CD5 and CD43.

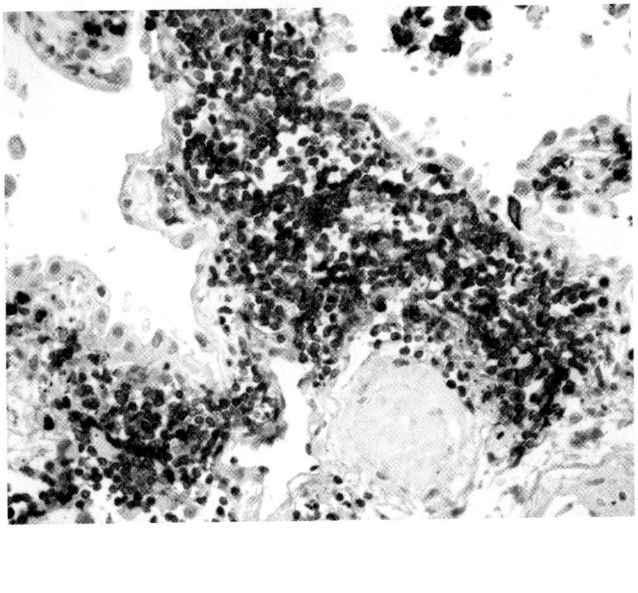

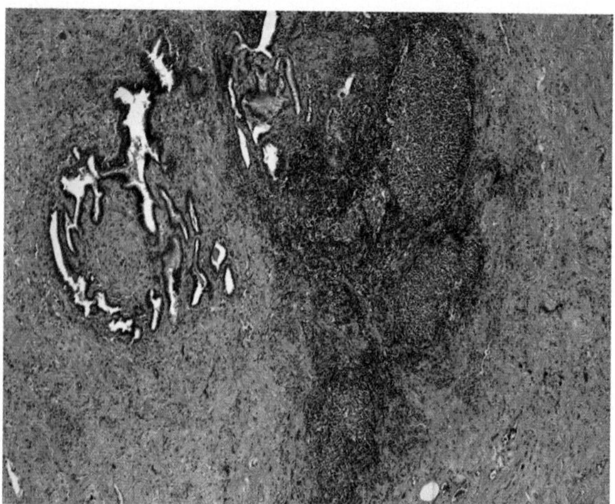

Figure 12.20 Follicular lymphoma, with peribronchial nodules and associated fibrosis. Note the near absence of phagocytic macrophages and thus lack of the usual "starry sky" pattern seen in normal reactive follicles.

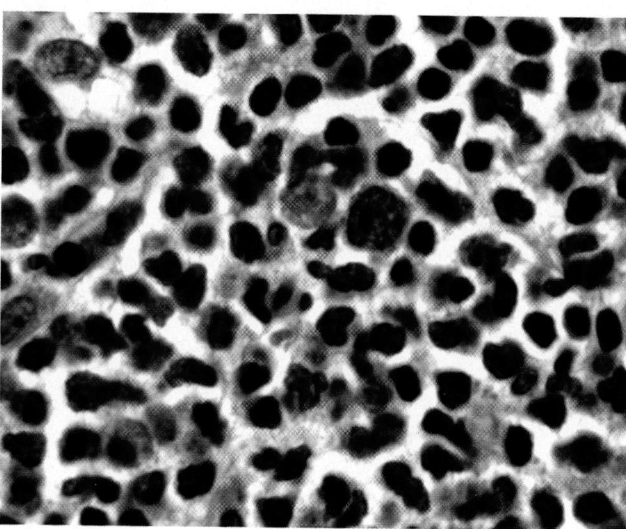

Figure 12.21 Follicular lymphoma, with predominantly small- to intermediate-sized cells with irregular nuclei, and scattered large cells.

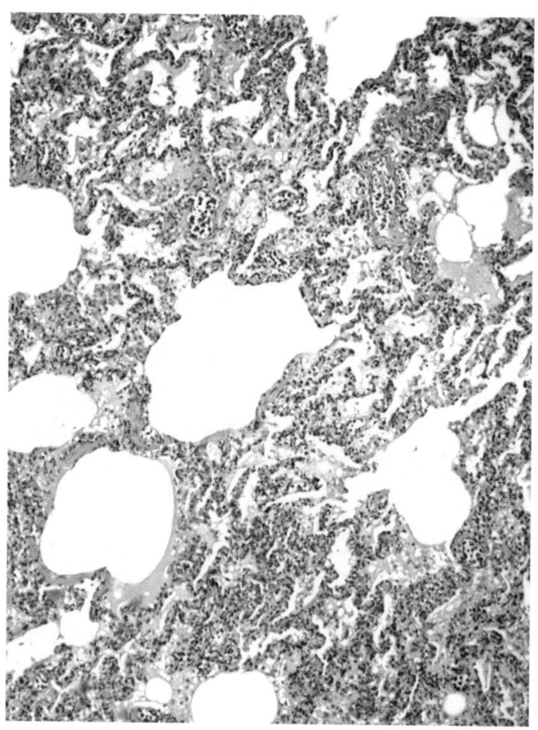

Figure 12.22 Intravascular large B-cell lymphoma showing a subtle interstitial infiltrate at low power.

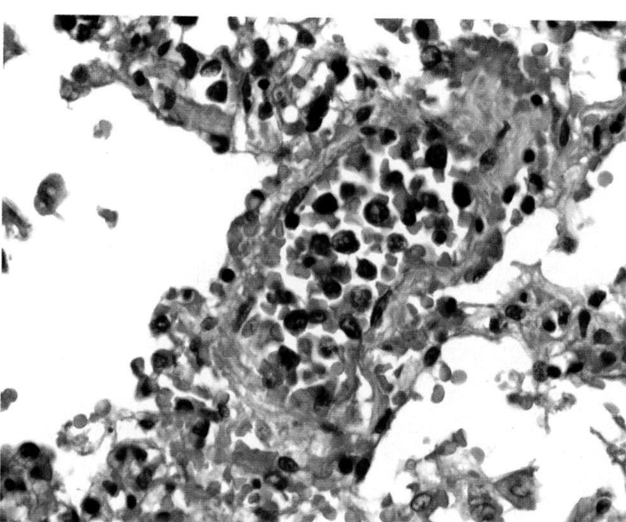

Figure 12.23 Intravascular large B-cell lymphoma, with atypical large lymphocytes within a small vessel.

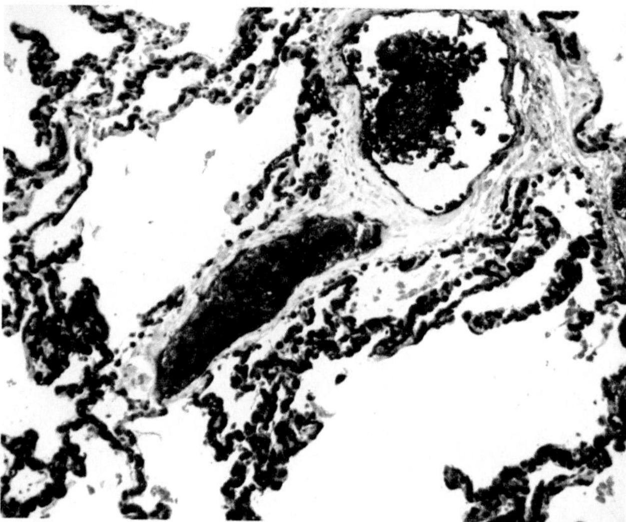

Figure 12.24 Intravascular large B-cell lymphoma immunostain for CD20, highlighting malignant B cells within small vessels and interstitial capillaries.

Subpart 5.3

Secondary Hodgkin Disease

▶ Jeffrey Jorgensen and Rodolfo Laucirica

Systemic Hodgkin lymphoma frequently involves the lung during the course of the disease, either by direct extension from the mediastinum or in the form of disseminated metastatic disease. It may recur in the lung just outside the field of radiation therapy of a mediastinal primary. Recurrent Hodgkin lymphoma may show increased numbers and greater pleomorphism of the HRS cells, and some cases show a reduction in accompanying inflammatory background cells.

Histologic Features:

See the discussion of primary Hodgkin lymphoma for additional details of the clinical, morphologic, and immunophenotypic findings.

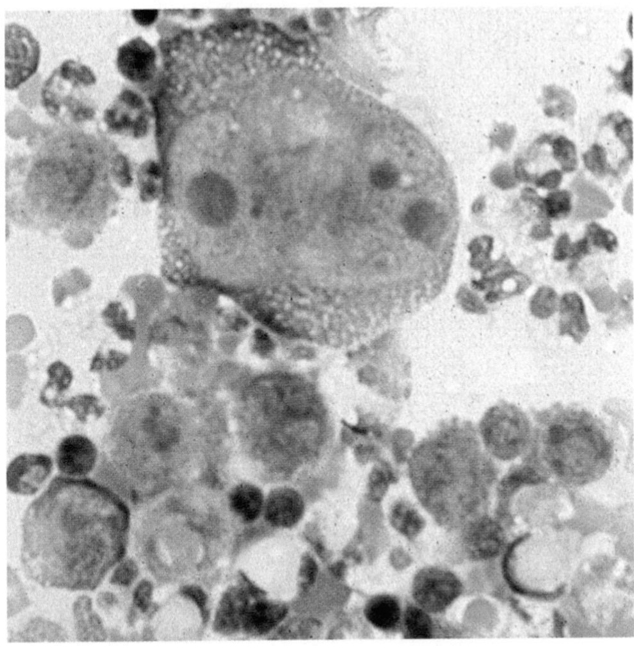

Figure 12.25 Pleural fluid cytology showing Reed-Sternberg cell and a mixture of lymphocytes and neutrophils in mixed cellularity Hodgkin disease.

Figure 12.26 Nodule containing a polymorphous infiltrate, delimited by dense sclerosis.

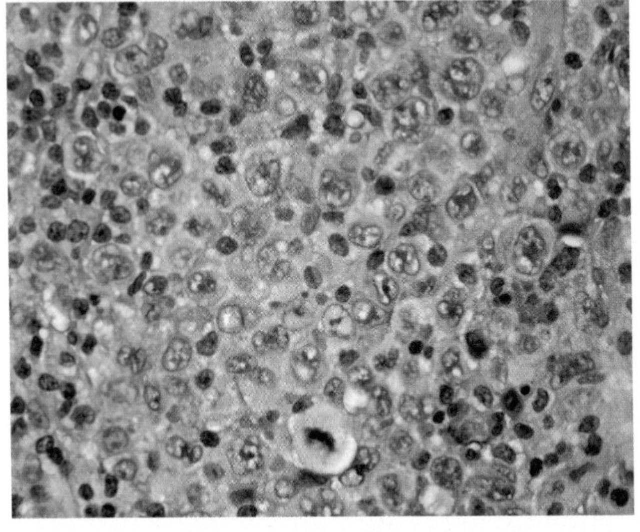

Figure 12.27 Pleomorphic mononuclear Hodgkin cells predominate in this field.

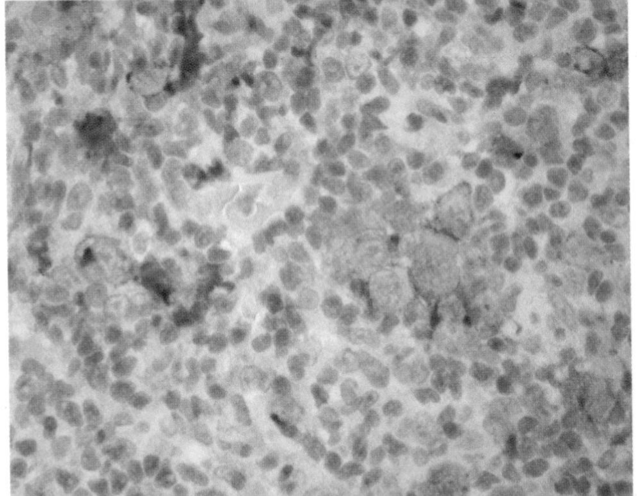

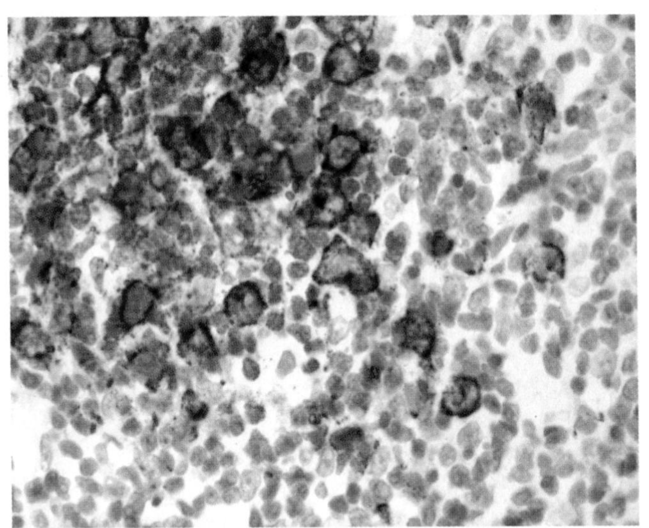

Figure 12.28 CD30 immunostain (**A**) and CD15 immunostain (**B**), both demonstrating a membrane and paranuclear Golgi staining pattern of Hodgkin and Reed-Sternberg cells. This case is unusual; most cases show more extensive staining for CD30 than for CD15.

Subpart 5.4

Systemic T-Cell Lymphoma

▶ Jeffrey Jorgensen

Mycosis fungoides (MF) is a mature T-cell lymphoma that presents in the skin. In late-stage cases, the lung is the second most common site of involvement beyond the skin. Pulmonary symptoms may result. There may be a nodular and/or diffuse infiltrate.

PTCLs often involve multiple nodal and extranodal sites, particularly the skin but also including the lungs.

Histologic Features:

- Usually infiltration in a lymphatic distribution, along bronchovascular bundles and septa.
- Varying degrees of cytologic atypia; MF cells are generally small with convoluted cerebriform nuclei, but in late stages may include large cells with vesicular chromatin and prominent nucleoli.
- PTCLs, particularly the angioimmunoblastic subtype, may show a polymorphous inflammatory background including histiocytes, plasma cells, and eosinophils.
- MF and PTCL may be associated with granulomatous inflammation.
- Tumor cells may show loss or quantitative alterations in T-cell markers (CD2, CD3, CD5, CD7, CD43, or CD45RO).
- Tumor cells are immunopositive for CD4 in nearly all cases of MF and in most PTCLs, whereas infrequent PTCL cases are $CD8^{+}$, $CD4^{+}CD8^{+}$, or $CD4^{-}CD8^{-}$.
- Flow cytometric immunophenotyping of fresh material is more sensitive than immunoperoxidase studies on paraffin sections for identifying aberrations in T-cell markers.
- Diagnosis may require analysis of T-cell receptor gene rearrangements by polymerase chain reaction.

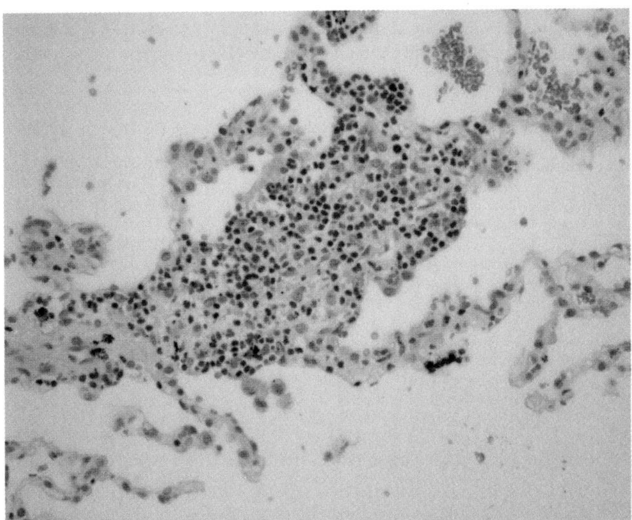

Figure 12.29 Mycosis fungoides with focal interstitial infiltration by small lymphocytes.

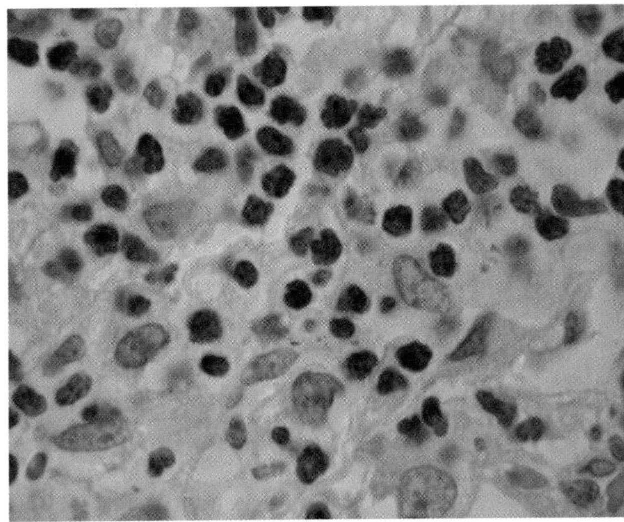

Figure 12.30 Mycosis fungoides with atypical small lymphocytes having convoluted, "cerebriform" nuclei.

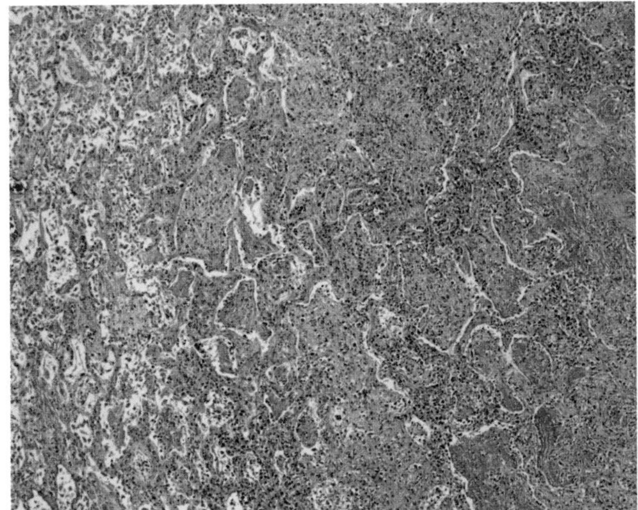

Figure 12.31 Mycosis fungoides with large cell transformation showing interstitial infiltration with associated organizing pneumonia.

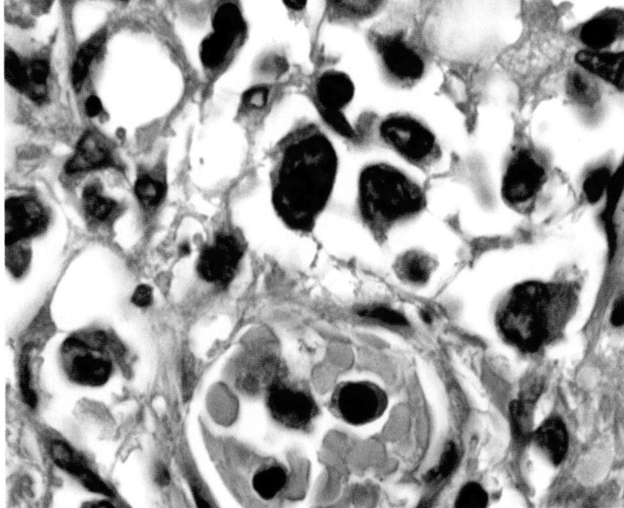

Figure 12.32 Mycosis fungoides with large cell transformation showing pleomorphic intermediate-sized to large cells.

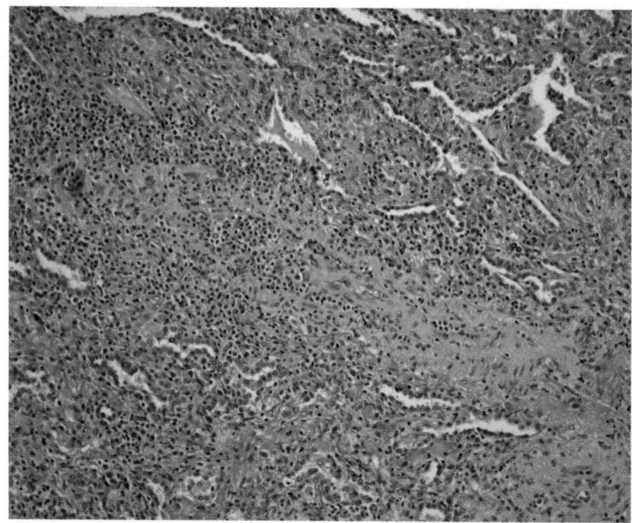

Figure 12.33 Peripheral T-cell lymphoma with a dense interstitial lymphoid infiltrate and associated fibrosis. This case showed angioinvasion, a common and nonspecific finding in large cell lymphomas in the lung.

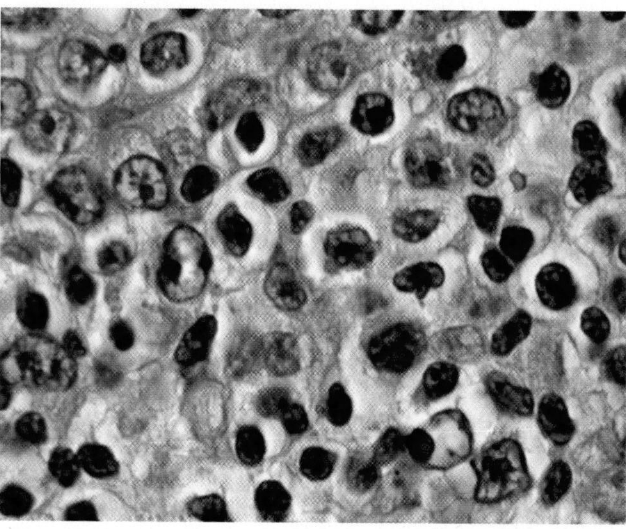

Figure 12.34 Peripheral T-cell lymphoma showing a spectrum of intermediate-sized to large atypical lymphocytes with oval to irregular nuclei, many with clear cytoplasm; an eosinophil is present.

Subpart 5.5

Multiple Myeloma and Related Conditions

▶ Jeffrey Jorgensen

Multiple myeloma may rarely infiltrate the lung, most often in late-stage disease. Primary plasmacytoma of the lung is even more rare. The lung may also be involved by secondary amyloidosis in myeloma or in other B-cell lymphoproliferative disorders including MALT lymphoma. Light-chain deposition disease may also cause pulmonary nodules, when myelomas or other B-lineage neoplasms secrete light chains, which polymerize but do not form β-pleated sheets.

Although lymphoplasmacytoid lymphoma may infiltrate the lung, many previously reported cases probably are best classified as MALT lymphomas with extensive plasmacytic differentiation. Regardless of classification, the presence or absence of associated Waldenstrom macroglobulinemia, with hyperviscosity and other manifestations of the secreted IgM paraprotein, may be the most significant clinical factor.

Histologic Features:

- Nodules or sheets of plasma cells in a lymphangitic pattern or forming large masses.
- Plasma cells may show atypical features, including nuclear enlargement and anisonucleosis, binucleation or multinucleation, and/or prominent nucleoli.
- Amyloid deposition is common, forming nodules or in a diffuse septal pattern.
- Histiocytes and multinucleated giant cells may be seen in association with amyloid deposits, and calcification is common.
- Rare cases show light-chain deposition.
- Plasma cells immunopositive for immunoglobulin κ or λ light chain, with monoclonal staining in infiltrating myeloma and plasmacytoma.

- Some cases of amyloidosis may show reactive, polyclonal plasma cell infiltrates (with amyloid deposition due to extrapulmonary myeloma or other B-lineage neoplasms).
- Amyloid deposits are Congo red positive, with apple-green birefringence under polarization.
- Amyloid deposits are often immunopositive for light chain, most often κ.
- Light-chain deposition disease shows Congo red-negative deposits.

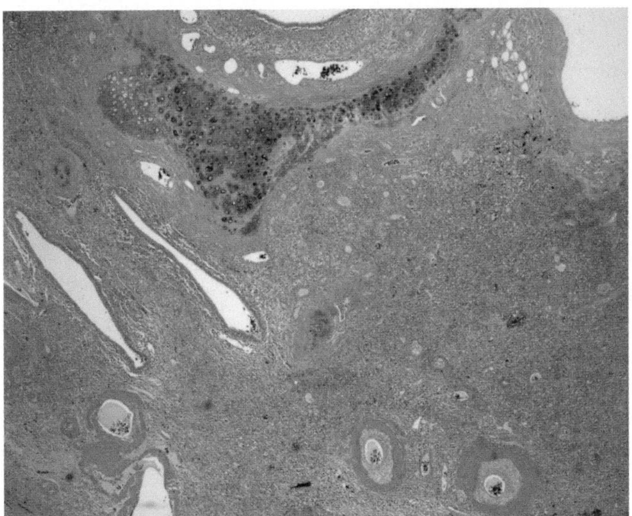

Figure 12.35 Plasmacytoma showing effacement of pulmonary parenchyma, destruction of bronchial cartilage by sheets of plasma cells, and deposition of amorphous eosinophilic material in vessel walls; this case did not show marrow involvement at presentation.

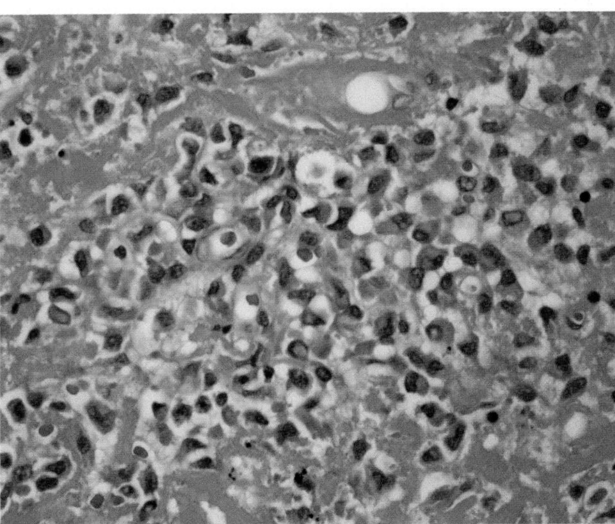

Figure 12.36 Plasmacytoma with atypical features including nuclear enlargement and occasional binucleation; Dutcher bodies (nuclear pseudoinclusions) are also present.

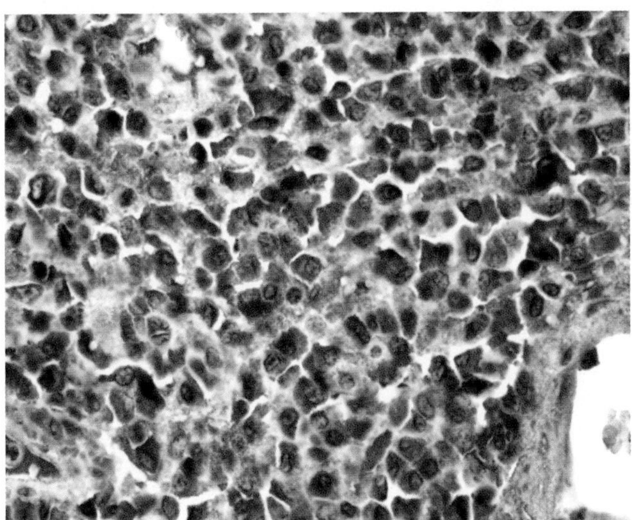

Figure 12.37 Immunostain for immunoglobulin κ light chain showing monoclonal cytoplasmic expression.

Other Cancers of the Lung

13

These cancers are extremely rare as primary tumors of the lung and are much more likely to be encountered as metastases or locally invasive tumors from other primary sites. A primary site outside of the lung must be excluded before classifying these tumors as primary lung tumors.

Part 1

Malignant Melanoma

▶ Alvaro C. Laga, Timothy Allen, and Philip T. Cagle

Primary pulmonary malignant melanoma (PPMM) is extremely rare. Diagnosis requires rigorous exclusion of metastatic melanoma by a thorough history and extensive physical examination. Metastatic melanoma is often multiple and bilateral, and involves lung parenchyma and/or pleura. PPMM often arises in the bronchus and is detected as a pigmented lesion on bronchoscopy. In contrast, peripheral nodular melanoma is almost always metastatic.

The histology of PPMM, similar to melanoma from other sites, generally shows large polygonal discohesive cells with abundant eosinophilic cytoplasm containing variable amounts of melanin pigment. Tumor cell nuclei are generally moderately enlarged with dense chromatin, prominent nucleoli, and occasional intranuclear cytoplasmic inclusions. Scattered mitotic figures are often present. Differential diagnosis includes poorly differentiated neoplasms, both primary and metastatic. Carcinoid tumors (see Chapter 10, Part 6) may contain melanin pigment but are generally synaptophysin and chromogranin positive, unlike melanoma. Clear cell "sugar" tumors or PEComas (see Chapter 25, Part 2) are generally positive for S-100 and HMB-45 and are usually peripheral lesions, not endobronchial, that are strongly positive for glycogen on periodic acid–Schiff (PAS) stain.

Cytologic Features:

- Mixture of epithelial and spindle cells with occasional mitotic figures and binucleate cells.
- Epithelial cells are large and polyhedral, with abundant cytoplasm.
- Epithelial cells have large eccentric nuclei with prominent nucleoli and occasional intranuclear cytoplasmic inclusions.
- Spindle cells show elongated cytoplasm and oval nuclei with macronucleoli.
- Occasionally, large irregular melanin granules are present in a few cells.

Histologic Features:

- Centrally located with an endobronchial component.
- Large polygonal discohesive cells with variable amounts of melanin pigment.
- Moderately enlarged nuclei with dense chromatin and prominent nucleoli.
- Occasional intranuclear cytoplasmic inclusions.
- Scattered mitotic figures.
- Generally S-100 and HMB-45 immunopositive.

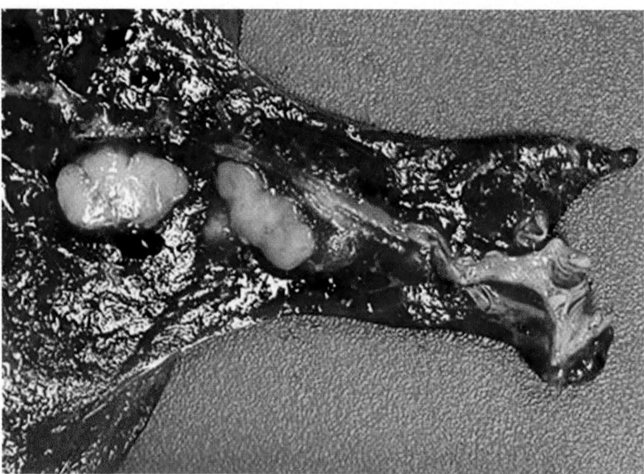

Figure 13.1 Gross figure of malignant melanoma showing a circumscribed yellow-tan mass.

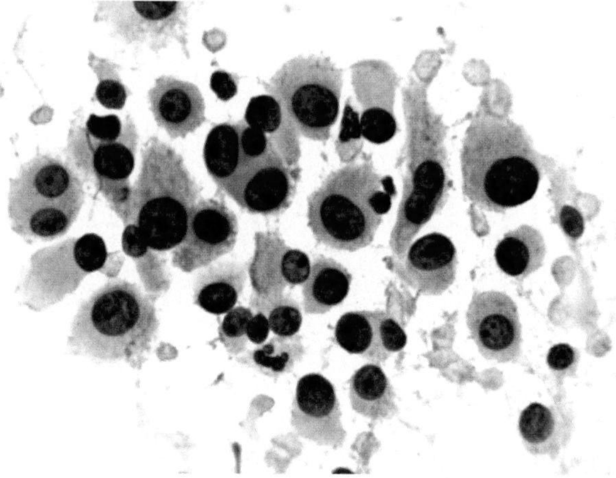

Figure 13.2 Cytology figure showing predominantly epithelial-like cells with large nuclei with dense chromatin and prominent nucleoli. A binucleate cell is present, and one cell contains melanin pigment within its cytoplasm.

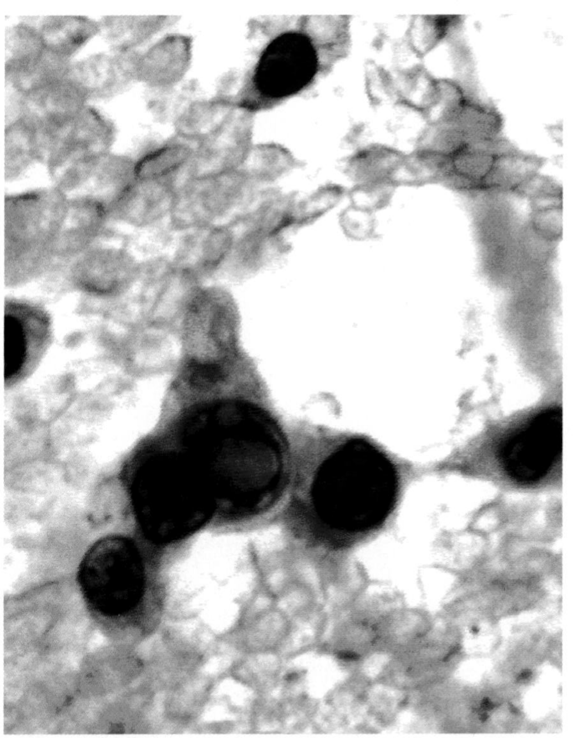

Figure 13.3 Cytology figure showing a prominent intranuclear cytoplasmic inclusion.

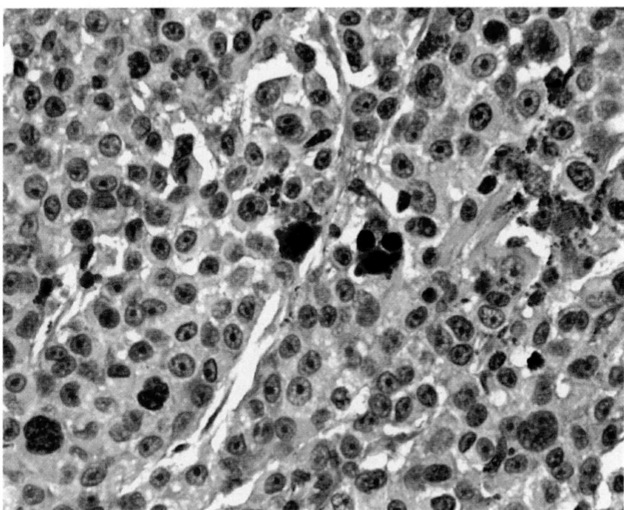

Figure 13.4 Medium power of malignant melanoma showing melanin pigment and a sheet of cells with abundant cytoplasm, enlarged nuclei, and prominent nucleoli. Scattered binucleate cells are present.

Part 2

Pleuropulmonary Thymoma

▶ Cesar Moran

Thymomas are tumors more commonly located in the anterior mediastinum. However, in unusual circumstances, these tumors can be located in other ectopic areas including pleura and lung. When these tumors are located within the lung parenchyma or along the pleural surface, they may pose problems in the clinical and radiologic differential diagnosis.

Clinically, all patients described in the literature were adult individuals without history of myasthenia gravis. The patients had symptoms of fever, cough, chest pain, or shortness of breath or were asymptomatic, and their neoplasm was discovered from a routine chest x-ray examination. Grossly, when the tumors are in an intrapulmonary location, they are indistinguishable from other more common intrapulmonary tumors. Similarly, when these tumors are located along the pleural surface, they can mimic malignant mesotheliomas. Surgical resection of these tumors appears to be the treatment of choice.

Histologic Features:

- Intrapulmonary or pleural-based thymomas share similar morphologic characteristics as their counterparts in the anterior mediastinum.
- The tumor may show a biphasic cellular population composed of epithelial cells and lymphocytes arranged in a lobular pattern separated by thin fibroconnective tissue.
- In some cases the histology is that of spindle cells with sprinkling of lymphocytes. Immunohistochemical studies play little role in their diagnosis; however, epithelial markers such as keratin may be helpful in arriving at a correct interpretation.
- Other immunohistochemical markers, including neuroendocrine markers, are negative in tumor cells.
- Electron microscopy may be helpful in finding evidence of epithelial differentiation.

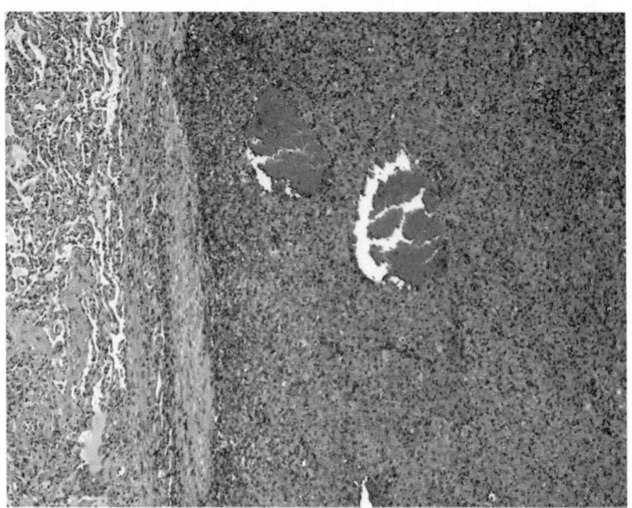

Figure 13.5 Low power of an intrapulmonary thymoma shows a cellular proliferation well demarcated from adjacent lung parenchyma.

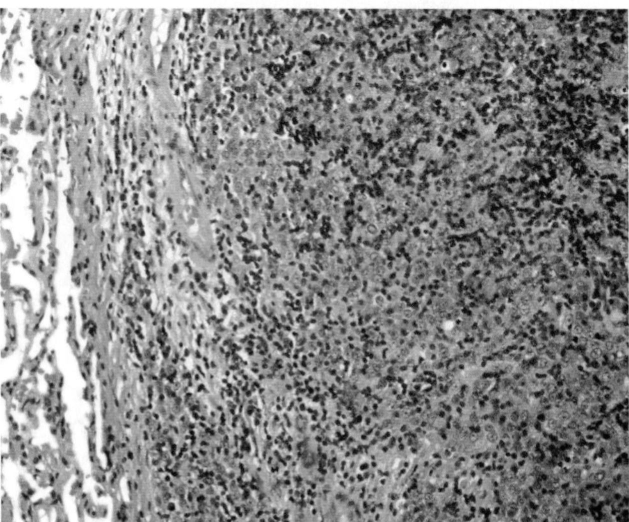

Figure 13.6 Intrapulmonary thymoma showing the characteristic biphasic cell population of lymphocytes and epithelial cells.

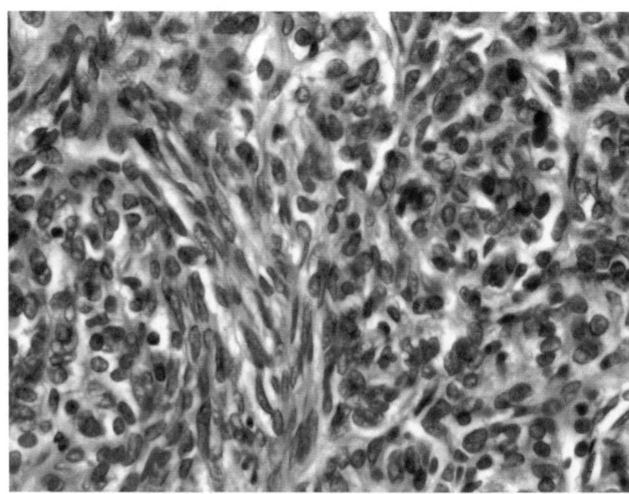

Figure 13.7 High power of an intrapulmonary thymoma shows spindle cells and interspersed lymphocytes.

Metaplastic, Dysplastic, and Premalignant Lesions

14

Metaplastic, dysplastic, and other premalignant proliferations often are precursors to lung cancers. These lesions are important to recognize for diagnostic purposes, for their importance in understanding the development of cancer, and for potential early therapeutic interventions. Premalignant lesions include squamous dysplasia and carcinoma *in situ,* atypical adenomatous hyperplasia, diffuse idiopathic pulmonary neuroendocrine cell hyperplasia, and bronchiolar columnar cell dysplasia.

Part 1

Squamous Metaplasia and Dysplasia and Carcinoma *In Situ*

Squamous metaplasia, squamous dysplasia, and carcinoma *in situ* are lesions of the bronchial epithelium that precede invasive carcinoma. Squamous metaplasia, the physiological repair process of injured bronchial epithelium, is reversible, whereas squamous dysplasia and carcinoma *in situ* are specific preneoplastic lesions. The spectrum of histologic changes representing the stepwise progression of airway epithelium toward invasive carcinoma is often not identified in individual lung carcinoma cases.

Subpart 1.1

Squamous Metaplasia

▶ Alvaro C. Laga, Timothy Allen, and Philip T. Cagle

Squamous metaplasia is a frequent epithelial alteration of the tracheobronchial mucosa. Its histogenesis may be related to chronic inflammation and injury of the bronchial epithelium, which leads to replacement of the normal ciliated columnar epithelium by a squamous epithelium. Therefore, squamous metaplasia may be seen in purely inflammatory settings such as infection or bronchiectasis. Squamous metaplasia may also be a preneoplastic lesion. In this situation, squamous metaplasia may be the result of exposure to tobacco smoke, in which case it is potentially a precursor after many years to the morphologic progression to bronchogenic carcinoma through varying degrees of dysplasia. Squamous metaplasia due to tobacco exposure may or may not progress to dysplasia and eventually carcinoma. Because of the "field effect" of tobacco smoke on the bronchial mucosa, multiple areas of squamous metaplasia may be seen in smokers, some of which may progress to dysplasia or eventually carcinoma, whereas others may not. Squamous metaplasia or varying degrees of dysplasia may be present at the margins of a carcinoma and a biopsy may be performed on it when one is not performed on the carcinoma itself. Early changes include a loss of the ciliated columnar epithelium, basal cell hyperplasia, and formation of a low columnar epithelium without cilia.

Cytologic Features:

- Small elliptical acidophilic squamous metaplastic cells with dark nuclei.
- Aggregates of cells with similarly sized nuclei and focal keratinization are characteristic.

Histologic Features:

- Mounds or aggregates of bland squamous epithelial cells lining the airways and/or airspaces.
- Necrosis, keratin pearl formation, and invasion of surrounding parenchyma do not occur.
- Regenerative atypical squamous metaplasia may occlude mucous bronchial glands with plugs of squamous epithelium.

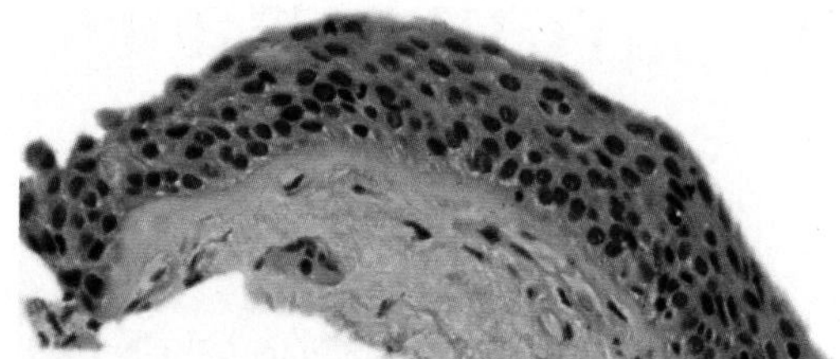

Figure 14.1 Squamous metaplasia shows bland squamous epithelial cells lining a portion of bronchial mucosa.

Subpart 1.2

Squamous Dysplasia

▶ Alvaro C. Laga, Timothy Allen, and Philip T. Cagle

Squamous atypia of the bronchial mucosa may be the result of inflammation or injury to the bronchial mucosa, or it may be a step in the morphologic progression from normal bronchial epithelium to carcinoma due to tobacco smoke exposure. In squamous dysplasia, cellular atypia progresses through mild, moderate, and severe dysplasia toward carcinoma *in situ*, analogous to the progression of squamous metaplasia through increasing degrees of dysplasia to carcinoma *in situ* seen with cervical carcinoma. With increasing degrees of squamous dysplasia, the degree of cytologic atypia increases and the degree of thickness of the squamous metaplasia exhibiting dysplasia increases. Similar to squamous metaplasia, squamous dysplasia may be multifocal in the bronchial mucosa of smokers, with some foci potentially progressing to more severe degrees of dysplasia or carcinoma over an extended period of time. As with squamous metaplasia, squamous dysplasia due to tobacco smoke does not always progress to carcinoma, and squamous dysplasia may be seen at the periphery of a carcinoma. On occasion squamous dysplasia at the margin of a carcinoma may be sampled on endobronchial biopsy rather than the adjacent carcinoma.

Cytologic Features:

- Mild dysplasia may show small aggregates of cells with slight size variation, maintained polarity, and inconspicuous nucleoli.
- In moderate dysplasia there is noticeable pleomorphism, and occasional cells may show loss of polarity. Nuclei are more hyperchromatic than in mild dysplasia but nucleoli are rarely found.
- In severe dysplasia there is an increased nuclear to cytoplasmic ratio greater than in moderate dysplasia, there is loss of cell polarity, nuclear chromatin is greatly increased in all cells accounting for marked hyperchromatism, and prominent nucleoli may be found occasionally.

Histologic Features:

- Mounds or aggregates of atypical (dysplastic) cells lining the airspaces.
- Mild dysplasia contains minimal architectural and cytologic changes, limited to the lower third of the epithelium, with rare to absent mitotic figures and vertically oriented nuclei.
- Moderate dysplasia shows partial maturation of squamous cells from the base to the luminal surface, with the basilar zone occupying approximately two thirds of the epithelium. It exhibits more cytologic atypia, with vertically oriented nuclei and mitotic figures present in the lower third of the epithelium.
- Severe dysplasia shows marked cellular pleomorphism with coarse chromatin and cell maturation and flattening present only in the upper third of the epithelium. Mitotic figures are present in the lower two thirds of the epithelium.
- Necrosis, keratin pearl formation, and invasion of surrounding parenchyma do not occur.

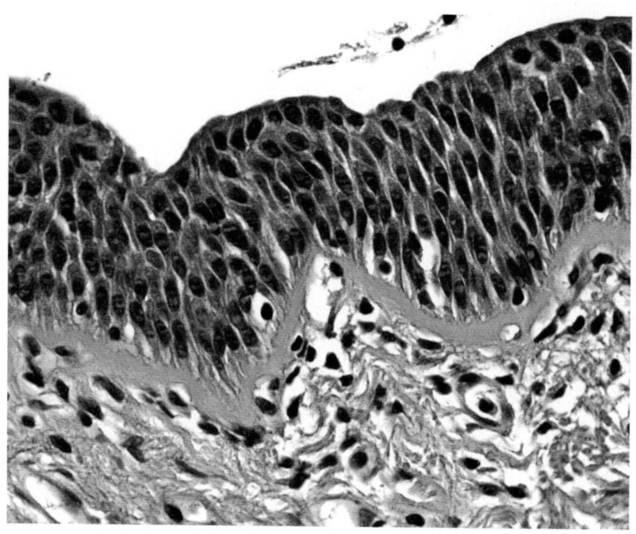

Figure 14.2 Moderate squamous dysplasia shows partial maturation of cells with vertically oriented nuclei.

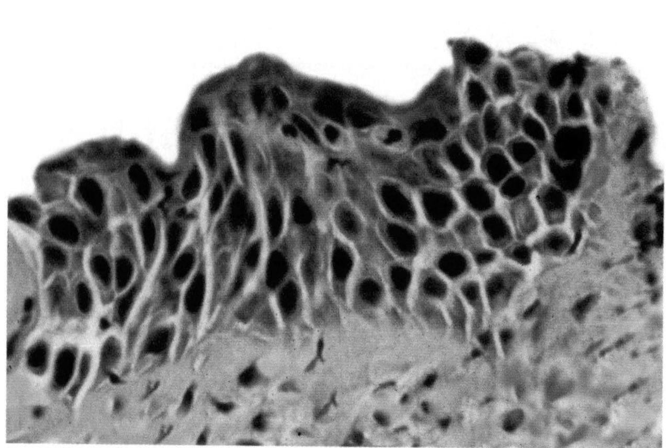

Figure 14.3 Severe squamous dysplasia consisting of marked cellular pleomorphism and coarse nuclear chromatin in at least two thirds of the epithelium.

Subpart 1.3

Carcinoma *In Situ*

▶ Alvaro C. Laga, Timothy Allen, and Philip T. Cagle

In carcinoma *in situ,* cellular atypia has advanced from severe dysplasia to a full-thickness mucosal abnormality, with an intact basement membrane (no invasion). Grossly, bronchial mucosa may show slight granularity and papillation, or it may be indistinguishable from normal mucosa. Carcinoma *in situ* may overlap considerably with severe squamous dysplasia, and a range of dysplastic findings may occur in any specific case. Eventually, carcinoma *in situ* may invade the underlying submucosa as a superficially invasive carcinoma and then beyond as an invasive carcinoma.

Cytologic Features:

- Marked nuclear size and shape variation.
- The nuclear membrane often shows irregularity, infolding, and thickening.
- The nuclear-to-cytoplasm ratio is very high, and the cells are less cohesive than the cells of severe dysplasia.
- Many single cells or loose aggregates are noted in cytologic preparations.

Histologic Features:

- Carcinoma *in situ* is characterized by full-thickness mucosal atypia with intact underlying basement membrane.
- Cytologic atypia is marked, and cellular maturation is absent.
- Mucosal thickening may occur, and bulbous masses of atypical cells may be present.
- Carcinoma *in situ* may extend into submucosal gland ducts.

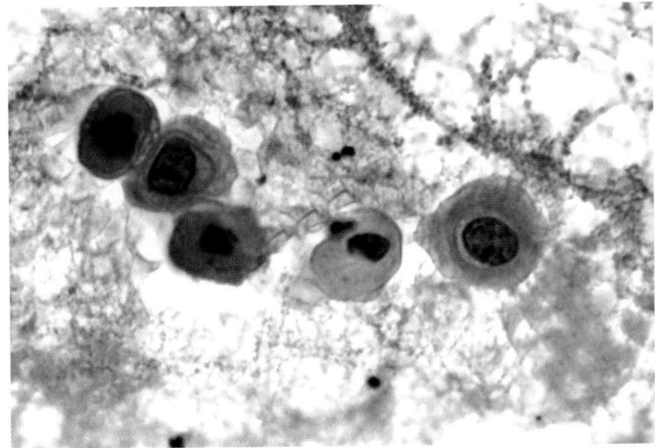

Figure 14.4 Cytology figure of carcinoma *in situ* shows single cells with a high nuclear to cytoplasmic ratio, irregular nuclear membrane, and large and prominent chromatin clumps.

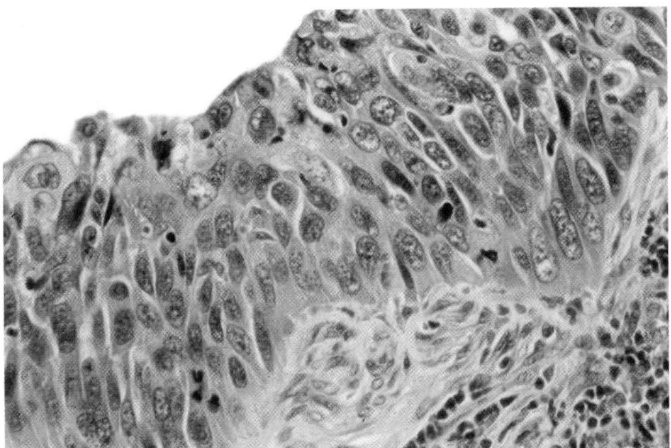

Figure 14.5 Carcinoma *in situ* shows full-thickness mucosal atypia with markedly pleomorphic cells and mitotic figures throughout, without invasion.

Part 2

Squamous Papilloma and Papillomatosis

▶ Alvaro C. Laga, Timothy Allen, and Philip T. Cagle

Squamous papillomas are rare endobronchial lesions, usually solitary and generally benign, that have been associated with human papilloma virus. Most are exophytic, but inverted variants very rarely occur. Exophytic squamous papillomas are generally wartlike lesions that often protrude into the bronchial lumen. Most present with airway obstruction, which may be incidental, and peripheral lesions may produce incidental cavitary solitary masses. Histologically, squamous papillomas consist of benign squamous epithelium overlying fibrovascular cores. The epithelium may show focal cytologic atypia and koilocytic viral changes. In some cases, squamous papillomas may have foci of squamous dysplasia or carcinoma *in situ* and may give rise to papillary squamous cell carcinomas. Differentiation of squamous cell papillomas from low-grade papillary squamous cell carcinomas may be difficult in some cases. Extension of the squamous epithelium of a papilloma along the mucosa of an underlying seromucinous gland duct and seromucinous gland should not be mistaken for invasion.

Papillomatosis of the larynx and tracheobronchial tree is rare and is a much more aggressive lesion typically occurring in children. Involvement of the upper respiratory tract, including the larynx, is much more common than involvement of the lung. In contrast to solitary squamous papilloma, papillomatosis consists of multiple papillomas (may be synchronous and/or metachronous), and cytologic atypia is increased. Carcinoma develops in up to 3% of papillomatosis patients. Invasive papillomatosis, with extension of squamous papillomas into lung parenchyma, may produce significant morbidity due to airway obstruction and alveolar filling.

Histologic Features:

- Fine papillae lined by bland, nonkeratinizing, or minimally keratinizing squamous epithelial cells.
- Squamous epithelial cells, often multilayered, line fibrovascular stalks containing a minimal amount of chronic inflammatory cells.
- May contain focal areas of condylomatous atypia.
- Multiple lesions with a greater degree of cytologic atypia are seen in papillomatosis.
- Invasive papillomatosis consists of extension of squamous epithelial lesions into lung parenchyma, with generally bland cytologic features.

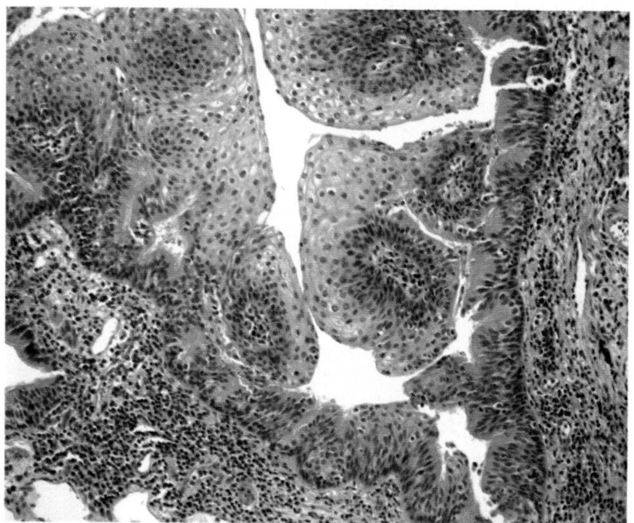

Figure 14.6 Squamous papilloma with papillae containing fibrovascular stalks and lined by nonkeratinizing squamous epithelial cells.

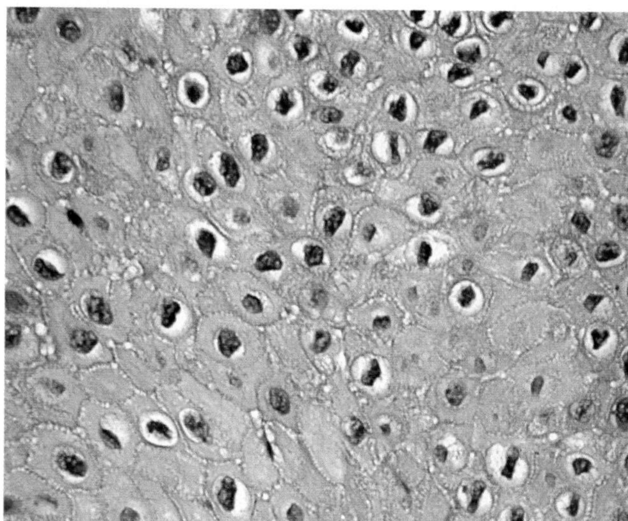

Figure 14.7 Higher power of papilloma squamous epithelium with focal condylomatous atypia.

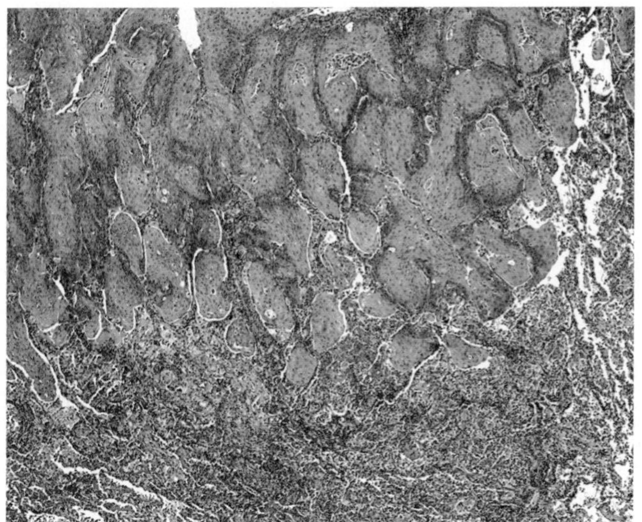

Figure 14.8 Low power of invasive papillomatosis with squamous epithelium extending through alveolar spaces.

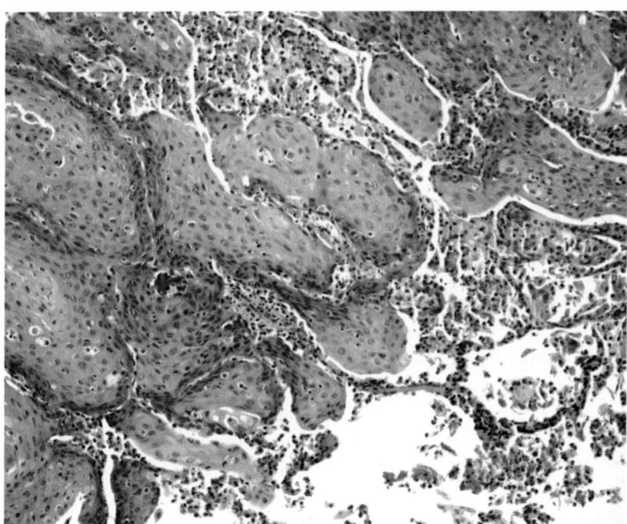

Figures 14.9 Medium power of invasive papillomatosis shows nests of squamous epithelium filling alveolar airspaces.

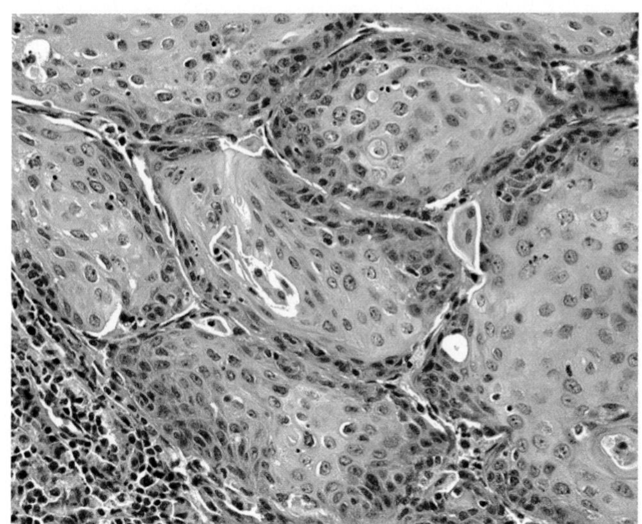

Figure 14.10 Higher power of invasive papillomatosis consisting of nests of cytologically bland squamous epithelium within alveolar spaces.

Subpart 2.1

Glandular Papilloma and Mixed Squamous and Glandular Papilloma

▶ Ilkser Akpolat

Glandular papillomas are extremely rare benign endobronchial polyps that may produce obstructive symptoms. These tumors consist of fibrovascular papillary cores lined by benign columnar glandular epithelium or goblet cells.

Mixed squamous and glandular papillomas, formerly known as *transitional papillomas,* are extremely rare benign endobronchial lesions. They may present with obstructive symptoms. These polyps consist of fibrovascular cores lined by both benign squamous epithelium and benign columnar goblet cell epithelium.

Histologic Features:

- Papillary endobronchial neoplasm consisting of thick fibrovascular cores lined by glandular goblet cell epithelium for glandular papillomas or a mixture of squamous and glandular epithelium for mixed papillomas.
- One third or more of the second epithelial component must be present in mixed papillomas.
- In glandular papillomas, the glandular epithelium consists of mucinous pseudostratified columnar or cuboidal cells, both ciliated and nonciliated.
- Cytologic atypia, mitoses, or necrosis may be focal and represent small foci of carcinoma.
- Fibrovascular cores can have a scattered lymphoplasmacytic infiltrate.

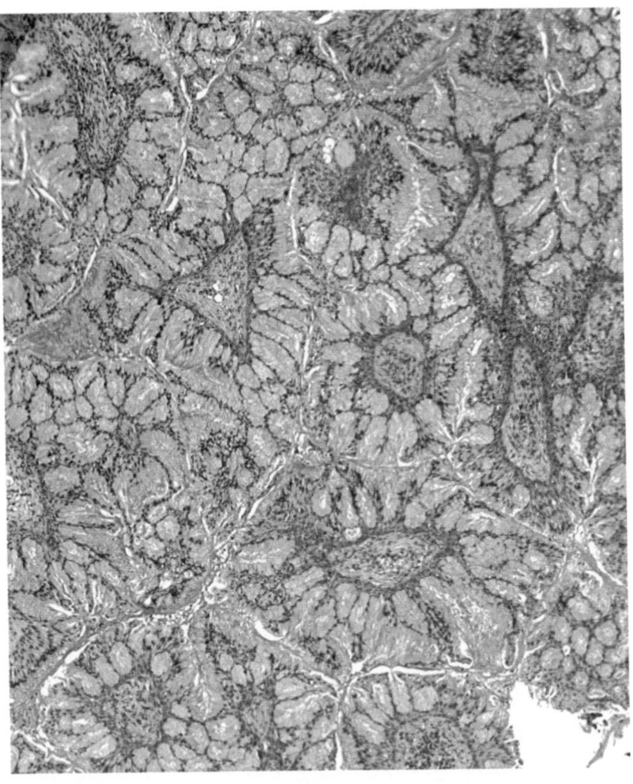

Figure 14.11 Low power shows glandular papilloma within a bronchus composed of multiple papillary fibrovascular cores lined by goblet cells.

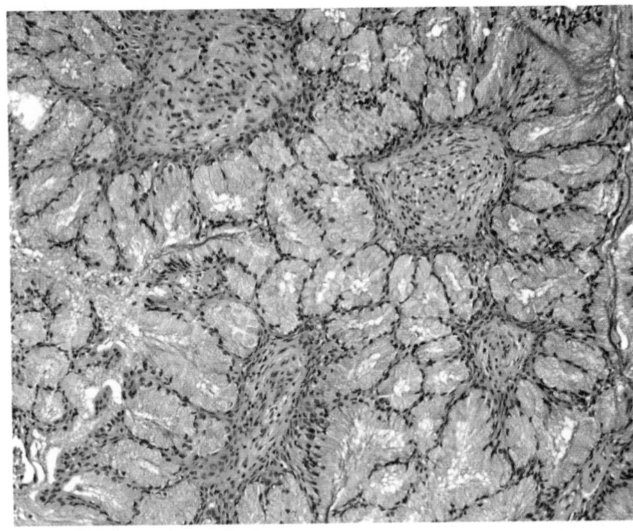

Figure 14.12 Higher power of glandular papilloma shows fibrovascular cores lined by goblet cells.

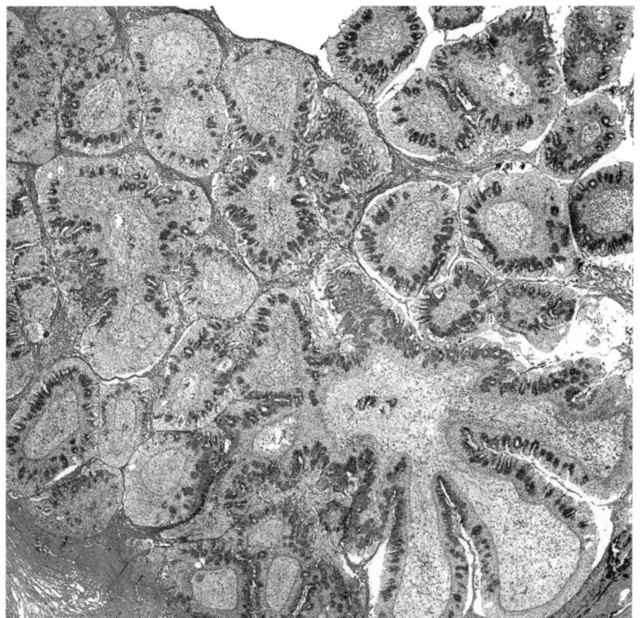

Figure 14.13 Low power of a mixed squamous and glandular papilloma in a large bronchus shows both squamous cell and glandular components lining multiple papillary fibrovascular cores.

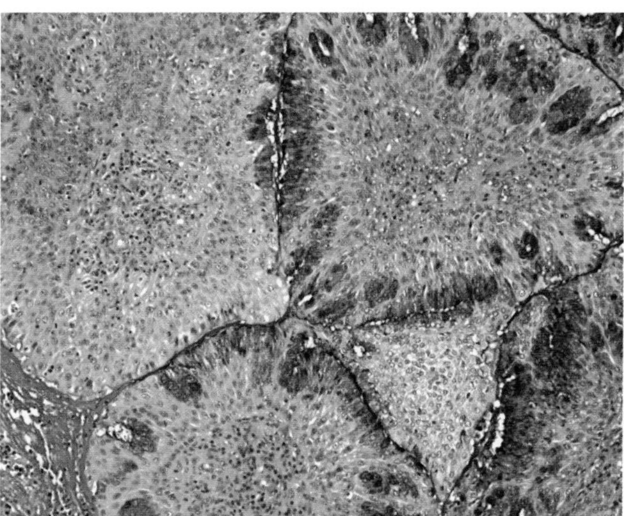

Figure 14.14 Thick fibrovascular cores are surrounded by squamous epithelium with overlying goblet cells in this section of a mixed papilloma.

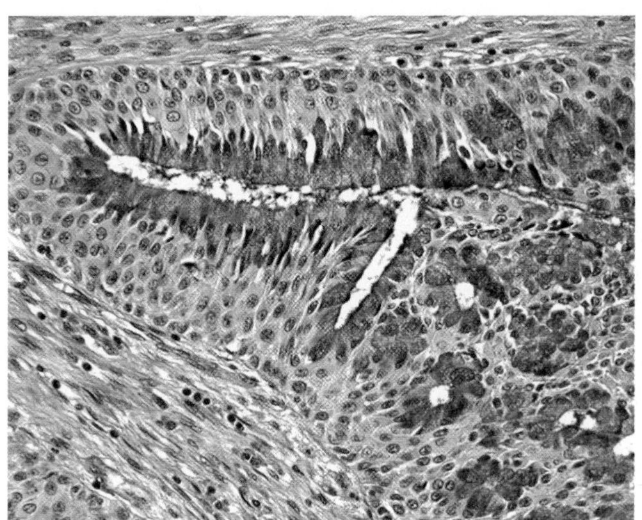

Figure 14.15 Higher power of a mixed papilloma shows both squamous epithelial component and glandular goblet cell component in a mixed papilloma.

Part 3

Atypical Adenomatous Hyperplasia

▶ Armando Fraire

Now recognized by the World Health Organization as a preneoplastic process, atypical adenomatous hyperplasia (AAH) is regarded as a precursor lesion of pulmonary adenocarcinoma (AD) and in particular a precursor lesion of bronchioloalveolar carcinoma. AAH is most often single but can be multiple. Conventionally AAH is regarded as a lesion less than 0.5 cm. Cellularity and cytologic atypia are variable. Some authors separate AAH into low and high grades. Low-grade AAH tends to have continuous rows of cuboidal cells with no intercellular gaps. Some lesions may show a mix of low and high grades of atypia.

Evidence for the preneoplastic nature of AAH is derived from (i) its frequent association with adenocarcinoma and (ii) objective data including comparative analysis of AAH and AD that reveals progressive increments of mean nuclear area by morphometry; alterations of cell cycle regulation as measured by the Ki-67 cell proliferation marker; acquisition of oncofetal protein expression such as CEA; demonstration of p53 accumulation; loss of heterozygosity at 3p, 9p, and 17p; k-*ras* mutations at codon 12; and evidence of monoclonality based on analysis of the X chromosome-linked polymorphic marker, the HUMARA (Human Androgen Receptor) gene.

Histologic Features:

High Grade

- Focal proliferation of atypical cells along preexisting alveolar framework.
- Atypical cells are cuboidal to low columnar but may be hobnailed or peg shaped.
- Occasional gaps between proliferating cells.
- Individually, cells have a high nuclear-to-cytoplasm ratio, dense nuclear chromatin, and may or may not have inconspicuous nucleoli.
- Absence of tufting or micropapillary formations.
- Mild fibrotic thickening of interalveolar septa.

Low Grade

- Architecturally, low-grade AAH does not differ from high-grade AAH.
- Cytologically, cells lining the alveolar surfaces are more homogenous and mostly cuboidal, and show no intercellular gaps.

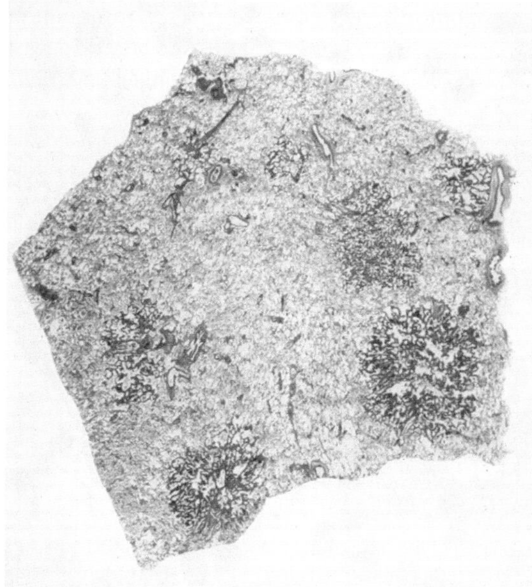

Figure 14.16 Multiple AAH lesions measuring 0.4 to 0.7 cm.

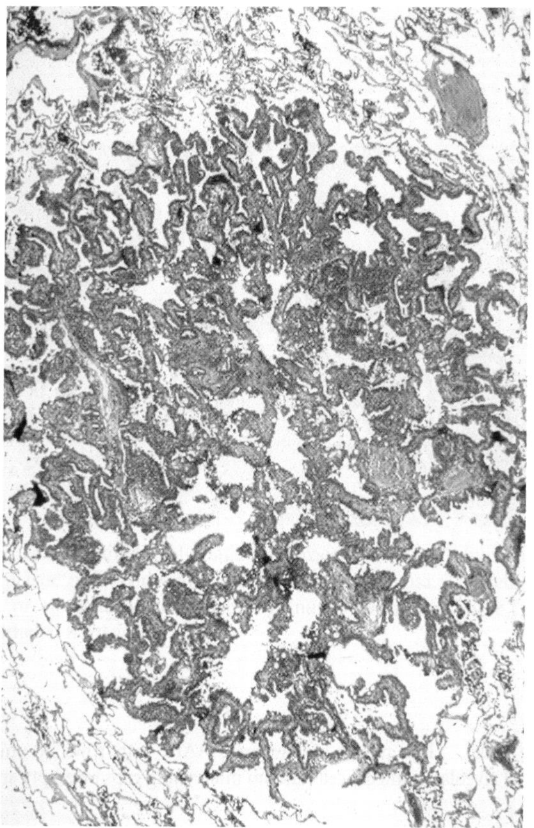

Figure 14.17 Low power of medusa headlike configuration of AAH, with normal architecture in the surrounding lung.

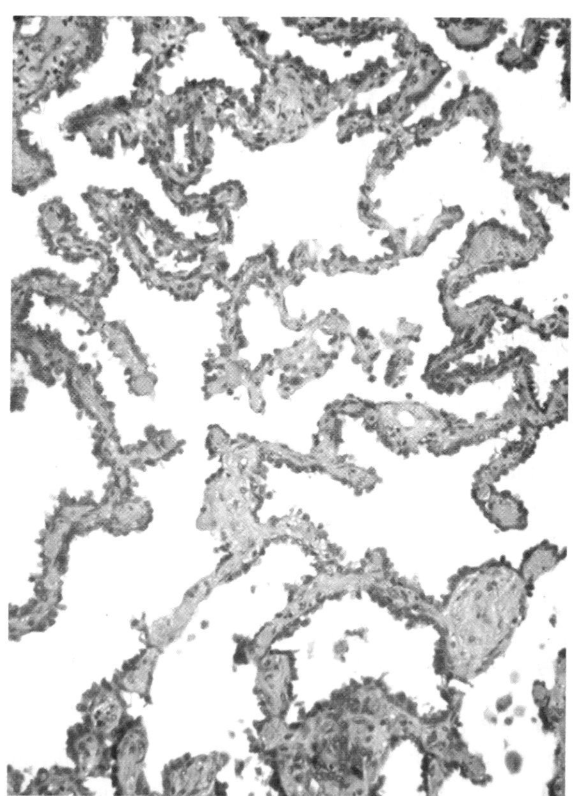

Figure 14.18 Medium power of AAH showing mild thickening of alveolar septa.

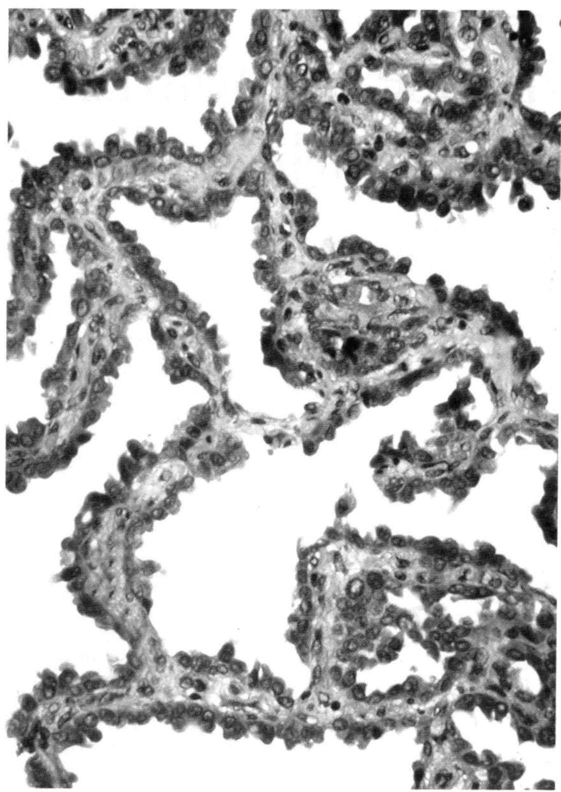

Figure 14.19 High power of high-grade AAH, with peg-shaped cells containing dense nuclear chromatin and empty spaces between cells.

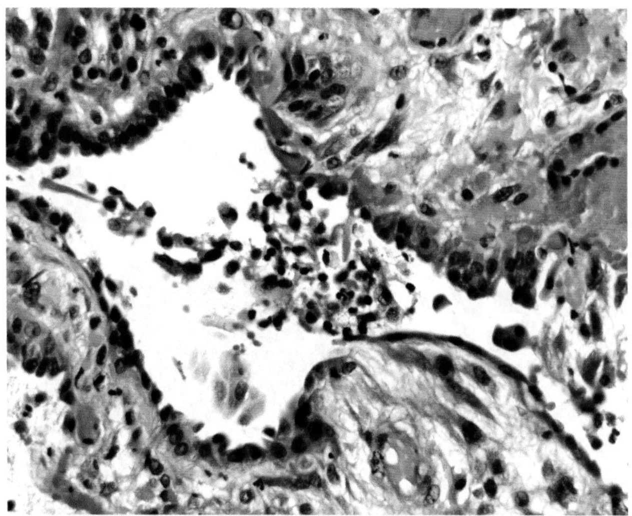

Figure 14.23 Low-grade BCCD showing loss of organization of bronchiolar epithelium and cytologic atypia in the basal cells.

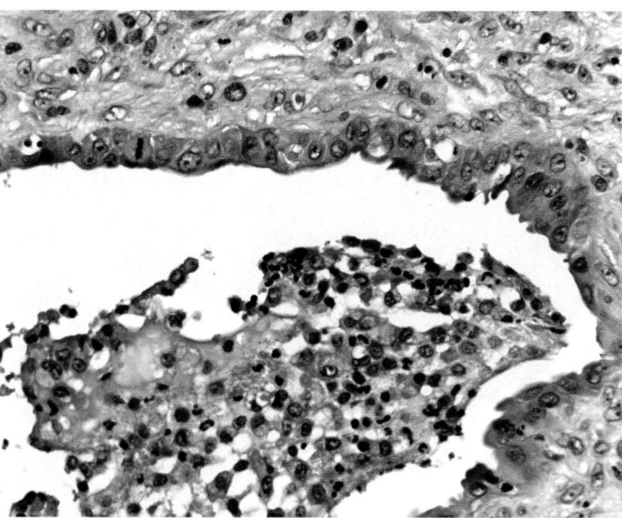

Figure 14.24 High-grade BCCD showing cytologic atypia and loss of organization of the epithelium.

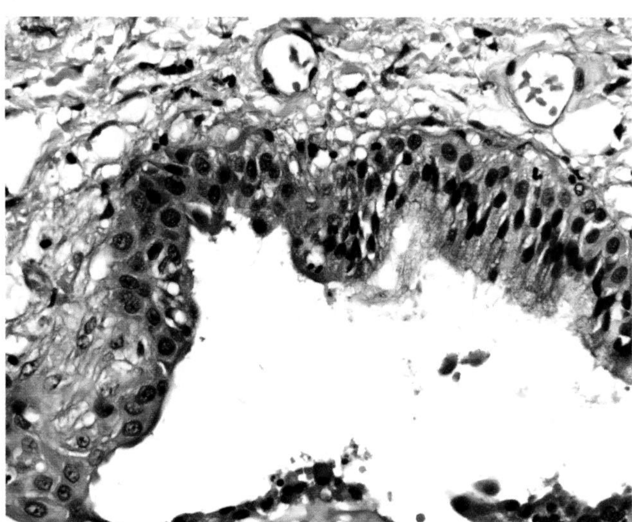

Figure 14.25 Low-grade BCCD on the *right* merging with high-grade BCCD on the *left*.

Cancers of the Pleura

15

Cancers often metastasize to the pleura, particularly metastatic carcinomas, but also metastatic sarcomas, lymphomas, and other types of cancer. Some cancers, particularly lung carcinomas, may also invade the pleura by direct extension. Diffuse malignant mesothelioma is the most common primary tumor of the pleura, but it is relatively rare compared to metastatic cancers. Other primary neoplasms of the pleura are very rare.

Part 1

Diffuse Malignant Mesothelioma

▶ Alvaro C. Laga, Timothy Allen, Carlos Bedrossian, Bruno Murer, and Philip T. Cagle

Diffuse malignant mesothelioma (DMM) of the pleura is a relatively rare tumor most commonly observed in adult males over age 50 years. The majority of DMMs are related to asbestos exposure and develop several decades after initial exposure. There is often a history of pleuritic pain and shortness of breath. Pleural effusions often occur and may be bloody and voluminous. Grossly, DMMs grow on the pleural surfaces initially as masses or multiple nodules that eventually circumferentially encase the lung in a rindlike fashion. DMMs can invade the underlying lung tissue or underlying chest wall or spread as metastases. DMM is a very aggressive tumor; traditionally, almost all patients die of the disease within 2 years of diagnosis. DMMs have three basic histologic types: epithelial, sarcomatous, and mixed or biphasic. Variations of these basic histologic types can be observed. The pathologist should be aware of the many patterns that DMM can present for diagnostic recognition, although most of them do not have any clinical significance.

Clinically, radiographically, and pathologically, many other neoplasms with pleural extension or pleural metastases can mimic DMM. Adenocarcinomas particularly mimic epithelial mesotheliomas, and spindle cell neoplasms can mimic sarcomatous mesotheliomas. A multimodal approach including conventional histology and immunohistochemistry provides the most reliable differentiation of DMM from other types of cancer. Electron microscopy may be useful particularly for epithelial mesotheliomas. It can be difficult to differentiate reactive mesothelial hyperplasia from epithelial mesothelioma and organizing

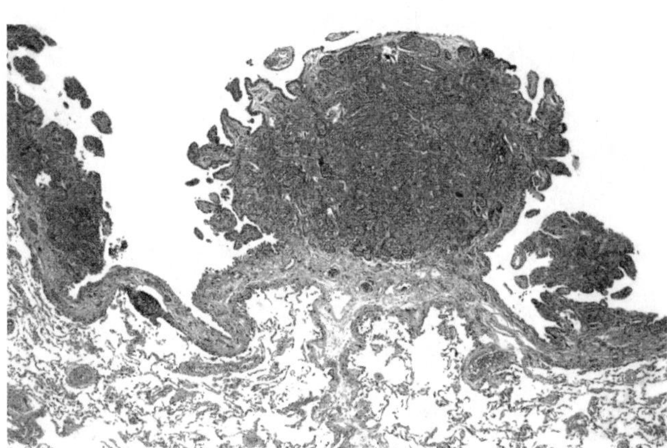

Figure 15.7 Tumor nodules of early-stage tubulopapillary DMM are observed on the visceral pleural surface; this is not a reactive hyperplasia.

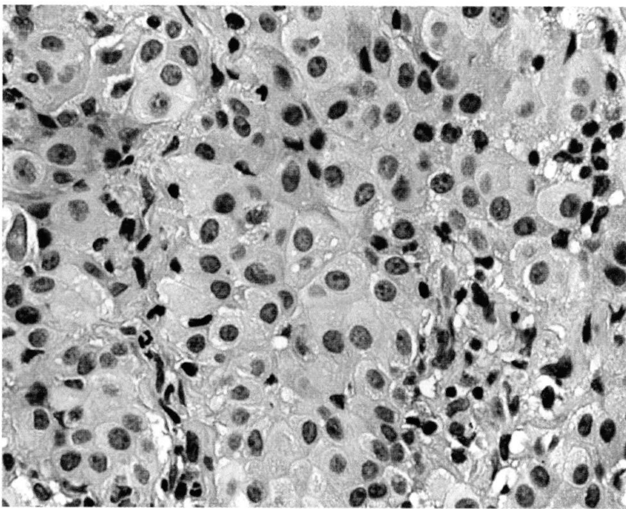

Figure 15.8 Sheets of cytologically bland epithelial DMM cells have regular, oval, eccentric nuclei, abundant cytoplasm, and distinct cell borders.

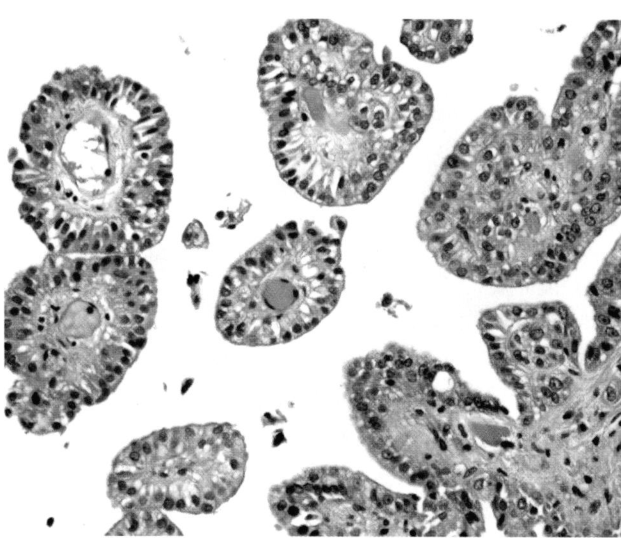

Figure 15.9 Fibrovascular cores are lined by epithelial DMM cells in a papillary DMM; biopsies limited to such areas should not be mistaken for well-differentiated papillary mesothelioma (see Chapter 15, Part 3).

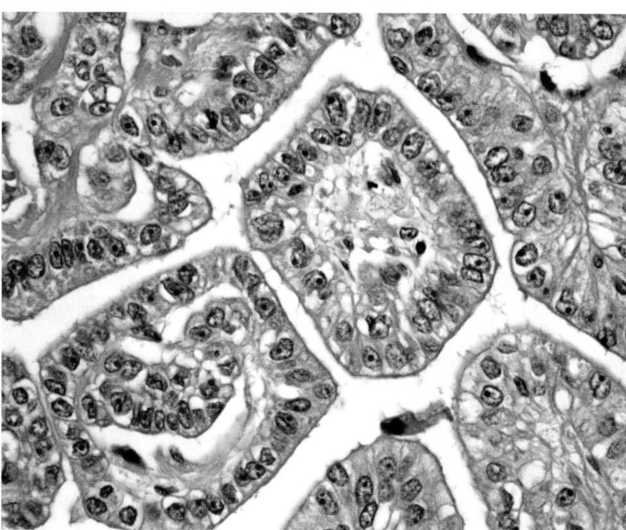

Figure 15.10 High power of fibrovascular cores lined by cuboidal malignant epithelial cells in papillary DMM.

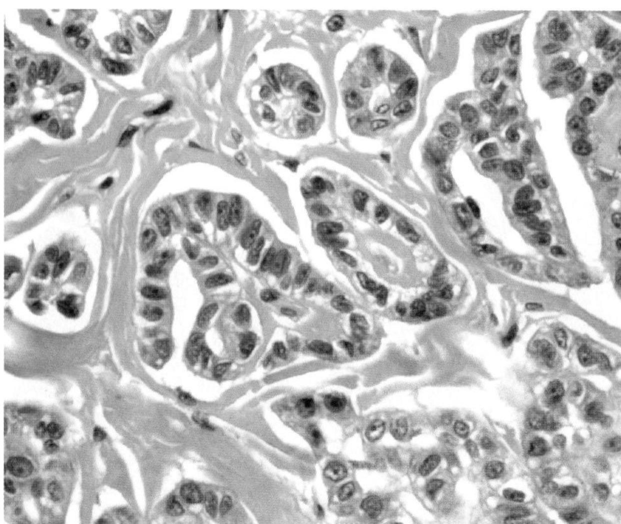

Figure 15.11 Small tubules lined by cuboidal malignant cells in tubulopapillary DMM.

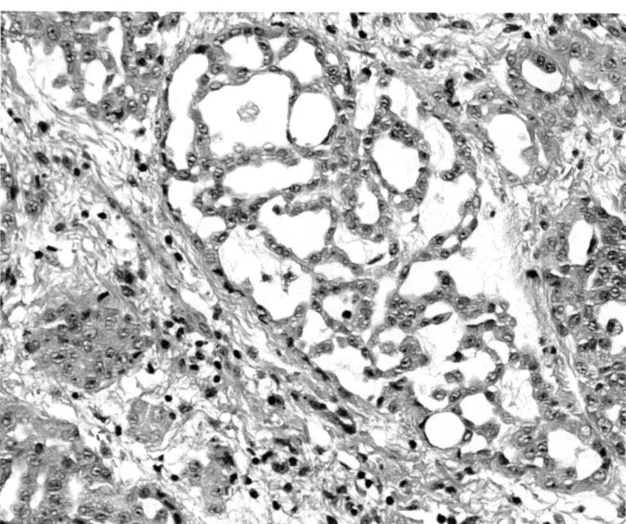

Figure 15.12 Tubular structures arranged in a complex pattern in tubulopapillary DMM.

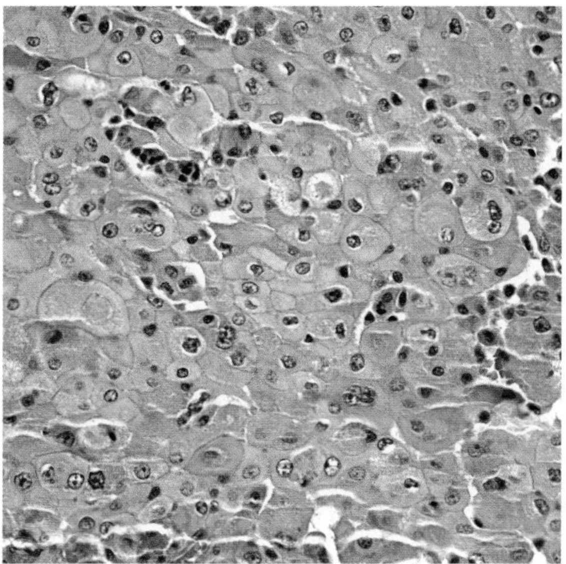

Figure 15.13 Deciduoid DMM consists of epithelial cells with plump pink cytoplasm and sharp cell borders resembling decidual cells in pregnancy.

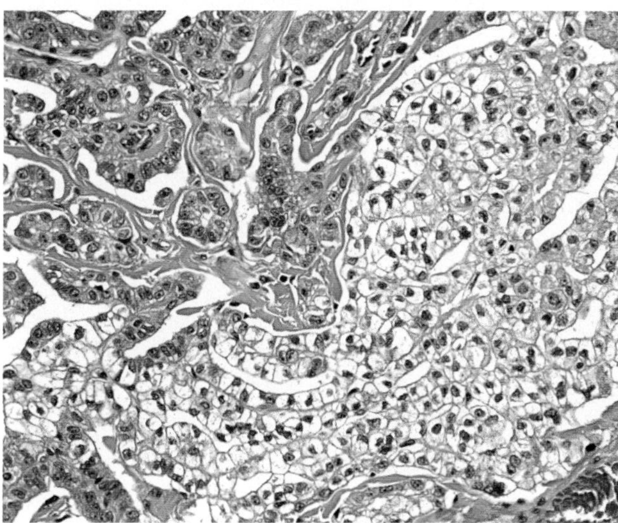

Figure 15.14 Medium power of a tubulopapillary DMM with an area composed of clear tumor cells.

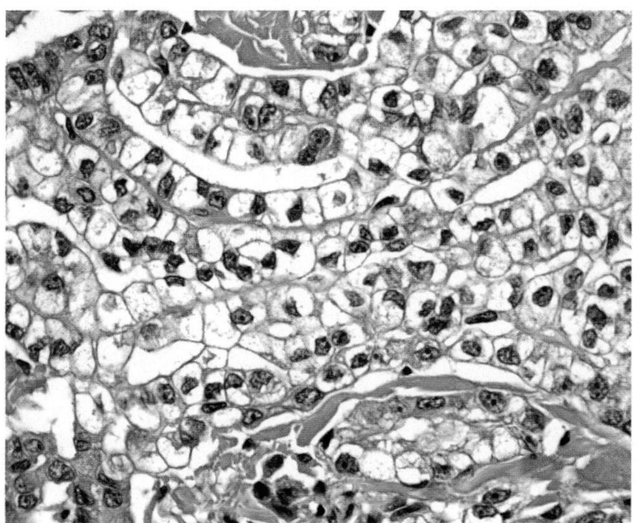

Figure 15.15 Higher power of clear cells from Figure 15.14 shows DMM cells with clear cytoplasm arranged in cords and tubular structures.

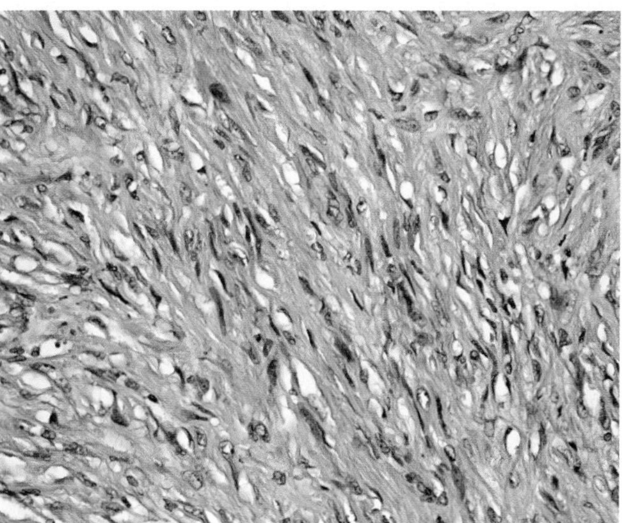

Figure 15.16 Sarcomatous DMMs are composed of malignant spindle cells and resemble sarcomas on H&E-stained sections.

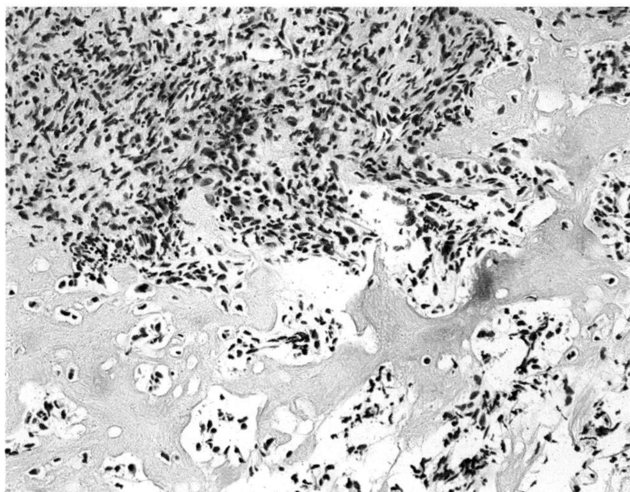

Figure 15.17 Sarcomatous DMM may have heterologous elements such as the malignant osteoid in this sarcomatous DMM.

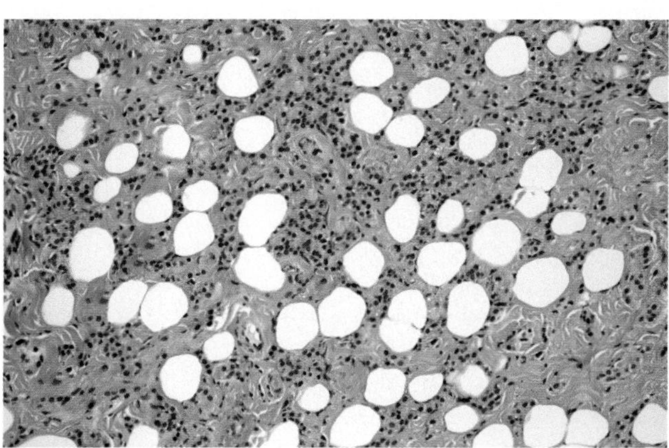

Figure 15.18 Invasion of DMM into underlying fat produces an appearance of holes (residual fat cells) resembling Swiss cheese.

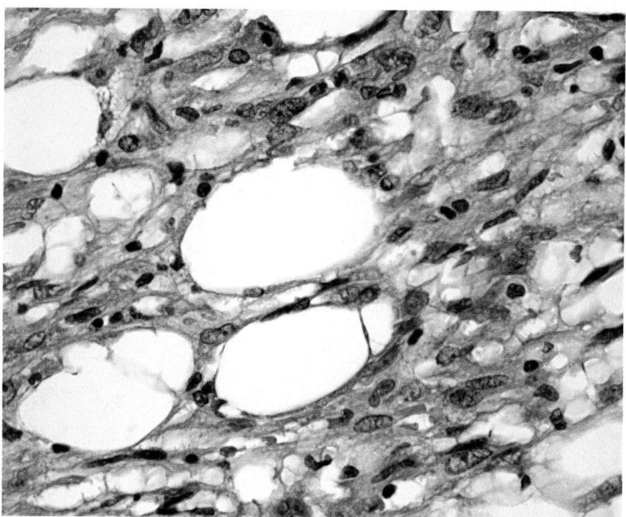

Figure 15.19 Spindle cells of sarcomatous DMM are observed invading adipose tissue.

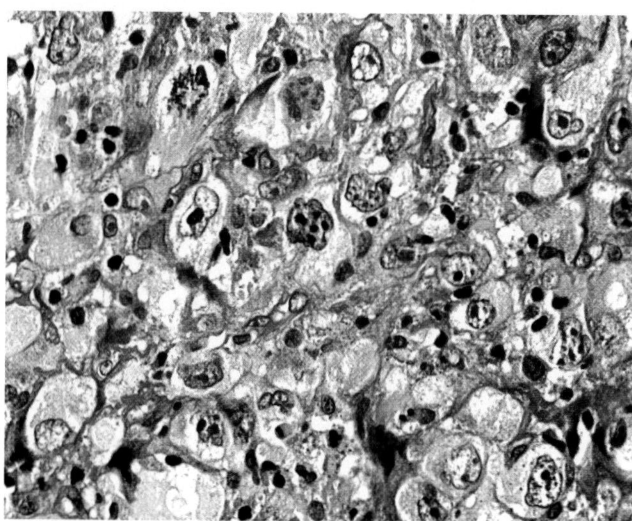

Figure 15.20 Pleomorphic DMM composed of anaplastic polygonal cells with pleomorphic nuclei, large and multiple nucleoli, and mitosis.

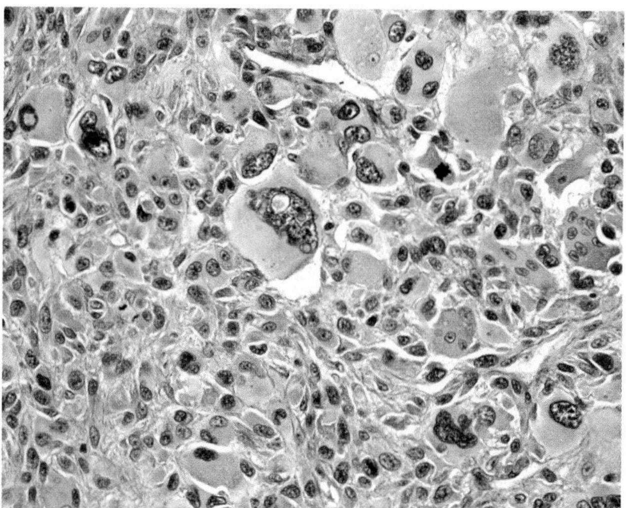

Figure 15.21 Tumor giant cells and multinucleated cells in a pleomorphic DMM.

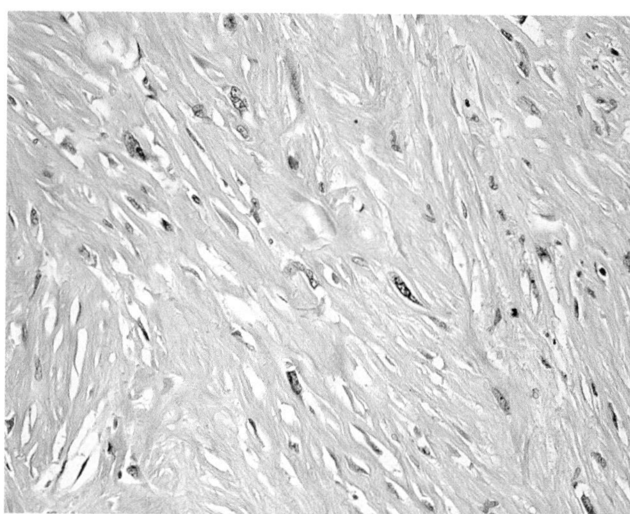

Figure 15.22 Desmoplastic DMM shows a few atypical spindle cells of sarcomatous DMM in a dense collagenized stroma.

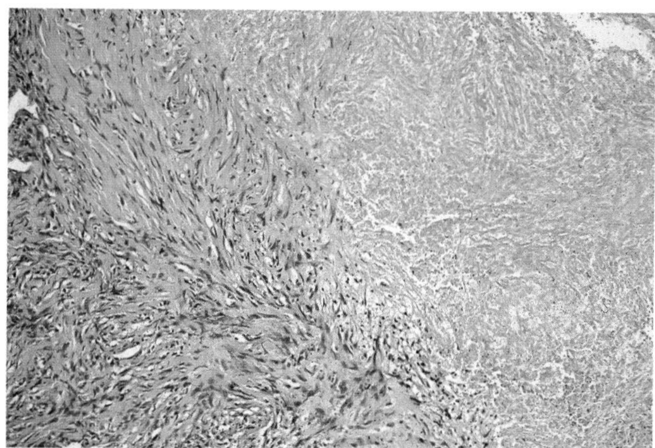

Figure 15.23 Bland necrosis in a sarcomatous DMM is "clean" ischemic necrosis lacking basophilic cellular debris and neutrophils.

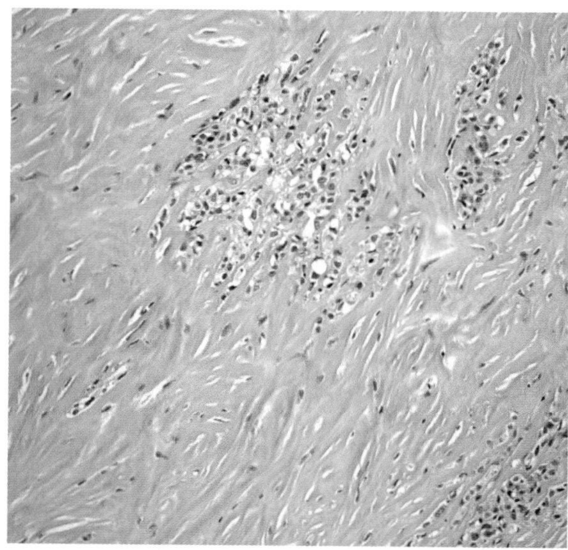

Figure 15.24 Desmoplastic DMM with a few clusters of epithelial cells in a dense collagenized stroma.

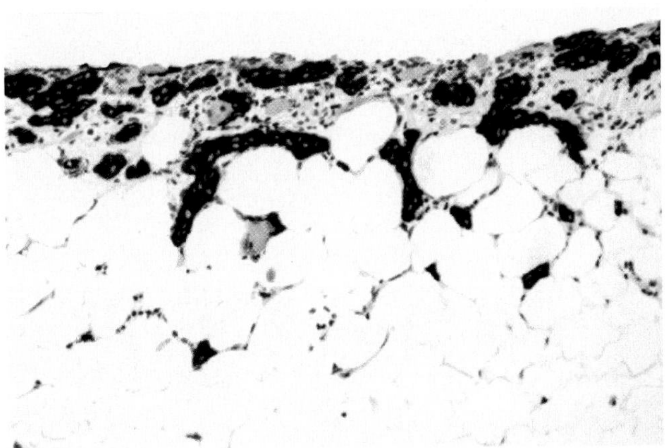

Figure 15.25 Keratin stain highlights mesothelioma cells superficially invading into adipose tissue from the pleural surface, confirming that the cells are malignant, in a very early mesothelioma.

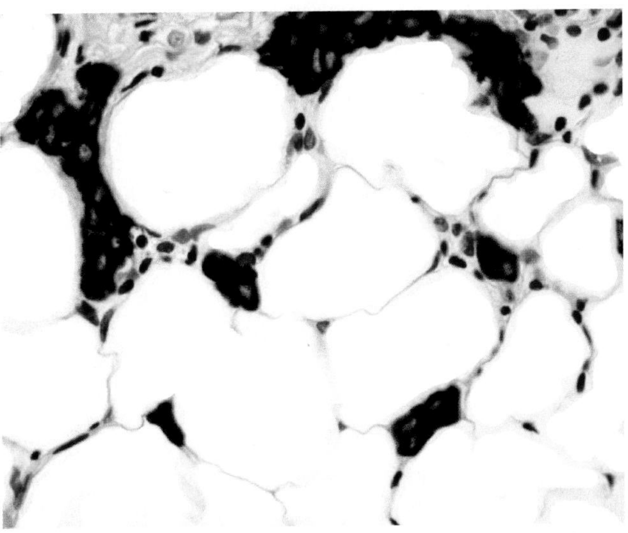

Figure 15.26 Higher power shows keratin-positive DMM cells among adipose tissue in early superficial invasion.

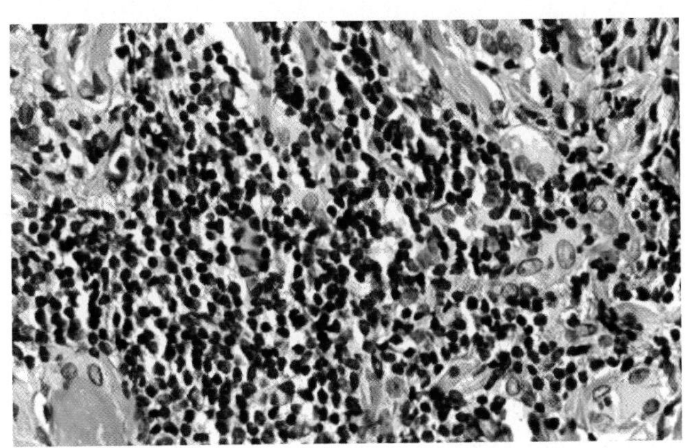

Figure 15.27 Rarely DMM cells may be obscured by intense lymphocytic infiltrates as in this example; chronic inflammation by itself does not confirm a reactive process and exclude malignancy; on occasion DMM with intense inflammatory infiltrates may resemble lymphoma on H&E stain; keratin immunostains may assist in identifying the mesothelioma cells.

Part 2

Localized Malignant Mesothelioma

▶ Alvaro C. Laga, Timothy Allen, and Philip T. Cagle

Localized malignant mesothelioma (LMM) is an extremely rare, recently recognized entity characterized by a discrete, circumscribed pleural mass that is either sessile or pedunculated but has histologic and immunohistochemical features identical to DMM. It is often found incidentally. Radiographic and gross information are required for proper diagnosis. LMM may recur and metastasize, ultimately killing the patient, but it does not spread over the pleura in the manner characteristic of DMM. Differential diagnosis includes DMM, solitary fibrous tumor, and other primary and metastatic neoplasms of the pleura.

Histologic Features:

- Nodular, discrete, well-circumscribed, pedunculated, or sessile mass arising from visceral or parietal pleura.
- Histologically, immunohistochemically, and ultrastructurally identical to DMM.
- Epithelial, sarcomatous, and biphasic patterns similar to those seen with DMM.
- Immunopositive for mesothelial markers such as calretinin and immunonegative for carcinoma markers.

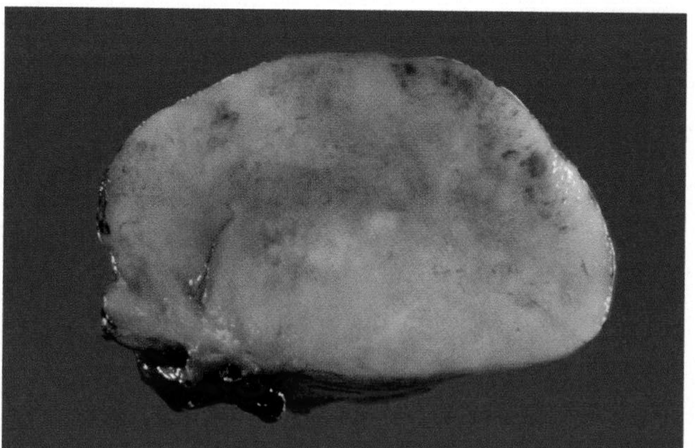

Figure 15.28 Gross figure of LMM showing a well-circumscribed tumor mass.

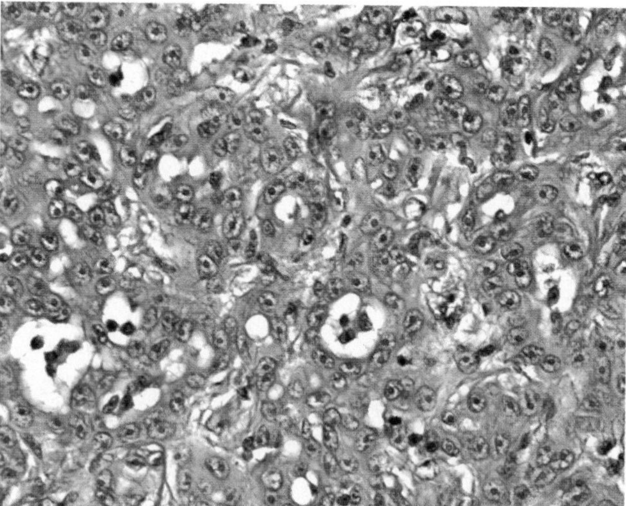

Figure 15.29 Epithelial LMM with cells containing vesicular nuclei and prominent nucleoli.

Part 3

Well-Differentiated Papillary Mesothelioma

▶ Alvaro C. Laga, Timothy Allen, and Philip T. Cagle

Well-differentiated papillary mesothelioma (WDPM) is a rare tumor that most often involves the peritoneum of women. However, very rarely WDPM may arise in a variety of serosal surfaces in both men and women, including the visceral and parietal pleura. WDPM is considered either a benign tumor or a tumor of equivocal or low malignant potential carrying a good prognosis with generally long survival. It is composed of fibrovascular cores lined by a single layer of bland mesothelial cells. WDPM may be localized or multifocal over the serosal surface and may recur. Localized WDPM typically follow a benign course and are typically cured by surgery. Most WDPMs are confined to the serosal surface but occasionally may exhibit superficial invasion, particularly when recurrent or after being present for extended periods of time. These occasional cases may eventually exhibit aggressive behavior and poorer prognosis. Although WDPM is typically benign, it is included in this section, because it must be differentiated from DMM and because of the superficial invasion reported in a few cases.

Areas resembling WDPM can sometimes occur in DMMs; therefore, it should be borne in mind that small biopsies fortuitously made of a WDPM-like area of a DMM can occur.

Histologic Features:

- WDPM is typically composed of papillae with fibrovascular cores lined by a single layer of bland cuboidal mesothelial cells, with no or very few mitoses.
- The fibrovascular cores may be myxoid and edematous.
- The lining mesothelial cells are immunopositive for keratin and mesothelial markers.
- WDPMs are typically confined to the serosal surface but occasionally long-standing or recurrent cases will exhibit focal superficial invasion, which may indicate a poorer prognosis.

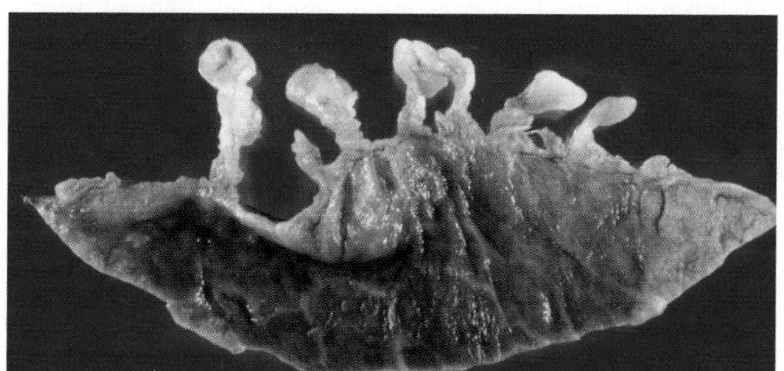

Figure 15.30 Gross figure of a wedge biopsy of lung tissue with papillary fronds of WDPM arising from the visceral pleural surface.

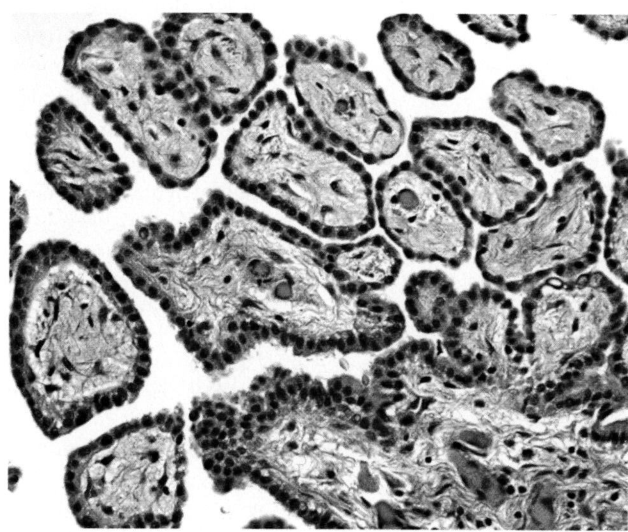

Figure 15.31 WDPM on pleural surface with multiple papillary fibrovascular cores lined by a single layer of bland cuboidal mesothelial cells.

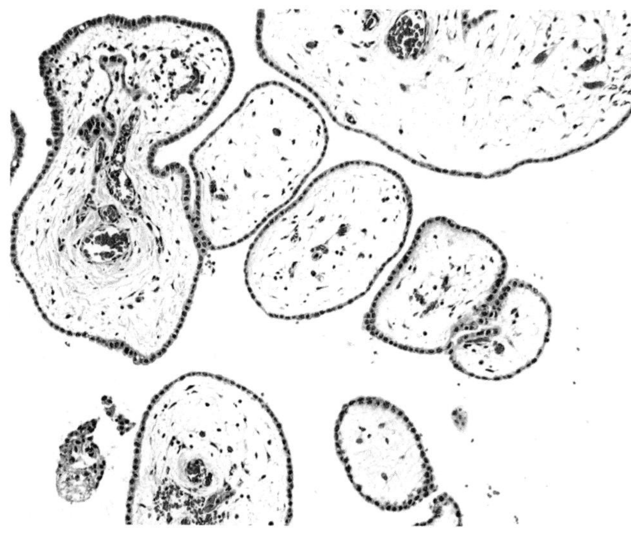

Figures 15.32 Pleural WDPM with papillary cores with edematous myxoid vascular stroma lined by single layer of bland, uniform cuboidal mesothelial cells.

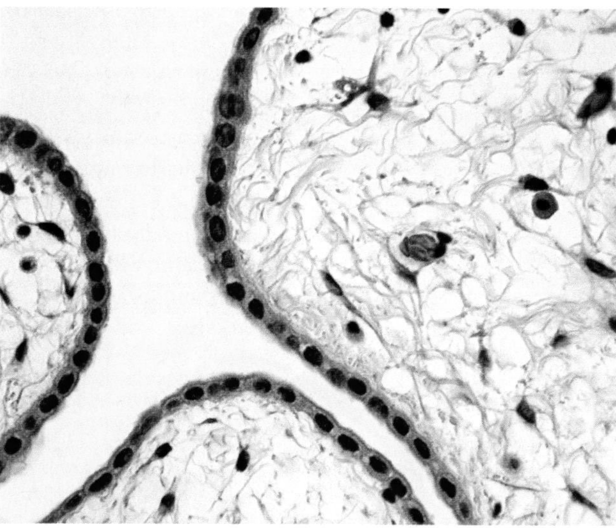

Figure 15.33 Higher power shows a single layer of very uniform, bland cuboidal mesothelial cells lining edematous myxoid cores.

Part 4

Synovial Sarcoma

▶ Alvaro C. Laga, Timothy Allen, and Philip T. Cagle

Synovial sarcomas of the extremities or other locations may metastasize to the pleura. Primary synovial sarcomas of the pleura occur mostly in young to middle-aged adults but have been reported in a wide age range. Most patients present with chest pain. Most primary pleural synovial sarcomas are localized or circumscribed neoplasms, but they may invade the chest wall and mediastinum. They may grow in a diffuse pattern over the pleural surface mimicking DMM grossly. Primary pleural synovial sarcomas exhibit the same histologic, immunohistochemical, and ultrastructural features as synovial sarcomas in other locations. Most primary pleural synovial sarcomas are of the biphasic type, although monophasic tumors also occur. Synovial sarcomas are typically immunopositive for keratin and calretinin and immunonegative for carcinoma markers, which, combined with their histologic appearance and gross distribution, may add to difficulties in distinguishing pleural synovial sarcomas from DMMs. The great majority of studied synovial sarcomas, primarily of the extremities in children, are reported to have a tumor-specific chromosome t(X;18)(p11.2;q11.2) translocation resulting in the production of fusion genes, and identification of these may be used to assist in diagnosis.

Cytologic Features:

- Monophasic synovial sarcomas show spindle cells with irregular nuclei and sparse cytoplasm.
- Biphasic synovial sarcomas contain an epithelial component consisting of an organoid pattern of moderately sized polygonal cells.

Histologic Features:

- Pleural synovial sarcomas are most often biphasic but may be monophasic.
- Both variants share a spindle cell population arranged in fascicles with uniform nuclei and pale cytoplasm in a background of collagenous stroma with a hyaline appearance.
- These spindle cells tend to be monomorphic, with variable mitotic activity, and are often associated with mast cells.
- Biphasic tumors contain glandular structures lined by well-differentiated cuboidal to columnar epithelium.
- Generally synovial sarcomas are immunopositive in the epithelial component for cytokeratin, EMA, CD56, and Bcl-2, often immunopositive for calretinin and CD99, and immunonegative for CD 34.

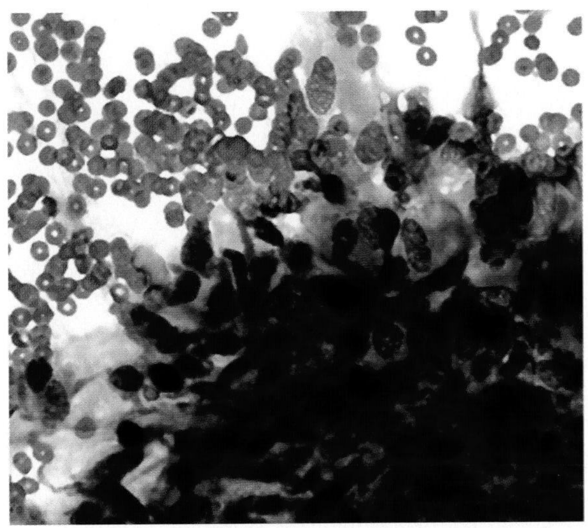

Figure 15.34 Cytology figure showing a cluster of spindle cells with irregular nuclei and sparse cytoplasm.

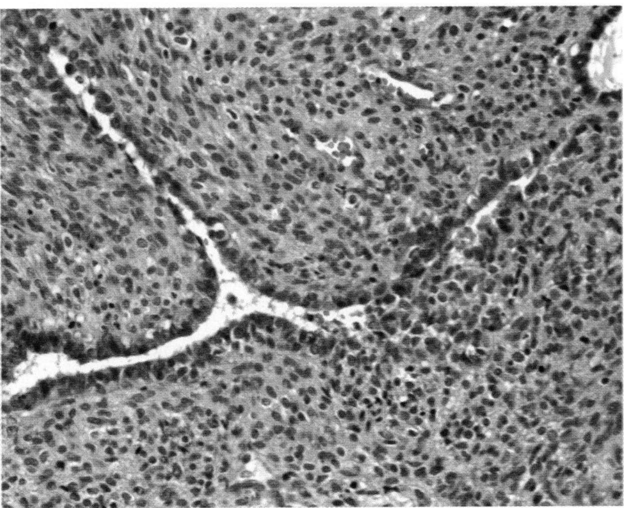

Figure 15.35 Biphasic synovial sarcoma with glandular structures surrounded by a cellular stroma.

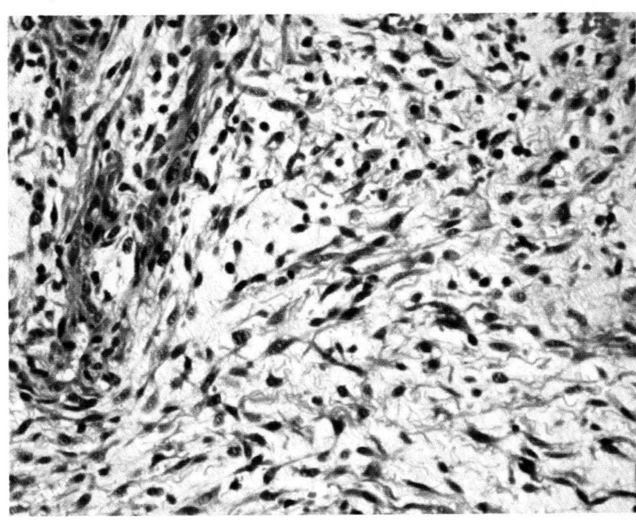

Figure 15.36 Pleural synovial sarcoma with myxoid stroma.

Part 5

Vascular Sarcoma

▶ Alvaro C. Laga, Timothy Allen, and Philip T. Cagle

Primary pleural vascular sarcomas are rare tumors that generally occur in adult men. The histology of primary pleural vascular sarcomas typically is epithelioid, ranging from epithelioid hemangioendothelioma-like tumors exhibiting low-grade nuclear features to high-grade epithelioid angiosarcomas. Although epithelioid hemangioendotheliomas of soft tissue and other organs are characteristically considered to be low-grade tumors, primary pleural vascular sarcomas, whether epithelioid hemangioendothelioma-like tumors or epithelioid angiosarcomas, are consistently aggressive neoplasms and typically cause death soon after diagnosis.

Some authors have noted an association between primary pleural vascular tumors and chronic pyothorax from pulmonary or pleural tuberculosis in Japanese patients. No such association has been confirmed in patients from western countries. Grossly, primary pleural vascular sarcomas may involve the pleural surface extensively and mimic DMM. In addition, these tumors may form a tubulopapillary pattern histologically, further mimicking DMM.

Cytologic Features:

Epithelioid Angiosarcoma

- Hemorrhagic background containing malignant endothelial cells arranged in loosely cohesive clusters.
- Large oval nuclei with prominent nucleoli.
- Cytoplasm may be angular.

Histologic Features:

Epithelioid Hemangioendothelioma

- Short strands or solid nests of rounded to slightly spindled endothelial cells within a hyaline or myxoid stroma.
- Tumor cells are polygonal or slightly spindled with bland nuclei.
- Small intracellular lumina may occur, forming clear spaces or vacuoles, some of which may contain red blood cells.
- Mitoses are infrequent.

Epithelioid Angiosarcoma

- Sheets and clusters of tumor cells showing large vesicular nuclei with occasional prominent nucleoli.
- Abundant eosinophilic cytoplasm with vacuoles.
- A tubulopapillary pattern similar to that of DMM may be present.

- Anastomosing vascular channels and atypical nuclear features such as enlarged nuclei and nucleoli or increased nuclear chromatin.
- Generally immunopositive with vimentin.
- Often immunopositive with one or more of the following: CD31, CD34, and factor VIII
- Often weakly and focally immunopositive with keratin.
- Type IV collagen, although not staining tumor cells themselves, may outline the presence of basal lamina around capillaries that may be otherwise difficult to identify on hematoxylin and eosin (H&E) stain, especially within solid areas of tumor.

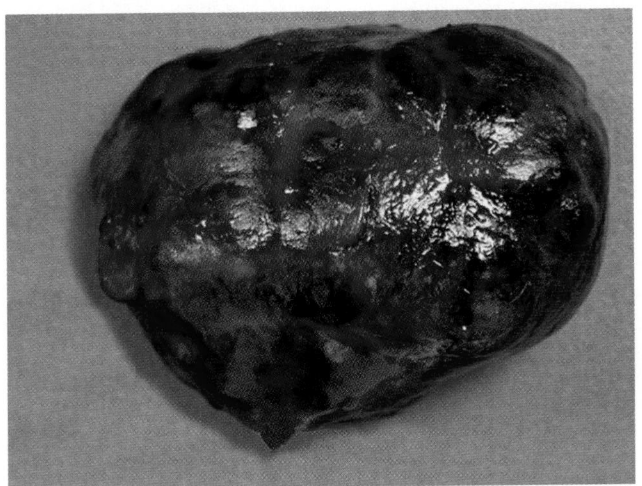

Figure 15.37 Gross figure of a primary pleural epithelioid angiosarcoma shows a hemorrhagic well-circumscribed mass.

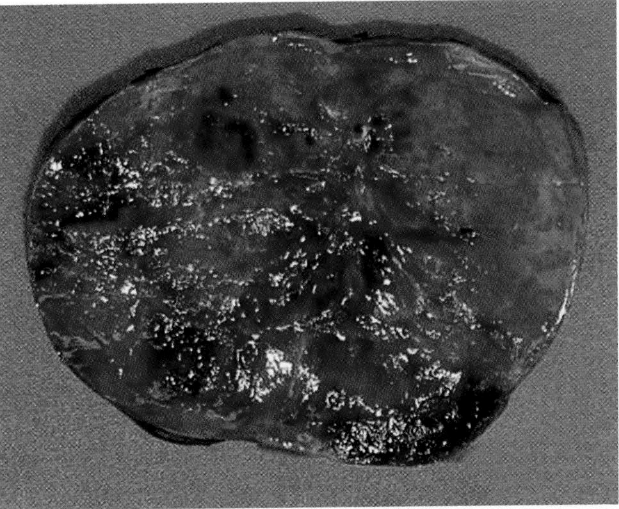

Figure 15.38 Gross figure of cut surface of a primary pleural epithelioid angiosarcoma shows hemorrhage and necrosis.

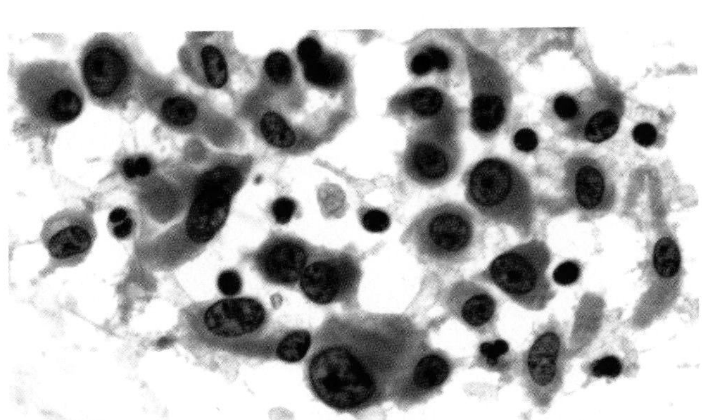

Figure 15.39 Cytology figure showing large oval nuclei with prominent nucleoli and abundant cytoplasm.

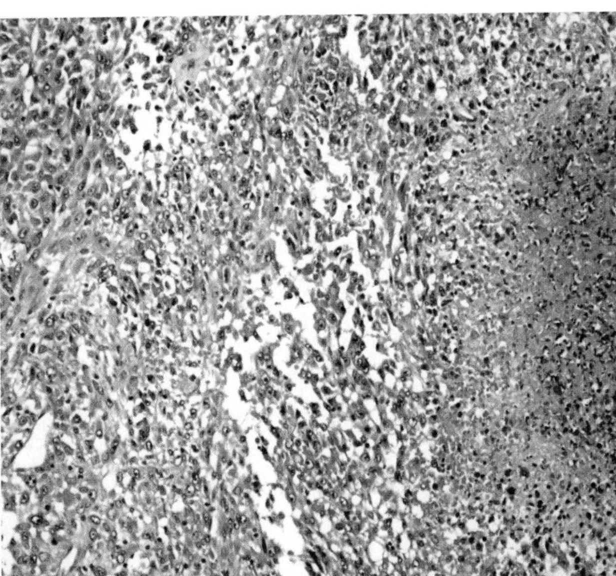

Figure 15.40 Low power of epithelioid angiosarcoma of the pleura showing tumor necrosis on the *right*.

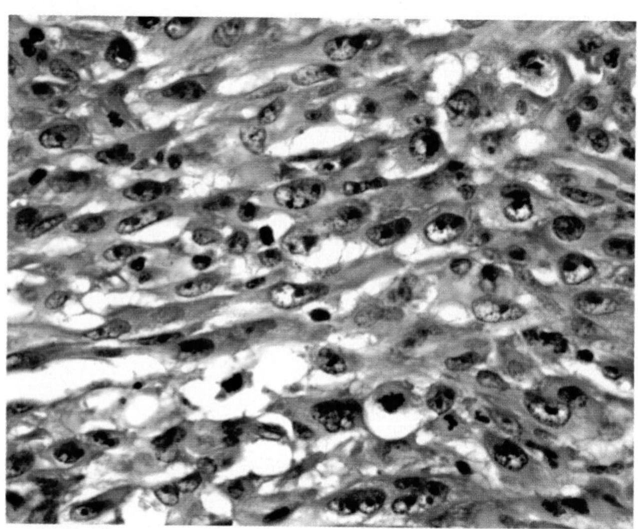

Figure 15.41 Higher power showing atypical epithelioid tumor cells in primary pleural epithelioid angiosarcoma.

Part 6

Malignant Solitary Fibrous Tumor

▶ Alvaro C. Laga, Timothy Allen, and Philip T. Cagle

Rare malignant variants of solitary fibrous tumors (SFT) can occur. Clinically, malignant SFTs present with chest pain, shortness of breath, and pleural effusion. Malignant SFTs typically measure more than 10 cm, are attached to the parietal pleura, mediastinum, or are inverted into the lung. They often recur locally, may metastasize, and may result in the patient's death. In some cases, the malignant tumors have the basic histopathology of SFTs but with cytologic pleomorphism, hemorrhage, tumor necrosis, and more than four mitoses per 10 high-power fields. In other cases, frank sarcomas can be seen arising from an area with histopathologic features of typical benign SFT. Inability to completely resect the tumor is associated with a poor prognosis.

Cytologic Features:

- Cytologic features on fine needle aspiration of solitary fibrous tumor with additional features of malignancy such as necrosis, mitotic figures, and nuclear pleomorphism.

Histologic Features:

- Cellular lesions composed of mitotically active spindled cells.
- Many of these tumors are overtly sarcomatous.
- Areas similar to those found in ordinary benign solitary fibrous tumors may be present
- These tumors are immunopositive for CD34 (>80%) and Bcl-2.
- Other useful immunomarkers include positive vimentin and negative keratin, EMA, actin, desmin, and S-100.

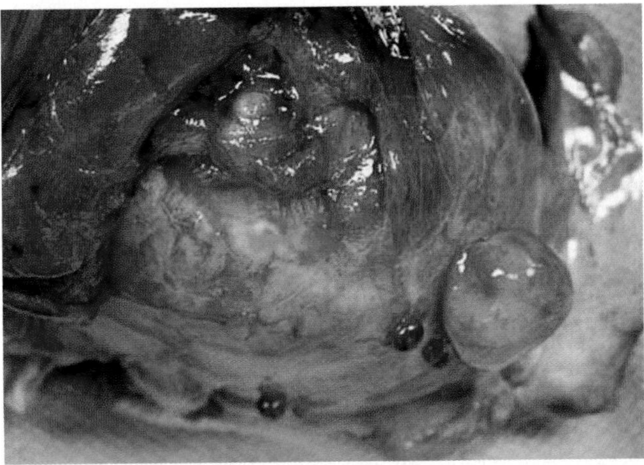

Figure 15.42 Gross figure of malignant solitary fibrous tumor consisting of a large multinodular pleural mass with lung at the *upper left corner*.

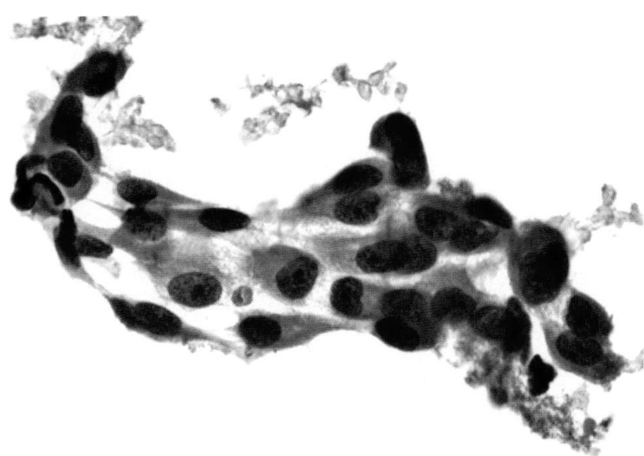

Figure 15.43 Cytology figure shows small cluster of cells with abundant cytoplasm, enlarged hyperchromatic nuclei, and occasional nucleoli.

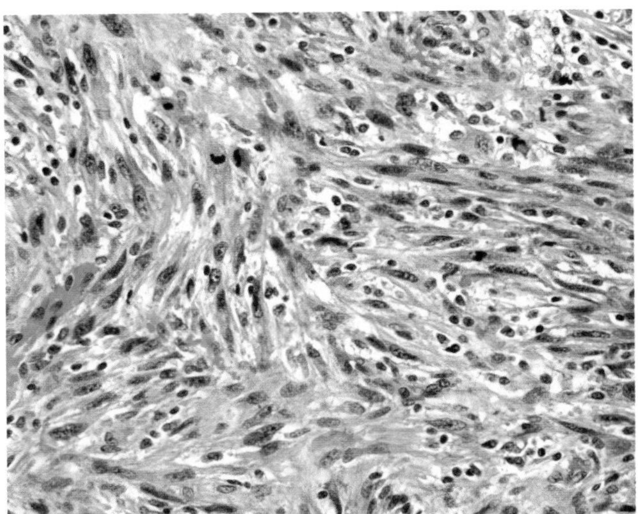

Figure 15.44 Malignant SFT with increased cellularity and increased mitotic figures.

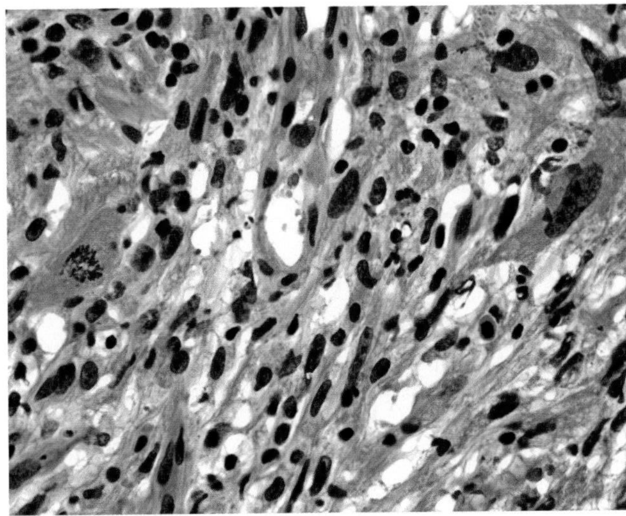

Figure 15.45 Higher power shows malignant solitary fibrous tumor with markedly atypical cells and mitoses.

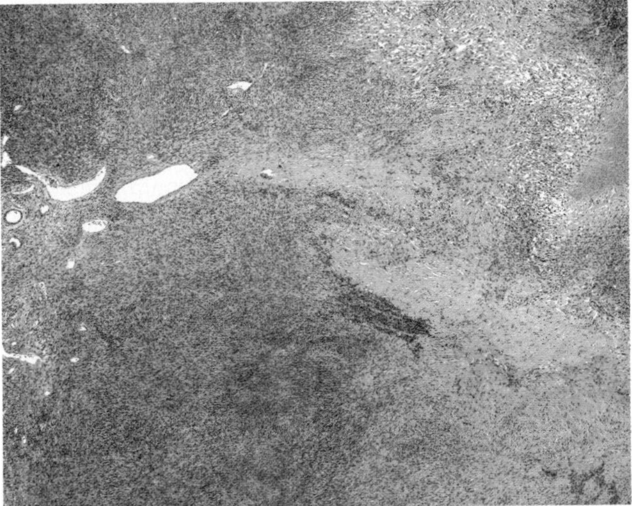

Figure 15.46 Malignant SFT arising in the setting of benign appearing solitary fibrous tumor, with tumor necrosis on the *right* and benign appearing component on the *left* edge.

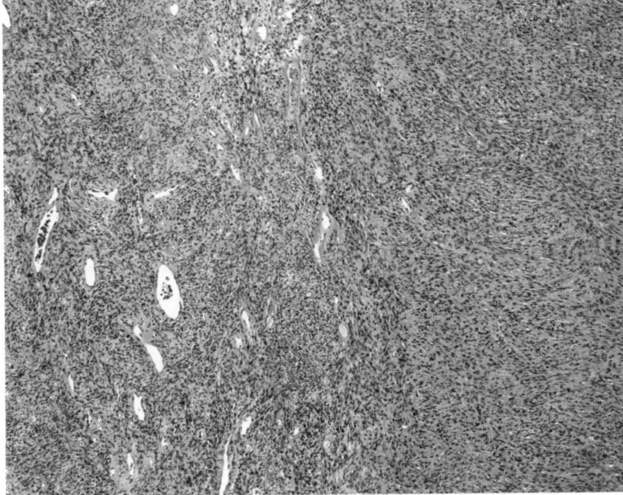

Figure 15.47 Medium power shows malignant SFT with increased cellularity on the *right* and benign appearing component on the *left*.

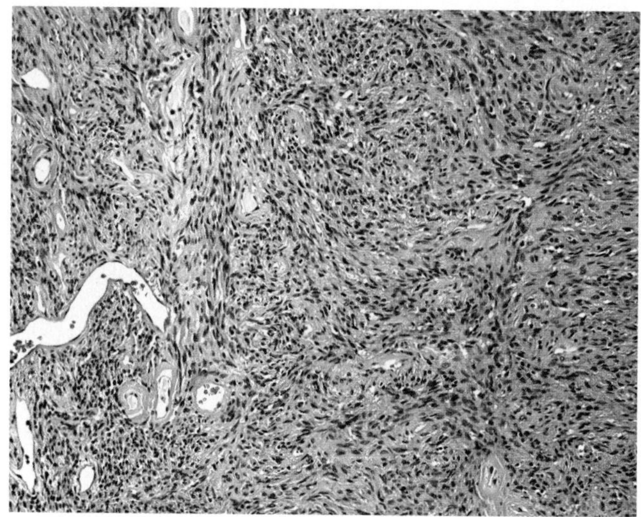

Figure 15.48 Higher power shows a sarcomatous area with increased cellularity, increased cell size, and nuclear pleomorphism on the *right* and a less cellular area with bland appearing cells and scattered blood vessels on the *left*.

Part 7

Pseudomesotheliomatous Carcinoma

▶ Alvaro C. Laga, Timothy Allen, and Philip T. Cagle

The term *pseudomesotheliomatous carcinoma* is used to describe carcinomas that grow over the pleural surface and encase the lung in a manner mimicking diffuse malignant mesothelioma (DMM). The term may be used loosely to refer to any carcinoma that metastasizes to the pleura and grows in this fashion, but primarily it has been used to describe peripheral lung adenocarcinomas that extend onto the pleural surface and grow along the pleural surface. The presumed primary site of these peripheral adenocarcinomas within the subpleural lung tissue may be small and difficult to identify, being overshadowed by the bulk of the tumor growing on the pleural surface. These adenocarcinomas can mimic DMM clinically, radiologically, and histologically. These tumors occur in older patients and are more frequent in men than in women. They present with chest pain, dyspnea, cough, and signs of an infiltrative pleural lesion. The most common radiographic finding is pleural effusion with or without pleural masses. Grossly, these tumors grow as pleural masses along the pleural surface encasing the lung. The prognosis for these tumors is poor, with high similarity to that of DMM. The findings described here refer to the traditional pseudomesotheliomatous adenocarcinomas, but it should be remembered that other cell types of carcinoma and primary sites of carcinoma other than the lung as well as cancers other than carcinomas can metastasize to the pleura and grow in a manner that grossly mimics DMM.

Histologic Features:

- Pleural infiltration by nests of cells that focally form glands or tubulopapillary structures.
- Psammoma bodies can be found, particularly in the papillary component.

- Isolated glands within a desmoplastic stroma are a common finding.
- The glandular lumens are frequently filled with periodic acid–Schiff (PAS)-positive, diastase-resistant mucin or intracytoplasmic vacuoles.
- These tumors show strong immunopositivity for polyclonal CEA and low-molecular-weight cytokeratins in the majority of cases; immunopositivity for Ber-EP4 Leu-M1 and B72.3 can be seen in some cases.
- The majority of cases express more than one of these markers.

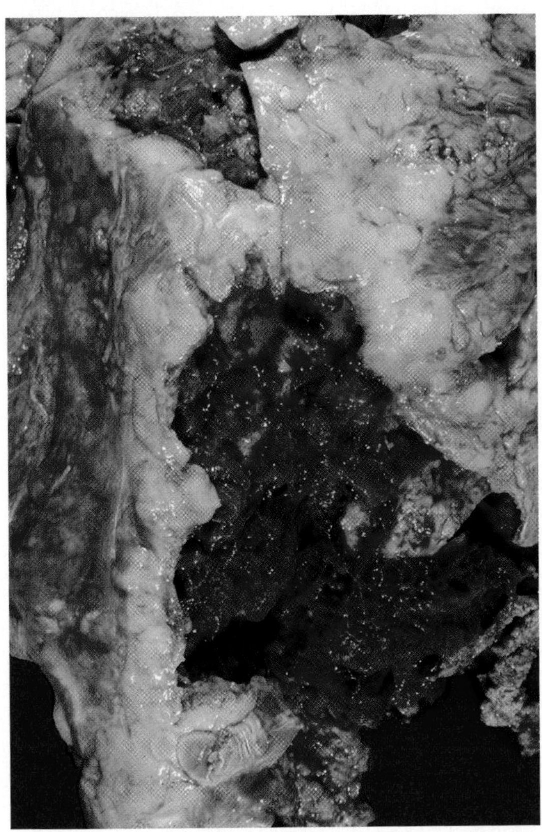

Figure 15.49 Gross figure shows rindlike spread of adenocarcinoma in a manner mimicking pleural DMM.

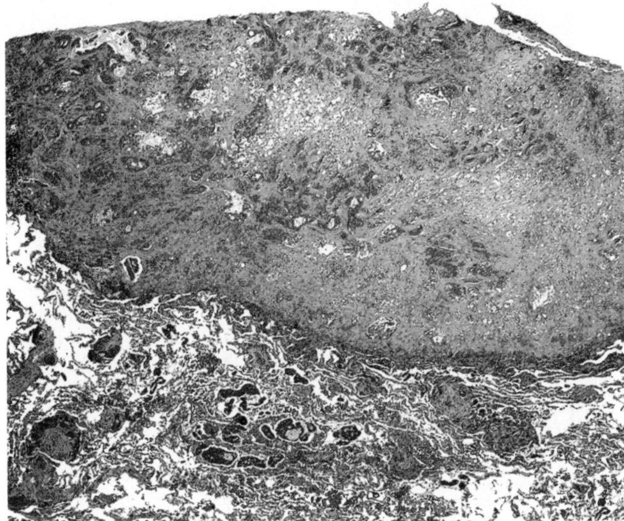

Figure 15.50 Section of rindlike tumor growing along the pleural surface.

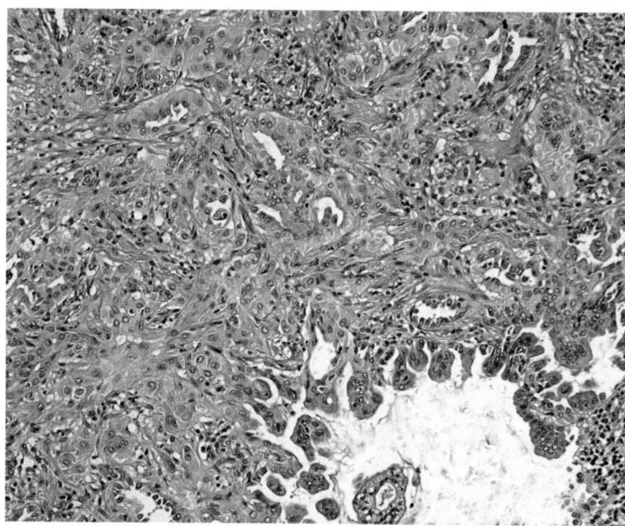

Figure 15.51 Medium power shows adenocarcinoma infiltrating desmoplastic pleura from a small subpleural primary adenocarcinoma with bronchioloalveolar type pattern on the *lower right*.

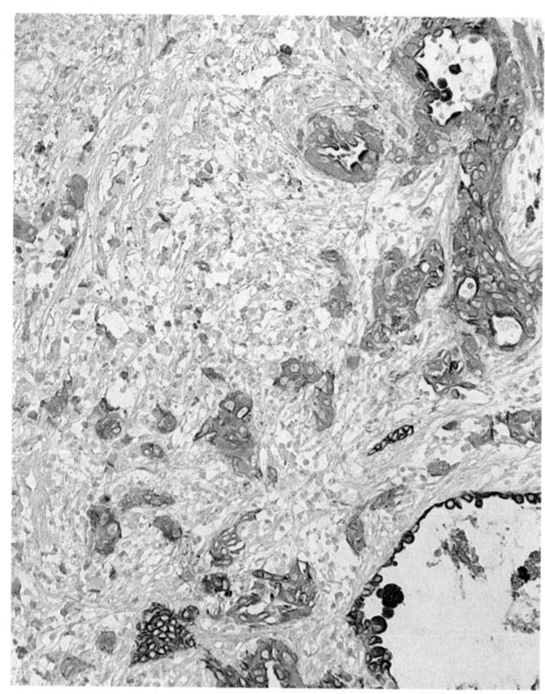

Figure 15.52 Keratin immunostain highlights the same tumor cells shown in Figure 15.51 with keratin-positive adenocarcinoma infiltrating the pleura from a keratin-positive small subpleural primary in the *lower right*.

Part 8

Primitive Neuroectodermal Tumor (Askin Tumor)

▶ Alvaro C. Laga, Timothy Allen, and Philip T. Cagle

Askin tumors are aggressive thoracopulmonary tumors of children, adolescents, and young adults. Askin tumors have many features in common with other members of the Ewing sarcoma family of tumors (Ewing sarcoma, peripheral primitive neuroectodermal tumor, and neuroepithelioma), including gene fusions between the EWS gene and a member of the ETS family of transcription factors.

Grossly, Askin tumor may be a single mass or multiple nodules involving the chest wall, pleura, and lung. The tumors consist of undifferentiated small round cells with scant cytoplasm arranged in nests and rosettes. The cells are typically immunopositive for synaptophysin and S-100 protein but often immunonegative for chromogranin.

Histologic Features:

- Cohesive small dark round undifferentiated cells with scant cytoplasm arranged in nests and rosettes.
- Generally immunopositive for synaptophysin, S-100, and neuron-specific enolase.

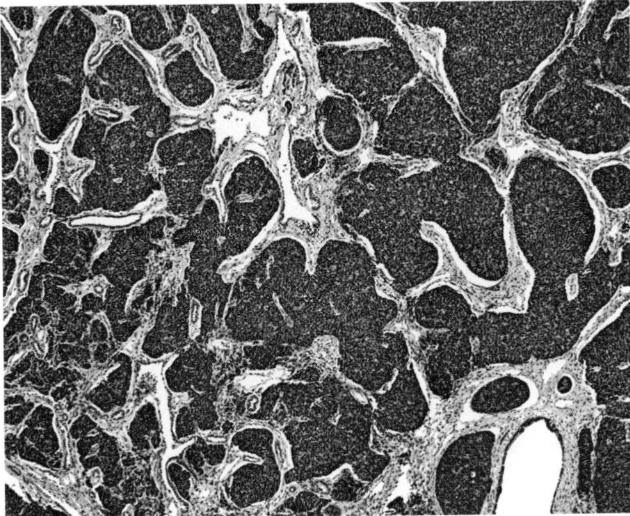

Figure 15.53 Askin tumor with nests of small dark cells and a fibrovascular stroma.

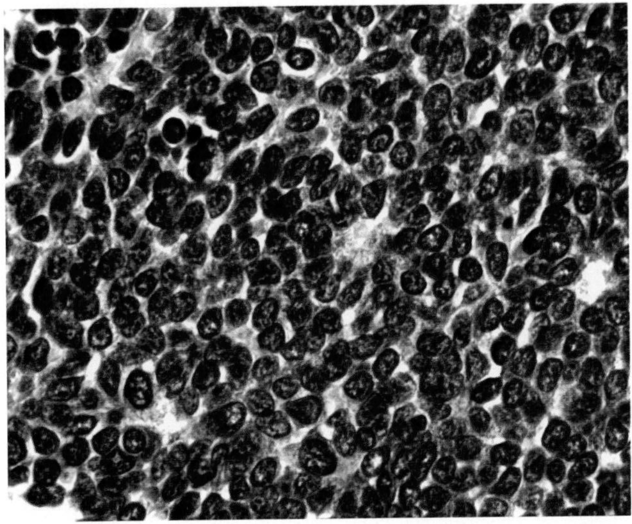

Figure 15.54 Higher power showing small round blue cells with hyperchromatic nuclei and scant cytoplasm, some of which form rosettes.

Part 9

Desmoplastic Small Round Cell Tumor

▶ Alvaro C. Laga, Timothy Allen, and Philip T. Cagle

Desmoplastic small round cell tumor (DSRCT) is a very rare primitive and highly aggressive malignancy that usually occurs in abdominal, pelvic, and paratesticular locations in adolescent and young adult males ages 15 to 35. Typically DSRCT spreads along the peritoneal surface, causing ascites and mimicking DMM of the peritoneum. DSRCT may spread to the pleura from the peritoneum. A handful of DSRCTs primary to the pleura have been reported. Of the primary pleural DSRCTs, most occurred in young adult males and most presented with pleural effusion. Most presented as nodular masses encasing the lung, one as studding of the pleural surface and one as a pedunculated mass.

Histologically, DSRCT consists of cords and nests of primitive small round malignant cells with scant cytoplasm within a fibrous stroma. Larger cells with rhabdoid features displaying more abundant cytoplasm and eccentric nuclei may be intermingled with the small round cells. Occasionally other features may be seen, including multinucleated sarcomatoid cells, large epithelioid cells with foci of anaplasia, or signet ring cells. Most DSRCTs are immunopositive for desmin, vimentin, keratin, epithelial membrane antigen, WT1, and neuron-specific enolase. DSRCTs have a characteristic chromosomal translocation that produces a chimeric or fusion transcript between the Ewing sarcoma gene and the Wilms tumor gene.

Histologic Features:

- The tumor is composed of irregular cell nests in a dense fibrous or hypercellular spindle cell stroma.
- The cells are of small to intermediate size with scant cytoplasm and nuclear molding.
- DSRCT usually shows immunohistochemical evidence of epithelial (cytokeratin-positive) and muscle (desmin-positive) differentiation.

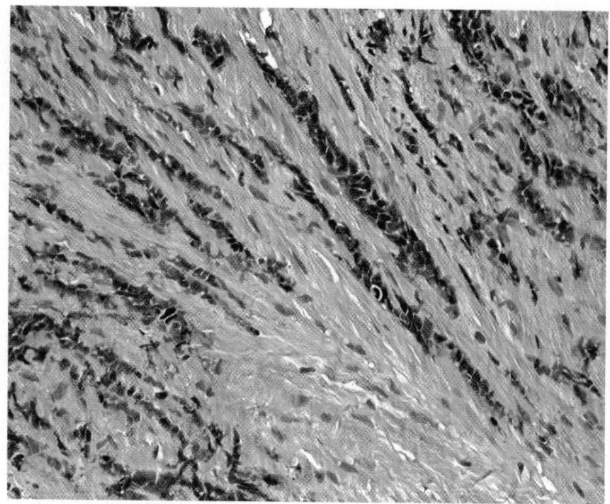

Figure 15.55 Cords of small round blue cells infiltrating dense fibrous stroma.

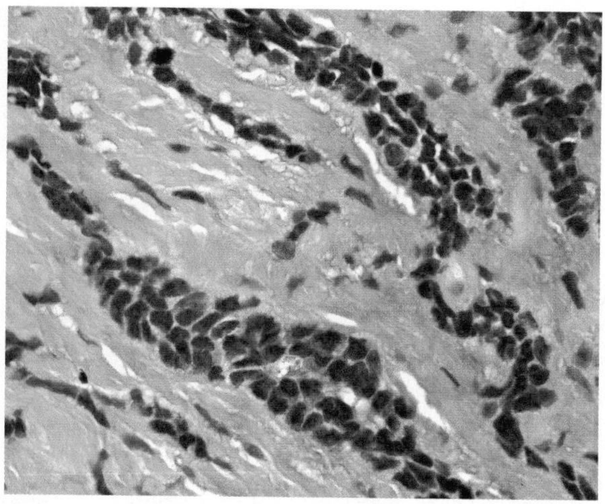

Figure 15.56 Higher power of small round blue cells showing scant cytoplasm and nuclear molding.

Part 10

Primary Effusion Lymphoma

▶ Jeffrey Jorgensen

Primary effusion lymphoma is a large B-cell lymphoma usually confined to the pleural, peritoneal, or pericardial cavity. Most cases are associated with immunodeficiency, most often caused by human immunodeficiency virus (HIV). The neoplastic B cells are infected by human herpes virus 8 (HHV-8, otherwise known as Kaposi sarcoma herpes virus [KSHV]). There is a strong association with Epstein-Barr virus (EBV). This is an aggressive process, with poor response to current therapy.

Cytologic Features:

- Large to very large cells, with oval to irregular to pleomorphic nuclei.
- Deeply basophilic cytoplasm, often abundant, with vacuoles in some cells.
- Some cases show paranuclear hofs (light-staining areas corresponding to Golgi apparatus), suggesting plasmacytic differentiation.
- Immunopositive for CD45 (leukocyte common antigen), the activation marker CD30, and the plasma cell associated markers CD38 and CD138.
- Usually immunonegative for B-cell markers and immunoglobulin light chains.
- HHV-8/KSHV is present, as determined by immunostaining or polymerase chain reaction.
- EBV is often present, best demonstrated by *in situ* hybridization.

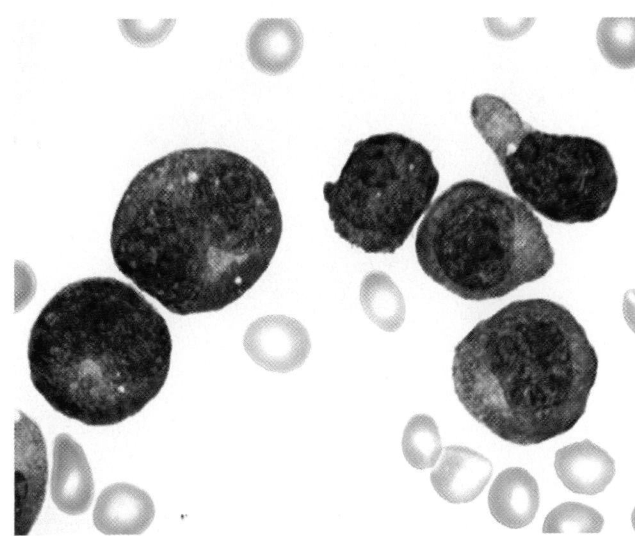

Figure 15.57 Large pleomorphic lymphoma cells with abundant basophilic cytoplasm, many with paranuclear hofs conferring a plasmacytoid appearance.

Part 11

Pleural Metastases

▶ Rodolfo Laucirica

Cancers often metastasize to the pleura because of the rich pleural lymphatic network. Pleural metastases commonly result in pleural effusions. Diagnosis of pleural metastases may be made based on exfoliative cytology, needle biopsy, or wedge (thoracoscopic or open) biopsy.

Metastatic cancers are overwhelmingly the most common cancers in malignant pleural effusions. In the United States, metastatic cancers cause about 200,000 pleural effusions each year compared to 1,500 malignant pleural effusions caused by DMM. Of the 200,000 malignant pleural effusions caused by metastatic cancers each year, about 60,000 are lung carcinomas, 50,000 are breast carcinomas, 40,000 are lymphoma, and 50,000 are from other primary sites, particularly gastrointestinal and genitourinary carcinomas.

Cancer cells in malignant effusions may be seen as individual cancer cells, in sheets of cells, in three-dimensional highly cellular balls called *morulae,* and in papillary or acinar structures. Psammoma bodies may be present in association with papillary tumors. Classic cytologic features of individual cancer cells in malignant effusions include enlarged cells with high nuclear-to-cytoplasmic ratios, coarse chromatin, enlarged and multiple nucleoli, irregular nuclear contours, and mitoses including atypical mitoses.

The most common cell type, regardless of organ of origin, is adenocarcinoma. Histopathologic identification of the primary site of a pleural metastasis depends on finding cytologic or histologic features characteristic of cancers from the primary site and on characteristic immunostain profiles.

Histologic Features:

- Histologic and immunohistochemical findings recapitulate those of the primary tumor.

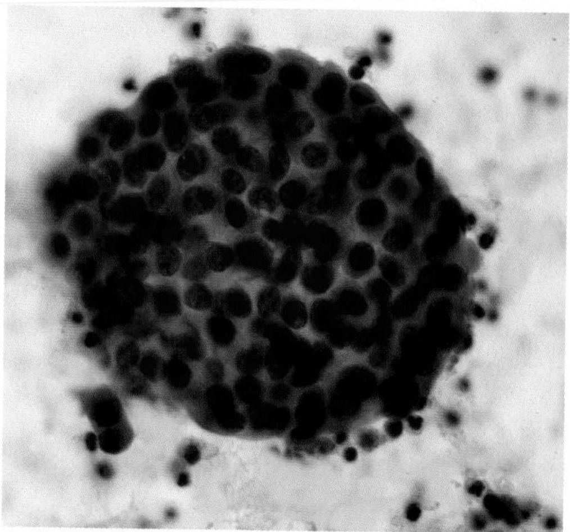

Figure 15.58 Spherical morulae are composed of densely packed cells, as seen in this cytology figure of a pleural effusion (H&E stain) from a patient with metastatic breast carcinoma.

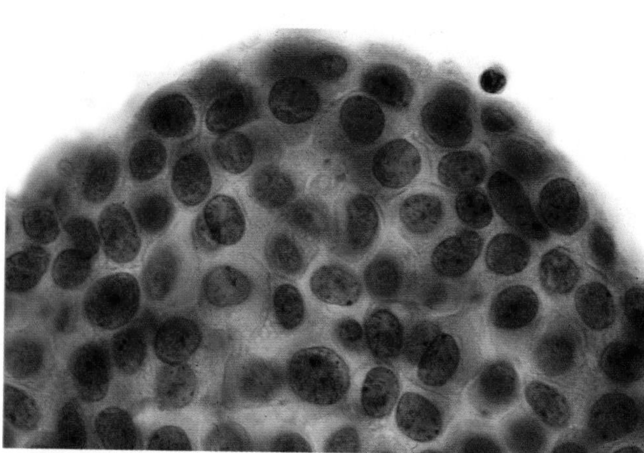

Figure 15.59 Higher power shows three-dimensional sphere or morula of metastatic breast carcinoma cells in pleural fluid (H&E stain).

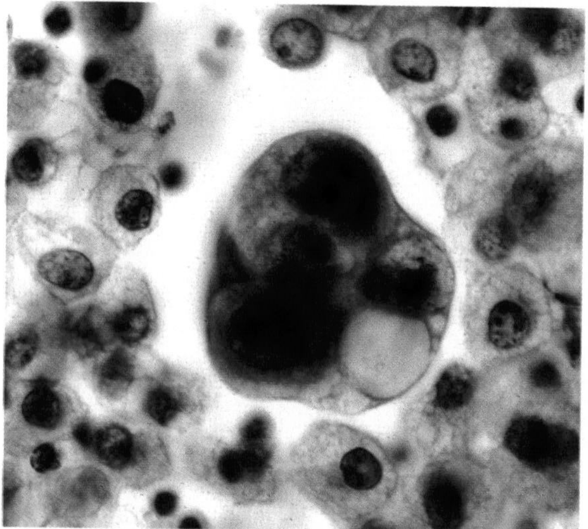

Figure 15.60 Metastatic adenocarcinoma in a pleural effusion (Papanicolaou stain) shows a cluster of malignant cells with enlarged nuclei, large nucleoli, and a cytoplasmic vacuole.

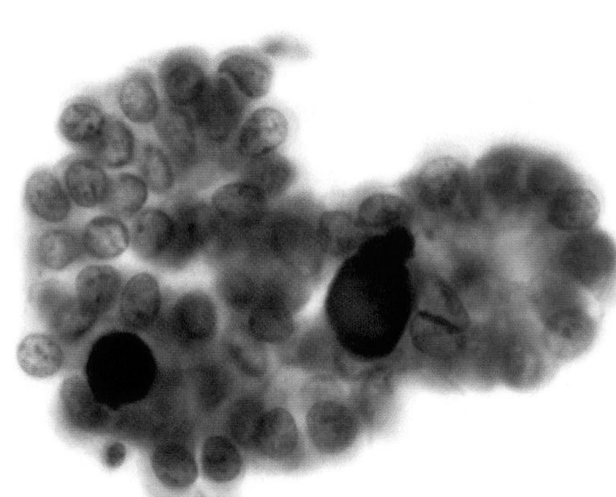

Figure 15.61 Serous papillary carcinoma of the ovary in a pleural fluid cytology figure (Papanicolaou stain) shows papillae composed of malignant cells containing psammoma bodies.

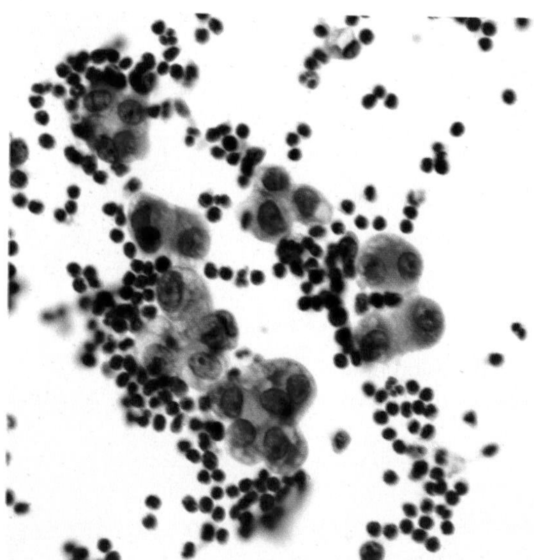

Figure 15.62 Cells of metastatic renal cell carcinoma in a pleural effusion (Papanicolaou stain) shows enlarged cells (compare to adjacent lymphocytes and neutrophils) with enlarged nucleoli and occasional cytoplasmic vacuole.

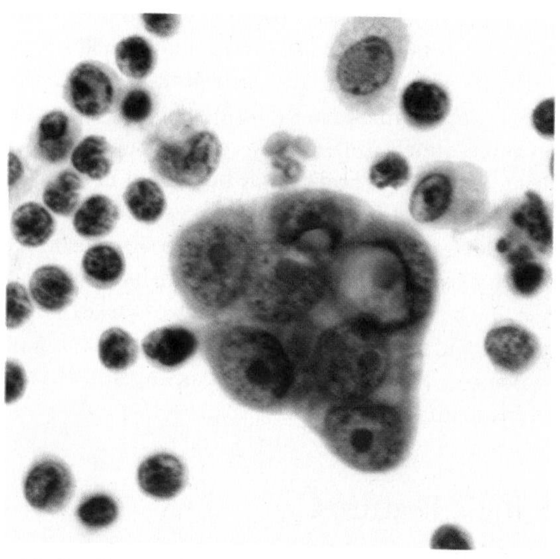

Figure 15.63 Cluster of metastatic endometrial carcinoma cells from pleural fluid (Papanicolaou stain) shows enlarged cells (compare to adjacent lymphocytes) with high nuclear-to-cytoplasm ratio and enlarged nucleoli.

Immunohistochemistry of Pulmonary and Pleural Neoplasia

16

▶ Alvaro C. Laga
▶ Nelson Ordonez

Many cancers metastasize to the lung and/or pleura, where they may mimic primary tumors of the lung and pleura radiologically, clinically, grossly, and histopathologically. Immunohistochemistry is a commonly used adjuvant technique for diagnosing primary versus metastatic neoplasms of the lung and pleura. Differentiation of cell type of primary lung tumors also may be an issue. Immunohistochemistry has largely replaced the use of histochemistry and electron microscopy as an adjunct in the diagnosis of pulmonary and pleural tumors. Most primary lung cancers can be diagnosed by histologic criteria alone. Immunohistochemistry cannot always determine the primary site or cell type of a cancer due to lack of a specific diagnostic marker for many cancers and to overlapping immunostaining patterns among different types of cancers. Results of immunostains depend on the quality of the tissue sample, techniques, and protocols; the antibodies and reagents used; proper controls; and correct interpretation of staining patterns. It is important to be aware that false-positive and false-negative results may occur. Interpretation of immunohistochemical stains should always be done in the context of the other clinical and pathologic findings.

Histologic Features:

Non–Small Cell Lung Carcinoma

- A variety of epithelial cell markers are expressed in primary non–small cell lung carcinomas, predominantly in adenocarcinomas.
- Lung primary adenocarcinomas are generally immunopositive with AE1/AE3, MOC-31, CK7, CEA, 35βH11, EMA, HMFG-2, Ber-EP4, and TTF-1, and often immunopositive with Leu-M1 and B72.3.
- Lung primary adenocarcinomas are generally immunonegative with CK20 and CK5/CK6.
- Lung primary squamous cell carcinomas are generally immunopositive with AE1/AE3, CK5/CK6, 34βE12, EMA, and HMFG-2, and often immunopositive with CEA (50%).
- Lung primary squamous cell carcinomas are generally immunonegative with Leu-M1, B72.3, Ber-EP4, TTF-1, and CK7.

Small Cell Lung Carcinoma

- Small cell lung carcinomas are generally immunopositive with CD56 (NCAM), TTF-1, NSE, AE1/AE3, pan-cytokeratin, and synaptophysin, and are occasionally immunopositive with chromogranin A.
- Small cell lung carcinomas, in the majority of cases, show a punctuate immunostaining pattern for pan-cytokeratin.

Large Cell Neuroendocrine Carcinoma

- Large cell neuroendocrine lung carcinomas are generally immunopositive with NSE, AE1/AE3, pan-cytokeratin, 35βH11, synaptophysin, and chromogranin A.

Epithelial Diffuse Malignant Mesothelioma

- Epithelial diffuse malignant mesotheliomas are generally immunopositive with AE1/AE3, WT1, CK7, CK5/CK6, HBME-1, calretinin, EMA, and HMFG-2.
- Epithelial diffuse malignant mesotheliomas are generally immunonegative with MOC-31, CEA, Leu-M1, B72.3, Ber-EP4, and TTF-1.

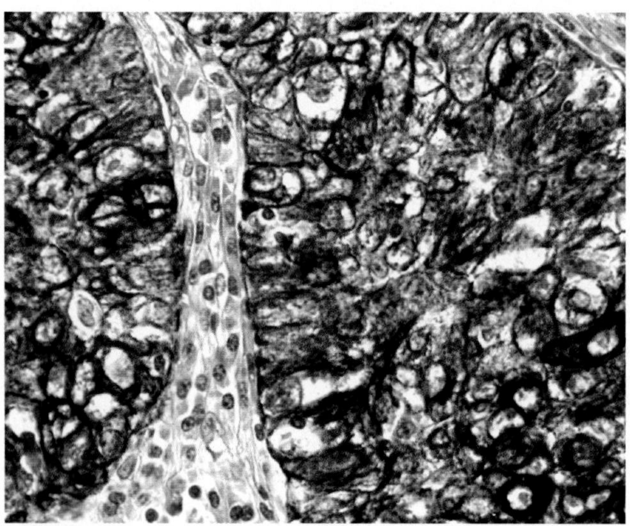

Figure 16.1 Pulmonary adenocarcinoma shows intense cytoplasmic staining with CK7 antibody.

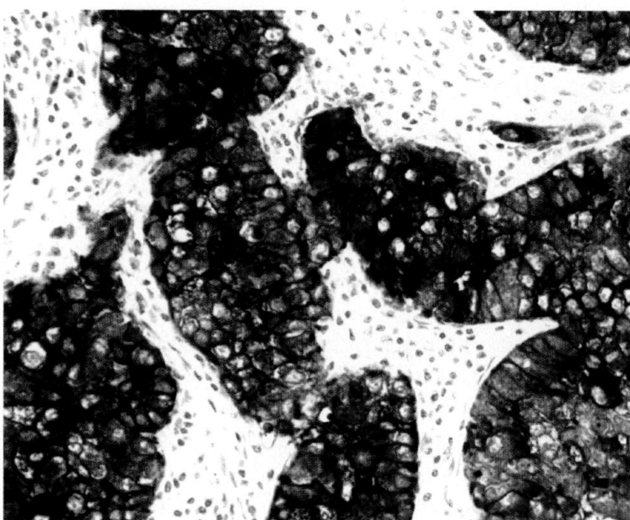

Figure 16.2 Intense cytoplasmic pattern of staining with CEA antibody in lung adenocarcinoma.

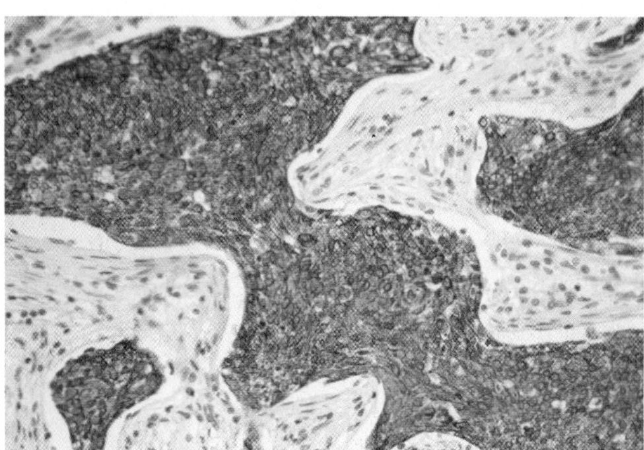

Figure 16.3 Squamous cell carcinoma shows strong cytoplasmic staining with CK5/CK6 antibody.

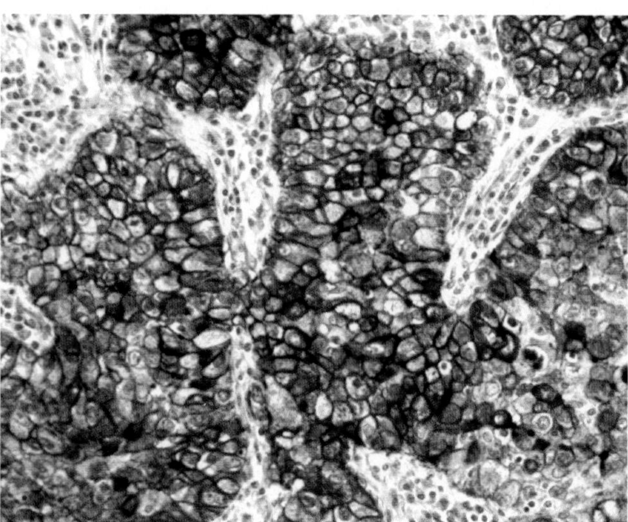

Figure 16.4 Pulmonary adenocarcinoma with cytoplasmic immunostaining pattern with Ber-EP4 antibody.

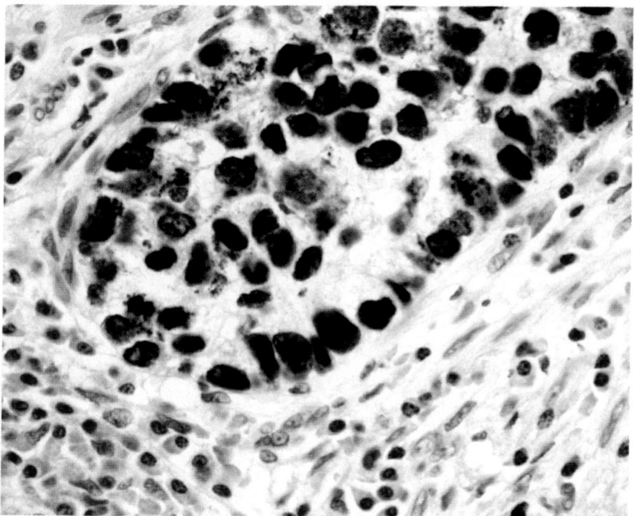

Figure 16.5 Intense nuclear staining with TTF-1 antibody in pulmonary adenocarcinoma.

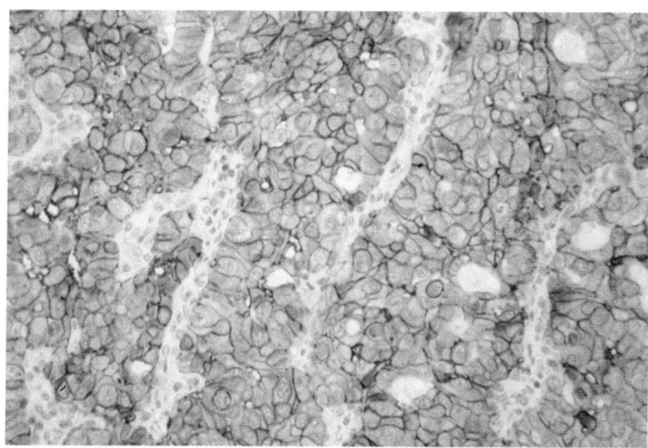

Figure 16.6 Poorly differentiated adenocarcinoma shows primarily membranous immunopositivity with MOC-31 antibody.

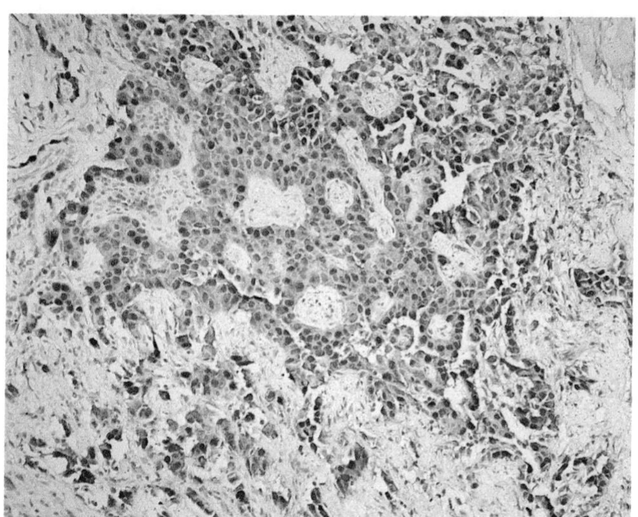

Figure 16.7 Epithelial mesothelioma shows classic cytoplasmic and nuclear immunostaining with calretinin antibody.

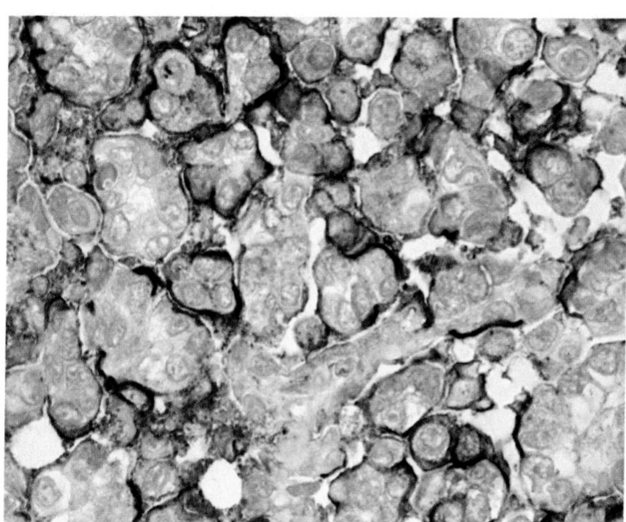

Figure 16.8 Epithelial mesothelioma with thick cell membrane immunostaining with HBME-1 antibody.

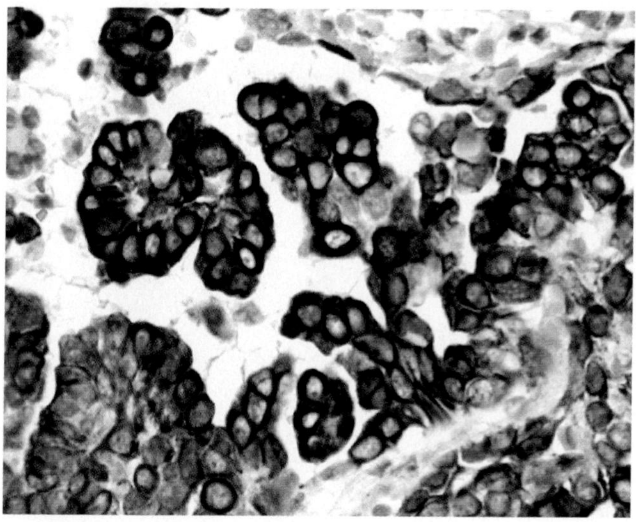

Figure 16.9 Epithelial mesothelioma shows positive immunostaining with CK5/CK6 antibody.

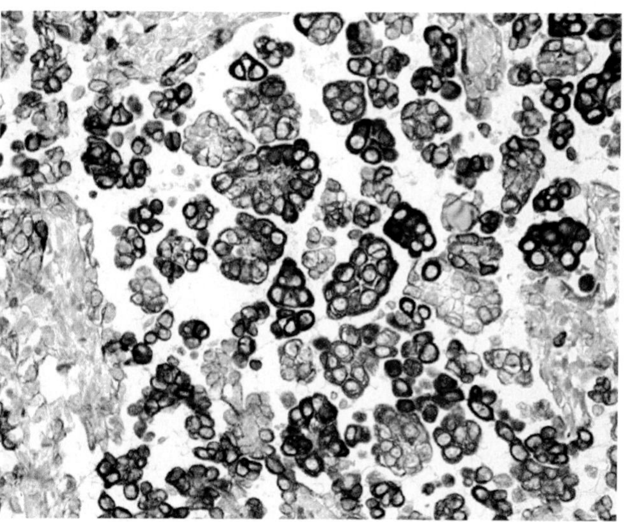

Figure 16.10 Epithelial mesothelioma shows positive immunostaining with CK7 antibody.

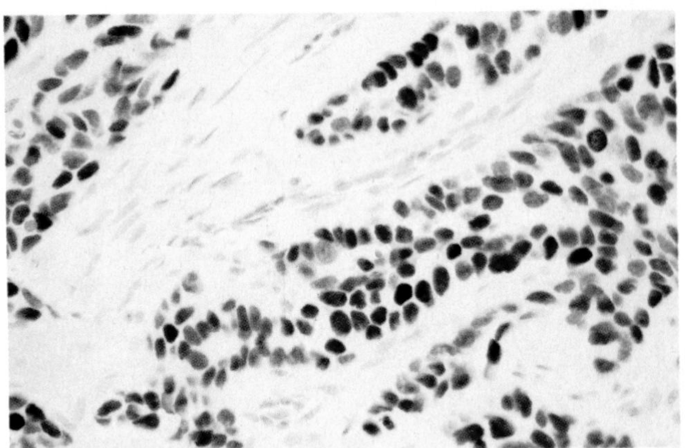

Figure 16.11 Epithelial mesothelioma shows positive nuclear staining with WT1 antibody.

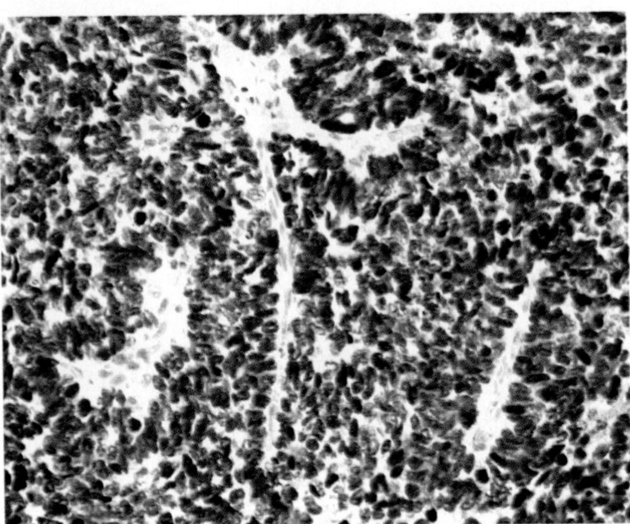

Figure 16.12 Small cell carcinoma of lung shows intense nuclear immunostaining with TTF-1 antibody.

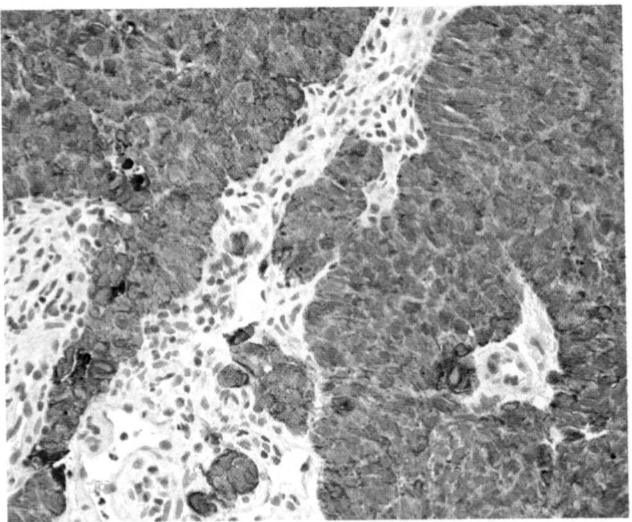

Figure 16.13 Small cell carcinoma shows punctate stippled immunostaining pattern with pan-cytokeratin antibody.

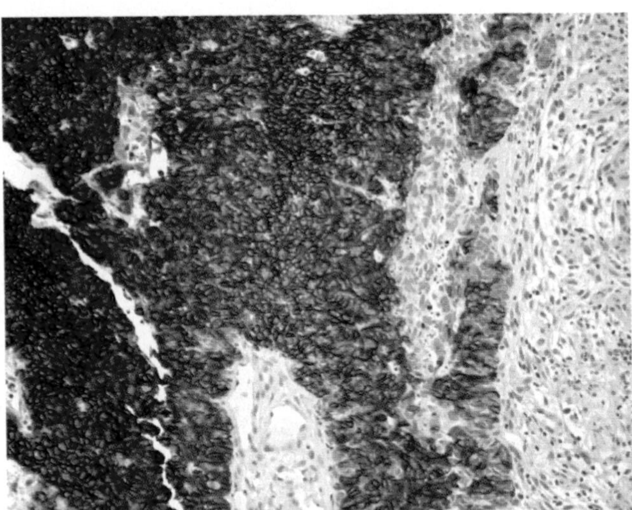

Figure 16.14 Small cell carcinoma of lung shows intense immunostaining with CD56 (NCAM) antibody.

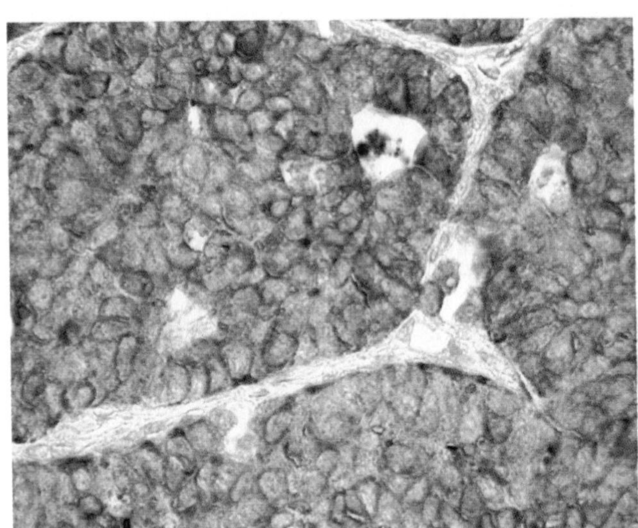

Figure 16.15 Large cell neuroendocrine carcinoma of lung shows positive immunostaining with synaptophysin antibody.

Section 4

Benign Neoplasms

Hamartoma

17

▸ Donna Coffey
▸ Hakan Cermik
▸ Mary Ostrowski

Hamartomas are the most common benign pulmonary neoplasm. They are usually solitary asymptomatic peripheral masses discovered incidentally as "coin lesions" on chest x-ray film. They are composed of mature mesenchymal elements, most often mature cartilage, but they also can be composed of adipose tissue, fibrous or fibromyxoid tissue, smooth muscle, and/or bone with or without bone marrow. The typical chondromatous hamartoma may have calcifications that gives rise to a characteristic "popcorn calcification" appearance on chest x-ray film. They have been called *mesenchymomas,* reflecting the observation that they are neoplasms with genetic mutations and are not true "hamartomas." Entrapped pulmonary epithelium, often entrapped in cleftlike spaces between lobules of cartilage, may be present. The majority are intraparenchymal, and a small minority (about 10%) are endobronchial. Grossly, hamartomas generally range from 1 to 3 cm and are very sharply demarcated so that they can often be "shelled" out by the surgeon. The color and texture depend on the histologic composition. As expected, because most are chondromatous, the majority have a cartilaginous appearance and texture on gross examination. Endobronchial hamartomas are polypoid and are typically composed of adipose tissue as the majority constituent.

Cytologic Features:

- Typically fragments of cartilage, a fibrillary stromal matrix, and benign epithelial cells on fine needle aspiration.

Histologic Features:

- Hamartomas are composed mostly of mature hyaline cartilage, but they also may be composed of adipose tissue, fibrous or fibromyxoid tissue, smooth muscle, and/or occasionally bone with or without bone marrow.
- Entrapped pulmonary epithelium may be present, lining slitlike clefts between lobules of cartilage or other elements.

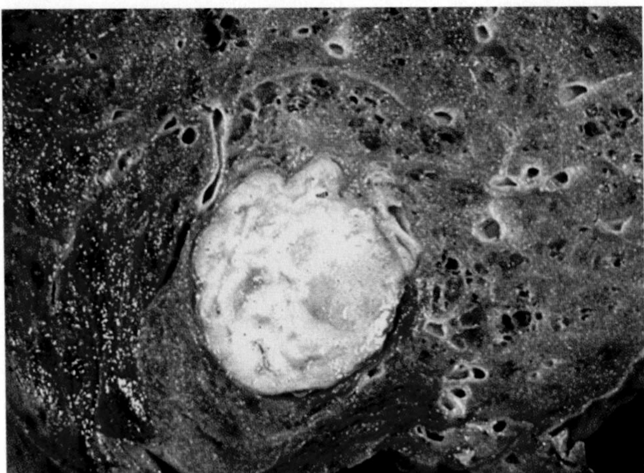

Figure 17.1 Gross figure of a pulmonary hamartoma shows a well-demarcated firm mass with prominent cartilaginous component.

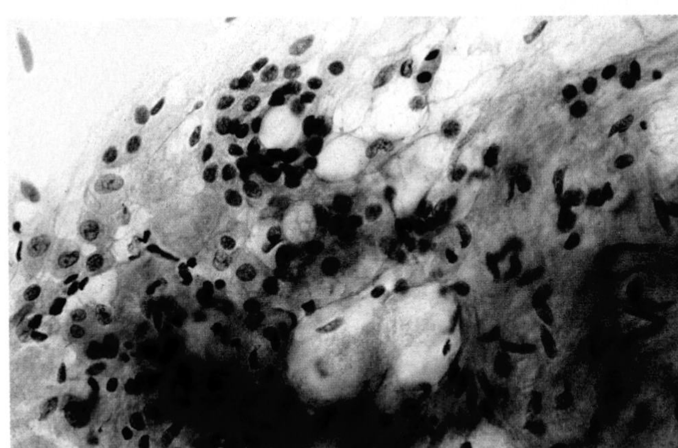

Figure 17.2 Fine needle aspiration shows a fibrillary stromal matrix and benign epithelial cells.

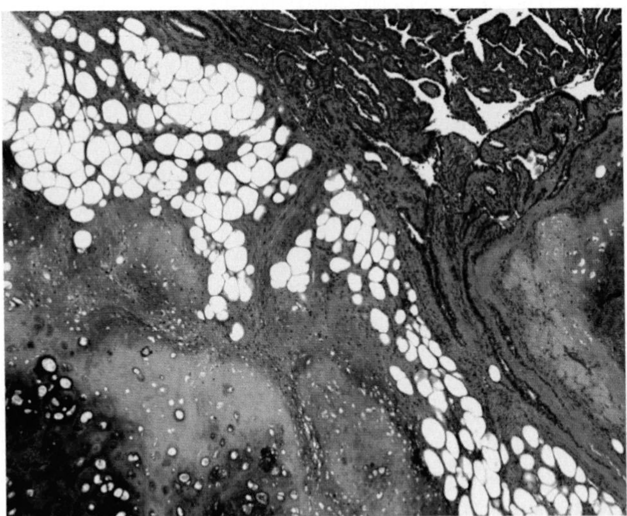

Figure 17.3 Hamartoma containing predominantly a mixture of mature cartilage and adipose tissue, with invaginations of pulmonary epithelium.

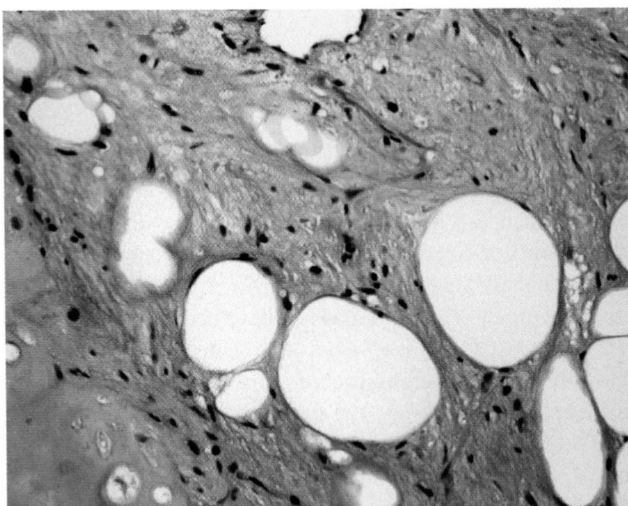

Figure 17.4 Higher power shows adipose tissue, cartilage, and myxoid stroma.

18

Solitary Fibrous Tumor

▶ Alvaro C. Laga
▶ Timothy Allen
▶ Philip T. Cagle

Solitary fibrous tumors (SFTs) are well-circumscribed spindle cell mesenchymal neoplasms with hemangiopericytoma-like pattern with characteristic branching vessels ("staghorn vessels") and other histologic patterns. Also known as *localized fibrous tumors*, SFTs are the most common benign pleural tumor. Most SFTs are attached to the visceral pleura, but they may be attached to the parietal pleura or may be intrapulmonary. Typically, SFTs are 5 to 10 cm in greatest dimension and may be found incidentally. Large benign SFTs may compress adjacent lung and other structures but, despite the sometimes distressing clinical presentation, do not invade these adjacent structures and are cured by resection. On the other hand, large size can be associated with malignancy, and careful sampling is recommended (see Chapter 15, Part 6). SFTs are occasionally multiple, which is why some investigators prefer calling them *localized fibrous tumors.* On cut section they typically have a fibrous appearance and consistency, usually off-white, firm, and often whorled. Hypoglycemia occasionally is seen with some patients.

Cytologic Features:

- On fine needle aspiration, the findings reflect the several histologic patterns of SFT depending on the tumor's histologic composition and the area sampled.
- Spindle cells in hemangiopericytoma-like or cellular pattern.
- Scant to moderate cellularity with a background of irregular ropy collagen fragments, few inflammatory cells, and singly dispersed or loose aggregates of cells within the collagen.
- Uniformly bland nuclei with evenly distributed, finely granular chromatin.

Histologic Features:

- Solitary fibrous tumors have a variety of patterns, including the "patternless pattern," hemangiopericytoma-like pattern, and cellular pattern.
- A solitary fibrous tumor may contain any or all of the above patterns.
- Typically immunopositive for Bcl-2, CD34, CD99, vimentin, and factor XIIIa, and immunonegative for S-100 and keratin.

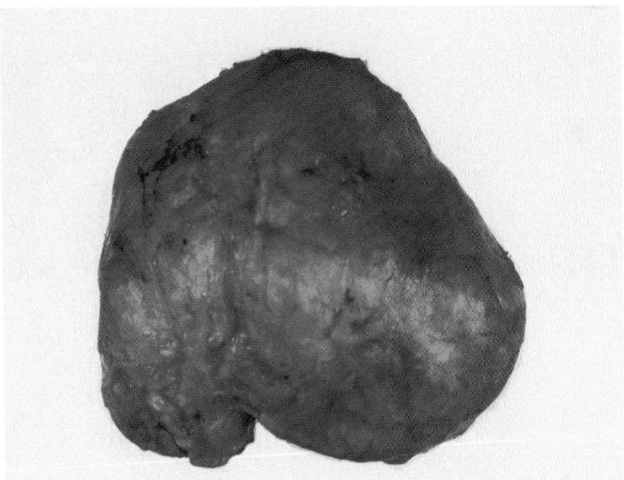

Figure 18.1 Gross figure of solitary fibrous tumor showing smooth outer surface.

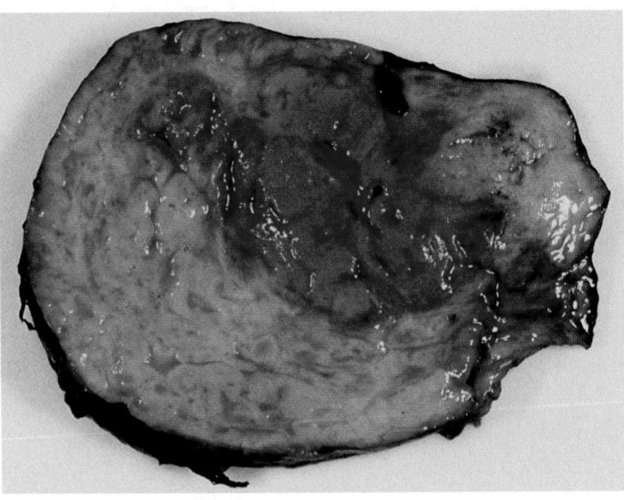

Figure 18.2 Cut section of solitary fibrous tumor shows a yellow-tan surface.

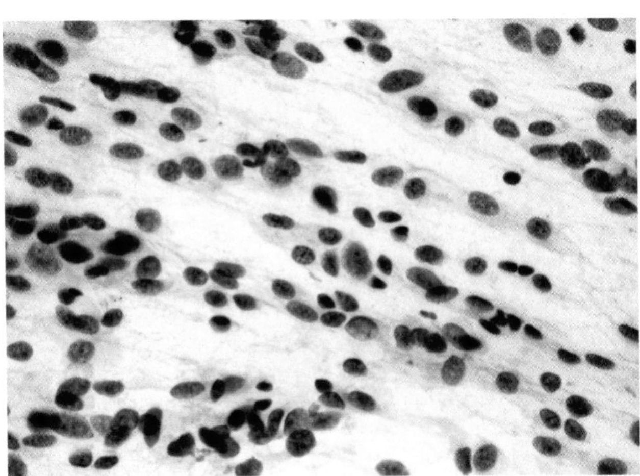

Figure 18.3 Cytology figure of solitary fibrous tumor showing relatively uniform bland nuclei without mitotic figures.

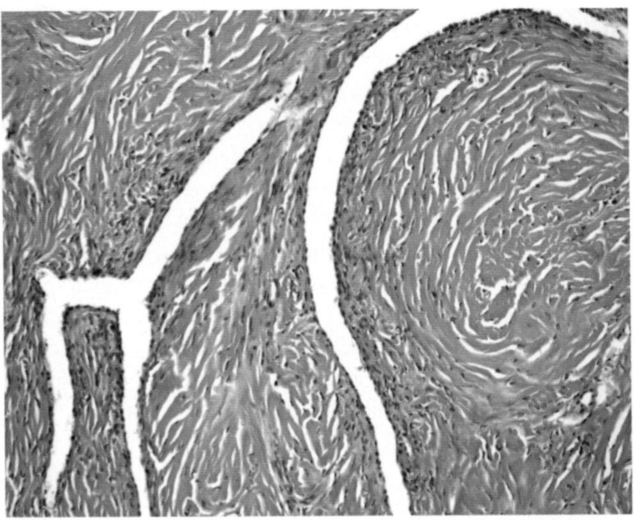

Figure 18.4 "Patternless pattern" of solitary fibrous tumor with inconspicuous cells within slitlike spaces.

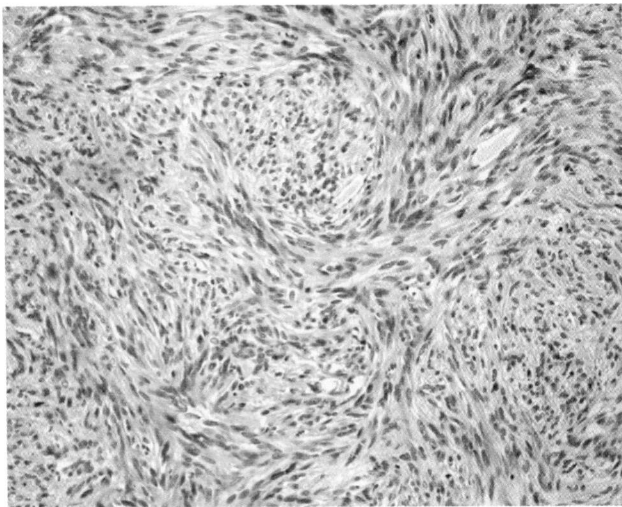

Figure 18.5 Cellular pattern of solitary fibrous tumor shows relatively bland cells without increased mitoses or necrosis.

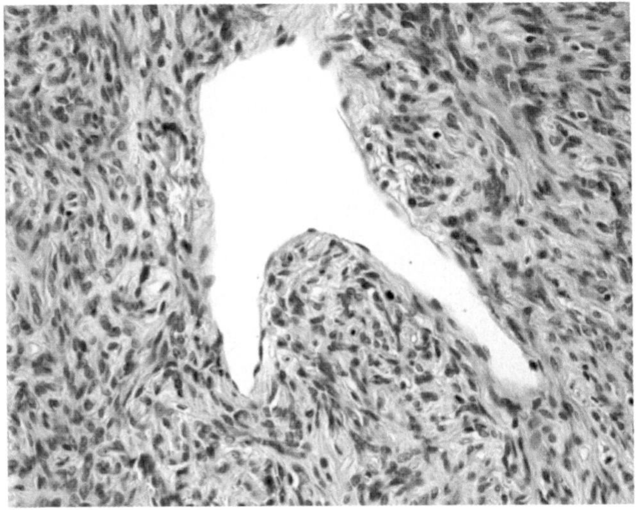

Figure 18.6 Hemangiopericytoma-like pattern with staghorn vessel.

Part 1

Desmoid Tumor

▶ Bruno Murer

Desmoid tumors of the pleura are generally associated with chest trauma or a previous thoracic surgery and can involve visceral or parietal pleura. Grossly, desmoid tumors are typically large firm masses with broad-based pleural attachments, with dense white, large irregular fascicles of fibrous tissue on cut surface. Differential diagnosis includes solitary fibrous tumor (generally CD34 and Bcl-2 immunopositive and β-catenin immunonegative), solitary neurofibroma (generally S-100 immunopositive), sarcomas and chronic pleuritis.

Histologic Features:

- A fibroproliferative process composed of fibroblasts, fibrocytes, and myofibroblasts set within a collagenous to myxoid stroma that possess uniformly bland nuclear features.
- Features of conventional desmoid tumor, including moderate cellularity with elongated, uniform bland fibroblasts arranged in long fascicles set in a fibrillar collagen matrix, often with loose mucoid character; numerous slitlike vessels with focal perivascular collection of lymphocytes.
- Generally immunopositive with vimentin and desmin.
- May be focally immunopositive with smooth muscle actin.
- Generally immunonegative for S-100, CD34, and EMA.
- Frequently exhibits nuclear overexpression of β-catenin.

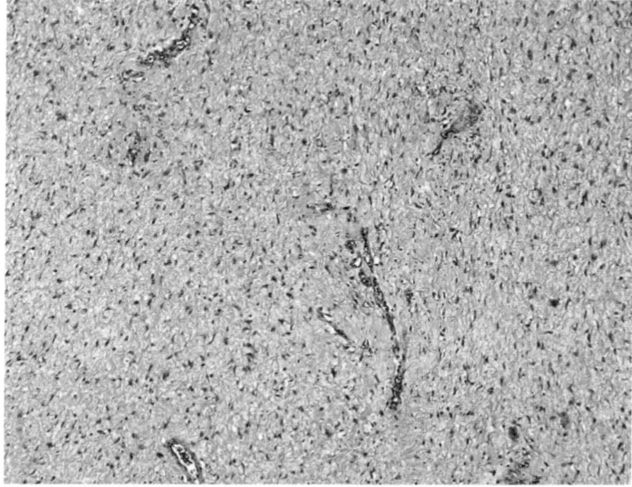

Figure 18.7 Low power of desmoid tumor shows elongated bland fibroblasts arranged within a loose mucoid fibrillar collagen matrix and slitlike vessels.

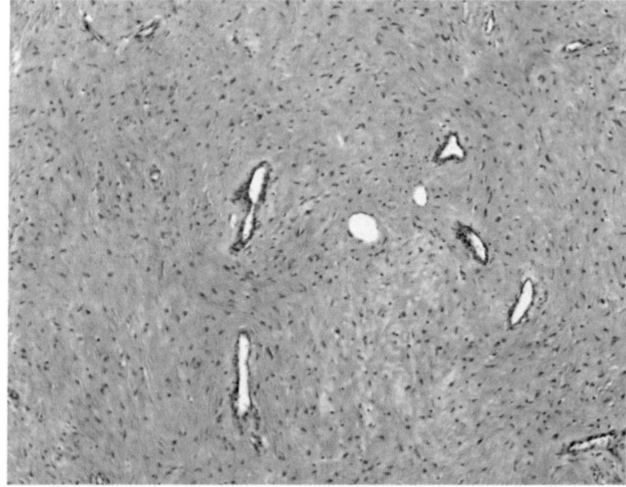

Figure 18.8 Uniform bland fibroblasts within a fibrillar collagen matrix, with several small vessels.

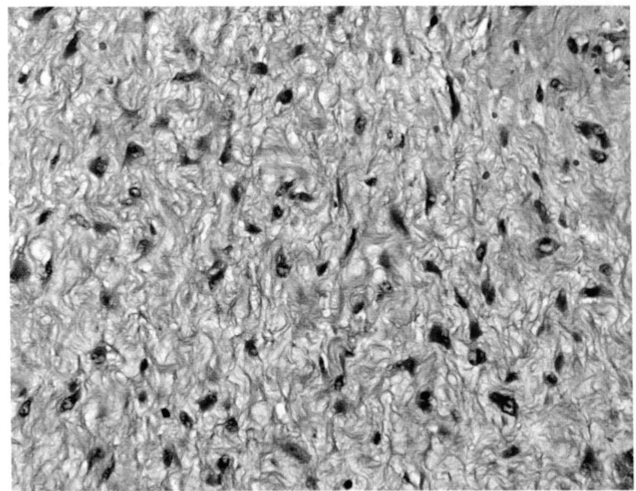

Figure 18.9 Higher power shows fibroblastic cells with bland nuclear features within a myxoid fibrillar stroma.

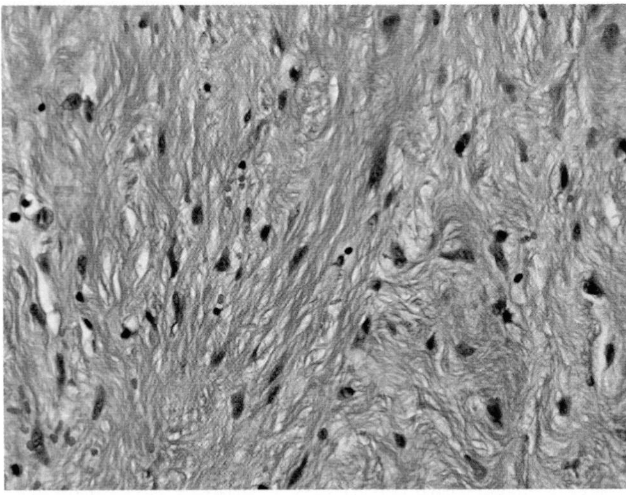

Figure 18.10 Higher power shows fibroblastic cells within a collagenous stroma.

19

Carcinoid Tumorlets

▶ Alvaro C. Laga
▶ Timothy Allen
▶ Philip T. Cagle

Carcinoid tumorlets are relatively common, generally incidental, pathologic findings. Although not typically identified grossly, carcinoid tumorlets have been described as gray-tan nodules measuring millimeters in size; 5 mm has been considered an arbitrary size for which carcinoid nodules should be termed *carcinoid tumors.* Carcinoid tumorlets may be seen in association with carcinoid tumors and/or neuroendocrine cell hyperplasia, and some schemes propose an evolution from neuroendocrine cell hyperplasia to tumorlet to carcinoid tumor. Differential diagnosis includes typical carcinoid, neuroendocrine cell hyperplasia, minute pulmonary meningothelial-like nodules (chemodectomas), small cell carcinoma, and lymphangitic metastases (see Chapter 10, Part 6 and Chapter 14, Part 4).

Histologic Features:

- Often peripheral and subpleural bronchiolocentric nodules with a fibrotic stroma containing neuroendocrine cells.
- Uniform cells with eosinophilic cytoplasm and oval to spindle-shaped nuclei with finely granular chromatin.

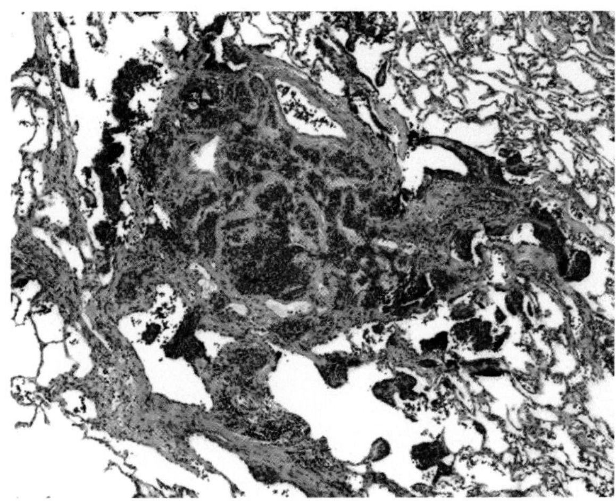

Figure 19.1 Lung parenchyma containing a carcinoid tumorlet composed of uniform cells with round to oval nuclei.

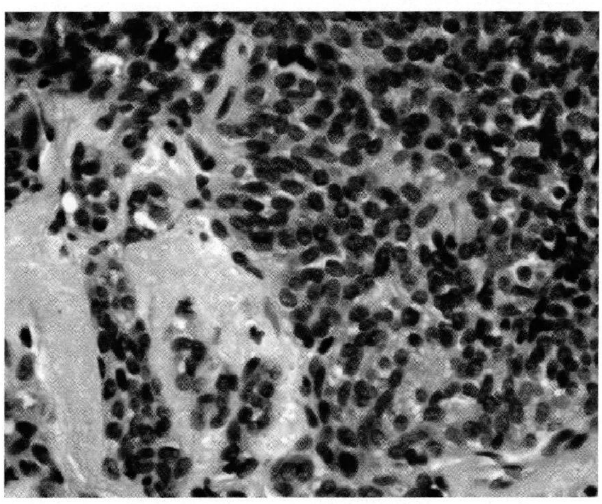

Figure 19.2 Higher power showing uniform cells with eosinophilic cytoplasm and round to spindled nuclei with finely granular chromatin.

20 Minute Meningothelial-Like Nodule (Chemodectoma)

▶ Alvaro C. Laga
▶ Timothy Allen
▶ Philip T. Cagle

Minute meningothelial-like nodules (MMLNs), previously called *chemodectomas*, are common, tiny, incidental interstitial nodular proliferations. MMLNs have diameters up to 1 to 3 mm. They may appear as grayish-tan nodules in the lung, including subpleurally. Both monoclonality and polyclonality have been demonstrated in MMLNs. It is not certain whether they are reactive or neoplastic, although investigators favor the former. Simultaneous occurrence of primary meningioma of the lung (see Chapter 24, Part 4, Subpart 4.5) and multiple MMLNs has been reported, and a possible pathogenetic relationship has been suggested. Differential diagnosis includes carcinoid tumorlet, metastatic carcinoma, interstitial fibrosis, and granuloma.

Histologic Features:

- Round or spindle-shaped cells in nests or "zellenballen" pattern, with eosinophilic and occasionally clear or vacuolated cytoplasm.
- Round to oval uniform nuclei, without "salt and pepper" features.
- Generally immunopositive for EMA and vimentin.
- Generally immunonegative for cytokeratin, S-100, NSE, actin, synaptophysin, and chromogranin A.
- Ultrastructurally resemble cells of meningiomas.

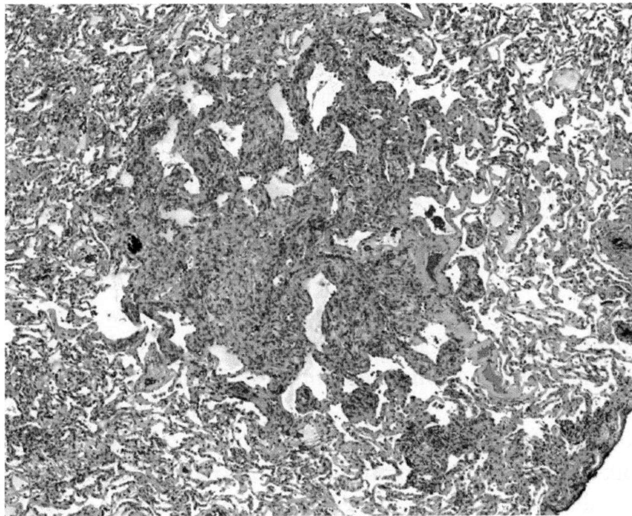

Figure 20.1 Subpleural MMLN shows localized proliferation of round to oval cells with eosinophilic cytoplasm.

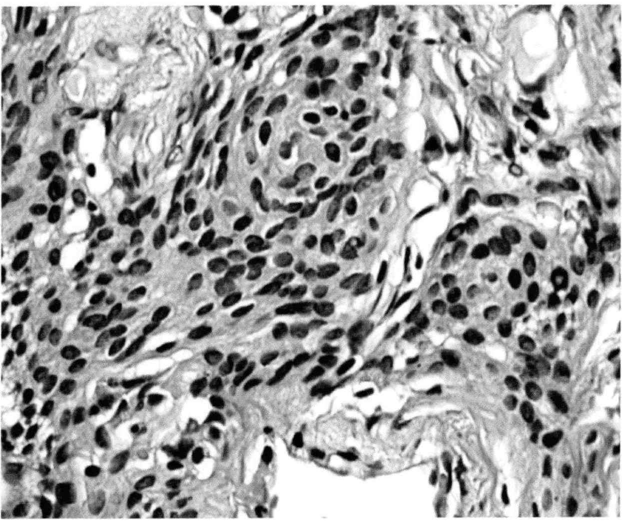

Figure 20.2 Higher power showing round to spindled cells in a "zellenballen" pattern, with bland nuclei.

- The solid pattern consists of sheets of round cells, with scattered cuboidal cells forming small tubules.
- The hemorrhagic pattern consists of large blood-filled spaces lined by epithelial cells or foci of hemorrhage with hemosiderin deposits, foamy macrophages, and cholesterol clefts sometimes surrounded by granulomatous and chronic inflammation.
- Round cells are immunopositive for TTF-1 and EMA and immunonegative for pan-cytokeratin.
- Surface cells are immunopositive for TTF-1, EMA, surfactant apoprotein A, and pan-cytokeratin.

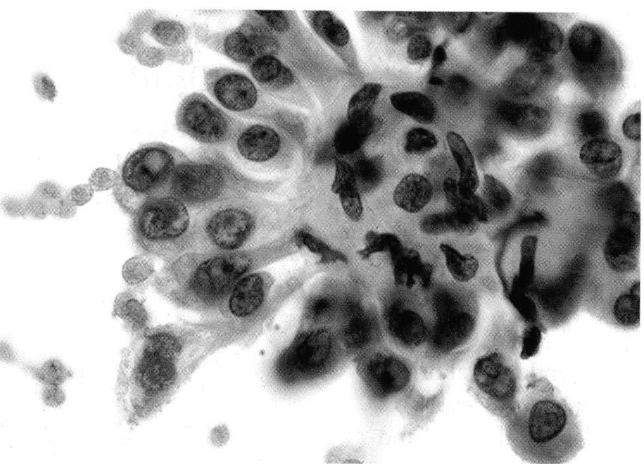

Figure 21.1 Cytology figure of sclerosing hemangioma showing loose fragment of cells with intranuclear cytoplasmic inclusion and surrounding red blood cells.

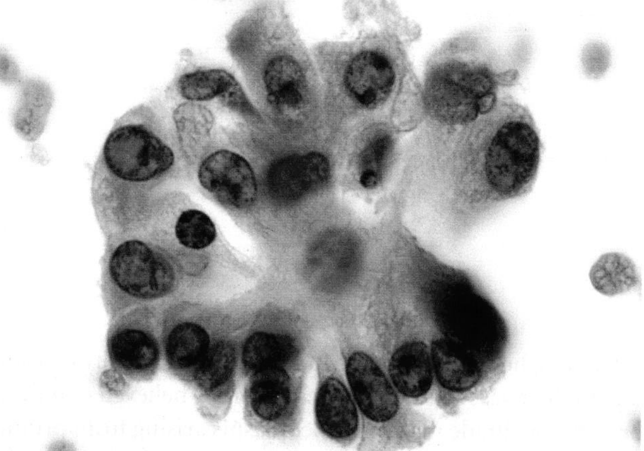

Figure 21.2 Cytology figure showing eccentric nuclei with evenly distributed finely granular chromatin and no obvious nucleoli.

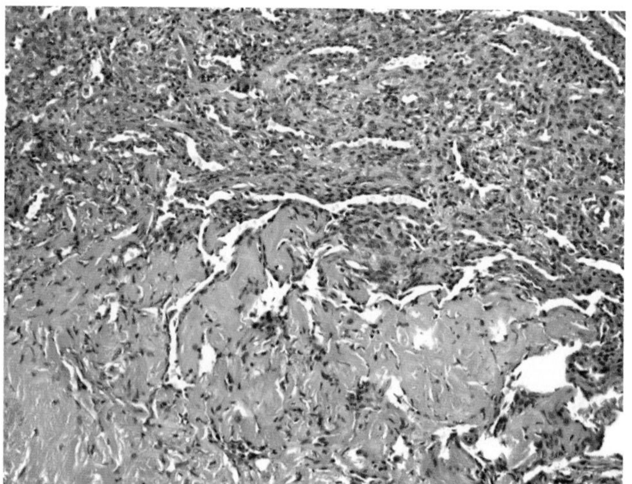

Figure 21.3 Sclerosing hemangioma with sclerosing pattern at *bottom*.

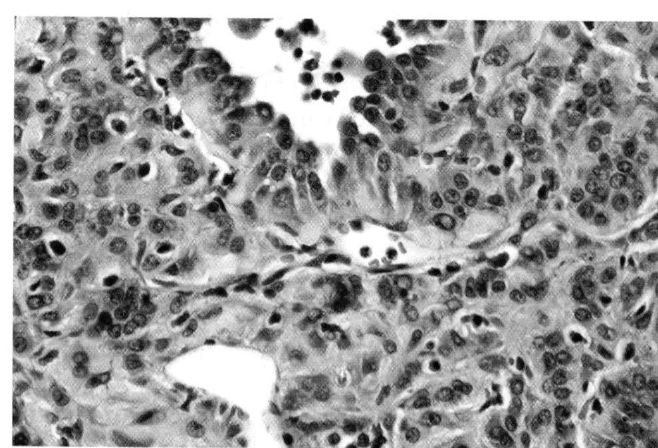

Figure 21.4 Higher power showing bland polygonal cells with round to oval nuclei and intranuclear cytoplasmic inclusions.

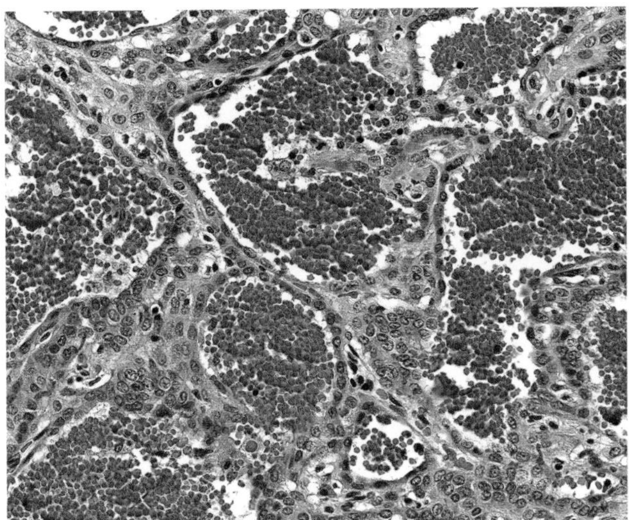

Figure 21.5 Hemorrhagic pattern with blood-filled spaces lined by epithelioid cells.

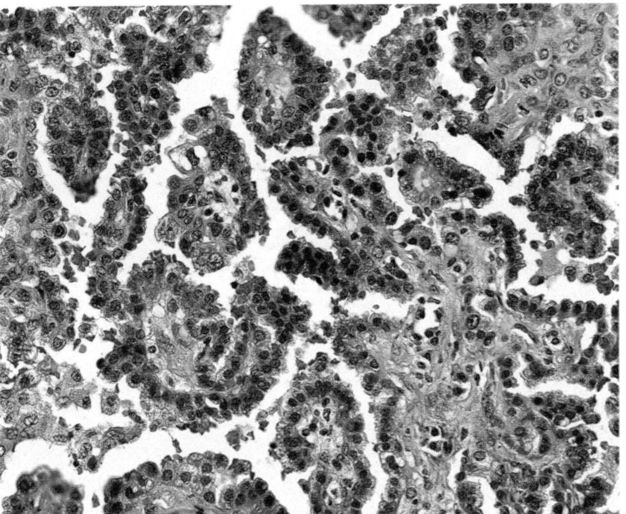

Figure 21.6 Papillary pattern has papillary projections lined by cuboidal surface cells.

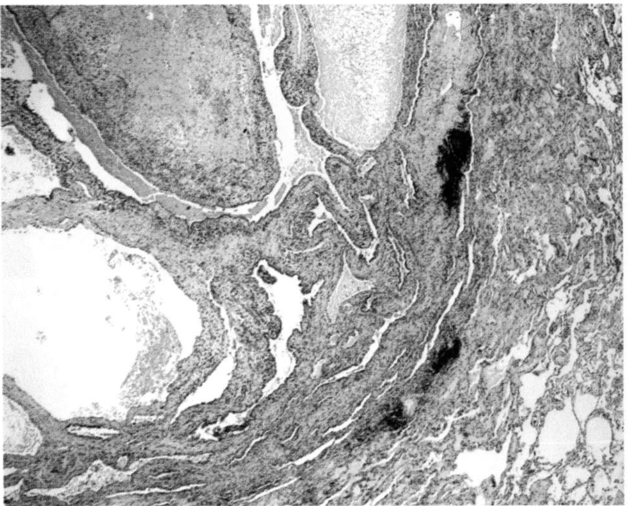

Figure 22.1 Alveolar adenoma with cystic spaces surrounded by intervening septa of variable thickness; cystic spaces are larger centrally.

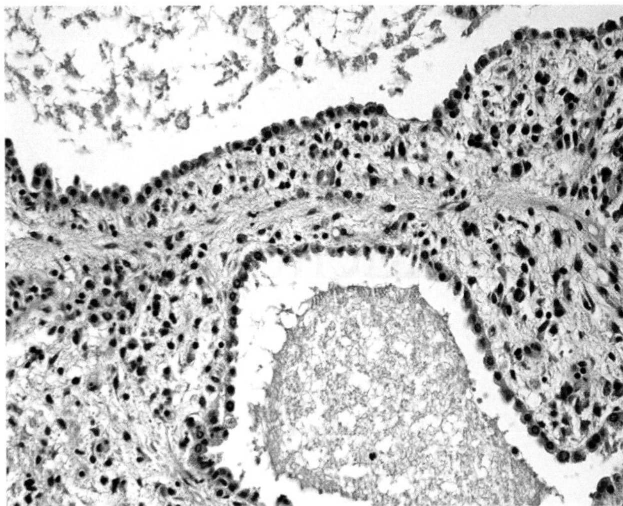

Figure 22.2 Higher power showing cuboidal to hobnail cells lining the cystic spaces.

Part 2

Papillary Adenoma

▶ Bruno Murer

Papillary adenomas are rare benign papillary neoplasms consisting of cells of type II cell origin, with Clara cells occasionally admixed. Papillary adenomas generally arise as 1- to 4-cm peripheral well-circumscribed solitary nodules.

Histologic Features:

- Usually well circumscribed tumors, but infiltrative growth has been reported.
- Papillary growth pattern sometimes mixed with solid areas.
- Branching papillae, with fibrous cores lined by bland cuboidal to columnar cells with round to oval nuclei containing fine chromatin.
- Occasional eosinophilic intranuclear inclusions.
- Mitoses, necrosis, and intracellular mucin are absent.
- Immunopositivity for cytokeratin, TTF-1, surfactant apoprotein, and CEA.

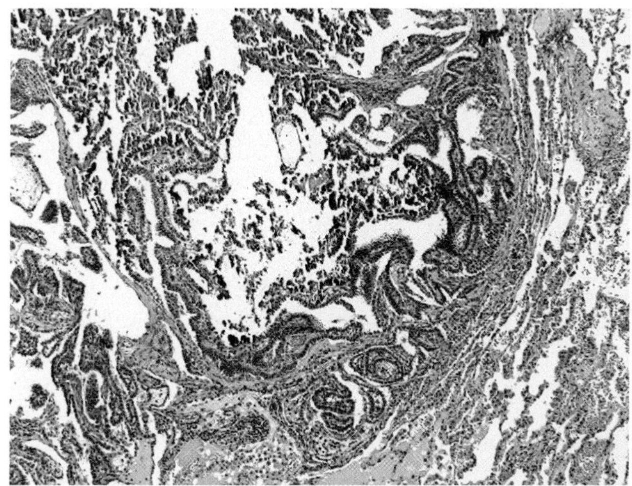

Figure 22.3 Well-circumscribed papillary adenoma compressing surrounding lung parenchyma.

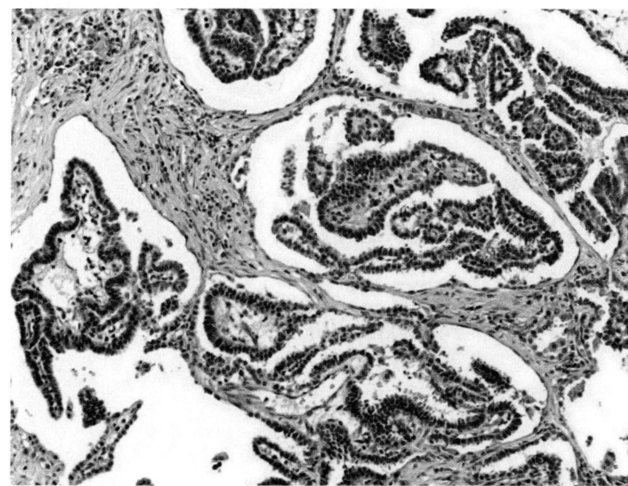

Figure 22.4 Medium power shows complex branching papillae lined by cuboidal to columnar cells and central fibrous cores.

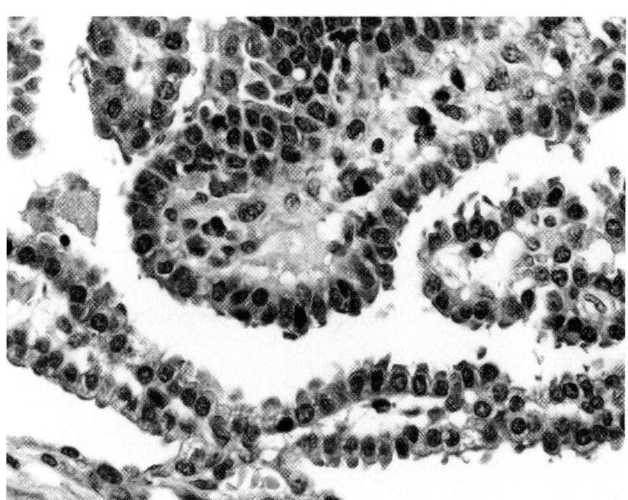

Figure 22.5 High power shows bland cuboidal cells with round to oval nuclei and fine chromatin lining fibrous cores.

Part 3

Mucinous Cystadenoma

▶ Alvaro C. Laga, Timothy Allen, and Philip T. Cagle

Mucinous cystadenomas are exceptionally rare benign tumors that typically arise as solitary nodules in adults. Differentiation from mucinous cystadenocarcinoma may be very difficult; however, histopathologic features of mucinous cystadenocarcinomas, including lepidic spread of the epithelium into the surrounding parenchyma, marked cytologic atypia, prominent pseudostratification of the lining epithelium, and mucus extravasation into surrounding tissue are absent in mucinous cystadenomas.

Histologic Features:

- Unilocular cysts with fibrous walls lined by well-differentiated columnar mucinous epithelium with hyperchromatic nuclei.
- The cysts contain abundant mucus.
- Mild nuclear atypia, focal cellular stratification, and rare mitoses may occur.
- Micropapillary fronds, necrosis, and severe cytologic atypia are absent.
- Foreign body giant cell reaction and chronic inflammation may be prominent around areas of denuded epithelium.

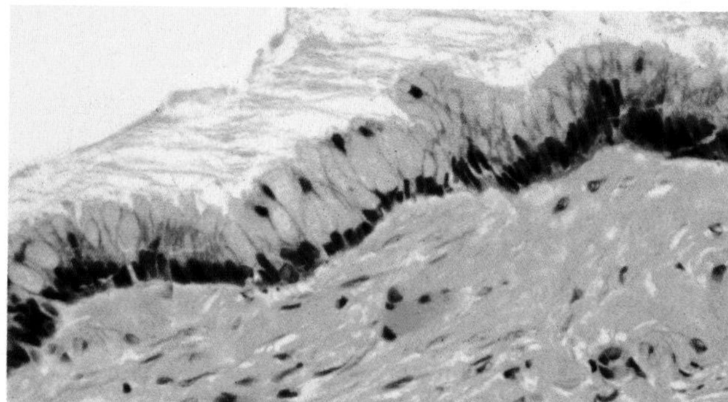

Figure 22.6 Cyst wall of mucinous cystadenoma lined by well-differentiated columnar mucinous epithelium with minimal atypia.

23 Seromucinous Gland Neoplasms

Seromucinous gland neoplasms are uncommon neoplasms that arise from the bronchial glands. They include true mucous gland adenomas as well as tumors similar to those found in the salivary glands.

Part 1

Mucous Gland Adenoma

▶ Bruno Murer

Mucous gland adenomas are extremely rare benign soft polypoid endobronchial tumors of the tracheobronchial seromucinous glands. Patients generally present with symptoms of airway obstruction, and radiographic studies demonstrate a coin lesion. Low-grade mucoepidermoid carcinoma may closely mimic mucous gland adenoma; however, unlike low-grade mucoepidermoid tumors, mucous gland adenomas do not contain an intermediate cell or squamous cell component.

Histologic Features:

- Mucous-filled cystic glands; nondilated microacini, glands, tubules, and papillae also may be seen.
- Cystic glands are lined by columnar to flattened mucus-secreting cells.
- Spindle cell stroma with occasional hyalinization and lymphoplasmacytic infiltrate.
- Oncocytic and clear cell change as well as focal ciliated epithelium may be seen.

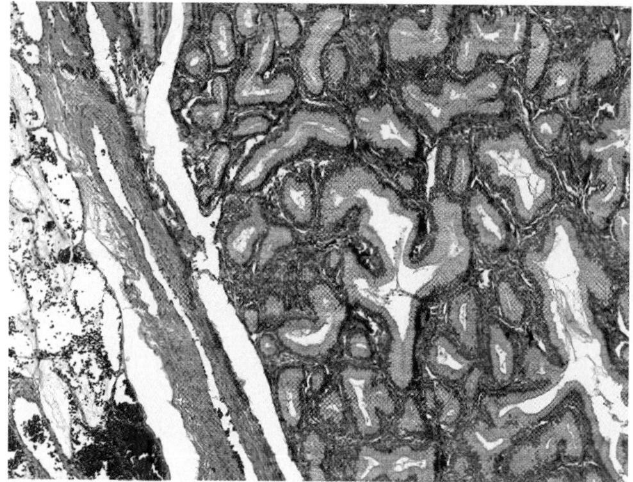

Figure 23.1 Low power of mucous gland adenoma showing a well-circumscribed lesion containing dilated and irregular glandular spaces, some of which contain mucin.

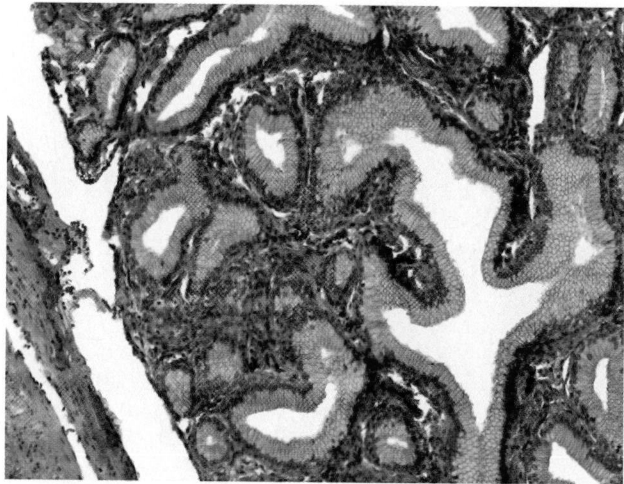

Figure 23.2 Higher power of mucous gland adenoma showing irregular glands lined by mucus-secreting cells.

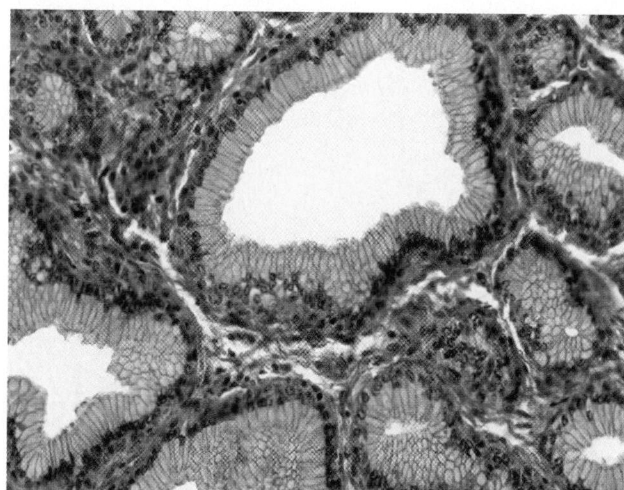

Figure 23.3 Glandular spaces lined by columnar cells with apical mucin and spindle cell stroma.

Part 2

Salivary Glandlike Tumors

Epithelial bronchial neoplasms that demonstrate submucosal seromucinous glandtype differentiation analogous to salivary gland neoplasms are uncommon. These include oncocytoma and pleomorphic adenoma, among others. Mucoepidermoid carcinoma and adenoid cystic carcinoma are illustrated in Chapter 10, Parts 14 and 15, respectively.

Subpart 2.1

Oncocytoma

▶ Alvaro C. Laga, Timothy Allen, Carlos Bedrossian, and Philip T. Cagle

Oncocytomas are benign epithelial endobronchial neoplasms that typically are 1- to 3-cm well-circumscribed soft exophytic nodules. The intensely eosinophilic granular appearance of the cytoplasm is due to increased numbers of mitochondria in the cytoplasm. Differential diagnosis includes oncocytic carcinoid, granular cell tumor, and acinic cell carcinoma.

Cytologic Features:

- Oncocytes both singly and in sheets, with distinct cell borders, round nuclei, and abundant red or green granular cytoplasm.

Histologic Features:

- Oncocytomas are composed of small nests of polygonal cells containing granular eosinophilic cytoplasm.
- Generally immunonegative for S-100.
- Ultrastructurally lack neurosecretory granules.

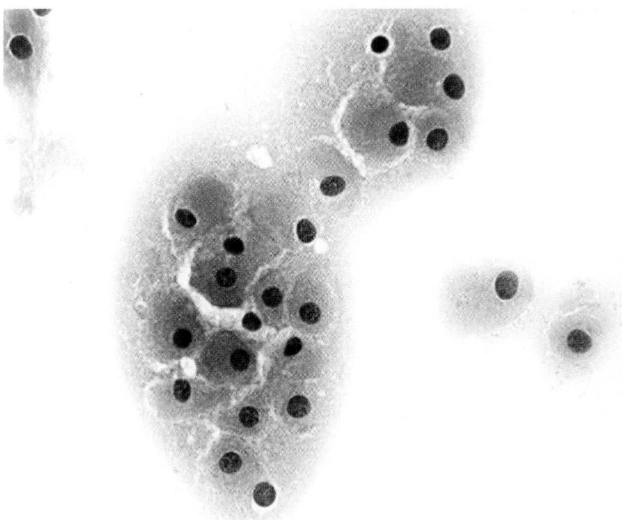

Figure 23.4 Cytology figure showing a cluster of oncocytes, with round nuclei and abundant granular cytoplasm.

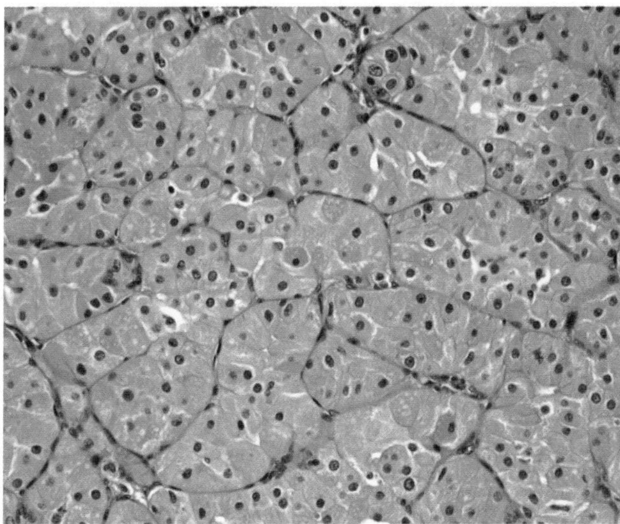

Figure 23.5 Nests of polygonal cells with granular eosinophilic cytoplasm and small round nuclei.

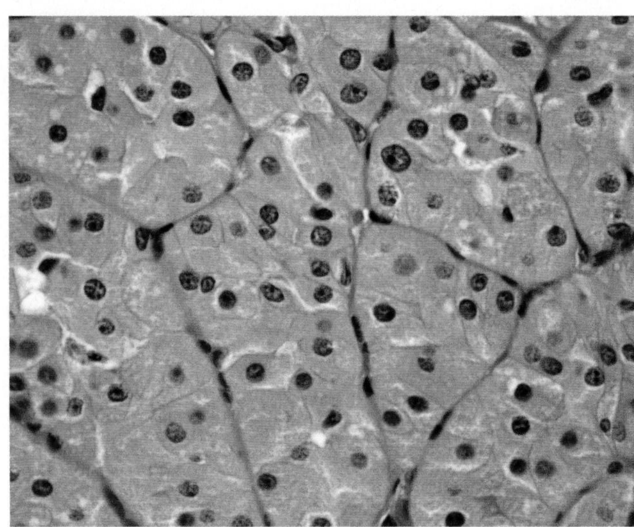

Figure 23.6 Higher power showing bland nuclear features and granular cytoplasm within a delicate fibrovascular stroma.

Subpart 2.2

Pleomorphic Adenoma

▶ Alvaro C. Laga, Timothy Allen, and Philip T. Cagle

Pleomorphic adenomas are benign neoplasms with mixed epithelial and mesenchymal components that may be endobronchial or intraparenchymal. Tumors are typically 2- to 16-cm soft to rubbery polypoid gray-white nodular masses. Endobronchial lesions are generally associated with a major or secondary bronchus and present with obstructive symptoms. Peripheral lesions are not intimately associated with airways and usually are an incidental finding on chest x-ray examination. Features including large size, poor circumscription, high mitotic rate, frankly malignant cytologic features, necrosis, and invasion indicate malignant behavior.

Histologic Features:

- Pulmonary pleomorphic adenomas are biphasic with mixed epithelial and mesenchymal elements; they do not often show either a prominent glandular component or prominent chondroid stroma.
- Sheets, trabeculae, or islands of epithelial and/or myoepithelial cells in a myxoid matrix.
- When present, ducts consist of an outer layer of myoepithelial cells and an inner layer of epithelial cells with scant periodic acid–Schiff-positive material.

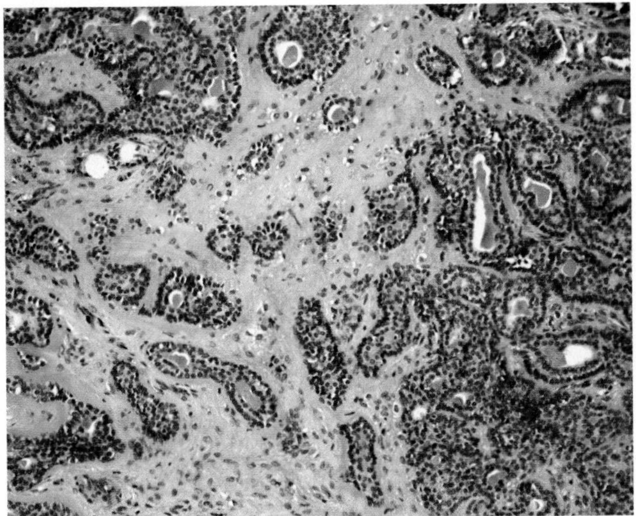

Figure 23.7 Pleomorphic adenoma with branching ductal structures in a myxoid stroma.

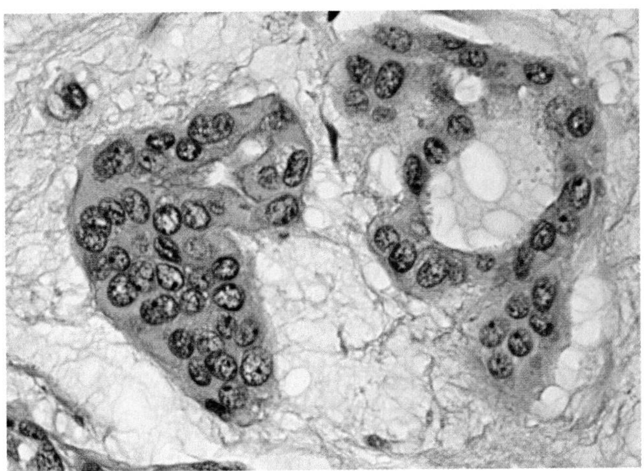

Figure 23.8 Higher power of pleomorphic adenoma showing columnar cells lining the ductal structures.

24 Rare Mesenchymal Tumors

Mesenchymal neoplasms including leiomyoma, lipoma, chondroma, and a variety of neural tumors rarely occur as primary lung neoplasms. Their histopathologic features are similar to those of the same tumors in other locations.

Part 1

Leiomyoma

▶ Donna Coffey

Leiomyomas primary to the lung are rare endobronchial or parenchymal neoplasms. Endobronchial leiomyomas may present with obstructive symptoms. Differential diagnosis includes hamartomas, low-grade leiomyosarcomas (primary and metastatic), spindle cell carcinoid, and solitary fibrous tumor.

Histologic Features:

- Leiomyomas are composed of intersecting bundles of smooth muscle.
- Generally immunopositive for desmin and actin.

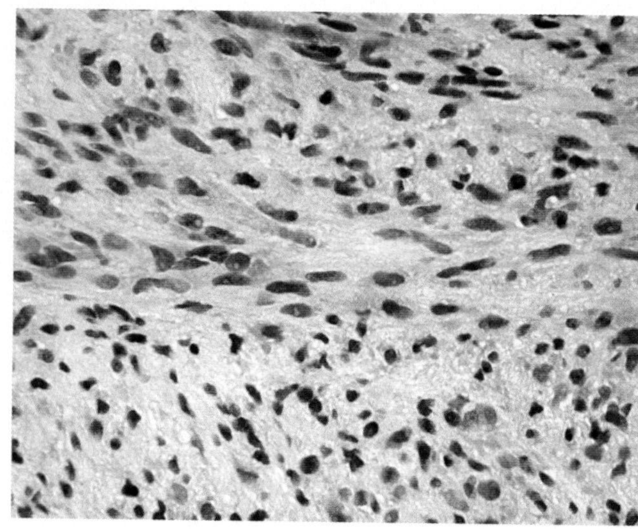

Figure 24.1 Leiomyoma with bundles of smooth muscle cells.

Part 2

Lipoma

▶ Alvaro C. Laga, Timothy Allen, and Philip T. Cagle

Pulmonary lipomas are rare predominantly endobronchial neoplasms that may, due to their polypoid nature, occlude the bronchial lumen. Differential diagnosis includes lipomatous hamartoma.

Histologic Features:

- Lipomas consist of mature adipose tissue.

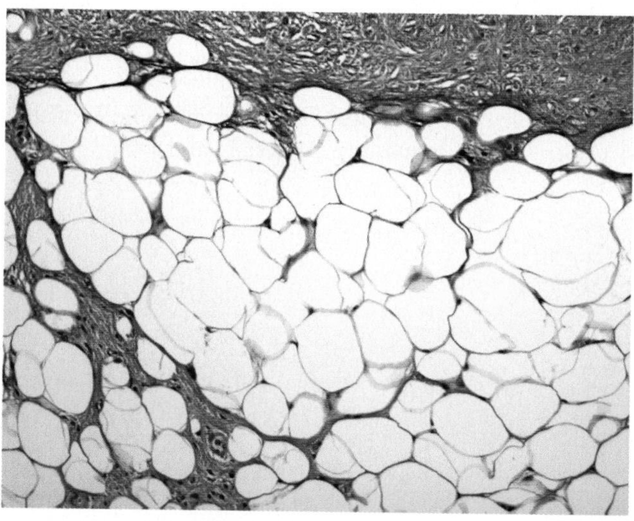

Figure 24.2 Pulmonary lipoma consisting of mature adipose tissue.

Part 3

Chondroma

▶ Helmut Popper

Chondromas are benign tumors composed of hyaline cartilage. They have been reported in association with the Carney triad, which consists of gastric stroma sarcoma, paraganglioma, and pulmonary chondroma. They are generally asymptomatic and may present radiologically with "popcorn" calcification.

Histologic Features:

- Well-defined lobular masses composed of hypocellular hyaline cartilage.
- No features of malignancy.
- Components of hamartoma such as adipose tissue and entrapped respiratory epithelium are absent.

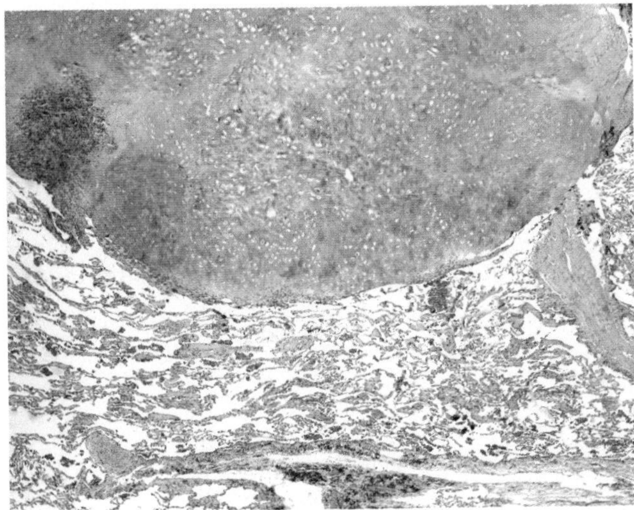

Figure 24.3 Chondroma of the lung shows cartilage lacking adipose tissue, entrapped respiratory epithelium, or other components of a hamartoma.

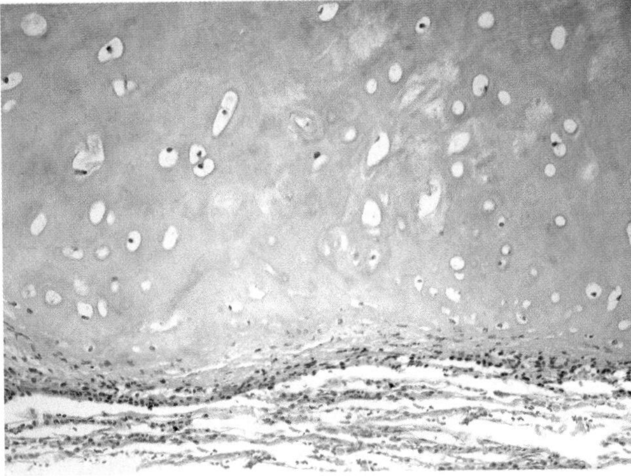

Figure 24.4 Higher power of benign cartilage with no invasion of surrounding compressed lung tissue.

Part 4

Neural and Related Tumors

Primary pulmonary neural neoplasms include granular cell tumor, Schwannoma, neurofibroma, and ganglioneuroma. All of these are very rare as lung primaries. Meningioma primary in the lung is extremely rare, although minute meningothelial-like nodules (see Chapter 20) are common by comparison. Rarely meningioma may metastasize to the lung. All of these tumors exhibit the same histopathology as neural and related tumors in other locations.

Subpart 4.1

Granular Cell Tumor

▸ Alvaro C. Laga, Timothy Allen, Carlos Bedrossian, Philip T. Cagle, and Roberto Barrios

Granular cell tumors are very rare mesenchymal neoplasms believed to be of Schwann cell origin. Most are incidental findings in young to middle-aged adults. They average about 1 cm in diameter, and most are endobronchial neoplasms, often situated near points of bifurcation. They may exhibit a papillary or a smooth endobronchial surface.

Cytologic Features:

- Polygonal epithelioid cells with abundant granular cytoplasm and small uniform nuclei.

Histologic Features:

- Circumscribed, but may be locally infiltrative.
- Round to oval and spindled tumor cells contain abundant periodic acid–Schiff (PAS)-positive eosinophilic cytoplasm.
- Nuclei are small, with finely granular chromatin and occasional small nucleoli.

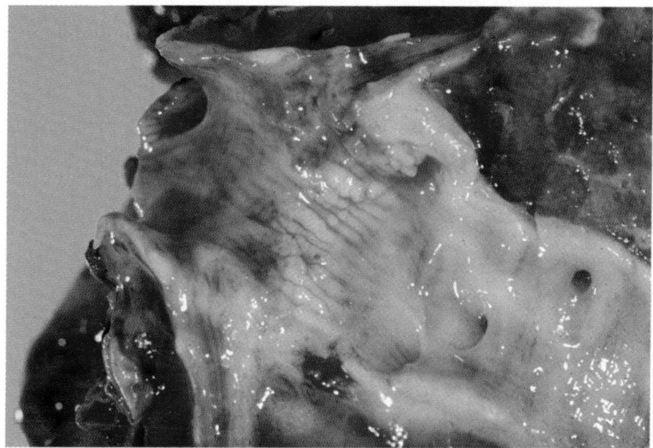

Figure 24.5 Gross figure of granular cell tumor showing papillary endobronchial tumor near bifurcation.

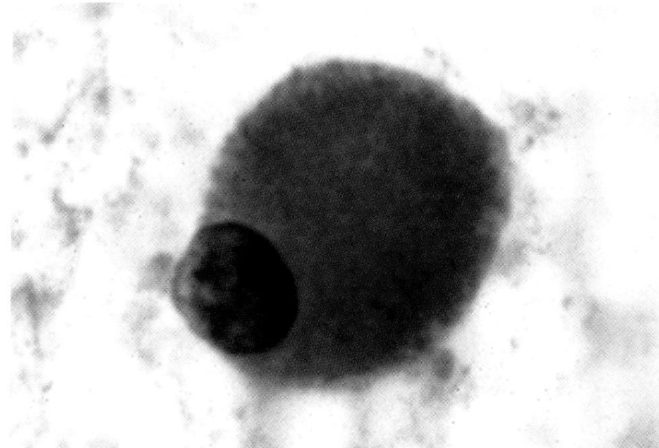

Figure 24.6 Cytology figure showing granular cell with abundant granular cytoplasm and small nucleus.

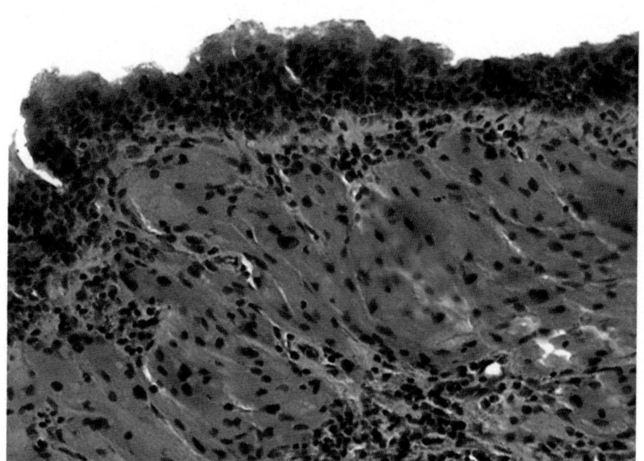

Figure 24.7 Endobronchial granular cell tumor with granular tumor cells underlying bronchial mucosa.

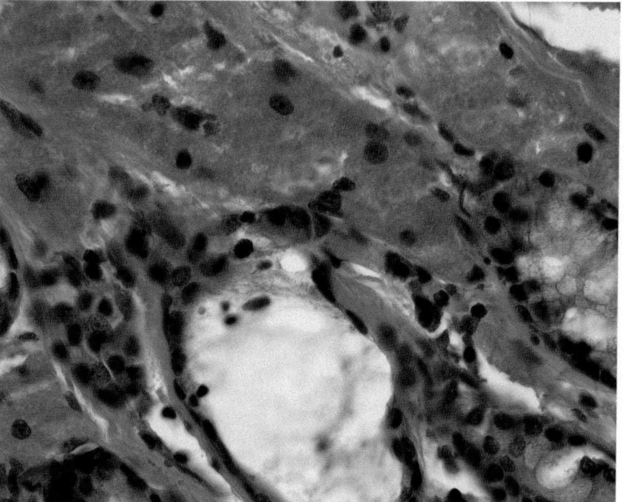

Figure 24.8 Higher power of endobronchial granular cell tumor showing eosinophilic cytoplasm and small central nuclei.

Subpart 4.2

Schwannoma

▶ Alvaro C. Laga, Timothy Allen, and Philip T. Cagle

Schwannomas are rare primary pulmonary neoplasms that histologically and immunohistochemically resemble extrapulmonary Schwannomas. They generally occur as asymptomatic solitary masses, except for endobronchial tumors, which may cause obstructive symptoms.

Histologic Features:

- Schwannomas show a mixture of Antoni A and Antoni B growth patterns.
- Antoni A growth pattern consists of elongated spindle cells arranged in dense palisades of elongated spindle-shaped nuclei, with zones of cytoplasmic processes without nuclei, termed *Verocay bodies.*
- Antoni B growth pattern consists of less dense cellularity with loosely arranged cells with microcysts and myxoid change.
- Generally immunopositive for S-100.

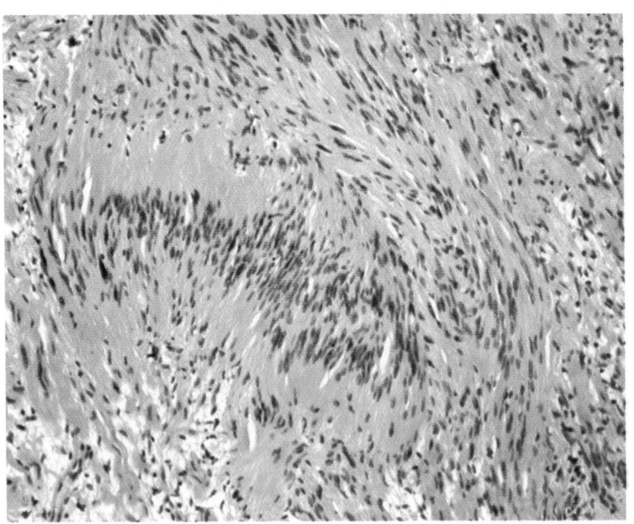

Figure 24.9 Schwannoma with Antoni A growth pattern.

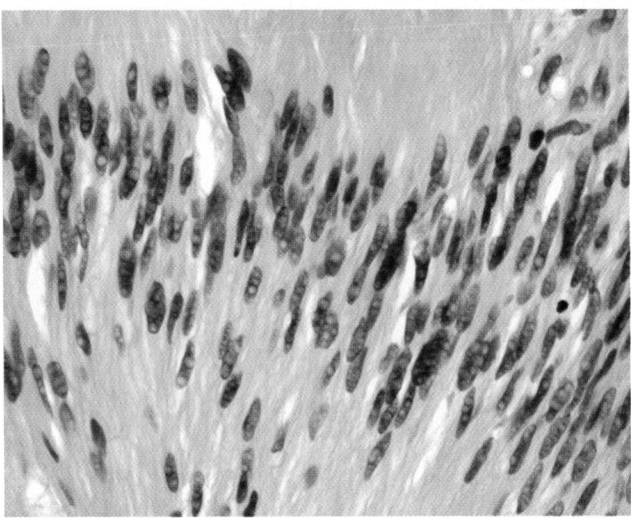

Figure 24.10 Higher power of Antoni A growth pattern with Verocay body.

Subpart 4.3

Neurofibroma

▸ Alvaro C. Laga, Timothy Allen, and Philip T. Cagle

Neurofibromas occur rarely in the lung in association with neurofibromatosis as single or multiple pulmonary lesions.

Histologic Features:

- Loose myxoid stroma with low cellularity.
- Mixture of Schwann cells with elongated nuclei and pink cytoplasmic extensions, large fibroblastic cells, and scattered inflammatory cells.

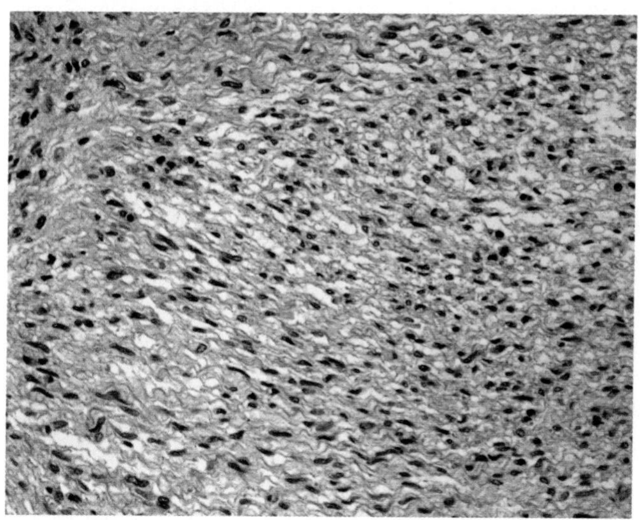

Figure 24.11 Neurofibroma shows a proliferation of cells with elongated wavy nuclei within a myxoid stroma.

Subpart 4.4

Ganglioneuroma

▶ Alvaro C. Laga, Timothy Allen, and Philip T. Cagle

Ganglioneuromas are rare benign neoplasms that arise from the sympathetic nervous system, most often in the posterior mediastinum. Primary pulmonary ganglioneuromas are extremely rare.

Histologic Features:

- Ganglioneuromas contain mature ganglion cells within a loose neurofibroblastic stroma, with variable amounts of intervening collagen.

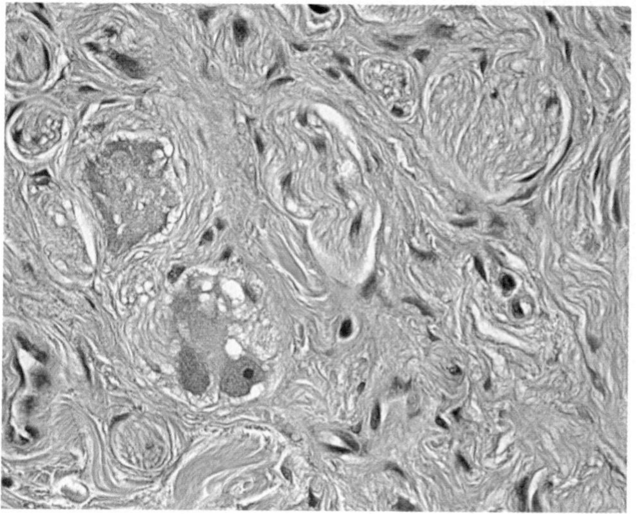

Figure 24.12 Ganglioneuroma with ganglion cells within a loose stroma.

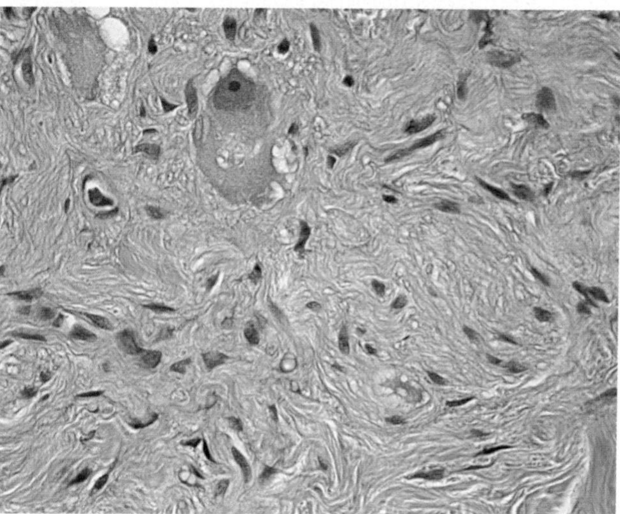

Figure 24.13 Ganglioneuroma with ganglion cells within a loose stroma.

Subpart 4.5

Meningioma

▶ Alvaro C. Laga, Timothy Allen, and Philip T. Cagle

Meningiomas may very rarely occur in the lung as metastases or extremely rarely as primary pulmonary neoplasms. Primary pulmonary meningiomas generally occur in adults and typically are asymptomatic. A careful examination to exclude primary meningioma of the meninges should be performed before proposing a primary origin in the lung. A case of primary pulmonary meningioma in association with multiple minute meningothelial-like nodules (see Chapter 20) has been reported and suggested to indicate a possible pathogenetic relationship.

Histologic Features:

- The histologic features of meningiomas in the lung are similar to those of primary central nervous system meningiomas, with whorls of meningothelial cells and sometimes psammoma bodies.

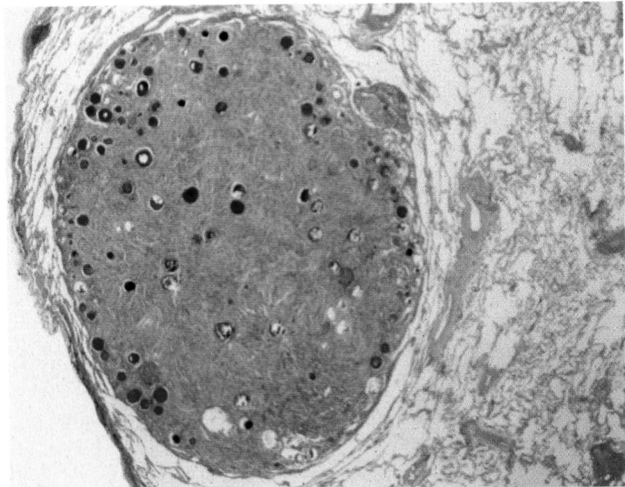

Figure 24.14 Low power of oval subpleural mass consists of meningioma with psammoma bodies within lung parenchyma.

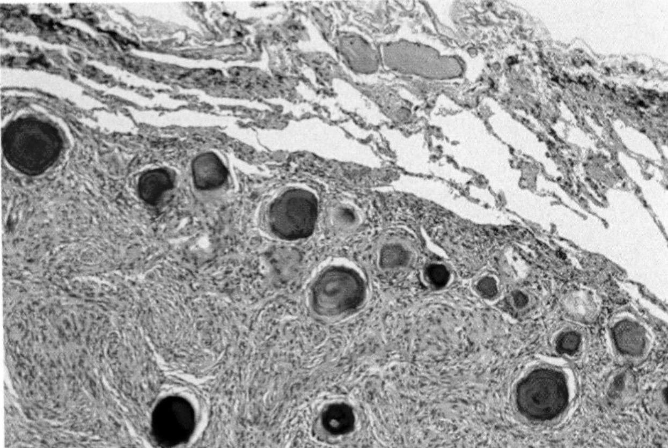

Figure 24.15 Whorls of meningioma cells and psammoma bodies with lung parenchyma adjacent to the meningioma.

Lymphangioleiomyomatosis

25

▸ Jaishree Jagirdar

Lymphangioleiomyomatosis (LAM) is a rare interstitial lung disease that typically occurs in women of childbearing age. It is characterized by widespread abnormal proliferation of smooth muscle in the lung, mediastinal and retroperitoneal lymph nodes, and the major lymphatic ducts. It rarely occurs in males. Approximately 30% of patients with tuberous sclerosis (TS) have LAM. Patients present with shortness of breath, cough, and recurrent pneumothorax. Chylothorax is present in 70% of cases of LAM. Angiomyolipomas may precede pulmonary manifestations and are present in about half of patients. Spirometry usually shows normal lung volumes in contrast to abnormally large lungs due to air trapping on chest x-ray examination.

Most patients with LAM die of progressive respiratory failure within 10 years. Hormonal manipulation has yielded mixed results. Lung transplantation has been used successfully, although recurrence of LAM may occur. The cells in the recurrence are of recipient origin.

Pathogenesis is unknown. Cyst formation in LAM may be from uninhibited action of matrix metalloproteinases (MMP-2 and MMP-9), which are capable of degrading both elastic tissue and collagen. The proliferative and invasive nature of LAM cells may be due, in part, to somatic mutations in the *TSC*-1 and *TSC*-2 genes on chromosomes 9q34 and 16p13, respectively. The abnormal smooth muscle cell in LAM may be related to the perivascular epithelioid clear cell. These cells give rise to a variety of tumors, such as angiomyolipomas, which are seen in LAM and are HMB-45 positive.

Grossly the lungs are diffusely enlarged with extensive cystic changes resembling honeycomb lung.

Histologic Features:

- Cystic spaces lined by variable number of haphazardly arranged spindle cells representing smooth muscle cells.
- Smooth muscle proliferation is around bronchioles, lymphatics, vessels, pleura, and interlobular septa.
- HMB-45 is positive and can be used to eliminate other causes of spontaneous pneumothorax.

	LAM	**TS**
1. Angiomyolipoma	47%–57%	80%
2. Sex	F	M
3. Cerebral involvement	55%	
4. Adenoma sebaceum	84%	
5. Chylothorax	70%	Rare
6. LAM	Yes	50%
7. MMPH	Not studied	Yes

MMPH, multifocal micronodular pneumocyte hyperplasia.

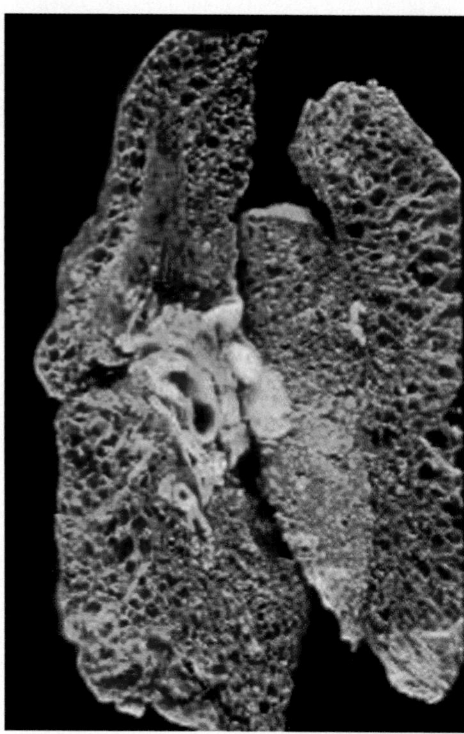

Figure 25.1 Gross figure of large lungs with a uniform distribution of cysts in upper and lower lobes and a beefy color.

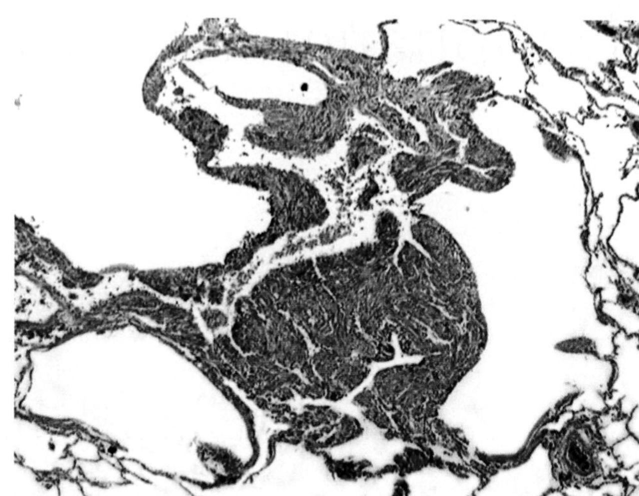

Figure 25.2 Cystic lymphatic space with smooth muscle proliferation.

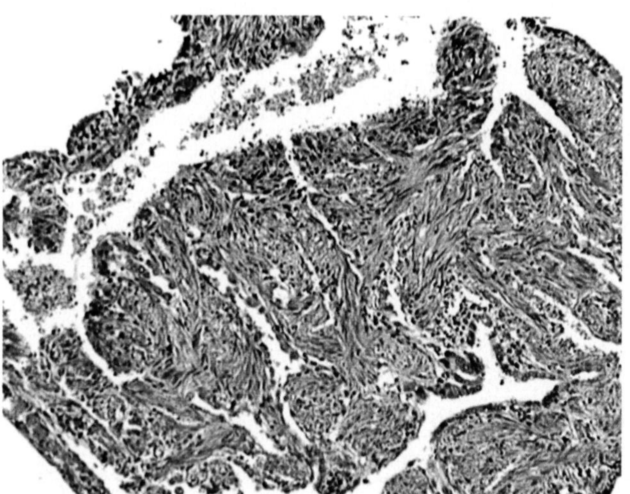

Figure 25.3 Haphazardly arranged abnormal smooth muscle.

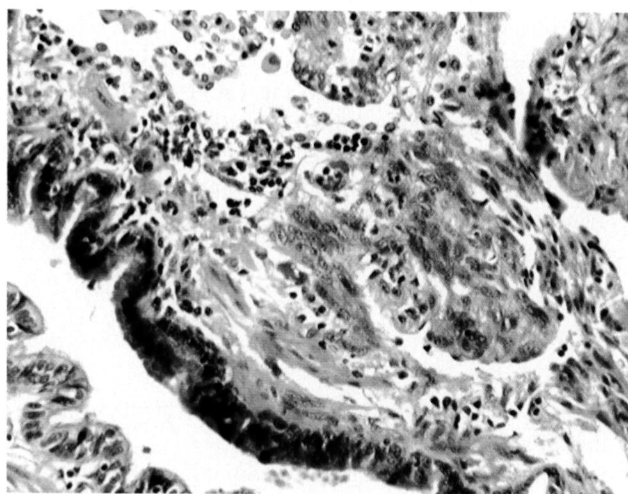

Figure 25.4 Higher power showing haphazardly arranged spindle cells beneath bronchiolar mucosa.

Part 1

Multifocal Micronodular Pneumocyte Hyperplasia

▶ Andras Khoor

Pulmonary manifestations of tuberous sclerosis include lymphangioleiomyomatosis and multifocal micronodular pneumocyte hyperplasia. The latter is a rare hamartomatous proliferation of type II cells, which can occur in both men and women.

Histologic Features:

- Multiple well-demarcated nodules are seen, which usually measure a few millimeters in greatest dimension but may be larger than 1 cm.
- The nodules are produced by proliferation of enlarged but cytologically benign type II cells along the alveolar septa.
- Proliferating type II cells are immunoreactive for keratin, epithelial membrane antigen, and various surfactant proteins and are negative for HMB-45.

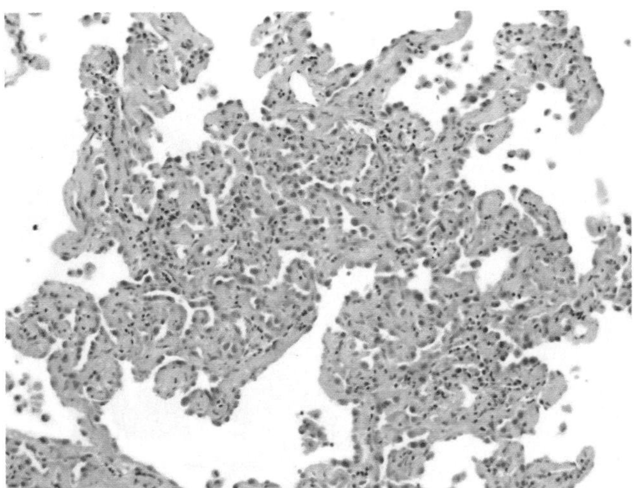

Figure 25.5 Medium power shows a well-demarcated nodule of multifocal micronodular pneumocyte hyperplasia.

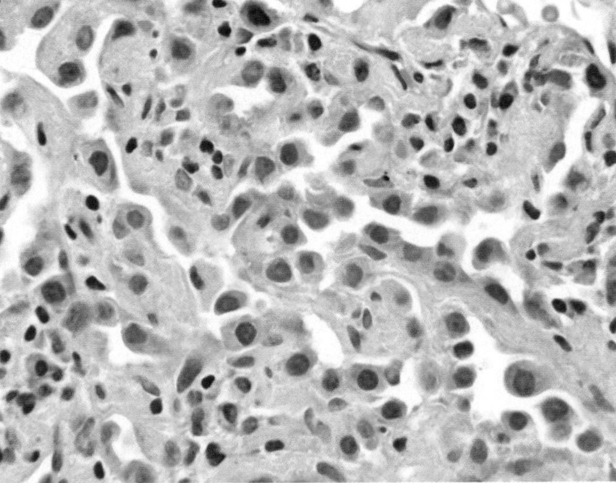

Figure 25.6 Higher power of the nodule shows enlarged type II cells.

Part 2

Clear Cell Tumor ("Sugar Tumor")

▶ Alvaro C. Laga and Roberto Barrios

Benign clear cell tumor of the lung is a rare benign primary pulmonary neoplasm, also called *sugar tumor* because of the high glycogen content of the cytoplasm of tumor cells. This neoplasm is believed to derive from the perivascular epithelioid cell (PEC), so these neoplasms have also been designated *PEComas.* They usually present as an incidental asymptomatic solitary coin lesion. Grossly, they are well-circumscribed masses with tan surfaces on sectioning. A rare association with tuberous sclerosis and other HMB-45–positive lesions (lymphangioleiomyomatosis and angiomyolipoma) has been noted.

Histologic Features:

- Rounded or oval cells with distinct cell borders and clear or eosinophilic cytoplasm.
- Strong diastase-sensitive periodic acid–Schiff positivity from glycogen-rich cytoplasm.
- Nucleoli may be prominent, but mitoses are usually absent.
- Thin-walled blood vessels without a muscular coat are characteristic.
- Abundant cytoplasmic glycogen is a characteristic ultrastructural feature, and melanosomes have been reported.
- Clear cell tumors show positive immunostaining for HMB-45.

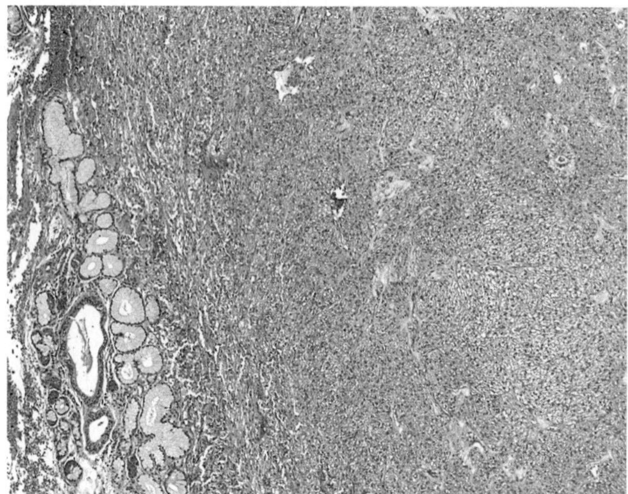

Figure 25.7 Low power shows a monotonous proliferation of cells abutting adjacent bronchial mucus glands.

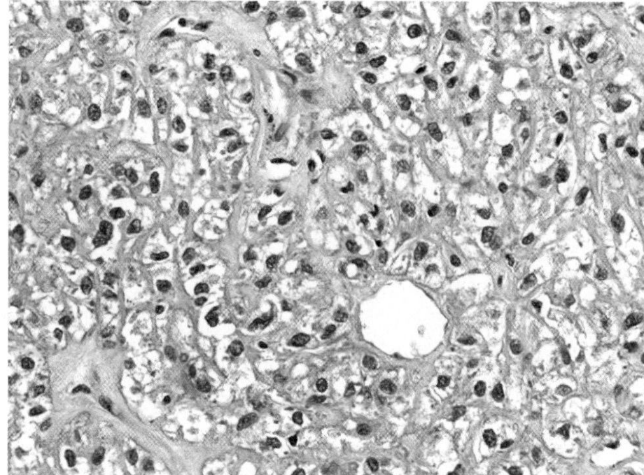

Figure 25.8 Cells with clear to eosinophilic cytoplasm and a central thin-walled blood vessel.

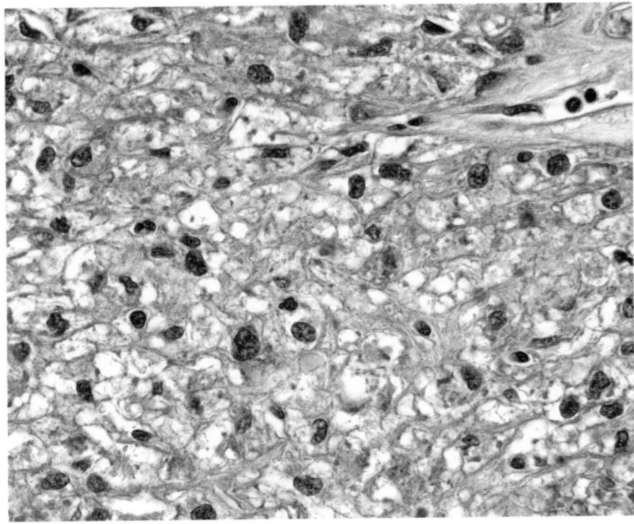

Figure 25.9 Higher power shows cells with clear to eosinophilic cytoplasm and mild nuclear atypia.

Pulmonary and Pleural Lymphangiomatosis

26

▶ Dani S. Zander

Lymphangiomatosis is a rare developmental abnormality of the lymphatics. The condition can be isolated to the lungs and pleura, but more commonly it involves other sites as well, particularly bones. It is usually diagnosed by age 20 years. Chylous pleural effusion is common and, when coexisting lytic bone lesions are present, should prompt consideration of this disorder. Radiographic studies reveal bilateral interstitial infiltrates that represent thickened interlobular septa and bronchovascular bundles, and pleural effusions. Hilar and mediastinal involvement is common. The disease progresses over time, leading to compression of adjacent structures and problems with continuing accumulation of chylous effusions.

Histologic Features:

- Anastomosing lymphatic channels of varying size and shape lined by flattened endothelial cells, expanding bronchovascular bundles, and interlobular septa and pleura.
- Bundles of spindle cells and collagen accompany lymphatic channels.
- Adjacent lung may show hemosiderin-laden macrophages in alveoli but does not manifest the cystic changes or smooth muscle cell proliferations typical of lymphangioleiomyomatosis.
- Immunohistochemistry for factor VIII-related antigen and CD31 highlights the endothelial cells.
- Differential diagnosis includes lymphangioma (solitary), lymphangiectasis, lymphangioleiomyomatosis, and Kaposi sarcoma.

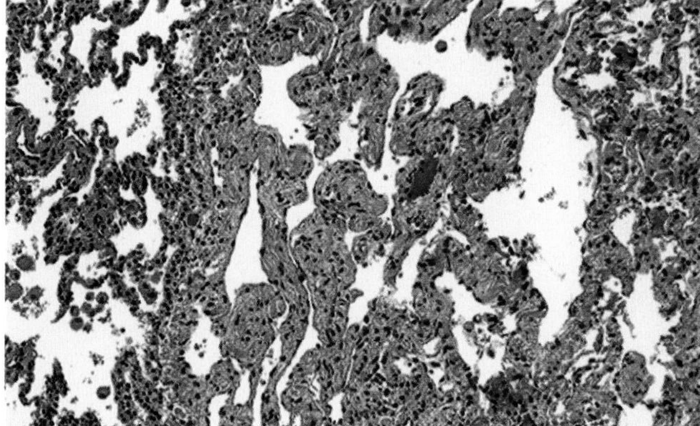

Figure 26.1 Histology. Anastomosing vascular channels lined by flattened endothelial cells and separated by collagenous stroma thicken the pleura.

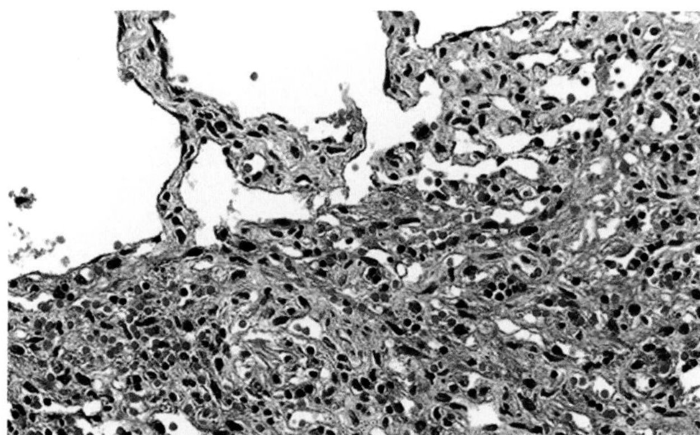

Figure 26.2 Histology. Large vascular channels with a flat endothelial cell lining lie on the *upper left,* and smaller channels lie *below* and to the *right,* separated by collagenous stroma with a small number of lymphocytes and red blood cells.

27 Glomus Tumor

▸ Donna Coffey

Glomus tumors are benign neoplasms derived from cells of the neuromyoarterial glomus or glomus body (malignant variants of this tumor [glomangiosarcomas] are discussed in Chapter 11, Part 16). Pulmonary glomus tumors are very rare and generally occur in middle-aged men. Approximately two thirds of patients are asymptomatic. Pulmonary glomus tumors may be peripheral or central and are generally well-circumscribed gray-tan masses. Differential diagnosis includes carcinoid tumor, hemangiopericytoma, smooth muscle tumors, paraganglioma, and primitive neuroectodermal tumors.

Histologic Features:

- Medium-sized to small cells in a monotonous pattern with round to oval nuclei.
- Nucleoli are inconspicuous.
- Variable cell borders, some distinct, yielding a "chicken wire" pattern.
- Rare mitotic figures.
- Generally immunopositive for vimentin, actin, and collagen type IV.
- Generally immunonegative for neuroendocrine markers.

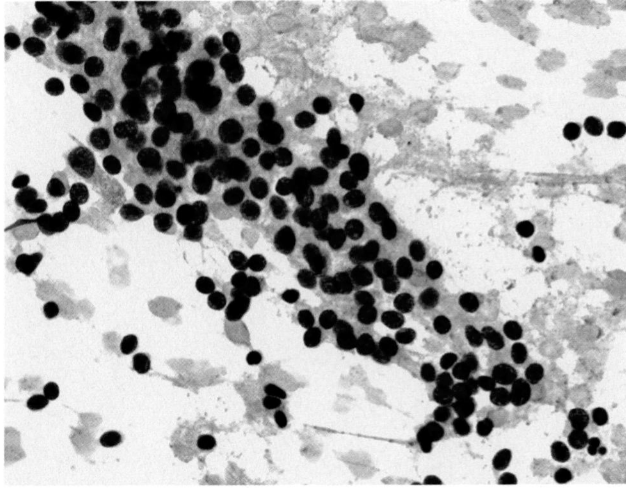

Figure 27.1 Cytology figure showing small to medium-sized cells with round to oval nuclei and inconspicuous nucleoli, and without mitotic figures.

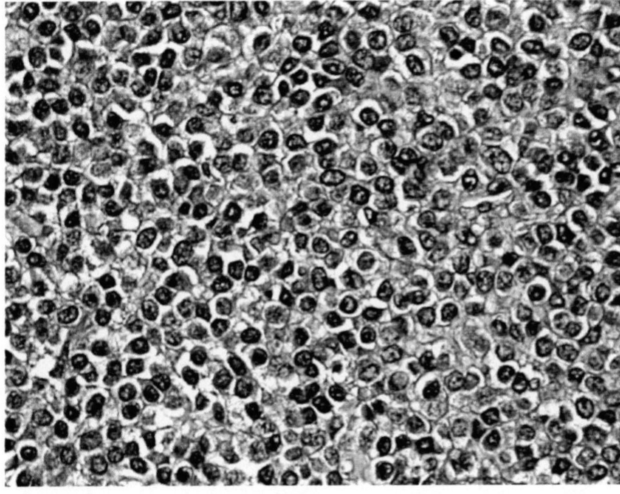

Figure 27.2 Glomus tumor with monotonous small to medium-sized cells lying in a "chicken wire" pattern.

28 Giant Cell Tumor

▸ Alvaro C. Laga
▸ Timothy Allen
▸ Philip T. Cagle

Primary giant cell tumor (GCT) of the lung, a tumor histologically resembling giant cell tumor of the bone, is extremely rare—only a few cases have been reported in the literature. In addition to the lung, primary GCT has rarely been reported in other extraosseous tissues, including pancreas, thyroid, skin, and soft tissue. In a series of five cases, including the case illustrated here, three occurred in men and two in women (age range 43–79 years, average 67 years). Prognosis was good with long survival, even in a patient with subsequent resected metastatic disease.

Histologic Features:

- Large numbers of multinucleated osteoclast-like giant cells interspersed frequently throughout the stroma.
- Stroma consists of spindle to oval cells with nuclei similar to those in multinucleated giant cells.
- Mitoses may be frequent.
- Sarcomatous foci may be present.
- Generally immunopositive for vimentin and CD68.
- Generally immunonegative for keratin.

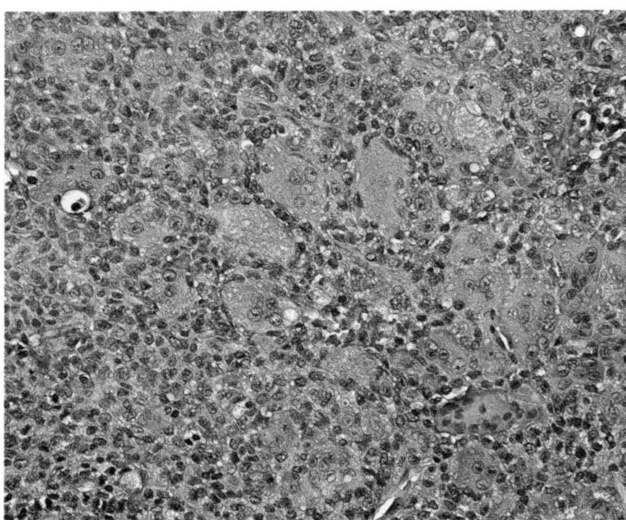

Figure 28.1 Multinucleated giant cells with scattered blood vessels and mononuclear stromal cells in this primary pulmonary GCT.

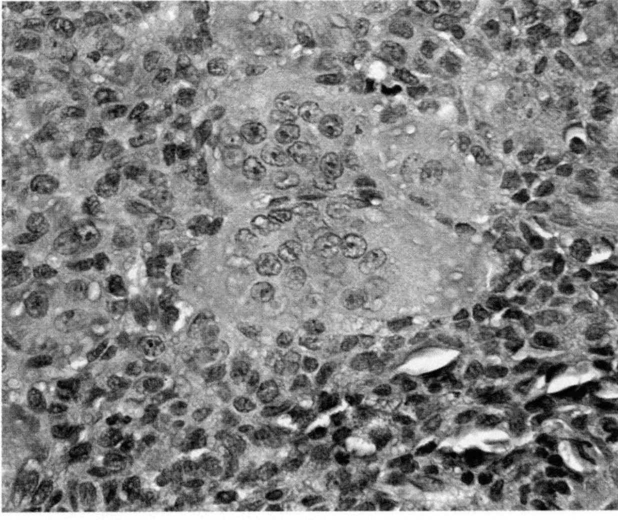

Figure 28.2 Higher power shows large numbers of nuclei within each giant cell.

Section 5

Histiocytoses

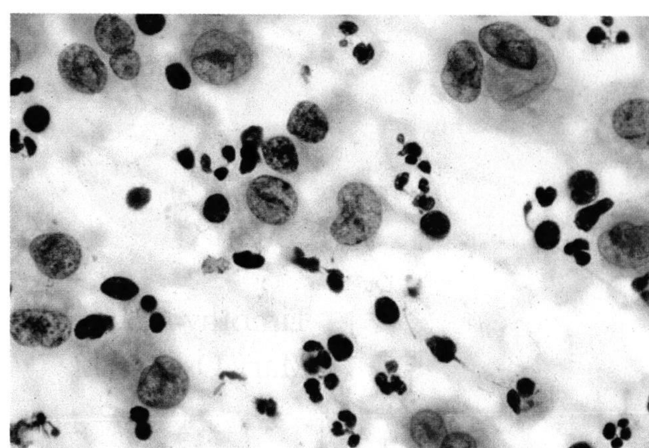

Figure 29.1 Cytology figure showing Langerhans cells with elongated, folded nuclei and pale cytoplasm with indistinct cell margins, scattered neutrophils, and eosinophils.

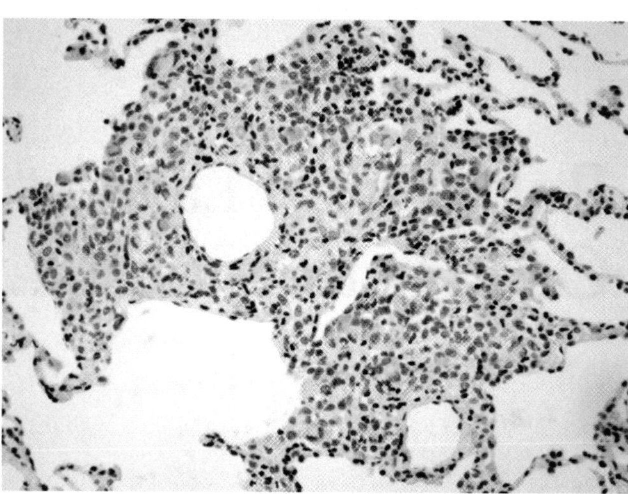

Figure 29.2 Early PLCH lesion, with interstitial infiltrate of Langerhans cells.

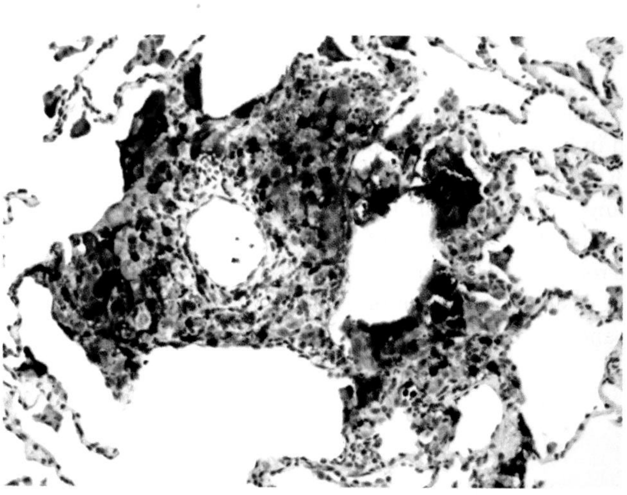

Figure 29.3 CD1a immunopositivity in Langerhans cells in an early PLCH lesion.

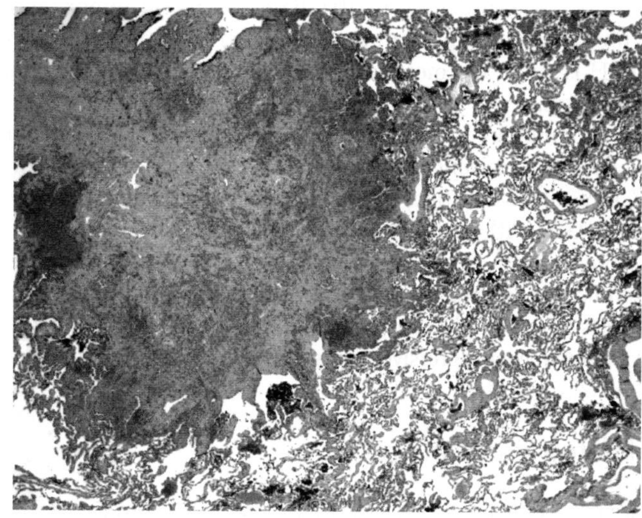

Figure 29.4 Characteristic stellate nodule with central scarring, active periphery, and relatively normal surrounding lung parenchyma.

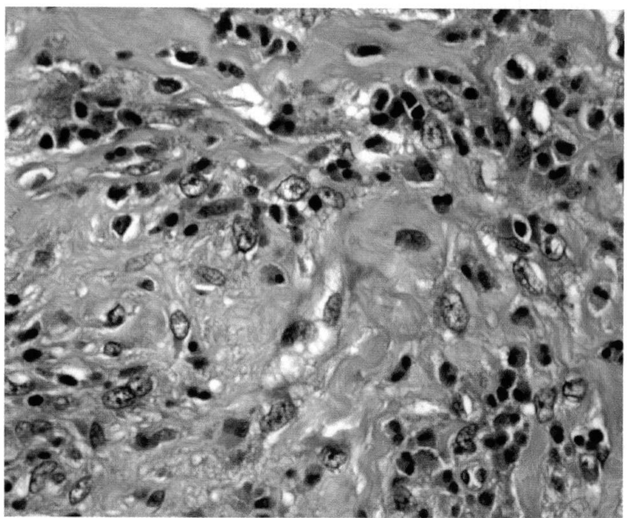

Figure 29.5 Higher power of Langerhans cells with characteristic nuclear folding and indistinct cell margins.

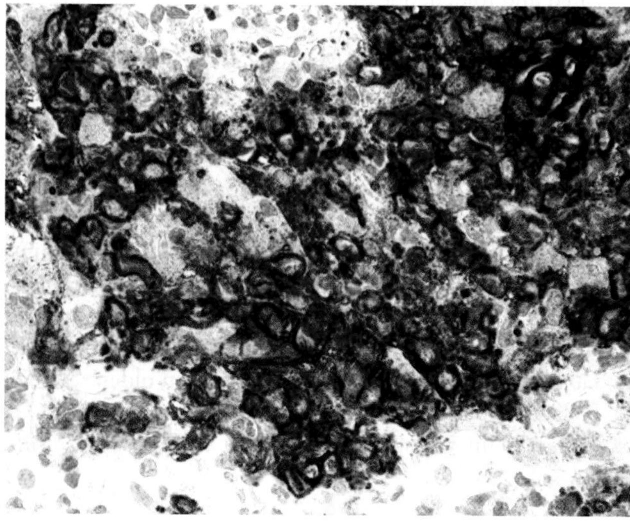

Figure 29.6 S-100 immunopositivity within a cluster of Langerhans cells.

Non-Langerhans Cell Histiocytoses

30

Non-Langerhans cell histiocytoses include a myriad of histiocytoses, many of which have primarily cutaneous manifestations. The following have been described in the lung.

Part 1

Erdheim-Chester Disease

▶ Timothy Allen

Erdheim-Chester disease is a rare nonfamilial histiocytic disorder of unknown etiology. It primarily affects adults middle-aged and older, and bone pain is the most common presenting symptom. It has characteristic long bone radiographic findings, namely, sclerotic changes in the diaphyses and metaphyses. Approximately half of cases have involvement of nonosseous tissue, and lung involvement occurs in approximately 20% of cases. Differential diagnosis includes pulmonary Langerhans cell histiocytosis, Rosai-Dorfman disease, and usual interstitial pneumonia.

Histologic Features:

- Accumulation of foamy or clear histiocytes with variable amounts of associated fibrosis and a variable lymphoplasmacytic infiltrate.
- Histiocytes and associated fibrosis and inflammation lie in a characteristic lymphangitic distribution: subpleural, intralobar septal, and bronchovascular.
- Generally immunopositive for CD68 and factor XIIIa and immunonegative for CD1a; S-100 immunostain is variably positive.

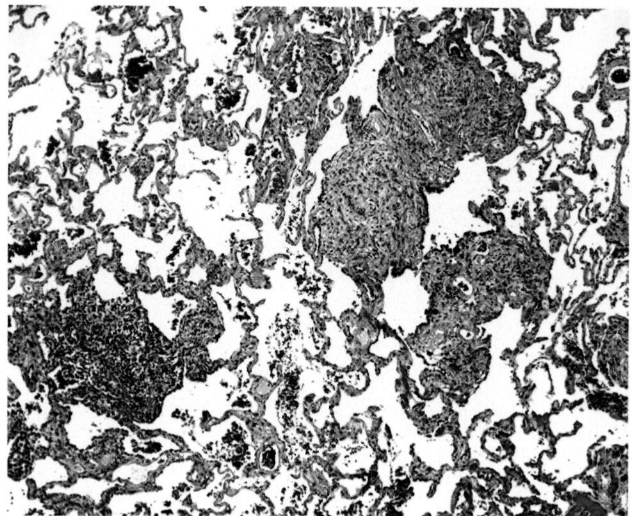

Figure 30.1 Lymphangitic distribution of histiocytes with associated fibrosis and inflammatory cells.

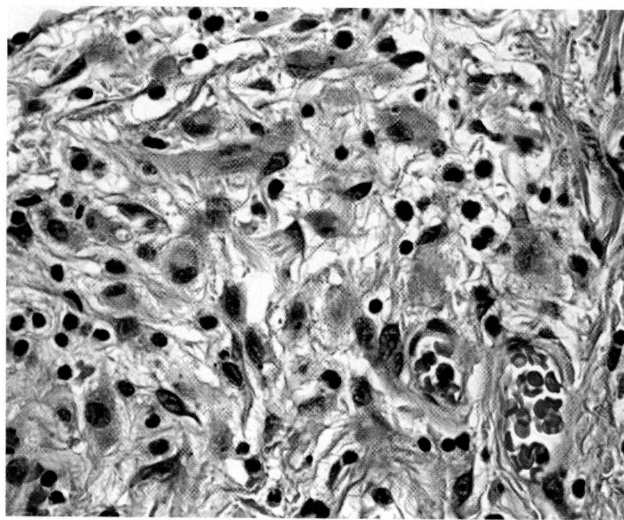

Figure 30.2 Higher power of foamy histiocytes within a background of fibrosis.

Part 2

Rosai-Dorfman Disease

▶ Dani S. Zander

Rosai-Dorfman disease, also known as *sinus histiocytosis with massive lymphadenopathy*, is a histiocytic proliferative disorder whose etiology is unknown. Although cervical lymph nodes are the most common site affected, it has now been described in most organs. Lower respiratory tract involvement is very rare and is often associated with a progressive and fatal course. Presentations include solitary or multiple mass lesions in the trachea, bronchi, or lung, and diffuse interstitial pulmonary involvement. Coexisting nodal involvement is usually present.

Histologic Features:

- Characteristic histiocytic cells have oval nuclei with one or more nucleoli and abundant eosinophilic cytoplasm; multilobated nuclei may be present.
- Mild nuclear cytoatypia may be present.
- Lymphocytes and other leukocytes in the cytoplasm of the Rosai-Dorfman cells (emperipolesis).
- Accompanying mixture of inflammatory cells and fibrosis; involved lung tissue also shows type II pneumocyte proliferation and foamy alveolar macrophages.
- Rosai-Dorfman cells usually positive for S-100, CD68, and CD14 and usually negative for CD1a.
- Differential diagnosis includes Hodgkin disease, Langerhans cell histiocytosis, lymphomatoid granulomatosis, Erdheim-Chester disease, malignant histiocytosis, carcinoma, melanoma, and fungal and mycobacterial infections.

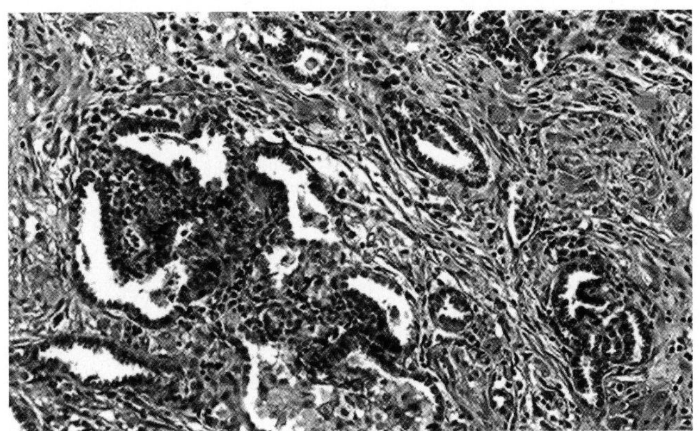

Figure 30.3 Interstitial widening caused by fibrosis and infiltration by Rosai-Dorfman cells and other leukocytes; alveoli are distorted and lined by cells with features of Clara cells and proliferating type II pneumocytes.

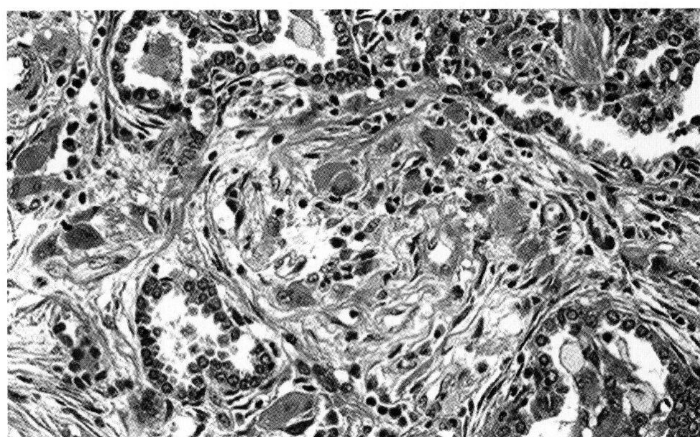

Figure 30.4 Interstitial and alveolar infiltrates of Rosai-Dorfman cells and other leukocytes, accompanied by interstitial fibrosis, type II pneumocyte proliferation, and foamy macrophages in alveoli.

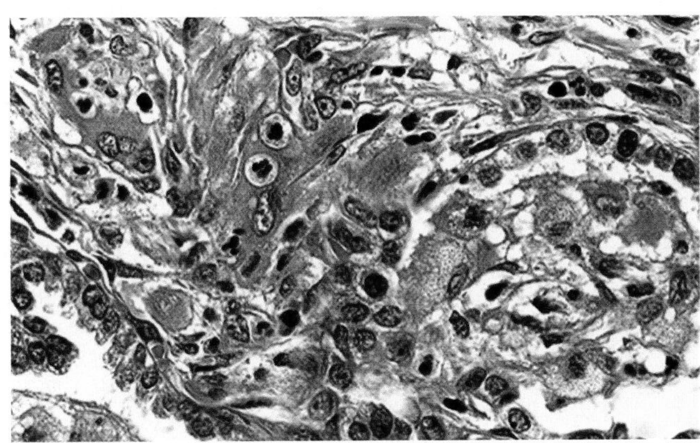

Figure 30.5 Large Rosai-Dorfman cells contain intracytoplasmic leukocytes.

Section 6

Benign and Borderline Lymphoid Proliferations

Lymphoid Interstitial Pneumonia

31

▶ Dani S. Zander

Lymphoid interstitial pneumonia (LIP) is a form of diffuse pulmonary lymphoid hyperplasia that rarely occurs as an idiopathic process. More commonly it arises in association with one of a large number of conditions, including infections (particularly Epstein-Barr virus, also *Pneumocystis carinii,* hepatitis B), collagen vascular diseases, acquired and congenital immunodeficiency syndromes, systemic or organ-specific autoimmune diseases, and exposure to certain drugs or toxins. LIP is more common in women than in men. It is diagnosed most often in middle-aged individuals but also is seen in children. Slowly worsening shortness of breath and cough are typical symptoms and may be accompanied by fever, weight loss, chest pain, arthralgias, anemia, and hypergammaglobulinemia. Corticosteroids often produce stabilization or improvement.

Histologic Features:

- Diffuse alveolar septal widening due to dense interstitial infiltrates of lymphocytes, plasma cells, and macrophages.
- T lymphocytes usually predominant, with aggregates of B lymphocytes forming germinal centers.
- Type II pneumocyte hyperplasia.
- Variably present findings are honeycombing, nonnecrotizing granulomas, alveolar organization, and alveolar macrophage accumulation.
- Lack of cytologic atypia and infiltration along lymphatic pathways suggesting lymphoma.
- Polyclonality indicated by immunohistochemical stains for T-cell and B-cell antigens, flow cytometry, and/or gene rearrangement studies.
- Differential diagnosis includes nonspecific interstitial pneumonia, follicular bronchiolitis, nodular lymphoid hyperplasia, small lymphocytic or mucosa-associated lymphoid tissue (MALT) lymphoma, chronic lymphocytic leukemia, lymphomatoid granulomatosis, hypersensitivity pneumonia, and graft versus host disease.

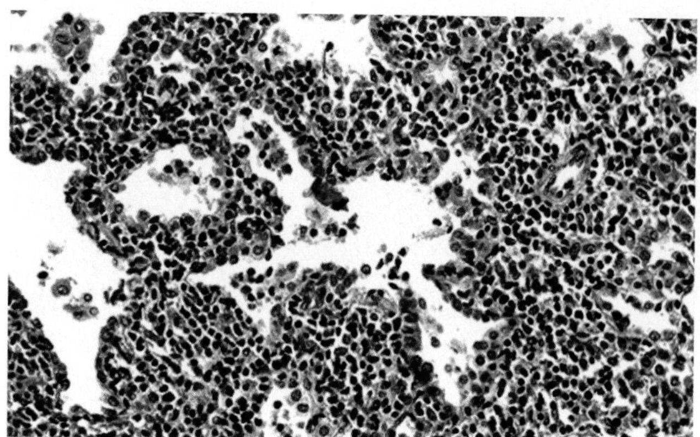

Figure 31.1 There is prominent interstitial widening by an infiltrate consisting predominantly of small lymphoid cells.

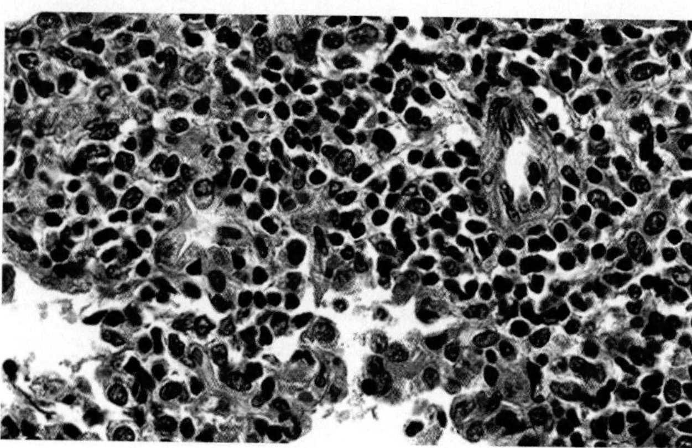

Figure 31.2 The small lymphoid cells lack cytologic atypia and are accompanied by a smaller number of macrophages and occasional plasma cells.

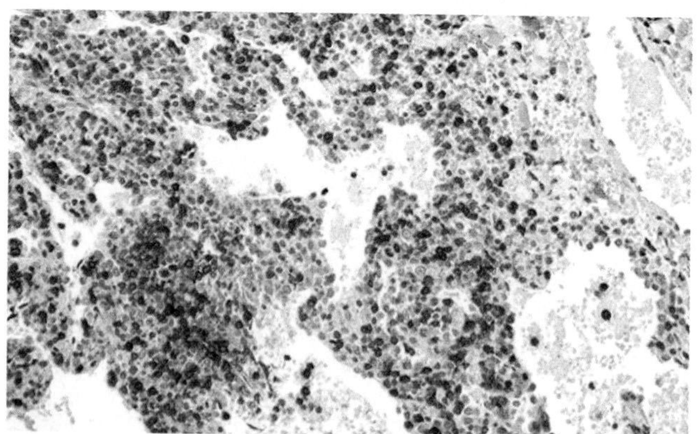

Figure 31.3 Immunohistochemistry for CD3. Most of the interstitial lymphocytes are T cells that express CD3; B cells, plasma cells, and macrophages do not stain.

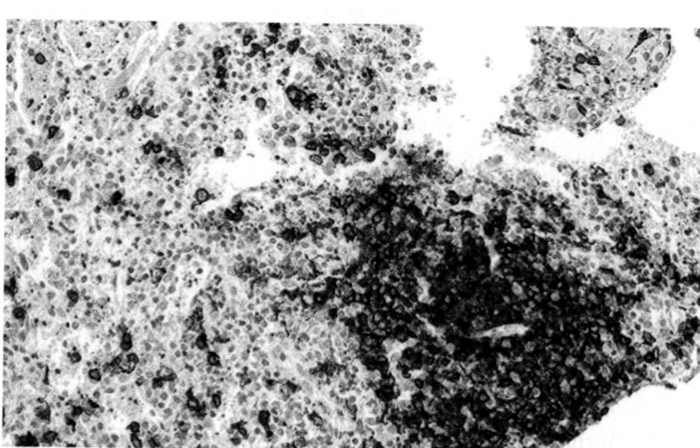

Figure 31.4 Immunohistochemistry for CD20. The infiltrate is partly composed of an aggregate of CD20-expressing B cells and scattered interstitial B cells.

32 Nodular Lymphoid Hyperplasia

▶ Dani S. Zander

Nodular lymphoid hyperplasia, also referred to as *pseudolymphoma,* is an uncommon nodular or localized reactive lymphoid proliferation. Most patients are between 50 and 80 years of age, and the lesion is usually discovered incidentally on routine chest radiograph. Solitary nodules are more common than multifocal lesions, and most examples range in size from 2.0 to 4.0 cm in greatest dimension. Surgical excision serves the purposes of diagnosis and therapy. In some cases, coexisting follicular hyperplasia in hilar, mediastinal, or paraesophageal lymph nodes is present.

Histologic Features:

- Well-circumscribed mass, usually subpleural.
- Prominent reactive germinal centers with mantle zones.
- Numerous interfollicular mature plasma cells that may have Russell bodies.
- Interfollicular fibrosis.
- Limited perilesional lymphangitic spread of lymphocytes and plasma cells is common.
- Uncommon associated findings are giant cells, organizing pneumonia and neutrophils, and plaquelike involvement of the pleura.
- Lymphoepithelial lesions are absent.
- Immunohistochemical stains for T-cell and B-cell antigens, flow cytometry, and/or gene rearrangement studies provide evidence of polyclonality.
- Differential diagnosis includes mucosa-associated lymphoid tissue (MALT) lymphoma, follicular bronchitis/bronchiolitis, lymphoid interstitial pneumonia, and inflammatory myofibroblastic tumor.

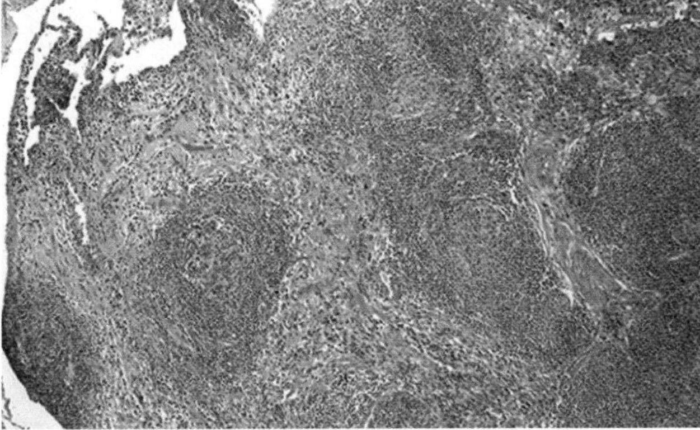

Figure 32.1 This well-demarcated lymphoid proliferation demonstrates multiple germinal centers with mantle zones and interfollicular fibrosis.

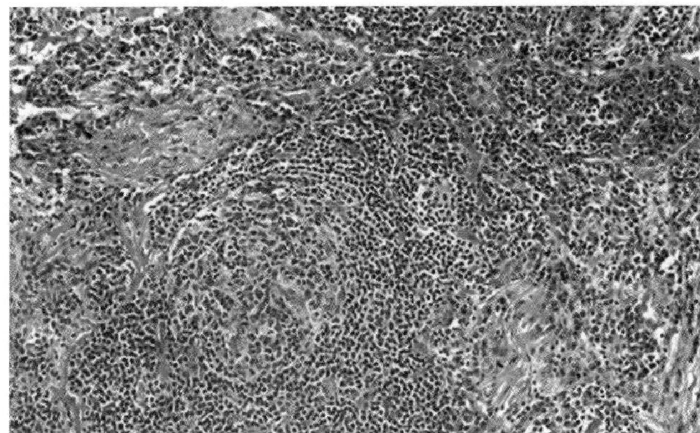

Figure 32.2 Germinal center with prominent mantle zone and numerous adjacent plasma cells.

Section 7

Focal Lesions and Pseudotumors

33

Apical Scars

▶ Alvaro C. Laga
▶ Timothy Allen

Apical scarring of the lung, often referred to as *apical caps*, is found predominantly in older men and is usually a bilateral process present in individuals of lower socioeconomic class that increases with age. Such changes of apical scarring are not restricted to the upper lobes. It also can occur in the superior segments of the lower lobes. Studies performed in the early 1900s proposed tuberculosis as a root cause, but closer analysis of the available literature showed that granulomatous inflammation was seen only in a minority of cases. The combination of infection and chronic ischemia seems to be the likely etiology, with some authors favoring the latter. The appearance of fragmented fibers resembling elastosis seen at high power is suggestive of ischemia.

Histologic Features:

- Grossly, apical scars (apical caps) are slightly depressed gray-white plaques with a pyramidal shape on cross section, with peripheral emphysematous change.
- Microscopically, distinct for their triangular shape with a broad base along the pleural surface and unique basophilia at high magnification.
- At high power, the basophilia resembles the fragmented connective tissue fibers of solar elastosis in the dermis.
- Alveolar pneumocytes at the junction of the apical scar and emphysematous lung are plump, hyperplastic, and hobnail shaped (not to be mistaken for scar carcinoma).

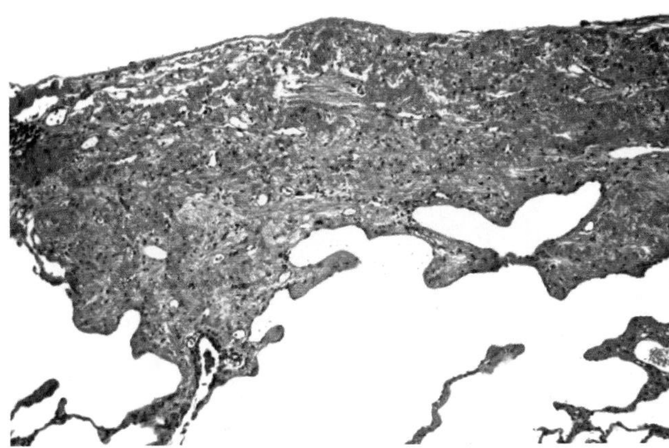

Figure 33.1 Subpleural scar with characteristic pyramidal shape.

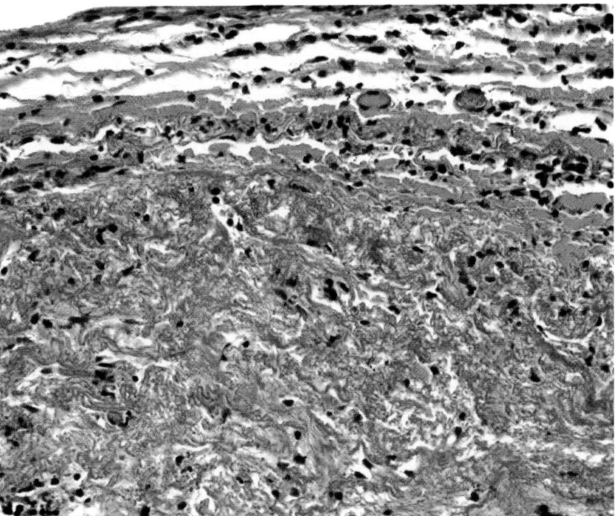

Figure 33.2 Higher power of subpleural scar showing basophilia within the scar composed of fragmented fibers resembling elastosis.

35

Dendriform Ossification

▶ Mary Beth Beasley
▶ Dani S. Zander

Dendriform ossification is a unique form of pulmonary ossification that is associated with various causes of pulmonary fibrosis. Most often diagnosed at autopsy, it can produce lacy-appearing shadows radiographically. Mature, linear branching, bone spicules lie in a connective tissue background that probably represents expanded alveolar septa.

Histologic Features:

- Mature lamellar bone with dichotomous branching.
- Bone marrow spaces containing hematopoietic cells and fat.
- Cartilage very rare.
- Associated fibrosis.

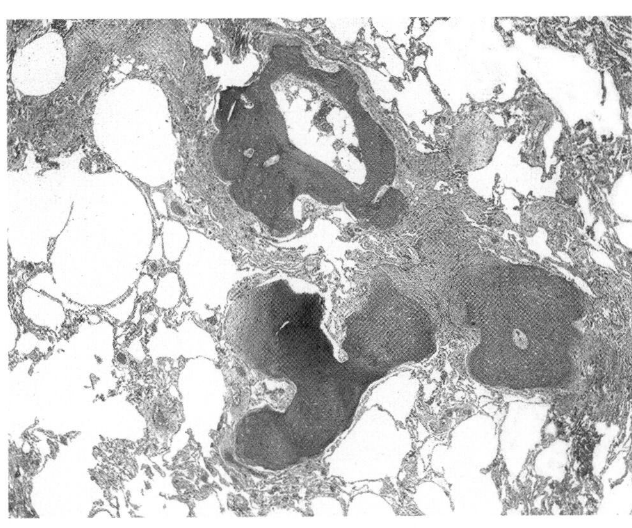

Figure 35.1 Branching bone spicules lie in fibrotically thickened alveolar septa.

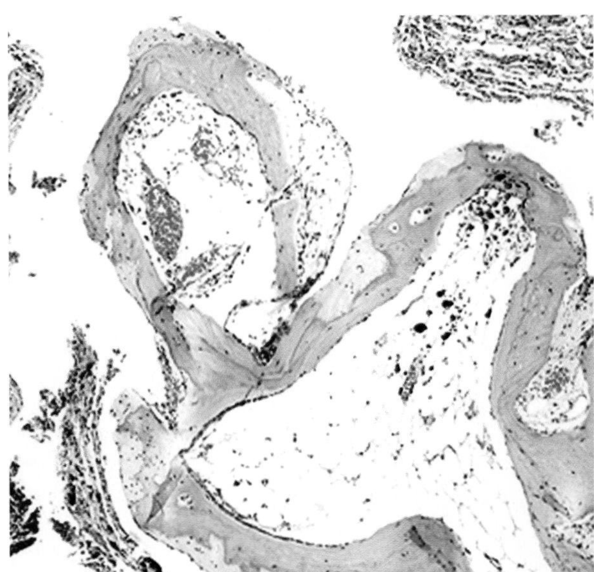

Figure 35.2 Mature bone spicules branch and contain marrow spaces.

Intrapulmonary Lymph Node

36

▶ Alvaro C. Laga
▶ Timothy Allen

Intrapulmonary lymph nodes are generally a normal finding. They are increasingly recognized with imaging techniques in heavy smokers and individuals with high dust exposure and, therefore, are biopsied. They are usually 10 mm or less in size. Intrapulmonary lymph nodes are usually peribronchial, septal, or subpleural; they are not usually found in the peripheral lung parenchyma.

Histologic Features:

- Ovoid or round, well-circumscribed lymph nodes.
- Lymphoid follicles, sinus histiocytes, and anthracotic pigment are common.
- Occasionally, small aggregates of lymphocytes can be seen along adjacent interlobular septa.

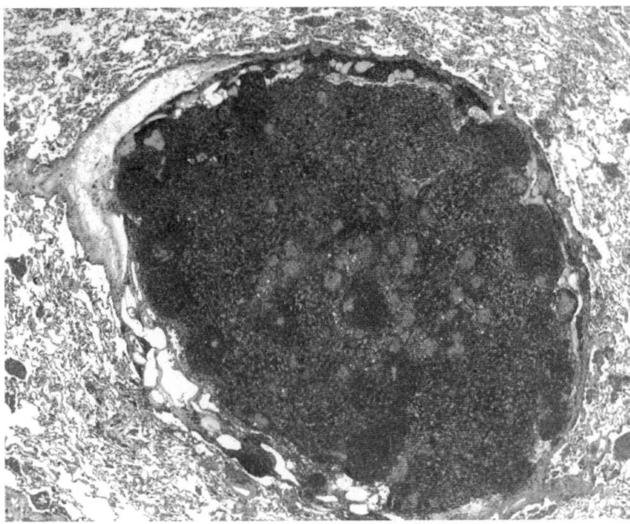

Figure 36.1 Intrapulmonary lymph node with surrounding normal lung parenchyma.

Inflammatory Pseudotumor/Inflammatory Myofibroblastic Tumor

37

- Handan Zeren
- Angela Shen
- Alvaro C. Laga
- Timothy Allen
- Philip T. Cagle

Many issues regarding inflammatory pseudotumor and inflammatory myofibroblastic tumor (IMT) are unresolved, including the usage of these terms. Different investigators have different concepts of these entities, and it appears that various lesions have been included under this diagnosis. Traditionally, in the lung, inflammatory pseudotumors were considered nonneoplastic reactive lesions. In the past, synonyms for inflammatory pseudotumor included plasma cell granuloma. However, even in years past, there were cases of so-called inflammatory pseudotumors of the lung that were multiple, recurrent, or locally invasive. In retrospect, many of the inflammatory pseudotumors with these more aggressive features were probably neoplasms. IMTs are distinctive lesions composed of myofibroblastic spindle cells accompanied by inflammatory cells; they occur primarily in soft tissues but occasionally in the lungs. IMTs have also been called *inflammatory pseudotumors.* There is disagreement among investigators as to whether or not any or all IMTs are neoplastic. Further confusion is added by inclusion of IMTs with frank clinical and pathologic malignant features as inflammatory fibrosarcomas. Because of the traditional classification of inflammatory pseudotumors as nonneoplastic, we discuss these entities in this section, fully recognizing that some of these are probably true neoplasms.

The following discussion concerns both the traditional nonneoplastic lesions in the lung and IMTs in the lung. IMTs are histologically distinctive and yet the pathologist is more likely to encounter wedge resections of traditional nonneoplastic inflammatory pseudotumors. It is recognized that some lesions overlap histologically or may not be specifically classifiable.

The term *inflammatory pseudotumor of the lung* was first introduced in the 1950s to characterize pulmonary masses with propensity to mimic a malignant process clinically and radiologically. Similar to focal organizing pneumonias, these lesions present as radiologic masses suspected of being malignancies and are found to be purely inflammatory on histopathologic examination. Based on the predominant histopathologic features, these lesions have been divided into three types: (i) organizing pneumonia pattern, (ii) fibrous histiocytic pattern (most common), and (iii) lymphohistiocytic pattern (least common). The etiology of inflammatory pseudotumors is unknown, but an antecedent pulmonary insult, usually infection, is found in about 20% of cases.

IMT represents a subgroup of the broad category of "inflammatory pseudotumors." Some authors believe IMT is a reactive inflammatory condition, whereas others believe it represents a low-grade mesenchymal malignancy. It presents as a well-defined mass on chest radiographs in the majority of cases. Grossly, IMTs consist of multilobular or bosselated tumors with a rubbery surface and a yellowish-white or gray appearance on sectioning. Pulmonary IMTs have been associated with viral infections including HHV-8. In most cases surgical excision is curative, with a minority of cases exhibiting recurrence, extrapulmonary invasion, and metastases. Some authors continue to use the terms *inflammatory pseudotumor* and *IMT* interchangeably. Other investigators suggest that IMTs that exhibit frank malignant behavior and/or histopathologic features of malignancy are best designated *inflammatory fibrosarcomas.*

Histologic Features:

- Traditional nonneoplastic inflammatory pseudotumors may show an organizing pneumonia pattern characterized by airspaces filled with plump fibroblasts and foamy histiocytes.
- Traditional nonneoplastic inflammatory pseudotumors may show a lymphohistiocytic pattern composed of a mixture of lymphocytes and plasma cells with only minimal fibrous tissue.
- IMTs are composed of spindle cells arranged in fascicles, with a prominent lymphocytic inflammatory infiltrate, often rich in plasma cells.
- Immunohistochemistry is generally positive for vimentin, desmin, smooth muscle actin, and muscle-specific actin in IMTs.
- Some cases of IMT are immunopositive for ALK-1 and p80.
- Ultrastructurally, IMTs show features of myofibroblastic differentiation: well-developed Golgi apparatus, abundant rough endoplasmic reticulum, and intracytoplasmic thin filaments and dense bodies.

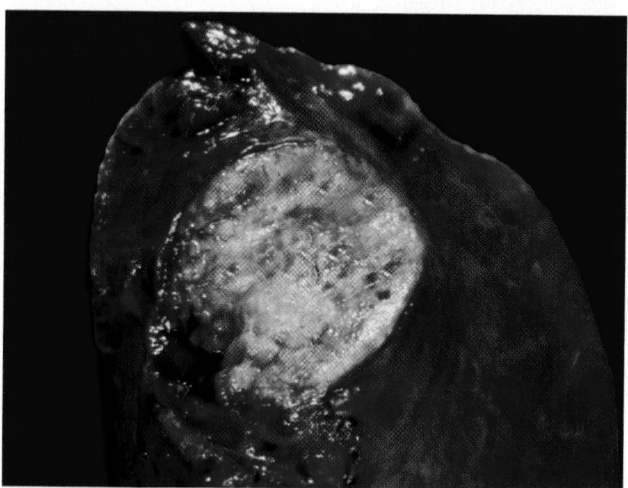

Figure 37.1 Gross figure of IMT showing a white-gray well-circumscribed mass.

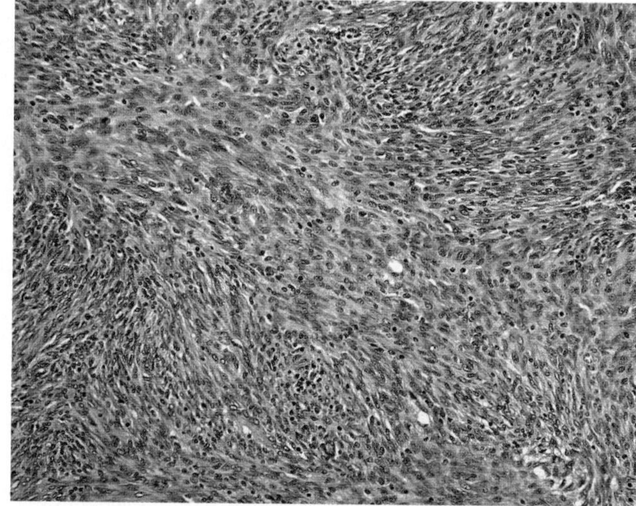

Figure 37.2 Fascicles of spindle cells with a mild lymphocytic infiltrate in an IMT.

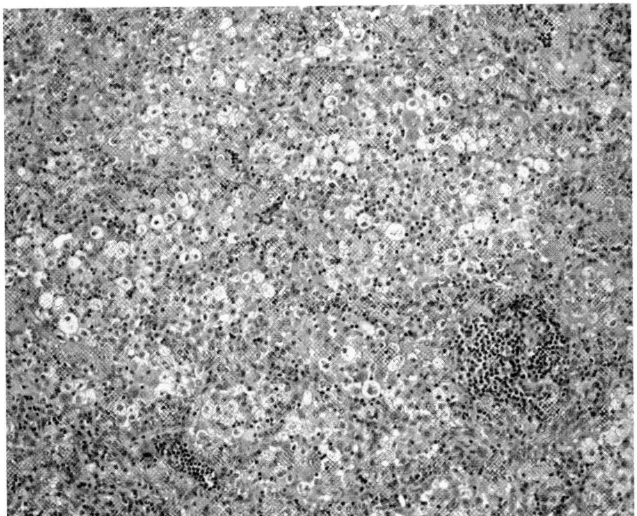

Figure 37.3 Foamy macrophages and pigment-laden macrophages with a lymphoplasmacytic infiltrate in the background in an IMT.

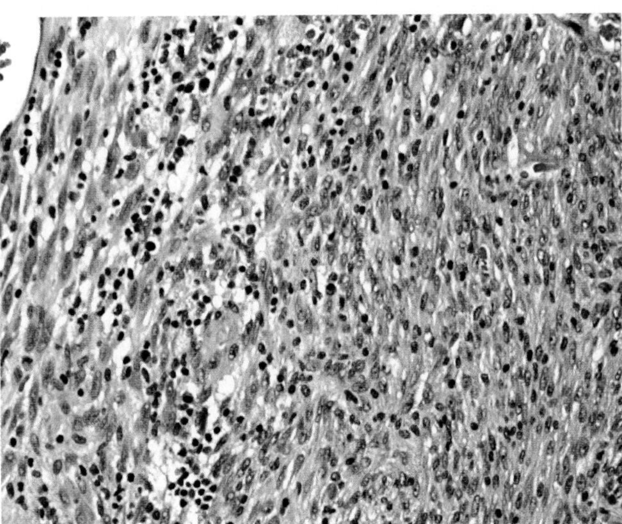

Figure 37.4 Higher power of IMT shows spindle cells with associated lymphoplasmacytic infiltrate.

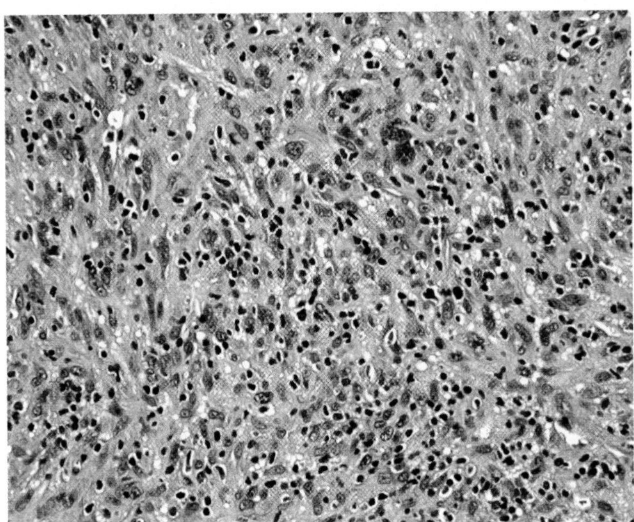

Figure 37.5 Pleomorphic spindle cells with infiltrate of lymphocytes and plasma cells and elsewhere increased mitotic rate (see Fig. 37.6) in an IMT-like neoplasm, which some investigators designate inflammatory fibrosarcoma.

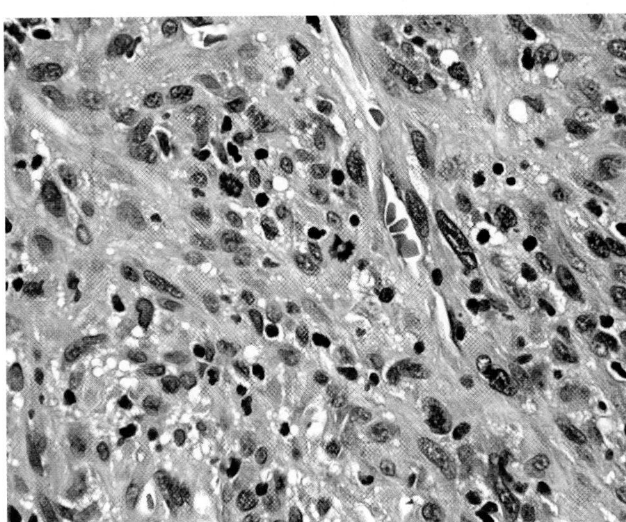

Figure 37.6 Occasional mitoses are present in this IMT-like neoplasm, which some investigators designate inflammatory fibrosarcoma.

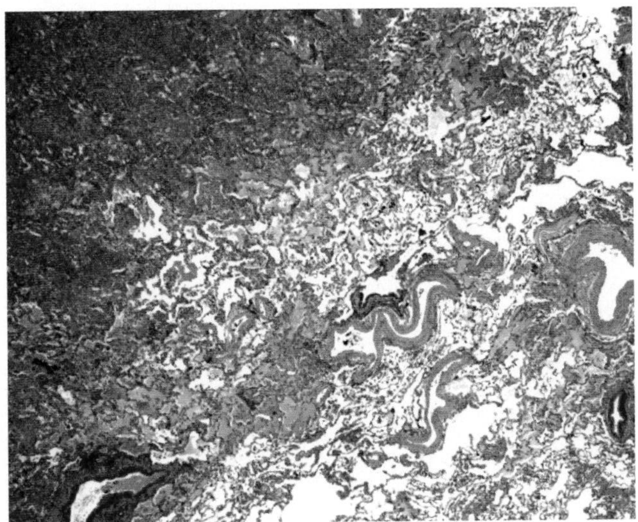

Figure 37.7 Low power of traditional nonneoplastic inflammatory pseudotumor shows relatively circumscribed demarcation of a discrete inflammatory/fibrotic mass from adjacent lung tissue in a lesion that presented as a lung mass radiologically and was removed to rule out cancer.

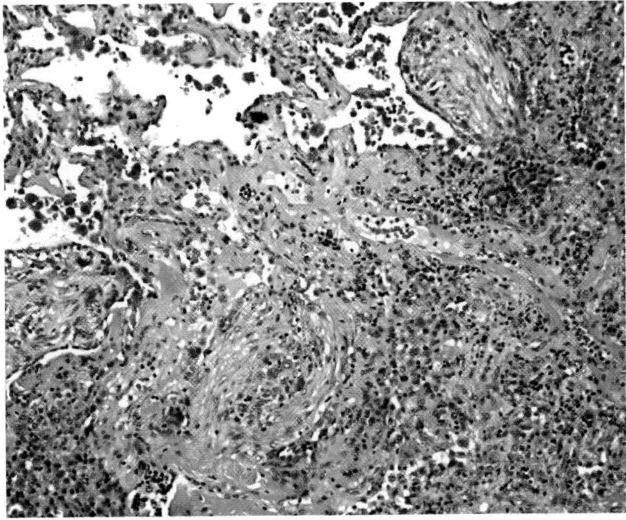

Figure 37.8 Higher power of margin of traditional nonneoplastic inflammatory pseudotumor shows foci of organizing pneumonia and inflammatory infiltrates.

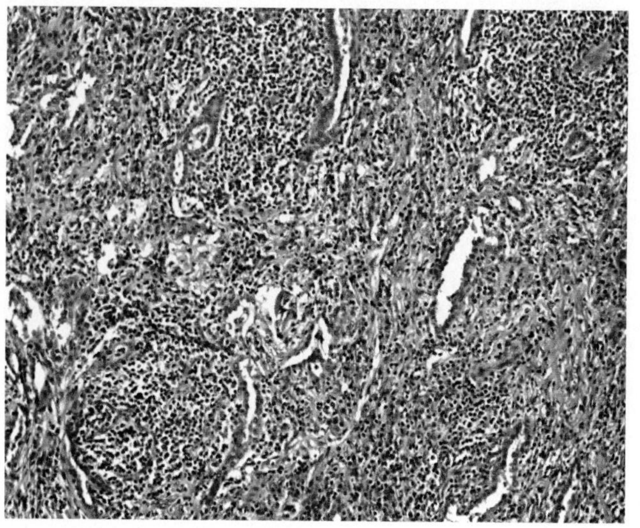

Figure 37.9 Traditional nonneoplastic inflammatory pseudotumor shows prominent lymphoid aggregates.

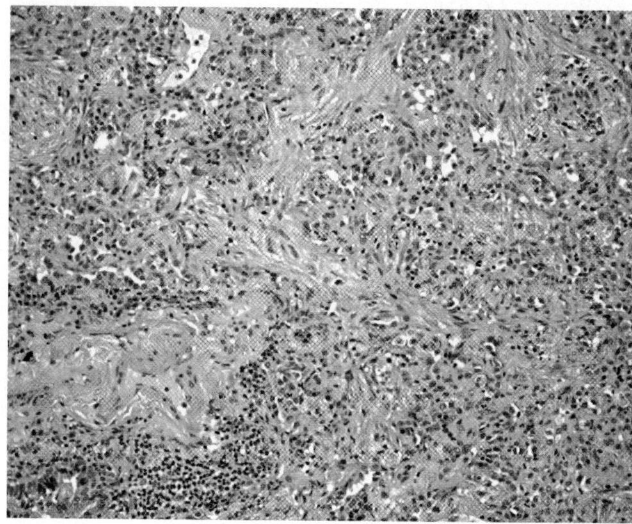

Figure 37.10 Traditional nonneoplastic inflammatory pseudotumor shows organizing pneumonia, fibrosis, and inflammatory infiltrates.

38

Rounded Atelectasis

▶ Alvaro C. Laga
▶ Dani S. Zander

Rounded atelectasis (also known as *folded lung* or *Blesovsky syndrome*) is an area of atelectatic lung subjacent to an area of localized pleural thickening, often with infolding or buckling of the fibrotic pleura. It may be unilateral or bilateral. The process appears as a subpleural mass lesion on chest x-ray film and may be mistaken for a neoplasm clinically or radiographically. It is strongly associated with a history of prior exposure to asbestos. It has a characteristic appearance on computed tomography of the thorax, including a pleural-based mass lesion, usually on the lower lung zones and posteriorly.

Histologic Features:

- Atelectasis adjacent to an area of pleural thickening with infolding of fibrotic pleura.
- Usually located in the lower lobes; may be bilateral.

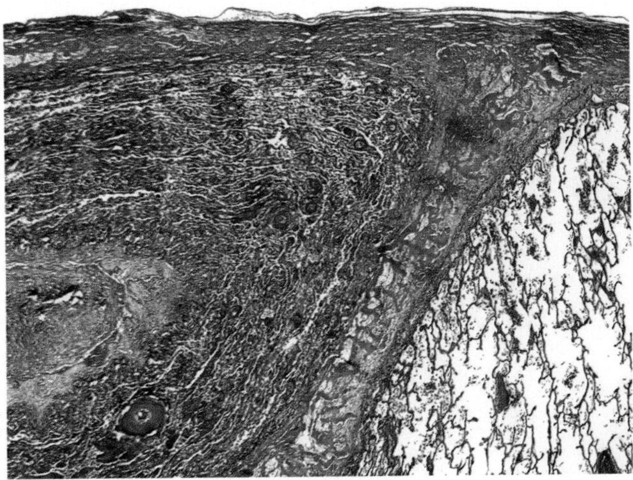

Figure 38.1 Normal alveolar parenchyma adjacent to thickened, infolded pleura with underlying atelectatic lung parenchyma. Elastic stain.

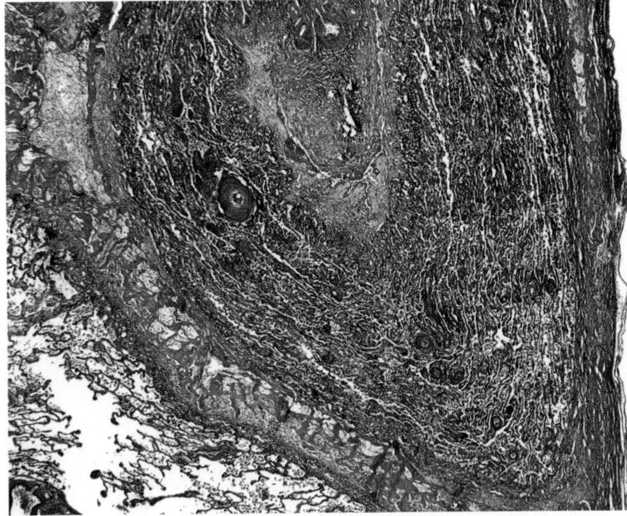

Figure 38.2 Normal alveolar parenchyma adjacent to thickened, infolded pleura with underlying atelectatic lung parenchyma. Elastic stain.

39 Nodular Amyloidosis

▶ Timothy Allen
▶ Mary Ostrowski

Nodular amyloidosis is a rare lesion that generally presents incidentally in adults as a 1- to 4-cm slow-growing nodule. The nodules are typically irregular hard yellow-gray nodules consisting of intrapulmonary masses of extracellular amyloid.

Cytologic Features:

- Acellular globules of amorphous material.
- Generally paucicellular background.

Histologic Features:

- Amorphous sheets of eosinophilic extracellular amyloid.
- Characteristic foreign body giant cell reaction accompanying the amyloid deposits.
- Lymphoplasmacytic infiltrate is generally present, most prominent at the periphery.
- Ossification and calcification occur frequently.
- Apple-green birefringence on Congo red stain.

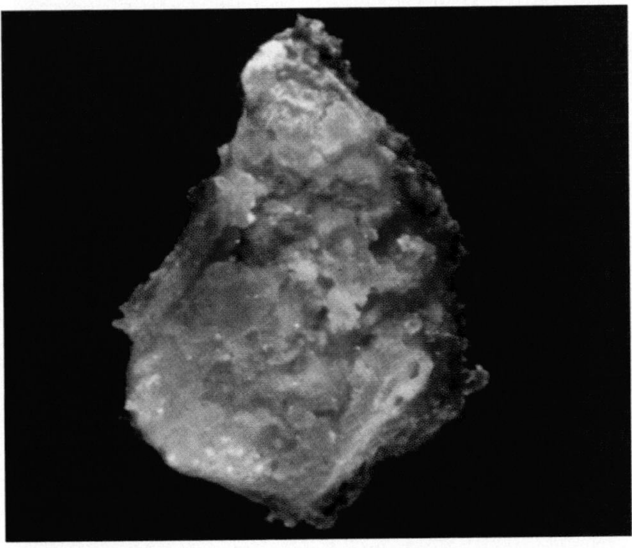

Figure 39.1 Gross figure of nodular amyloidosis.

Figure 39.2 Cytology figure showing amorphous amyloid material.

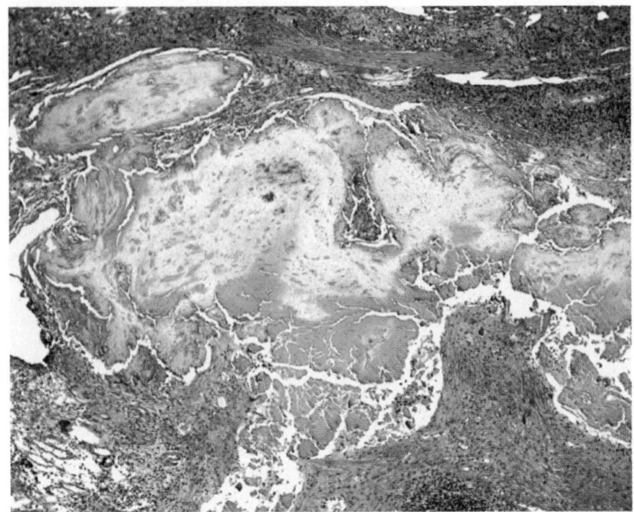

Figure 39.3 Nodular amyloidosis with waxy amorphous eosinophilic material with surrounding foreign body giant cell reaction and fibrosis.

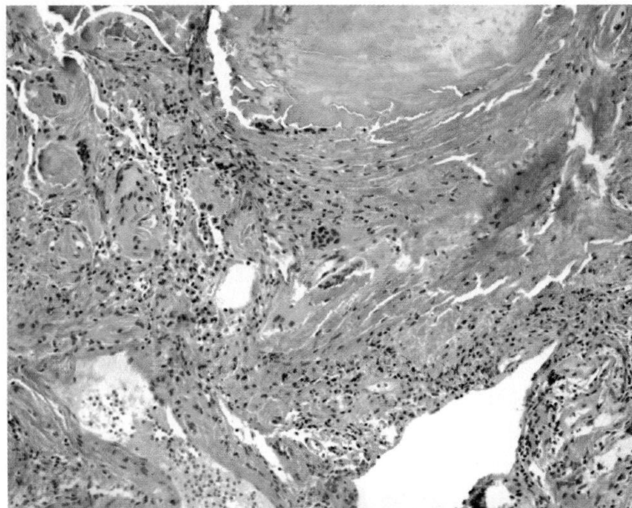

Figure 39.4 Higher power of amorphous amyloid and foreign body giant cell reaction.

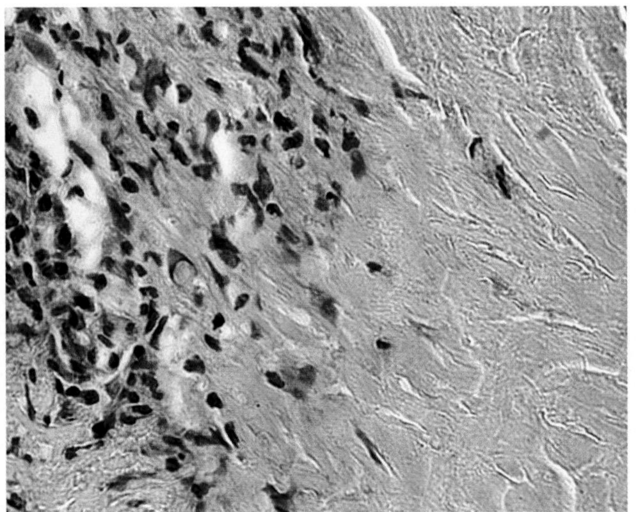

Figure 39.5 Amorphous waxy eosinophilic material characteristic of amyloid.

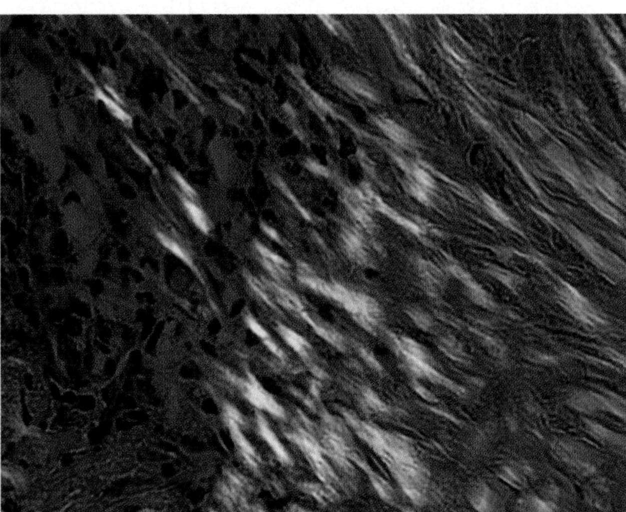

Figure 39.6 Apple-green birefringence on Congo red stain of amorphous sheet of amyloid from Figure 39.5.

Part 1

Tracheobronchial Amyloidosis

▶ Alvaro C. Laga, Timothy Allen, and Philip T. Cagle

Tracheobronchial amyloidosis, which is amyloidosis limited to the tracheobronchial system, frequently causes obstruction or constriction of airways. Recurrent pneumonia and bronchiectasis may occur.

Histologic Features:

- Amorphous sheets of eosinophilic extracellular amyloid in the submucosa.
- Multinucleated giant cells often identified.
- Calcification, chondrification, and ossification are generally present.
- Apple-green birefringence on Congo red stain.

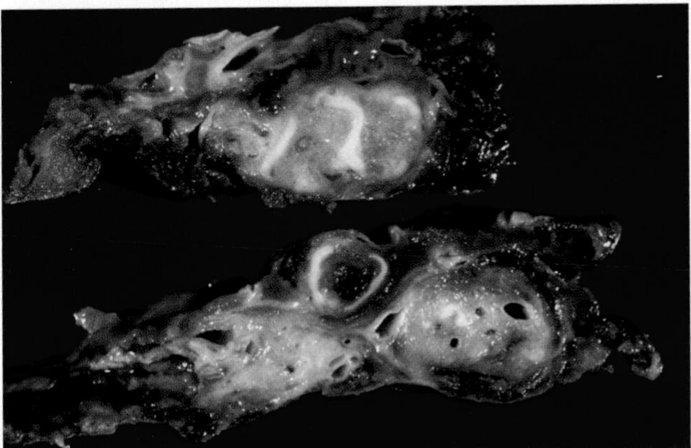

Figure 39.7 Gross figure of nodular amyloidosis showing yellow-brown nodules surrounding the bronchial cartilage and filling the bronchial lumens.

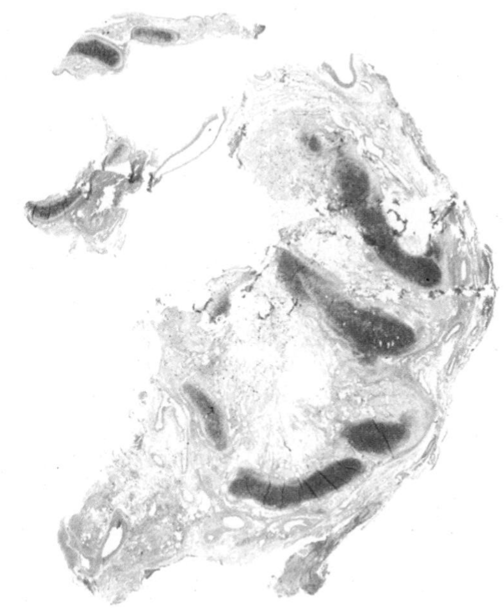

Figure 39.8 Amorphous eosinophilic material obstructs the bronchial lumen.

Section 8

Granulomatous Diseases

Infectious Granulomas

40

Infection is a common cause of granulomas. The most common infections resulting in granulomas are tuberculosis, fungi, and parasites.

Part 1

Tuberculosis

▶ Abida Haque

Tuberculosis is an infectious disease caused by *Mycobacterium tuberculosis* that is spread person to person via airborne droplets. Patients not previously exposed develop primary tuberculosis, characterized by the formation of a Ghon focus. Bacilli are carried by macrophages to lymph nodes, and hematogenous spread of disease may then occur. Most patients remain without symptoms and heal; however in some patients, disease advances into progressive primary tuberculosis. In some patients, disease progresses after a latency period (progressive post-primary tuberculosis). Progressive tuberculosis is typically symptomatic and may be complicated by tuberculous bronchopneumonia, military tuberculosis, and tuberculous empyema.

Histologic Features:

- Infection with *M. tuberculosis* is characterized by the formation of necrotizing granulomas.
- Rarely, there may be noncaseating granulomas.
- Tubercle bacilli are often difficult to find, and a careful search of the caseous areas in the center of the granulomas is required.
- Tubercle bacilli stain red with Ziehl-Neelsen stain or modified Kinyoun stain.

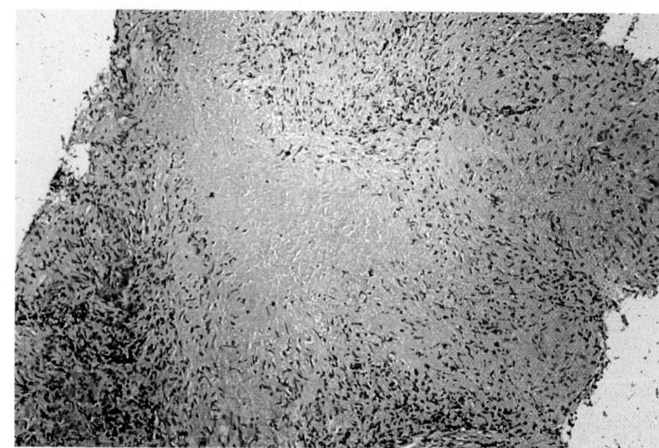

Figure 40.1 Granuloma with central caseation surrounded by histiocytes, lymphocytes and multinucleated giant cells suggestive of infectious granuloma.

Part 2

Fungi

▶ Abida Haque

Fungi are eukaryotic unicellular or filamentous organisms with chitinous cell walls. They lack chlorophyll and reproduce asexually and/or sexually. Immunocompromised patients are very susceptible to opportunistic fungal infections, and most fungi infecting the lungs are opportunistic fungi, such as *Candida, Aspergillus,* and *Cryptococcus,* among others.

Histologic Features:

- Granulomas often have necrosis.
- Multinucleated giant cells are frequent and often contain fungal organisms that are highlighted by special stains, such as Gomori methenamine silver and periodic acid–Schiff (PAS).
- Immunostains are helpful in patients who have undergone anti-fungal therapy, such as AIDS patients with *Pneumocystis carinii* infection.

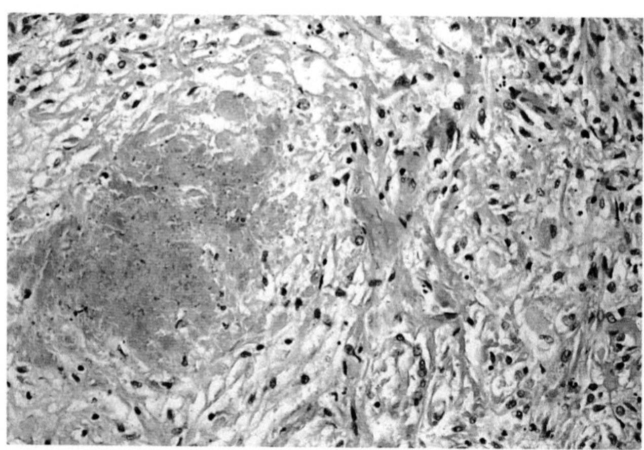

Figure 40.2 Granuloma with central caseation surrounded by macrophages, lymphocytes, and giant cells, suggestive of infectious granuloma.

Part 3

Parasites

▶ Abida Haque

Many parasites can migrate to the lungs and cause disease. Most parasites in the lung can be seen on routine hematoxylin and eosin stain.

Histologic Features:

- Granulomas often have eosinophils, along with macrophages, lymphocytes, plasma cells, and multinucleated giant cells.
- Careful search may reveal sections of parasites within the giant cells or macrophages.
- Special stains such as Giemsa, Movat pentachrome, and PAS are helpful in individual cases.

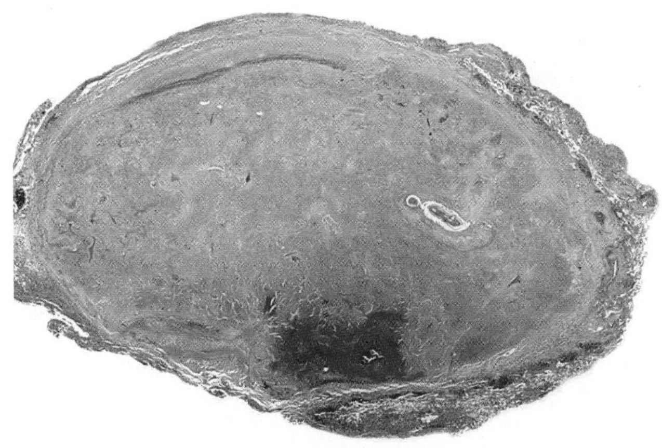

Figure 40.3 Large granuloma with bland necrosis and a section of a small wormlike structure that is consistent with *Dirofilaria immitis*.

Bronchocentric Granulomatosis

41

▶ Roberto Barrios

Bronchocentric granulomatosis is characterized by destructive, necrotizing bronchocentric and bronchiolocentric inflammation. Early lesions show partial epithelial erosion and replacement of the airway wall by epithelioid histiocytes around the lumen. More advanced lesions may show occasional presence of granulomas. Multiple causes have been associated with this histologic lesion, including infectious and noninfectious causes. It is thought that noninfectious cases represent an allergic response to the presence of aspergillus. The inflammatory process centers on the airways. There may be some secondary inflammation involving adjacent vessel walls. Primary vasculitis with necrosis of vessel walls is not seen, and vascular involvement is usually secondary to inflammation of airways in the vicinity.

In all cases, a series of special stains and cultures for microorganisms should be obtained. In biopsies from patients with allergic bronchopulmonary aspergillosis, nonviable hyphal fragments may be found in the lumen of some airways. The differential diagnosis should include primary vasculitis (Wegener's granulomatosis, Churg-Strauss angiitis), aspiration pneumonia, and rheumatoid nodules.

Histologic Features:

- Destruction of small bronchi and bronchioles due to a granulomatous and necrotizing inflammation.
- Early lesions may be nondestructive and consist of acute and chronic bronchiolitis.
- Airway wall is replaced by palisading of histiocytes with central necrosis in a "comedo-like" pattern.
- Eosinophils prominent in allergic bronchopulmonary aspergillosis and in some infections.
- Eosinophilic pneumonia may be associated in cases with allergic bronchopulmonary aspergillosis.
- Absence of true vasculitis or capillaritis differentiates bronchocentric granulomatosis from a primary vasculitis, but vessel involvement secondary to adjacent airway inflammation may be observed.

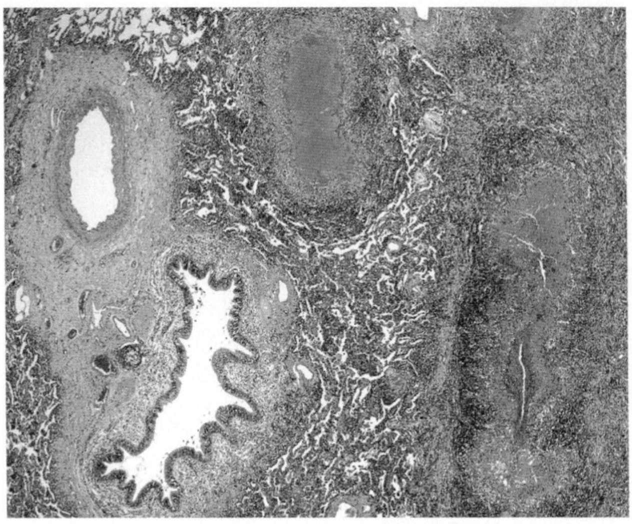

Figure 41.1 Characteristic destruction of the bronchial wall with central necrosis surrounded by palisading of histiocytes. A bronchus without destruction shows edema and inflammation. The vessel adjacent to the bronchi is not involved.

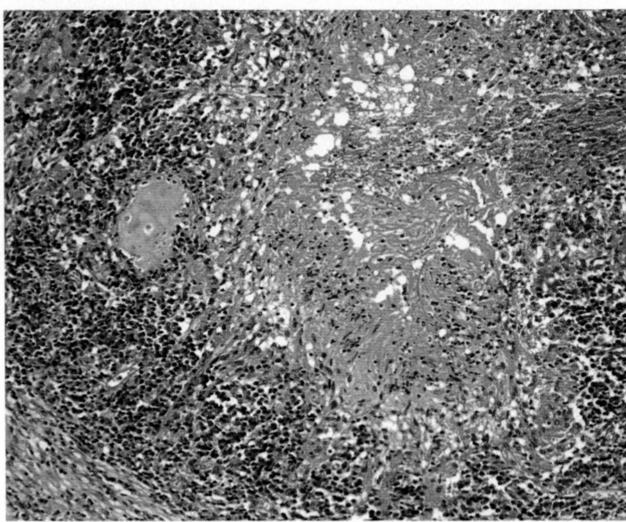

Figure 41.2 Higher power shows destruction of bronchial cartilage, central necrosis, and inflammation.

42

Pulmonary Hyalinizing Granuloma

▶ Alvaro C. Laga
▶ Timothy Allen
▶ Philip T. Cagle

Pulmonary hyalinizing granuloma is a rare nonneoplastic fibrosclerosing inflammatory lung condition. Lesions are often identified incidentally on routine chest radiography. Pulmonary hyalinizing granuloma generally occurs in adults, with no sex predilection. Symptoms may include cough, shortness of breath, fatigue, fever, chest pain, and, rarely, hemoptysis. About one fourth of patients are asymptomatic. Grossly, pulmonary hyalinizing granulomas are generally well-circumscribed peripheral lung nodules measuring 2 to 3 cm in diameter, with a tan homogeneous cut surface. They may be solitary or multiple.

Pulmonary hyalinizing granuloma is sometimes associated with sclerosing mediastinitis and retroperitoneal fibrosis. Most cases are associated with *Histoplasma* infection. An association with *Aspergillus* also has been reported. In occasional cases of pulmonary hyalinizing granuloma, the presence of a pulmonary mass and sclerosing mediastinitis may clinically mimic a lung cancer with mediastinal extension or metastasis. Differential diagnosis includes tuberculosis, histoplasmosis, inflammatory pseudotumor, nodular amyloidosis, rheumatoid nodule, Hodgkin's disease, Wegener's granulomatosis, and solitary fibrous tumor.

Cytologic Features:

- Scattered bundles of dense acellular collagen within a variable background of lymphoplasmacytic cells.

Histologic Features:

- Dense, acellular, hyalinized collagen bundles with a sparse lymphoplasmacytic infiltrate.
- Peripheral rim of chronic inflammatory cells.
- Obliterated vessels may be present.
- Often confluent, simulating silicotic nodules (but without silica particles on polarized light).
- Histoplasma organisms are often identified with Gomori methenamine silver stain.
- Histopathologic features of true granulomas (numerous epithelioid histiocytes) are not present.
- Silicates, silica, and other foreign materials are not observed on polarized light.
- Congo red may give false-positive stain.

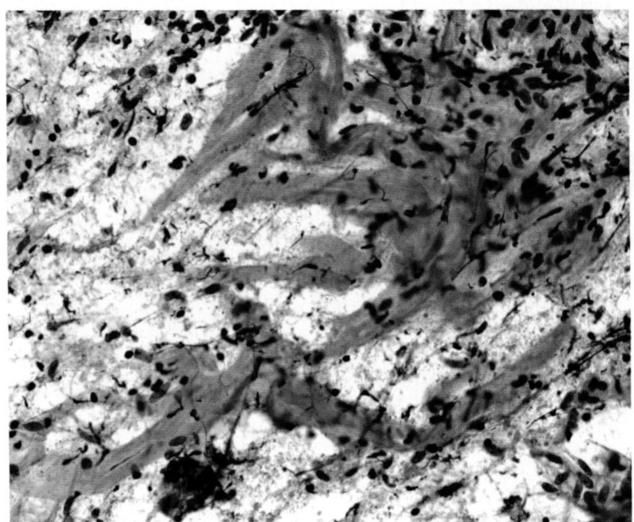

Figure 42.1 Fine needle aspiration shows bundles of hyalinized collagen with scattered inflammatory cells.

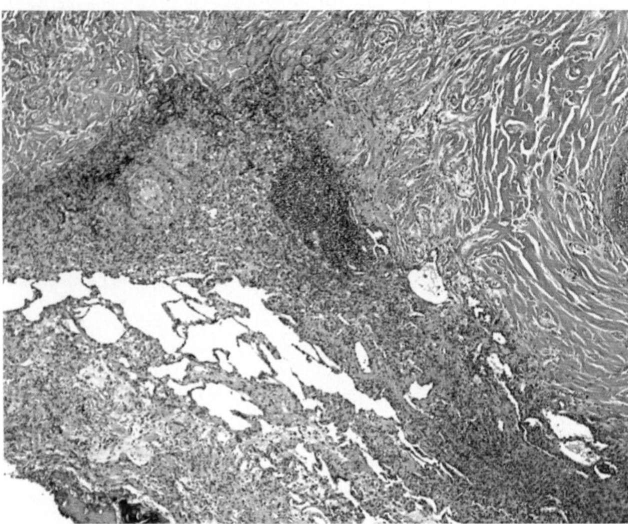

Figure 42.2 Low power shows nodular collagen bundles with peripheral chronic inflammatory infiltrate extending superficially into the surrounding lung parenchyma.

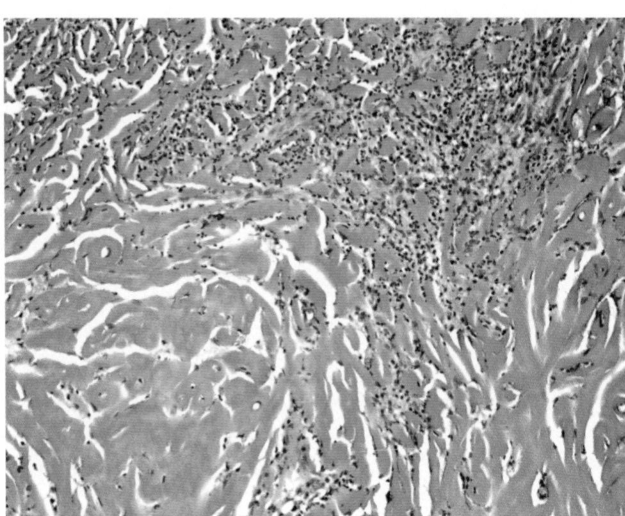

Figure 42.3 Higher power shows dense, acellular, hyalinized collagen bundles and scattered chronic inflammatory cells.

43 Sarcoidosis

Abida Haque

Sarcoidosis is a systemic disease of unknown etiology, characterized by formation of noncaseating granulomas in the lung, lymph nodes, and multiple other organs. Patients are often asymptomatic, with bilateral hilar lymphadenopathy or pulmonary reticulonodular infiltrates on chest radiograph. Lungs are involved in more than 90% of patients. Most patients demonstrate elevated serum angiotensin-converting enzyme, increased uptake of gallium, and skin anergy. Sarcoidosis is a diagnosis of exclusion; infectious causes for pulmonary granulomas should always be excluded, not only by special stains on the biopsy specimen but also by cultures.

Histologic Features:

- Granulomas are compact and discrete; they are found in the peribronchial, perivascular, and alveolar septal connective tissue, and the pleura.
- Granulomas consist of predominantly epithelioid cells with peripheral lymphocytes and multinucleated giant cells.
- Often the giant cells have inclusions, such as Schaumann bodies, asteroid bodies, and calcium oxalate crystals; all are nonspecific and may be seen in other diseases.
- In early stages of sarcoidosis, there may be interstitial and alveolar lymphocytic infiltrates without distinct granulomas (alveolitis).
- Foci of central necrosis are rare and often small, sometimes with apoptotic bodies.
- Gomori methenamine silver and Ziehl-Nielsen stains should be performed in all cases to exclude fungal and mycobacterial infection.
- Late stages of sarcoidosis exhibit partial or complete replacement of granulomas with fibrosis and associated bronchiectasis.

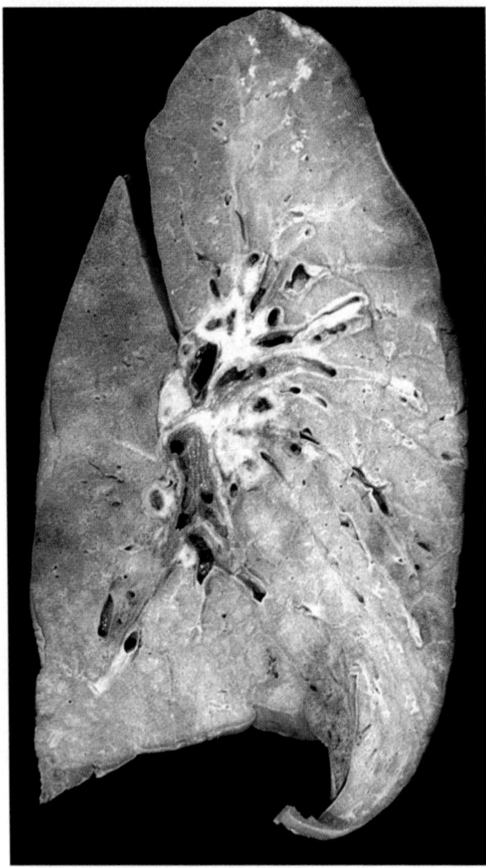

Figure 43.1 Gross figure showing focal pulmonary fibrosis and hilar lymphadenopathy.

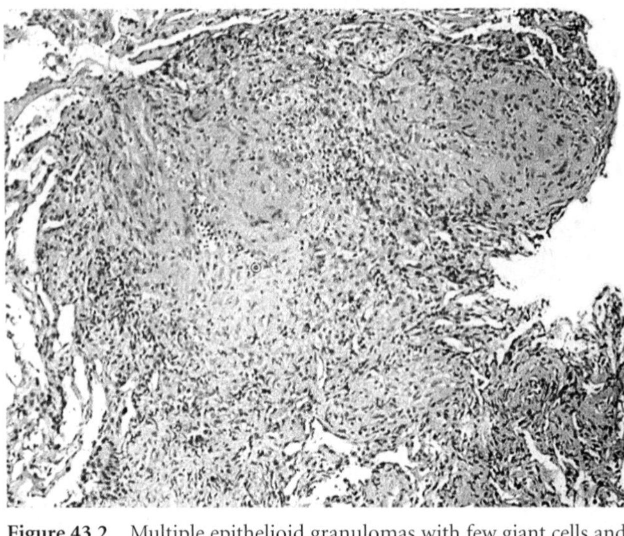

Figure 43.2 Multiple epithelioid granulomas with few giant cells and no necrosis.

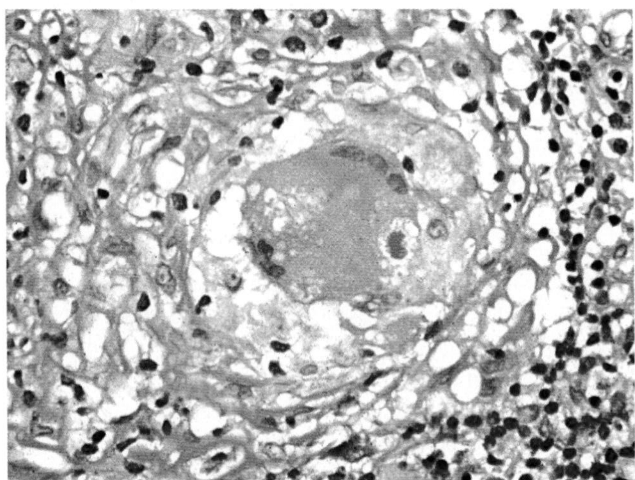

Figure 43.3 Multinucleated giant cell with asteroid bodies; these inclusions are characteristic, but not diagnostic, of sarcoidosis.

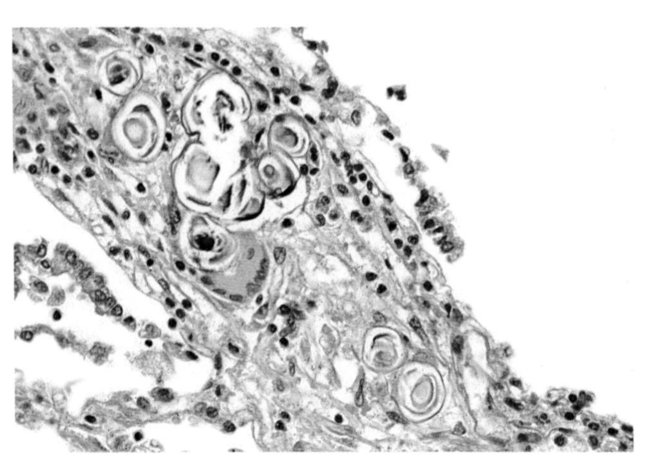

Figure 43.4 Schaumann bodies in the airway wall.

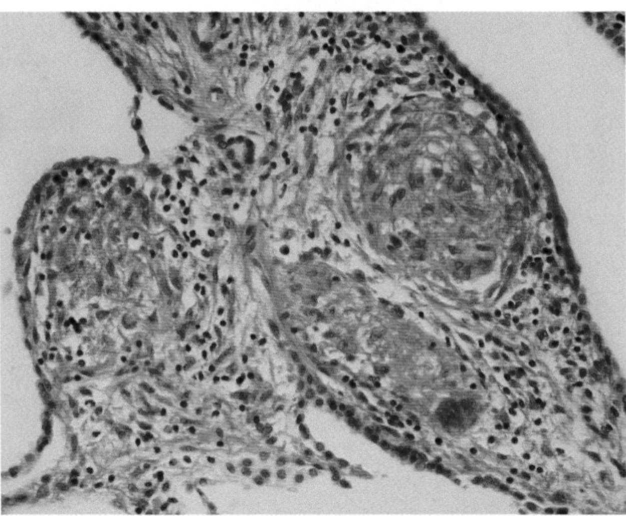

Figure 43.5 Higher power of noncaseating granulomas in alveolar wall.

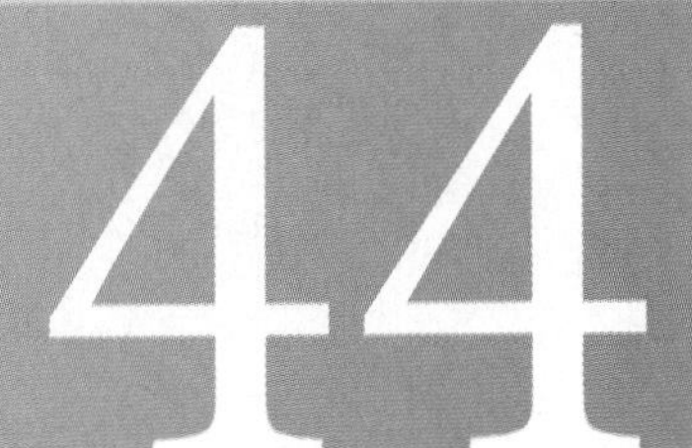

Necrotizing Sarcoid Granulomatosis

- Alvaro C. Laga
- Timothy Allen
- Abida Haque

Necrotizing sarcoid granulomatosis (NSG) is an unusual pulmonary lesion first described by Liebow and thought to represent a variant of Wegener's granulomatosis. In contrast to Wegener's granulomatosis, NSG contains well-formed granulomas in a lymphangitic distribution suggesting its relationship to sarcoidosis. Also, NSG has a better prognosis than Wegener's granulomatosis. The mean age of presentation is approximately 50 years, with a male-to-female predominance of 2:1. Presenting symptoms include cough, dyspnea, fever, and chest pain. Originally, the disease was thought to involve only the lungs; however, subsequent reports have demonstrated systemic disease with multiple organ involvement. Several reports suggest that NSG is a variant of nodular sarcoidosis. Grossly, the lesions of NSG are gray-white, well-circumscribed masses with central necrosis.

Histologic Features:

- Necrosis may appear suppurative, caseous, infarctlike, or fibrinoid, and palisading histiocytes frequently surround it.
- Vascular involvement in the form of granulomatous angiitis or lymphoplasmacytic angiitis.

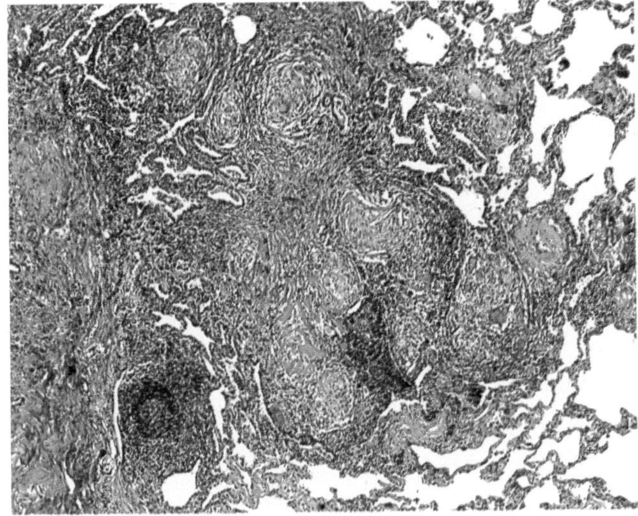

Figure 44.1 Low power showing well-formed granulomas.

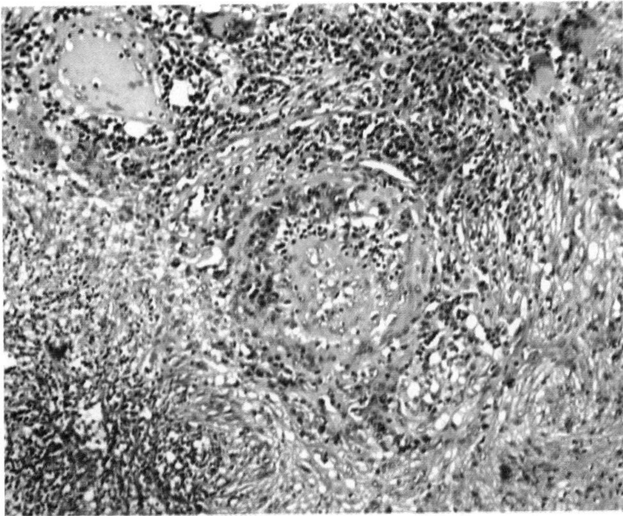

Figure 44.2 Medium power showing granulomatous angiitis and necrosis at *bottom left*.

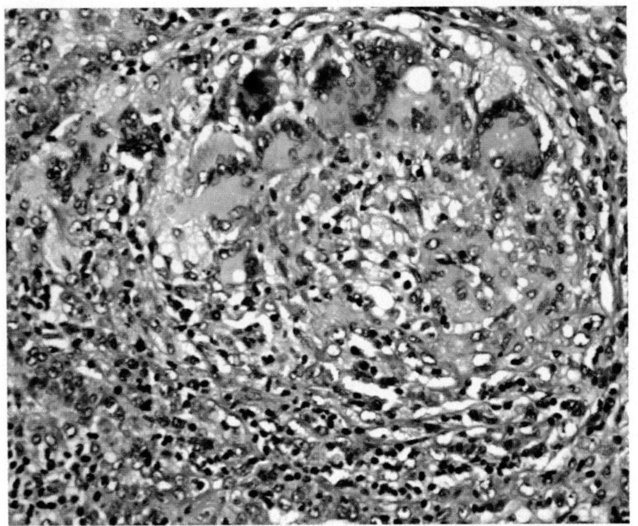

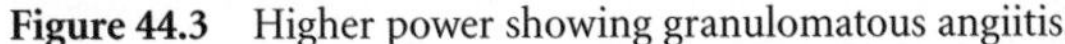

Figure 44.3 Higher power showing granulomatous angiitis.

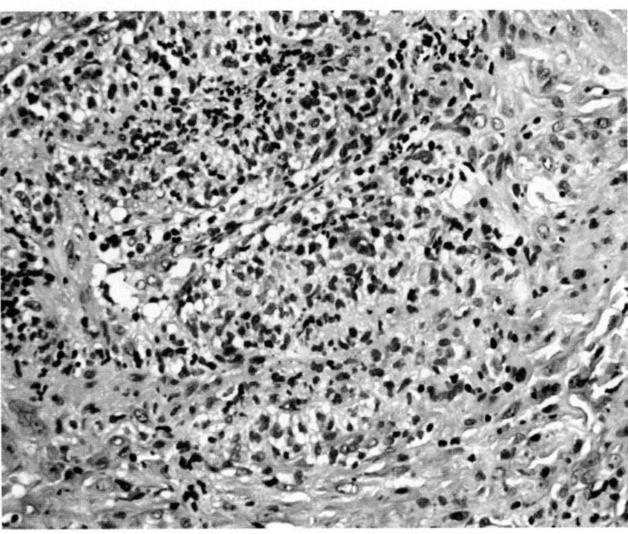

Figure 44.4 Higher power showing lymphoplasmacytic angiitis.

45 Sarcoidlike Reaction

▶ Abida Haque

Sarcoidlike epithelioid granulomas may be seen in thoracic lymph nodes draining areas of lung with carcinoma.

Histologic Features:

- These granulomas are identical to sarcoid granulomas; clinical history is essential for diagnosis.

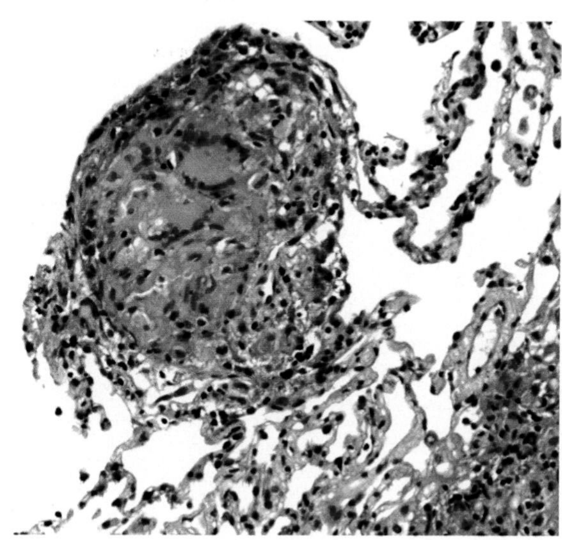

Figure 45.1 Small sarcoidlike granuloma is present in interstitium near a primary lung carcinoma.

46 Berylliosis

▶ Abida Haque

Beryllium is a lightweight metal used in the aerospace and electronic industries and in the manufacture of thermal couplings, atomic reactors, and fluorescent lights. Exposure to beryllium can result in acute or chronic disease. Acute berylliosis results from short-term exposure to high levels of soluble salts of beryllium, leading to a chemical pneumonitis with development of diffuse alveolar damage.

Chronic berylliosis manifests after several years of low-level exposure, resulting in granulomatous inflammation and pulmonary fibrosis later in the course of disease. Occupational history of beryllium exposure is essential for diagnosis. Diagnosis can be confirmed by demonstration of beryllium in the tissues using electron energy loss spectrometry (EELS), secondary ion mass spectrometry (SIMS), or laser microprobe mass analyzer (LAMMA). Differential diagnosis includes sarcoidosis and hypersensitivity pneumonitis.

Histologic Features:

- Epithelioid granulomas with asteroid bodies and Schaumann's bodies.
- Interstitial lymphocytic infiltrates are common; granulomas may be rare or absent in some cases.
- Peripheral airways show a greater nongranulomatous inflammation and alveolitis compared to sarcoidosis.
- Hilar lymph nodes usually not enlarged.

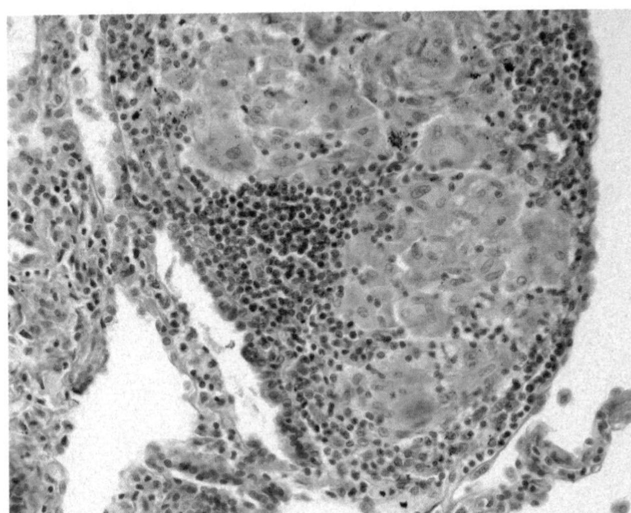

Figure 46.1 Noncaseating epithelioid granuloma adjacent to an airway.

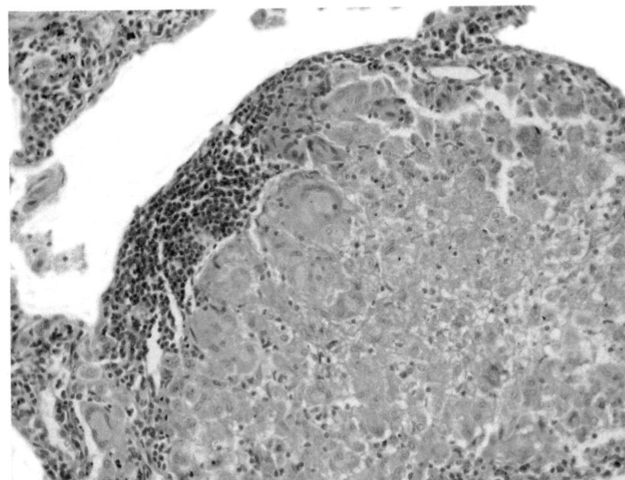

Figure 46.2 Epithelioid granuloma in the interstitium.

47 Foreign Body Granulomas

Foreign body granulomas may occur in the lung in the setting of intravenous drug abuse, chronic aspiration, and mineral oil aspiration, among other situations.

Part 1

Intravenous Drug Abuse

▶ Abida Haque and Carlos Bedrossian

Chronic intravenous drug abuse is associated with formation of foreign-body giant cell granulomas in the pulmonary alveolar interstitium and small vessels. Intravenous injection of unfiltered suspensions of drugs intended for oral use can result in formation of granulomas containing polarizable cellulose and talc in the lumen and walls of small to medium pulmonary arteries. Some of the common drugs used are methadone, propoxyphene hydrochloride, methylphenidate, tripelennamine, barbiturates, and pentazocine. Recently, several case reports of pulmonary granulomas following intravenous injection of pentazocine via parenteral nutrition catheters have been reported.

Histologic Features:

- Granulomas consist of lymphocytes, macrophages, and multinucleated giant cells containing small crystalline to platelike polarizable foreign bodies.
- Alveolar pulmonary capillaries and sometimes the small arterioles may show thrombosis associated with the birefringent crystalline deposits of talc.
- Granulomas may be associated with fibrosis.
- Pulmonary hypertensive changes, usually of mild degree, may be seen in chronic drug abusers.

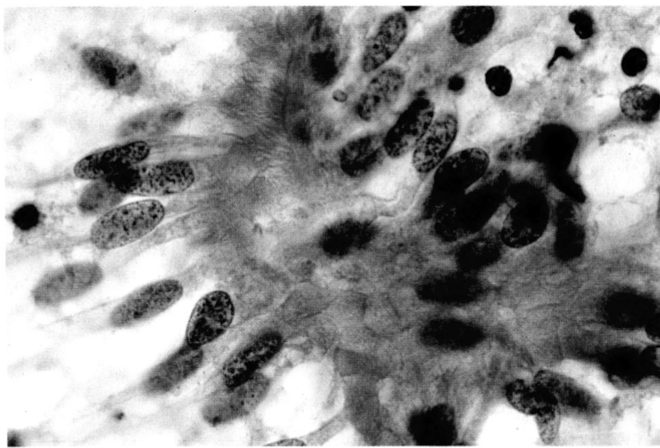

Figure 48.1 Fine needle aspirate cytology showing a small granuloma with palisading histiocytes.

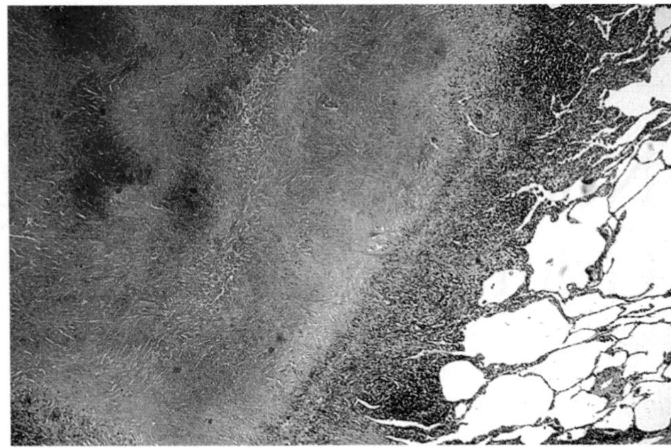

Figure 48.2 Rheumatoid nodule with central fibrinoid necrosis and peripheral palisading histiocytes with small collections of lymphocytes.

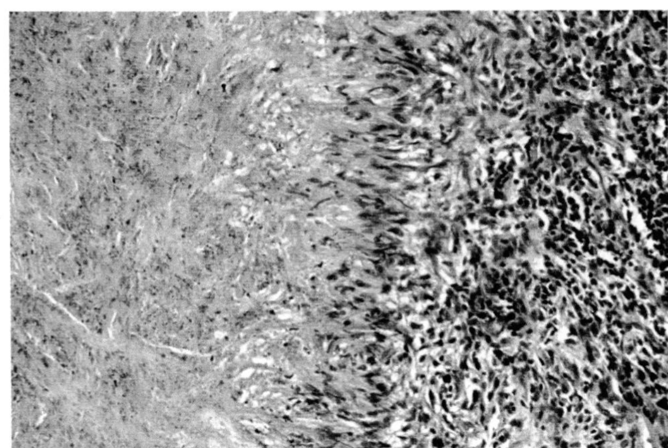

Figure 48.3 Higher power of palisading histiocytes.

Part 2

Malakoplakia

▶ Abida Haque and Mary Ostrowski

Malakoplakia is an unusual, granulomatous, often tumorlike inflammatory lesion associated with *Rhodococcus equi* infection in lungs of patients with acquired immunodeficiency syndrome or those immunosuppressed secondary to heart transplantation, lymphoma, or alcoholism. The lesion is caused by a defect in macrophage phagolysozyme function resulting in phagolysosomes being overloaded with bacteria and formation of Michaelis-Gutmann bodies (MGB).

Histologic Features:

- Nodules consist of sheets of foamy and granular histiocytes with eccentric nuclei, mixed with lymphocytes, plasma cells, and few neutrophils.
- The characteristic feature is the presence of MGB in the cytoplasm of histiocytes; these may be difficult to find, and a careful search is required if malakoplakia is suspected.
- Ultrastructurally, MGBs show a phospholysosomal core and a peripheral mineralized circle giving the characteristic targetoid appearance; the center may have intact or degenerating bacteria.
- Calcium stain (von Kossa) and Pearl iron stain differentiate these structures from fungi.
- Periodic acid–Schiff, with and without diastase, mucicarmine, colloidal iron, and Alcian blue, may also be used for diagnosis.

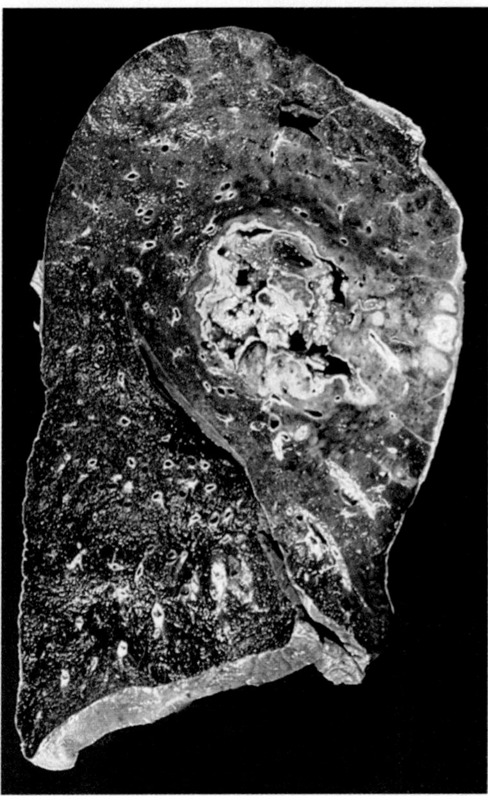

Figure 48.4 Gross figure showing consolidation surrounding a tumorlike nodule with central necrosis. Other cases may show only consolidation.

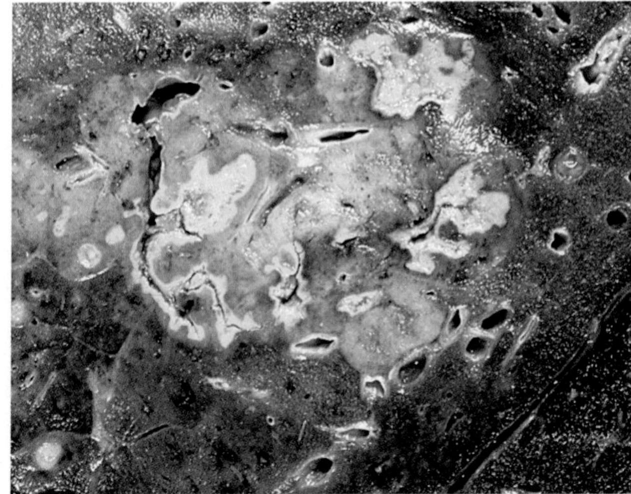

Figure 48.5 Higher power of the central necrotic area.

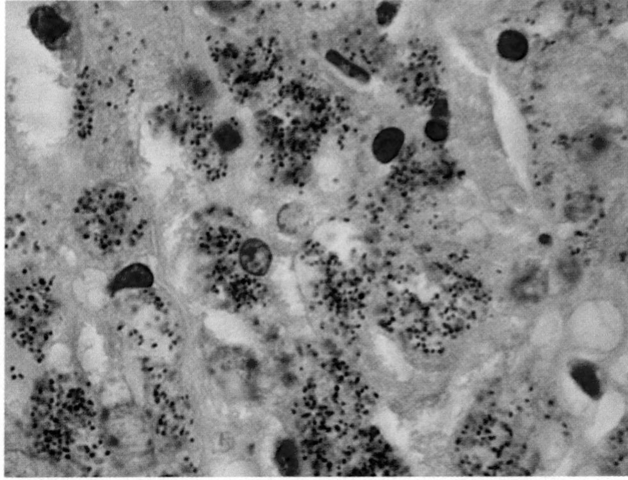

Figure 48.6 Gram stain showing the consolidated area with a dense lymphohistiocytic infiltrate containing intracellular Gram-positive coccobacilli of *R. equi.*

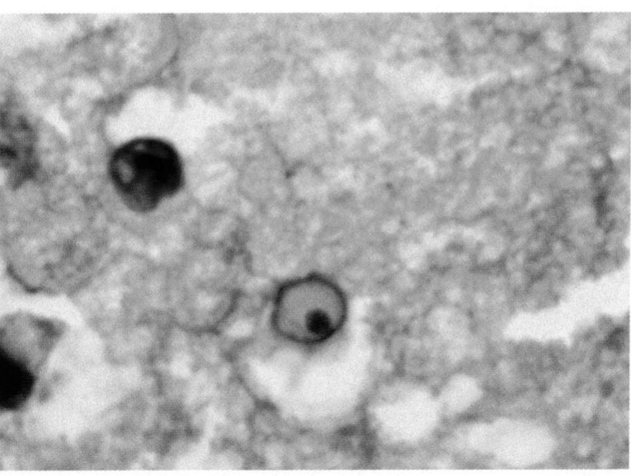

Figure 48.7 Macrophages with foamy cytoplasm and targetoid inclusion of MGB, which will stain with calcium (von Kossa) and iron (Pearl) stains.

Section 9

Diffuse Pulmonary Hemorrhage

Pulmonary Hemorrhage Without Vasculitis

49

Pulmonary hemorrhage without vasculitis is a common histologic finding. It may occur alone or in association with underlying conditions, including infections, diffuse alveolar damage, chronic passive congestion, arteriovenous abnormalities, and idiopathic pulmonary hemosiderosis.

Part 1

Hemorrhage Without Other Histologic Abnormalities

▶ Dani S. Zander

In lung biopsies, evidence of recent alveolar hemorrhage is extremely common and most often is a consequence of the biopsy procedure. The process of obtaining a biopsy of necessity interrupts vascular channels, causing release of blood into alveolar spaces. Coarse hemosiderin granules in the cytoplasm of macrophages, erythrophagocytosis, and evidence of acute lung injury or inflammation, however, are important clues that the hemorrhage predated the biopsy procedure and is a result of a pathologic process. Hemorrhage associated with a native or iatrogenic coagulopathy can appear identical to biopsy-induced hemorrhage, except for the additional finding of hemosiderin-laden macrophages. Nonprocedural trauma to lung tissue can also produce these same histologic changes but may be accompanied by other evidence of lung injury (necrosis, inflammation, hyaline membranes).

Occasionally the situation arises in which the patient has hemoptysis and blood in alveoli, but no other histologic abnormalities and no immunoglobulin deposition along the basement membrane are visible by immunofluorescence. Depending upon the history and chest radiograph findings, idiopathic pulmonary hemosiderosis may be considered, as well as the possibility that the lesion responsible for the hemorrhage was not sampled. Localized hemorrhage can be associated with neoplasms, localized infections, and thromboemboli that may not be represented in the biopsy. Blood in distal air spaces can also stem from small airway lesions (small neoplasms, vascular malformations, airway infections, and ulcerations) that may not be easily visualized during bronchoscopy or gross examination.

Histologic Features:

- Red blood cells and leukocytes in alveolar spaces.
- Hemosiderin-laden macrophages, erythrophagocytosis, evidence of acute lung injury, necrosis, and/or inflammation are clues that the hemorrhage stems from a pathologic process and not the biopsy procedure.

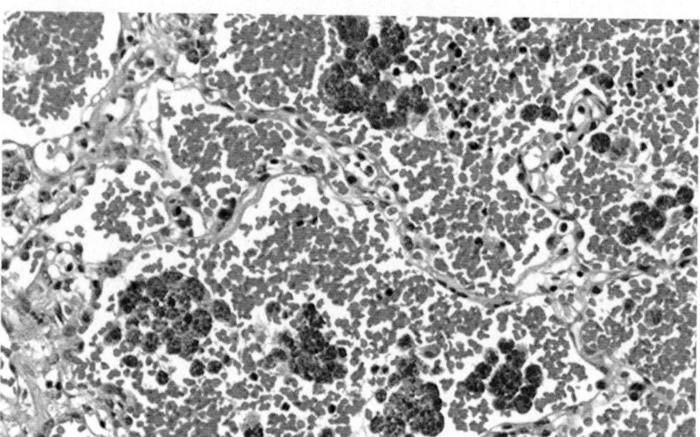

Figure 49.1 Hemosiderin-laden macrophages, indicating old hemorrhage, suggesting that the alveolar hemorrhage is a result of a pathologic process and not the biopsy procedure.

Part 2

Hemorrhage Associated with Infections

▶ Dani S. Zander

Some infectious agents and their products, as well as the host responses to certain infections, can lead to alveolar hemorrhage that is usually, but not always, localized to the areas involved by the infection. Some causes of hemorrhagic necrotizing pneumonias include *Pseudomonas aeruginosa, Klebsiella pneumoniae, Staphylococcus aureus,* and the herpes viruses (herpes simplex, varicella zoster, and cytomegalovirus). Angioinvasive fungi, such as *Aspergillus* sp and the Zygomycetes, cause hemorrhages as a consequence of their propensity for vascular invasion and for causing thrombosis. Additionally, granulomas can erode into blood vessels, occasionally causing significant hemorrhage. A rare and potentially fatal complication of cavitary tuberculosis, the Rasmussen aneurysm, is a pulmonary artery aneurysm caused by erosion of a tuberculous cavity into the artery. Rupture of the aneurysm leads to substantial, and sometimes fatal, hemorrhage.

Histologic Features:

- Several examples of infectious processes associated with hemorrhage are illustrated in the figures.
- Information about the histologic features of each type of infection is found in its specific part.

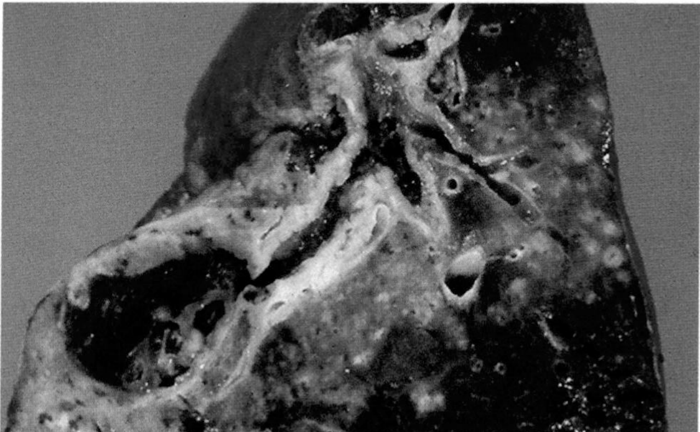

Figure 49.2 Gross figure of Rasmussen aneurysm showing a tuberculous cavity filled with blood. The source of the blood was a pulmonary artery into which the granuloma had eroded. The bronchus leading to the cavity has a nodular mucosal surface and a thickened wall, reflecting granulomatous bronchitis caused by *Mycobacterium tuberculosis.*

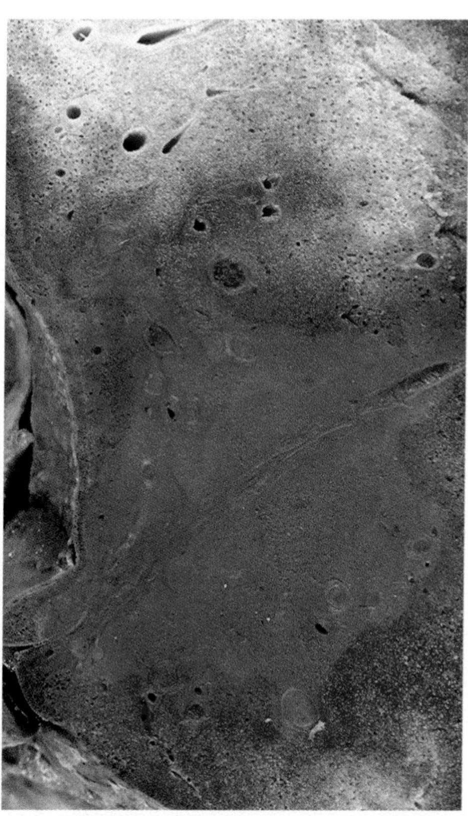

Figure 49.3 Gross figure of angioinvasive mucormycosis with extensive hemorrhage and infarction of the lung and multiple associated thrombi.

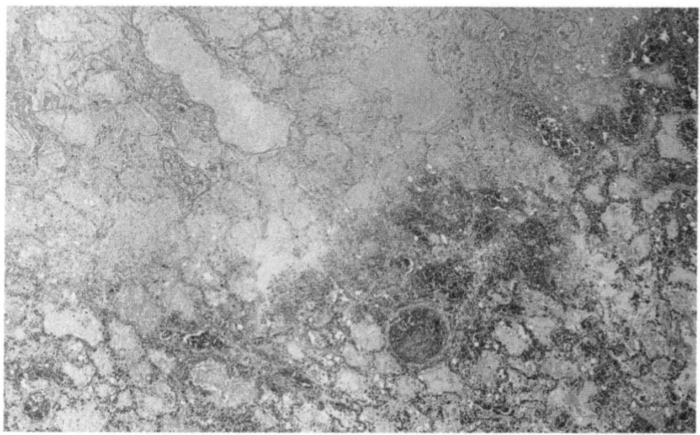

Figure 49.4 Hemorrhage and infarction secondary to angioinvasive mucormycosis, with recent coagulative necrosis and hemorrhage and a thrombus in a small vessel.

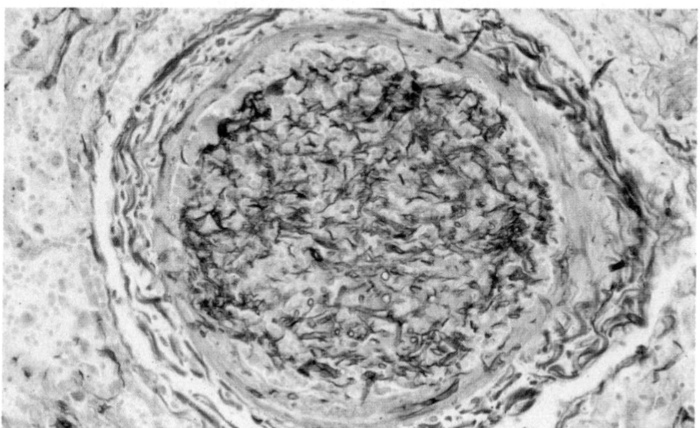

Figure 49.5 Angioinvasive mucormycosis showing a blood vessel obstructed by tangled fungal hyphae and fibrinous material, with hyphae extending through the vessel wall.

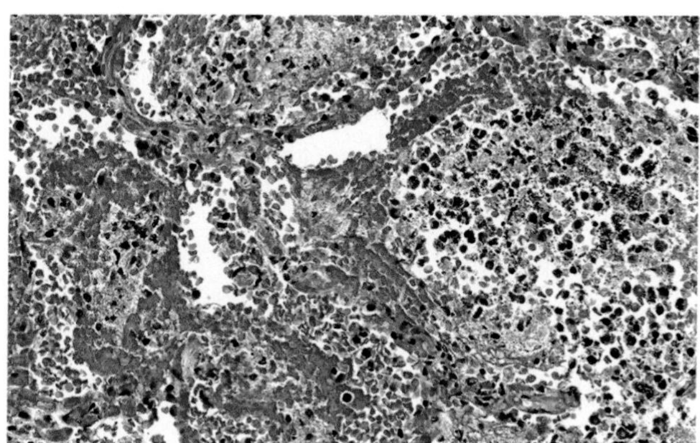

Figure 49.6 Necrotizing acute bronchopneumonia caused by *Staphylococcus aureus,* with an alveolar exudate consisting of degenerating inflammatory cells, fibrin, and numerous cocci associated with alveolar hemorrhage and alveolar septal necrosis.

Part 3

Hemorrhage with Diffuse Alveolar Damage

▶ Dani S. Zander

Diffuse alveolar damage accompanied by hemorrhage can be seen in multiple clinicopathologic settings. In many of these settings, additional histologic abnormalities are present to help point toward a particular process or group of processes. Histologic evidence of vasculitis and infections should be sought. Information about multisystem disease presentations, autoantibody serologies, drug (especially cytotoxic chemotherapeutic agents) and toxin exposures, and coagulation parameters may help to account for the observed findings.

Histologic Features:

- Red blood cells in alveolar spaces.
- Additional histologic abnormalities may be present, depending on the cause of the process.

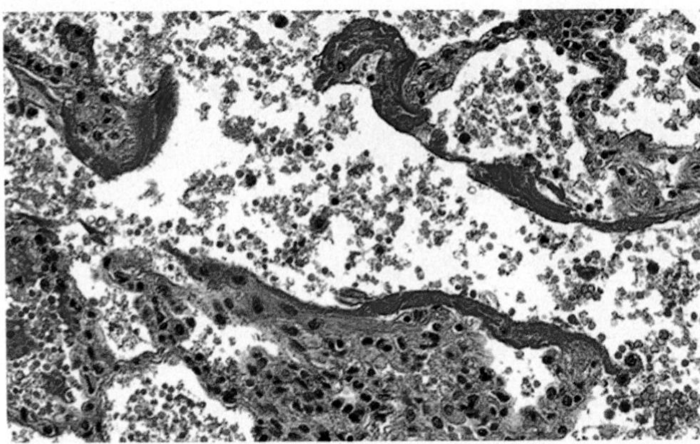

Figure 49.7 Hyaline membranes lining alveolar septa and alveolar spaces containing numerous red blood cells.

Part 4

Chronic Passive Congestion and Congestive Vasculopathy

▶ Dani S. Zander

Chronic passive congestion is a consequence of chronic pulmonary venous outflow obstruction, usually of cardiac origin. The impediment to pulmonary venous outflow causes elevation of pulmonary venous pressure, which is transmitted to the alveolar capillaries and the pulmonary arteries. Left ventricular failure and mitral valvular disease are the most common causes for this condition. Occasionally, however, the disorder results from congenital cardiac abnormalities, left atrial myxoma, or compression of the large pulmonary veins by a neoplasm, enlarged lymph nodes, or mediastinal fibrosis. Changes of chronic passive congestion also form part of the constellation of histologic findings seen in pulmonary venoocclusive disease.

Histologic Features:

- Alveoli contain hemosiderin-laden macrophages, congestion, interstitial and alveolar edema, and interstitial fibrosis and pneumocyte proliferation.
- Pulmonary veins show medial hypertrophy and arterialization and intimal fibrosis.
- Pulmonary arteries show medial hypertrophy and muscularization of arterioles, medial hypertrophy in muscular arteries, and intimal fibrosis.
- Lymphatic dilation.

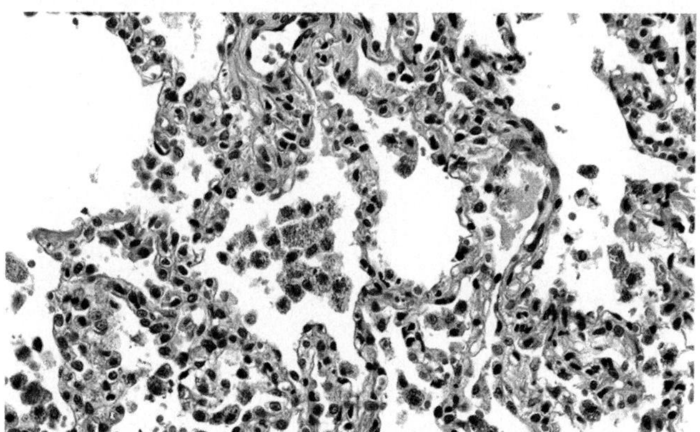

Figure 49.8 Alveoli with mild interstitial edema containing hemosiderin-laden macrophages and small numbers of red blood cells.

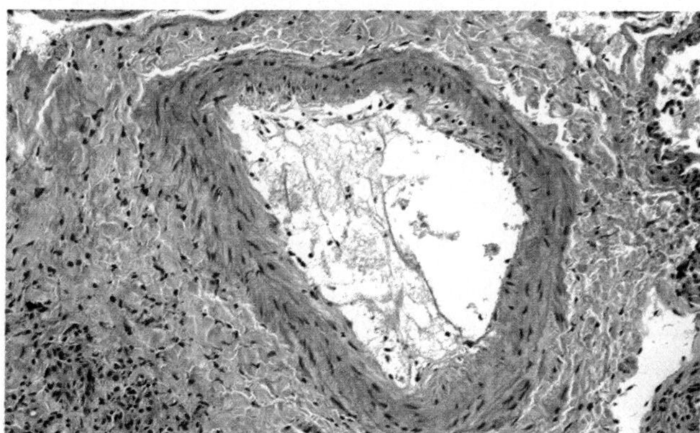

Figure 49.9 Dilated pulmonary vein with medial hypertrophy and adventitial fibrosis.

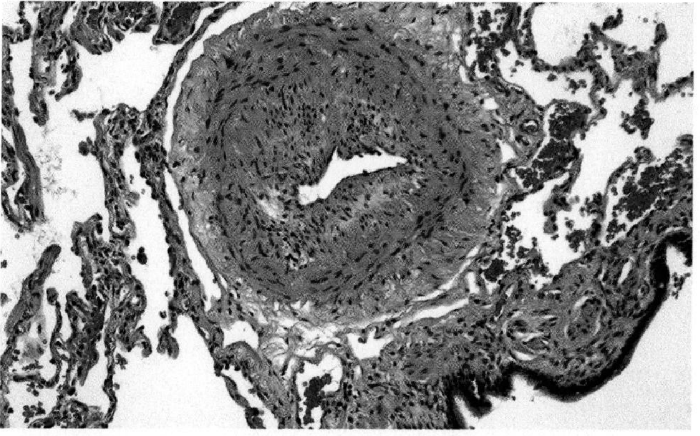

Figure 49.10 Muscular pulmonary artery with marked medial hypertrophy.

Part 5

Arteriovenous Malformation

▶ Dani S. Zander

Arteriovenous malformations occur in children and adults as isolated or multifocal lesions. Many are congenital and found in patients with Rendu-Osler-Weber syndrome. Pregnancy-related hemothorax and hemoptysis have been reported in several women with this syndrome. Other associations include alcoholism, trauma, and infection. The lesions may be visible as focal opacities on chest radiographs, but they can be clearly identified by arteriography. Coil embolization can be used to treat these lesions.

Histologic Features:

- Abnormally dilated blood vessels of varying sizes, often in a cluster.
- Blood vessels often have irregularly thickened walls.
- Hemorrhage and hemosiderin-laden macrophages may be present in adjacent lung tissue.
- Thrombosis may be present.

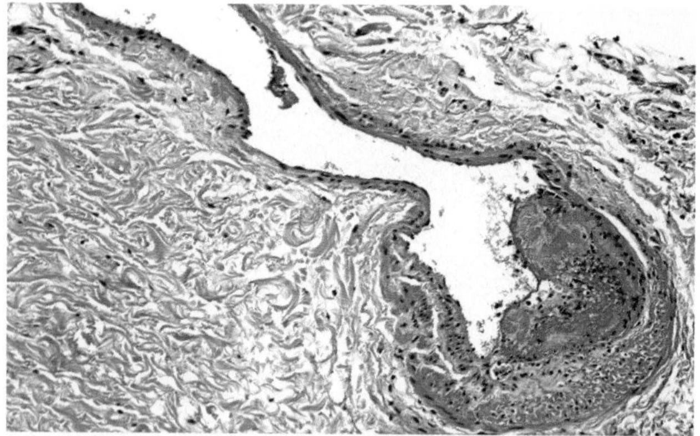

Figure 49.11 The vessel media varies markedly in thickness, and the vessel contains a fibrin thrombus.

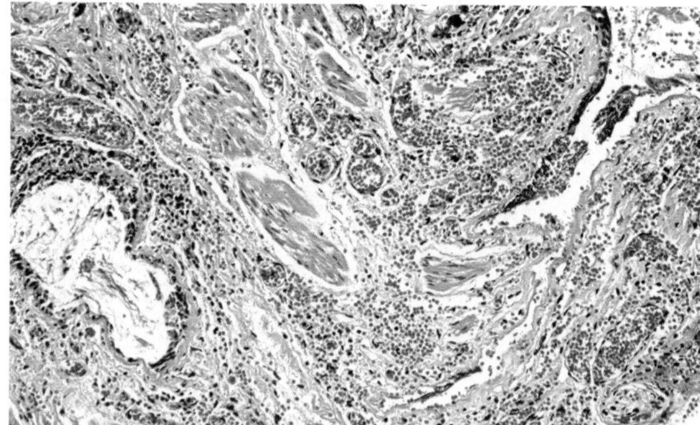

Figure 49.12 Bronchus of a patient with suspected Osler-Weber-Rendu syndrome who presented with hemoptysis during pregnancy shows multiple thin-walled channels filled with blood and hemorrhage in the bronchial mucosa.

Part 6

Idiopathic Pulmonary Hemosiderosis

▶ Dani S. Zander

Idiopathic pulmonary hemosiderosis primarily affects children and young adults; it is uncommon after the third decade of life. Symptoms include pulmonary hemorrhage, which is recurrent and intermittent, can be massive, and can lead to iron deficiency; cough; shortness of breath; and chest discomfort. The diagnosis is one of exclusion. Other causes of diffuse alveolar hemorrhage must be investigated and eliminated before applying this diagnosis. Other systemic abnormalities are absent, and there are no detectable antinuclear antibodies, antiglomerular basement membrane antibodies, or antineutrophil cytoplasmic antibodies. The trigger for this disorder is unknown, but described associations include celiac disease, autoimmune hemolytic anemia, IgA nephropathy, dermatitis herpetiformis, thyrotoxicosis, and sensitivity to cow's milk. Familial cases have been reported.

Cytologic Features:

- Bronchoalveolar lavage: hemosiderin-laden macrophages and red blood cells.

Histologic Features:

- Extensive alveolar red blood cells and/or hemosiderin-laden macrophages.
- Interstitial fibrosis and pneumocyte proliferation may be present with increasing duration of the disease.
- Iron deposition on alveolar septal elastic fibers.
- No evidence of small vessel vasculitis.
- No immunoglobulin or complement deposition visible by immunofluorescence.

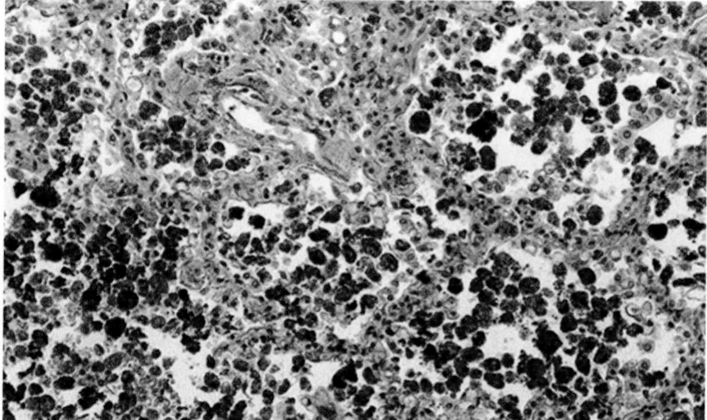

Figure 49.13 Alveolar spaces filled with numerous hemosiderin-laden macrophages. Mild interstitial fibrosis is present.

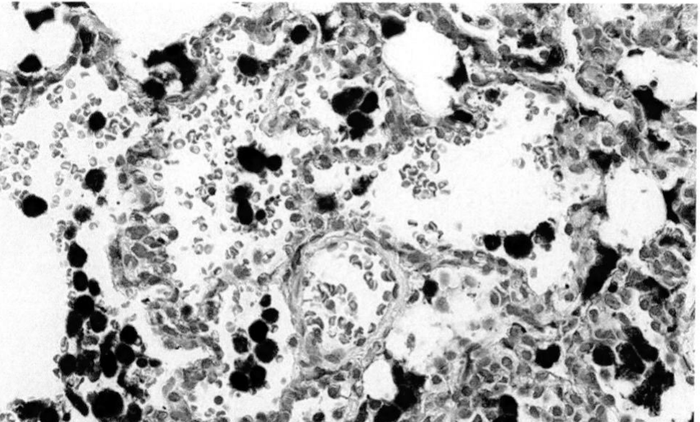

Figure 49.14 Prussian blue stain for iron (blue) highlighting the hemosiderin-containing macrophages. Red blood cells are present in alveoli.

Pulmonary Hemorrhage with Vasculitis

50

Pulmonary hemorrhage with vasculitis may occur in a variety of disorders, including collagen vascular disease, antiglomerular basement membrane antibody disease, Wegener's granulomatosis, Churg-Strauss syndrome, microscopic polyarteritis, and Behçet disease.

Part 1

Vasculitis in Collagen Vascular Diseases

▶ Dani S. Zander

Collagen vascular diseases represent an important category of causes of diffuse alveolar hemorrhage (DAH). Among the collagen vascular diseases, systemic lupus erythematosus is the most frequent cause of DAH, and the DAH may precede other disease manifestations. Other collagen vascular diseases associated with DAH include mixed connective tissue disease, rheumatoid arthritis, Henoch-Schönlein purpura, scleroderma, and polymyositis/dermatomyositis. Features of other systemic disease involvement and serologic studies for antinuclear antibodies, other autoantibodies, and rheumatoid factor, are usually helpful for diagnosis of specific conditions. Immune complexes are believed to play a role in the pathogenesis of alveolar hemorrhage.

Histologic Features:

- Extensive alveolar red blood cells and/or hemosiderin-laden macrophages.
- Small vessel vasculitis (also known as acute capillaritis, neutrophilic capillaritis, or necrotizing alveolitis), an intense neutrophil infiltrate in widened alveolar septa, sometimes associated with alveolar septal necrosis.
- Immunofluorescence shows granular deposits of IgG, IgM, IgA, and/or C3 in alveolar septal capillaries, interstitium, and other vessel walls.

highly associated with Wegener's granulomatosis and typically reflects specificity for proteinase 3. Occasionally a perinuclear immunofluorescence pattern (P-ANCA) may be demonstrated, but the P-ANCA pattern is more closely associated with other disorders. C-ANCAs are more common in patients with more active and more extensive disease. In patients with generalized disease that is active, in partial remission, or in complete remission, the frequencies of C-ANCAs are 84% to 99%, 50% to 71%, and 30% to 40%, respectively. In patients with limited disease, the corresponding frequencies for active disease, partial remission, and complete remission are 67%, 54%, and 32%. A positive ANCA result, however, does not mean that the patient has Wegener's granulomatosis. The diagnosis is most confidently made in the context of compatible clinical and pathologic findings, ideally supported further by the presence of C-ANCA. Exclusion of other processes that have overlapping clinical and histologic features, particularly infections, is also necessary.

Histologic Features:

Major Pathologic Manifestations

- Vasculitis.
  - Vessels involved: arteries, arterioles, veins, venules, alveolar capillaries.
  - Histologic changes:
    - Inflammation: neutrophilic, mononuclear cell, necrotizing granulomatous, non-necrotizing granulomatous, fibrinoid necrosis.
    - Cicatricial changes: intimal and medial fibrosis, intimal proliferation.
- Parenchymal necrosis: microabscess, geographic necrosis.
- Granulomatous inflammation: granuloma with central microabscess, palisading histiocytes, scattered giant cells, poorly formed granulomas, sarcoidlike granulomas (rare).

Minor Pathologic Manifestations

- Nodular interstitial fibrosis, organizing pneumonia, endogenous lipoid pneumonia, hemorrhage, eosinophil infiltration, lymphoid aggregates, xanthogranulomatous lesions, bronchiolitis (acute, chronic, or follicular), acute bronchopneumonia, bronchocentric granulomatosis, bronchial stenosis.

Differential Diagnosis

- Infections, especially mycobacteria, fungi, nocardia.
- Churg-Strauss syndrome.
- Lymphomatoid granulomatosis.
- Sarcoidosis.
- Necrotizing sarcoid granulomatosis.
- Bronchocentric granulomatosis.
- Rheumatoid arthritis (rheumatoid nodule, small vessel vasculitis).
- Other causes of small vessel vasculitis.

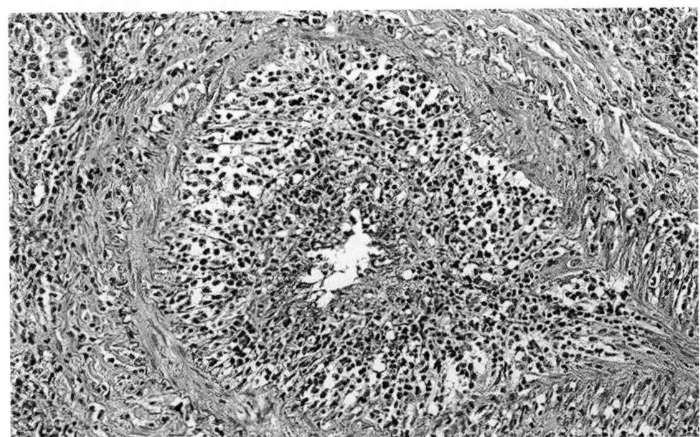

Figure 50.5 Medium-sized artery with vasculitis showing infiltration by a mixed population of inflammatory cells, with associated endothelial cell injury.

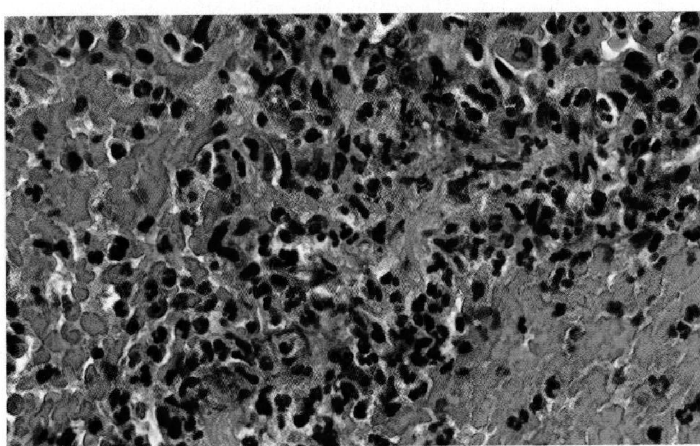

Figure 50.6 Small vessel vasculitis showing a dense, predominantly neutrophilic, infiltrate focused upon the alveolar capillary, with associated alveolar hemorrhage.

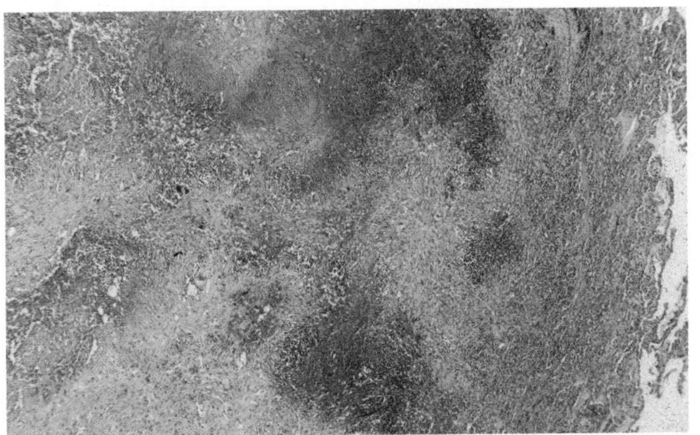

Figure 50.7 Large zones of geographic necrosis (basophilic) surrounded by inflammation.

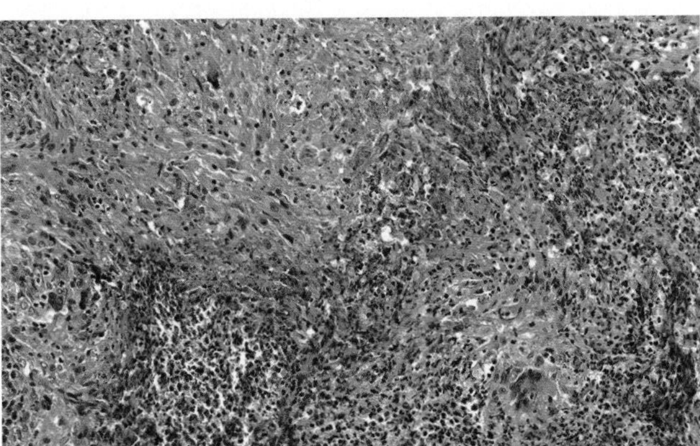

Figure 50.8 Areas of geographic necrosis containing abundant nuclear debris, mainly derived from neutrophils. Histiocytes and scattered multinucleated giant cells rim the necrotic focus.

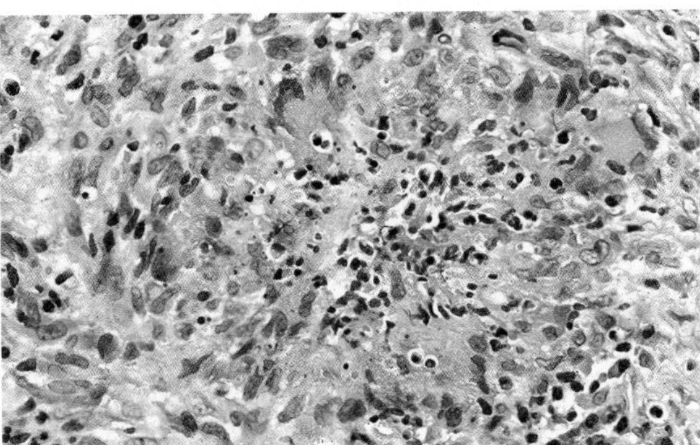

Figure 50.9 Small granuloma with neutrophils showing the beginnings of a microabscess.

Part 4

Churg-Strauss Syndrome

▶ Dani S. Zander

Churg-Strauss syndrome is a rare multisystem allergic disorder of unknown cause. Recent studies suggest that autoimmunity is involved in its pathogenesis, and 48% to 66% of patients with the syndrome have antineutrophil cytoplasmic antibodies (usually P-ANCA). Criteria for diagnosis have evolved from an emphasis on pathologic findings to a combination of features that are primarily clinical. A subcommittee of the American College of Rheumatology proposed two approaches to diagnosis: a traditional format classification and a classification tree. The traditional format classification system provides six criteria; satisfaction of four of these criteria is associated with a sensitivity of 85% and a specificity of 99.7% for diagnosis of Churg-Strauss syndrome. These criteria include the following:

- Asthma.
- Eosinophils >10% of the white blood cell differential count.
- Mononeuropathy or polyneuropathy.
- Nonfixed radiographic pulmonary infiltrates.
- Paranasal sinus abnormality.
- Extravascular eosinophil infiltration on biopsy.

The criteria included in the classification tree are asthma, eosinophilia >10% on differential white blood cell count, and history of documented allergy other than asthma or drug sensitivity. Presence of eosinophilia and a documented history of either asthma or allergy are associated with a sensitivity of 95% and specificity of 99.2% for diagnosis of Churg-Strauss syndrome.

The organ systems most often involved are the upper and lower respiratory tract, skin, and peripheral nerves. Other common sites include the kidneys, heart, gastrointestinal tract, and central nervous system. The spectrum of manifestations is broad and is discussed more extensively in the referenced articles. The disease is usually diagnosed in middle age and typically evolves through several phases. During the prodrome, patients experience allergic rhinitis, asthma, peripheral eosinophilia, and/or eosinophilic infiltrative disease in the lungs (eosinophilic pneumonia) or gastrointestinal tract. Patients identified during this phase usually respond well to corticosteroids and have an excellent prognosis. The time interval between this phase and development of vasculitis varies, but it can last for years (mean latency is 8 years). The vasculitic phase follows, offering the best opportunity for pathologic demonstration of vasculitis and clinical diagnosis of the condition. In the final postvasculitic phase, manifestations may include neuropathy, hypertension, asthma, and allergic rhinitis.

Corticosteroids are the first-line therapy for patients with Churg-Strauss disease. Tapering of the corticosteroid dose in some patients with asthma has been thought to "unmask" Churg-Strauss disease. Cyclophosphamide is also used with more severe or relapsing disease.

Cytologic Features:

- Bronchoalveolar lavage fluid often contains markedly increased numbers of eosinophils and Charcot-Leyden crystals; hemosiderin-laden macrophages also may be present.

Histologic Features: Prodromal Phase

- Extravascular tissue infiltration by eosinophils (may occur in any organ); in the lung, chronic eosinophilic pneumonia is common.
- Differential diagnosis includes allergic bronchopulmonary aspergillosis, chronic eosinophilic pneumonia, asthma, and peripheral blood eosinophilia without Churg-Strauss syndrome.

Vasculitic Phase

- Eosinophil-rich necrotizing or nonnecrotizing vasculitis involving small arteries, arterioles, venules, veins (may occur in any organ); occasionally capillaries are involved.
  - In the skin, a leukocytoclastic vasculitis is common.
  - Capillaritis occurs occasionally in the lung.
  - Hemosiderin-laden macrophages in the lung may reflect subclinical alveolar hemorrhage.
    - Necrotizing granulomas centered on necrotic eosinophils.
    - Extravascular tissue infiltration by eosinophils (may occur in any organ); in the lung, chronic eosinophilic pneumonia is common.
    - Differential diagnosis includes Wegener's granulomatosis and microscopic polyarteritis.

Postvasculitic Phase

- Healed vasculitis: small vessels are thrombosed and demonstrate loss of large portions of the elastic lamina (latter is uncommon with typical emboli).
- Eosinophils may be absent if steroid therapy has been successful.

Helpful Hints

- Steroid treatment alters the histology by suppressing eosinophil infiltration and causing eosinophil necrosis, which may make it difficult to identify the eosinophils in eosinophil abscesses; information about the existence of asthma, sinus disease, symptoms of neuropathy, and earlier peripheral blood eosinophilia may be invaluable for putting pathologic findings into perspective.
- Necrotic material in granulomas is usually eosinophilic, in contrast to Wegener's granulomatosis, where the necrotic material contains abundant neutrophil debris and is more basophilic.

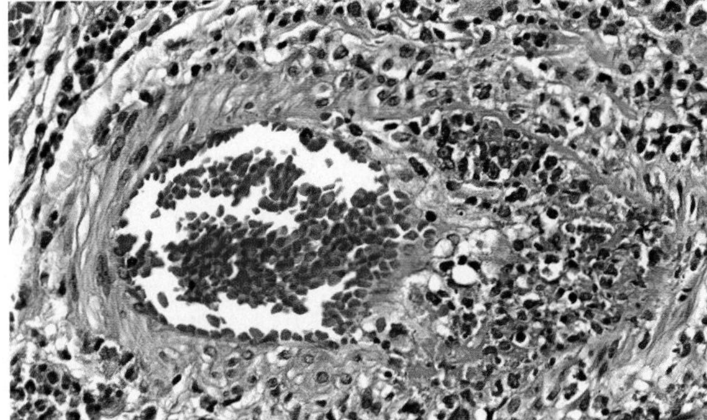

Figure 50.10 Necrotizing vasculitis, with a small vessel containing mural necrosis associated with a mixed inflammatory cell infiltrate containing eosinophils, which are also numerous around the vessel.

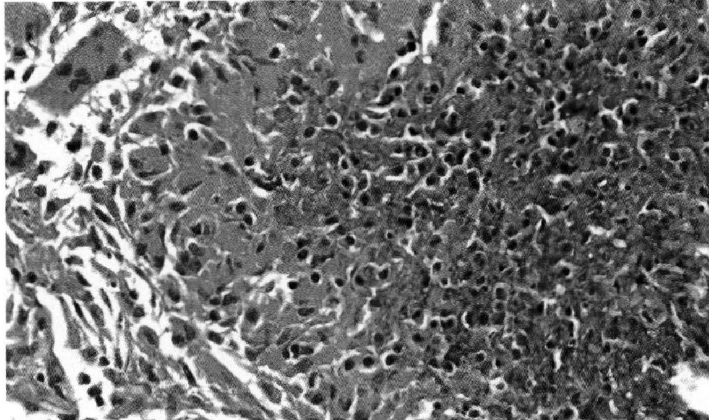

Figure 50.11 Necrotizing granuloma containing eosinophils, which are identifiable in the necrotic center of this granuloma.

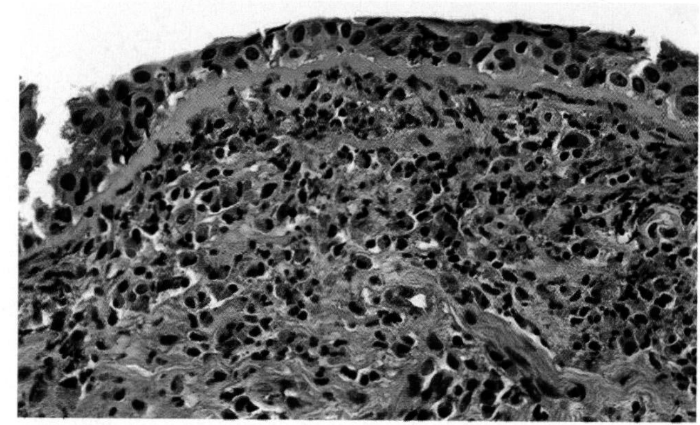

Figure 50.12 Asthma, with a bronchial wall containing a dense infiltrate of eosinophils and other inflammatory cells, basement membrane thickening, and metaplastic squamous epithelium lining the surface.

Part 5

Microscopic Polyarteritis

▶ Dani S. Zander

Microscopic polyarteritis is a multisystem necrotizing small vessel vasculitis with few or no immune deposits, which involves the lung in about 50% of patients. Most patients are middle aged or older adults. Disease onset usually progresses rapidly. Common manifestations include glomerulonephritis, dyspnea, cough, hemoptysis, fever, and arthralgias. Over 80% of patients have antineutrophil cytoplasmic antibodies (usually P-ANCA).

Histologic Features:

- Alveolar hemorrhage and fibrin.
- Depending upon chronicity, hemosiderin-laden macrophages and alveolar organization may be present.
- Small vessel vasculitis (neutrophilic capillaritis): patchy areas of prominent neutrophil infiltration into the interstitium; neutrophils often spill into adjacent alveolar spaces as well.
- Vasculitis may also affect arterioles and venules.
- Neutrophil nuclear debris is usually present.
- Diffuse alveolar damage may be present.
- Differential diagnosis includes acute pneumonia (bacterial, less often viral or fungal), early diffuse alveolar damage with hemorrhage, other causes of neutrophilic capillaritis (Wegener's granulomatosis, drug reactions, collagen vascular diseases, cryoglobulinemia, and other rare associated conditions).

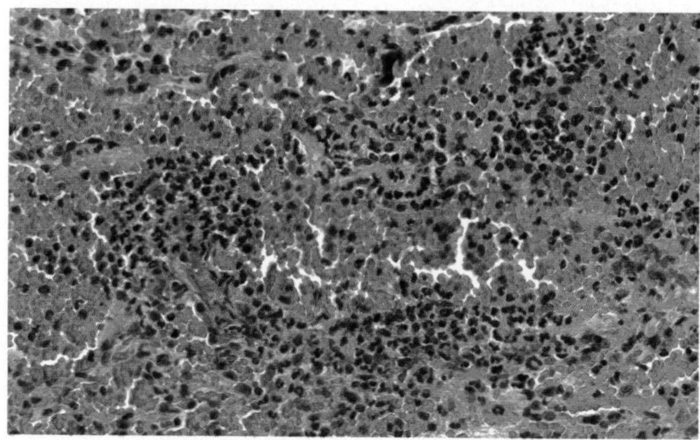

Figure 50.13 Alveolar septa permeated by neutrophils, which spill into alveolar spaces, and extensive alveolar hemorrhage.

Part 6

Behçet Disease

▶ Abida Haque and Dani S. Zander

Behçet disease is a multisystem disease with typical manifestations of recurrent aphthous stomatitis, uveitis, genital ulcers, synovitis, meningoencephalitis, and cutaneous vasculitis. This disorder has its highest prevalence in countries along the ancient "Silk Road" from Japan to the Middle East and Mediterranean, but cases have occurred worldwide. The etiology and pathogenesis of Behçet disease have not been fully outlined, but genetic and environmental factors appear to be important. HLA-B51 is linked to susceptibility to Behçet disease. Antigenic stimulation of T cells leading to cytokine production appears to play a role in the activation of neutrophils that is characteristic of this disorder. Antiendothelial cell antibodies have been demonstrated and may contribute to endothelial cell injury and predisposition to thrombosis. Circulating immune complexes have also been found in association with active pulmonary disease.

Histologic Features:

- Lymphocytic and necrotizing vasculitis involving pulmonary vessels of all sizes.
- Aneurysms of elastic pulmonary arteries, which may lead to bronchial erosions and arteriobronchial fistulas.
- Venous and arterial thrombosis.
- Pulmonary infarcts.
- Pulmonary hemorrhage.
- Perivascular adventitial fibrosis.
- Acute interstitial pneumonia.

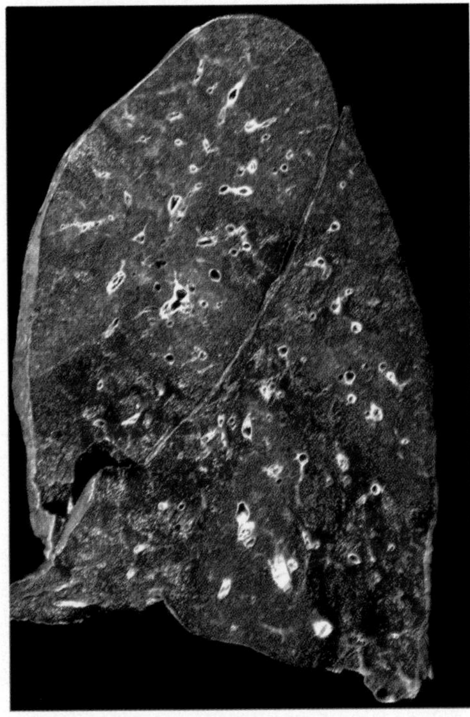

Figure 50.14 Gross figure showing irregular zones of parenchymal hemorrhage.

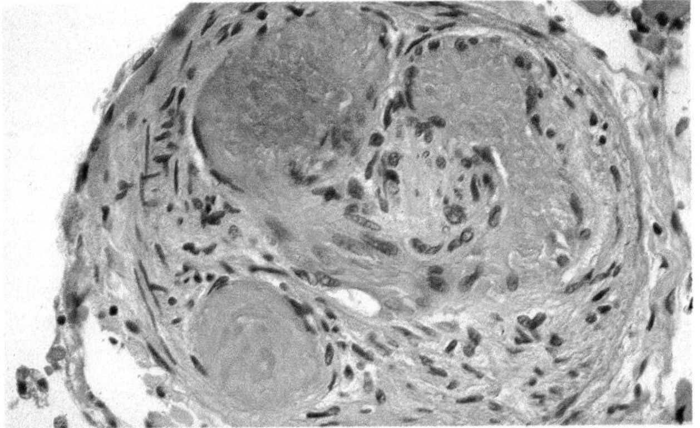

Figure 50.15 Recanalized vessel with recent thrombosis.

Section 10

Pulmonary Hypertension and Emboli

Primary Pulmonary Hypertension

51

▶ Abida Haque
▶ Dani S. Zander

Primary pulmonary hypertension is a disease of unclear etiology characterized by elevated pulmonary arterial pressure. The World Health Organization defines pulmonary hypertension as the presence of a systolic pulmonary artery pressure exceeding 40 mm Hg. Primary pulmonary hypertension is an uncommon disease that develops sporadically in most cases, and rarely occurs in a familial form linked with a mutation of the *PPH1* gene at chromosome 2q33. In a patient with pulmonary hypertension, exclusion of other recognized causes of pulmonary hypertension is necessary before considering a diagnosis of primary pulmonary hypertension. Primary pulmonary hypertension has a female predominance of 2:1 and can develop at any age. The initiating event in PPH is believed to be endothelial injury leading to intimal cellular proliferation, medial thickening, and plexiform and dilation lesions. The pathology is limited to pulmonary vessels and right heart.

Histologic Features:
Plexiform Lesions

- Capillary proliferations in the lumens of dilated small muscular pulmonary arteries near branch points, which often protrude outside the vessel wall through medial defects and may be associated with dilated distal arterial segments.

Angiomatoid Lesions

- Clusters of dilated thin-walled arterial branches.
- Medial hypertrophy of arteries.
- Muscularization of arterioles.
- Cellular intimal proliferation.
- Concentric laminar intimal fibrosis.
- Fibrinoid arterial necrosis.

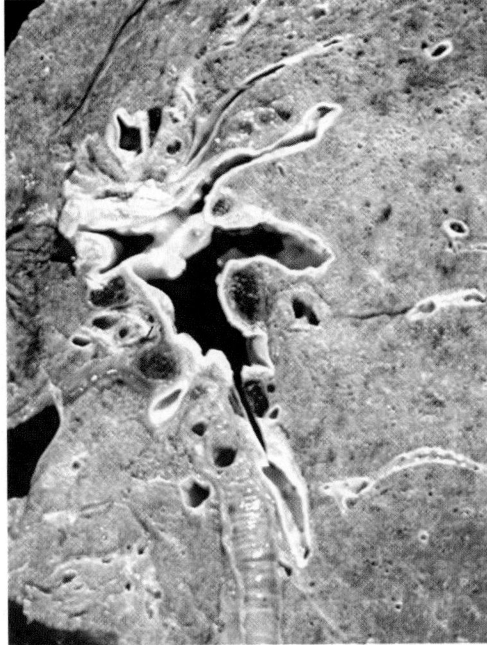

Figure 51.1 Gross figure showing a dilated and thickened pulmonary artery with yellowish atherosclerotic plaques. The lung parenchyma has a brownish-orange tinge from large collections of hemosiderin-laden macrophages indicating chronic alveolar hemorrhage.

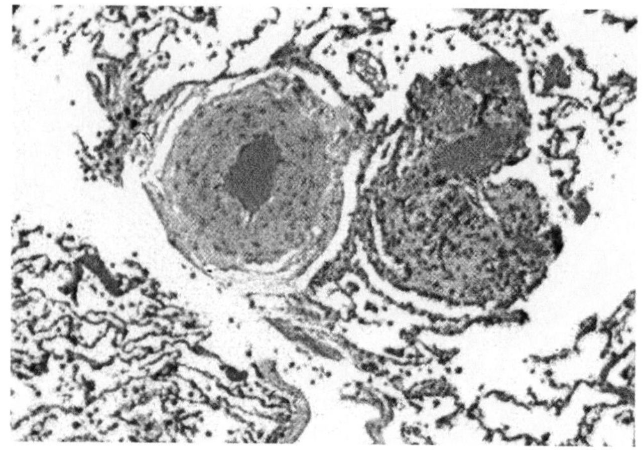

Figure 51.2 Small pulmonary artery with medial thickening on the **left,** and a plexiform lesion associated with dilatation lesion on the **right.**

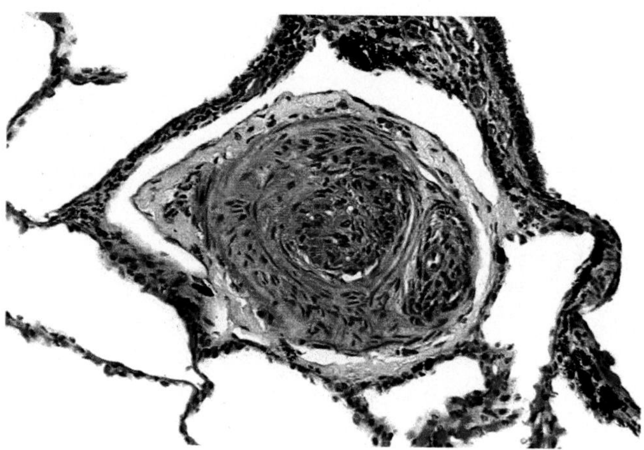

Figure 51.3 Higher power of a small pulmonary arteriole with plexiform lesion.

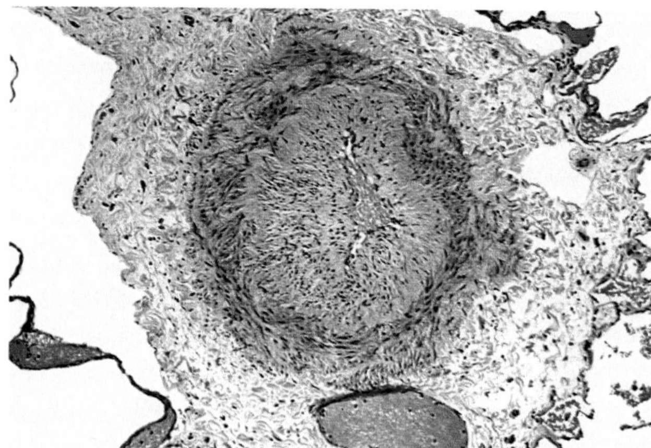

Figure 51.4 Small pulmonary artery with marked intimal thickening and fibrosis and mild medial thickening.

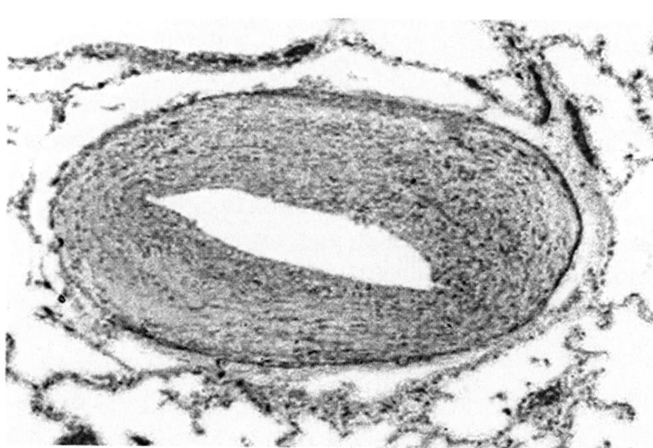

Figure 51.5 Movat stain of small pulmonary artery with marked medial hypertrophy and fibrosis.

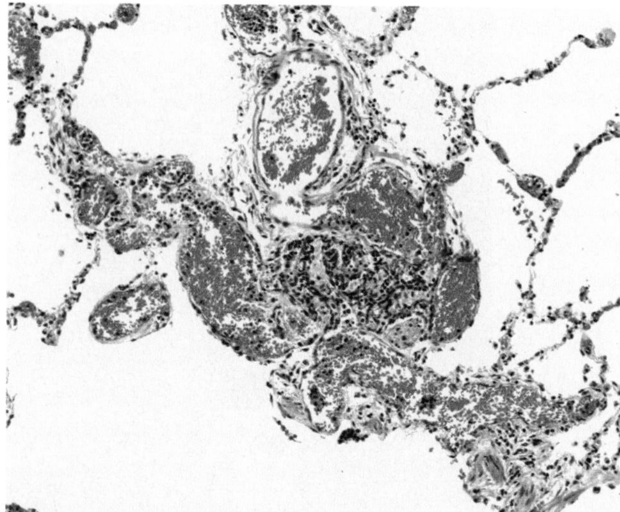

Figure 51.6 Plexiform lesion occupies the lumen of a dilated pulmonary artery and consists of a plexus of small-caliber vascular channels that open into dilated distal arterial branches. The dilated vessels show marked thinning of the media.

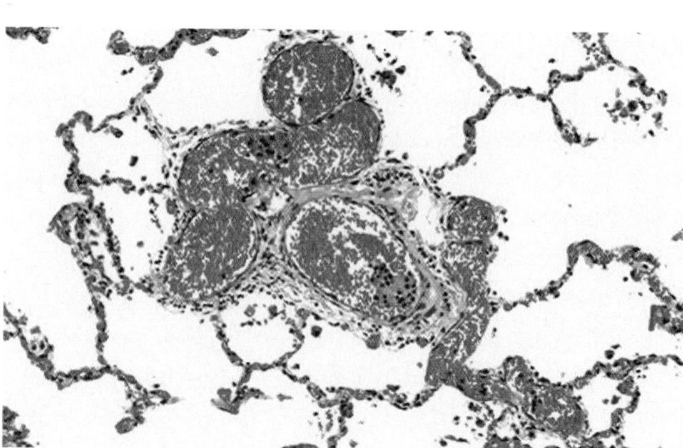

Figure 51.7 These arterial branches are dilated, resemble veins, and contain small platelet aggregates.

52 Secondary Pulmonary Hypertension

▶ Abida Haque
▶ Dani S. Zander

Pulmonary hypertension can develop as a complication of multiple disease processes and exposures, including the following:

- Congenital cardiac diseases with left-to-right shunt.
- Obstructive and interstitial lung diseases.
- Chronic pulmonary thromboembolic disease.
- Conditions associated with pulmonary venous outflow obstruction (left-sided cardiac disease, left-sided valvular disease, obstruction/compression of large pulmonary veins, pulmonary veno-occlusive disease).
- Sleep disordered breathing.
- Alveolar hypoventilation disorders.
- Chronic high altitude exposure.
- Collagen vascular diseases.
- Human immunodeficiency virus infection.
- Portal hypertension.
- Drugs and toxins.
- Persistent pulmonary hypertension of the newborn.
- Neonatal lung disease.
- Pulmonary amyloidosis.
- Sarcoidosis.
- Intravenous drug abuse.
- Schistosomiasis.
- Pulmonary capillary hemangiomatosis.

Histologic Features:

- Similar to primary pulmonary hypertension, including muscularization of arterioles, arterial medial hypertrophy, intimal proliferation and fibrosis in arteries, plexiform lesions, angiomatoid lesions, and fibrinoid necrosis of arteries in some of these conditions.
- Additional abnormalities characteristic of the predisposing process may be present.

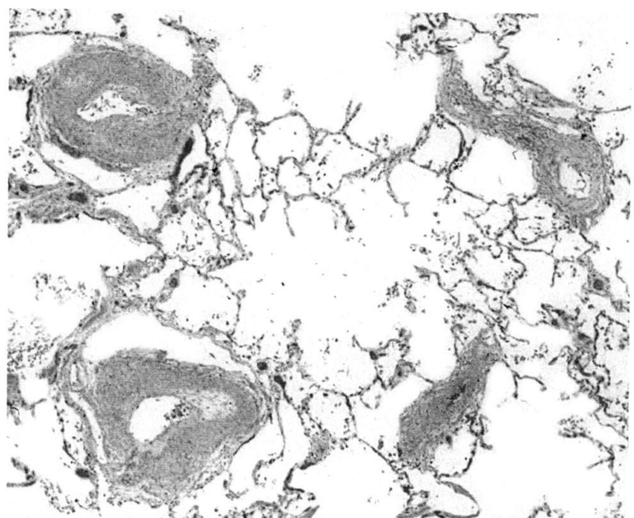

Figure 52.1 Small pulmonary arteries and arterioles with medial thickening in a young sickle cell anemia patient.

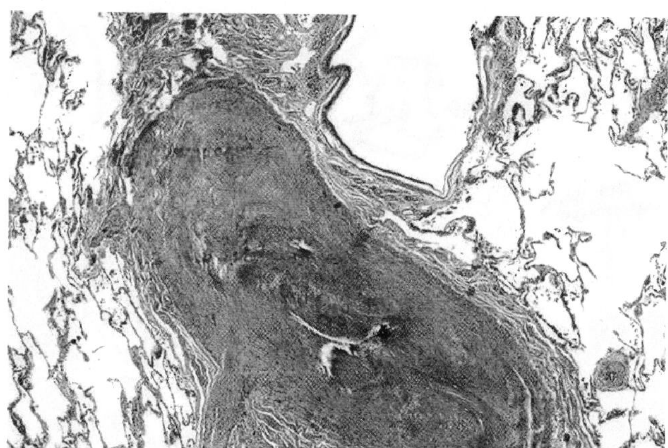

Figure 52.2 Medium-sized pulmonary artery showing marked intimal thickening and fibrosis with a resultant slitlike lumen.

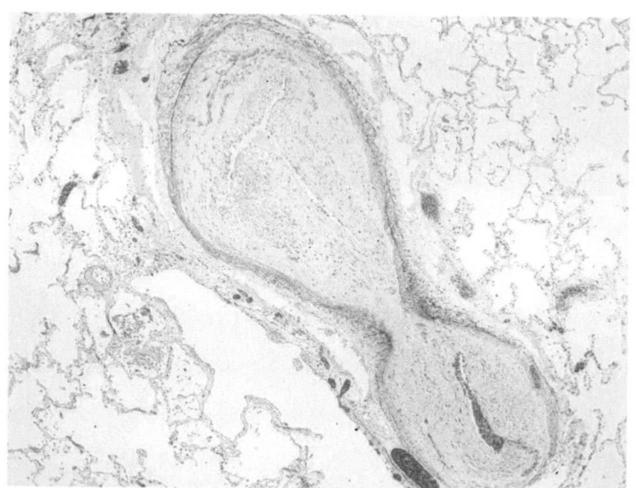

Figure 52.3 Movat stain of pulmonary artery branch with marked intimal thickening and fibrosis and a slitlike lumen.

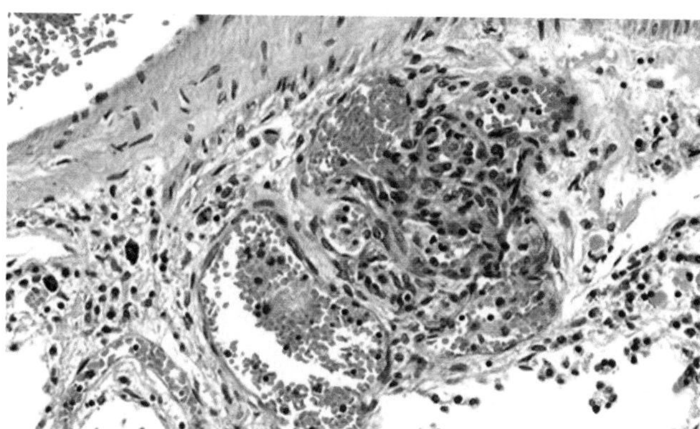

Figure 52.4 Plexiform lesion consists of a cluster of small-caliber vessels associated with dilated arterial branches.

Pulmonary Veno-Occlusive Disease

53

▶ Abida Haque
▶ Dani S. Zander

Pulmonary veno-occlusive disease is a rare, primary sclerosing disease of the pulmonary veins. Its etiology is unknown. Patients are most often in the first 3 decades of life, but the disorder can develop at any age. In adults, there is a male predominance of 2:1. The clinical presentation resembles that of primary pulmonary hypertension, and the diagnosis is often not suspected until late in the course of the disease. Although occasionally the process seems to develop rapidly, symptoms more often develop insidiously. The process follows a downhill course and has a very poor prognosis. Lung or heart-lung transplantation is necessary to prolong life. Some cases have followed use of chemotherapeutic agents, exposure to toxic agents, respiratory viral infections, and bone marrow and renal transplantation, suggesting that these conditions and agents may predispose to development of the disease. Other reported disease associations include scleroderma, human immunodeficiency virus infection, and malignancies. The pathogenesis is not well understood but is believed to involve thrombosis of pulmonary veins, leading to luminal fibrosis.

Histologic Features:

- Histologic abnormalities can be subtle; therefore, a careful search for the pathognomonic changes (obstructive intimal fibrosis in veins and venules) is essential.
- Elastic stains are very helpful for identification of venous luminal fibrosis.
- Intravenous fibrous septa or thrombi may be present.
- Medial hypertrophy may be present in veins.
- Patchy congestion and hemosiderin-laden macrophages, sometimes accompanied by extracellular hemosiderin and iron encrustation of blood vessel walls.
- Interstitial fibrosis and mild chronic inflammation may be present.
- Edema and fibrosis of interlobular septa may be present.
- Lymphatic dilation may be present.
- Pulmonary arteries and arterioles usually show hypertensive changes.

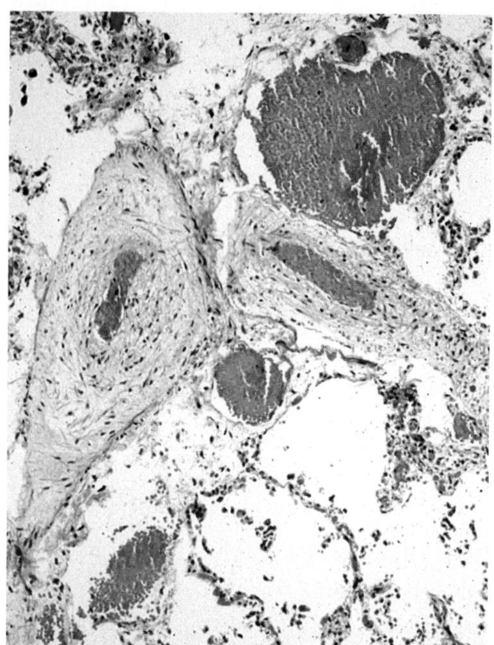

Figure 53.1 Venule demonstrating thickening of its wall due to intimal fibrosis. Adjacent lung parenchyma shows focal congestion and numerous hemosiderin-laden macrophages in alveoli. Mild interstitial fibrosis is also present.

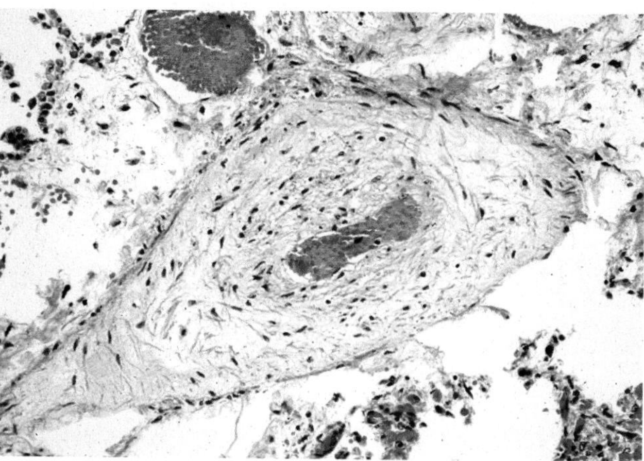

Figure 53.2 Vein having somewhat myxomatous fibrous intimal proliferation.

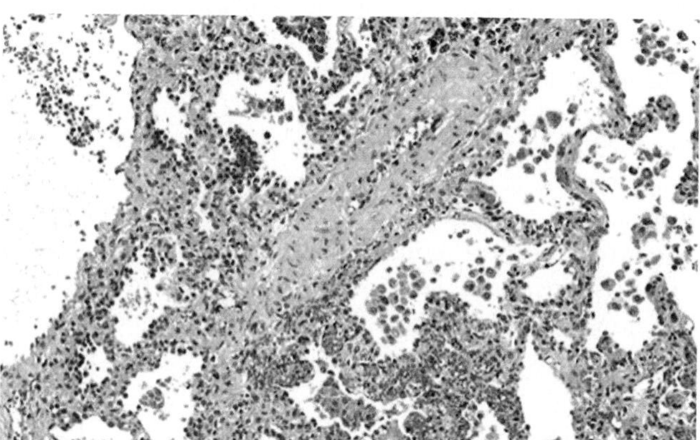

Figure 53.3 Thickened vein with adjacent interstitial fibrosis and hemosiderin-laden macrophages.

Pulmonary Capillary Hemangiomatosis

54

▶ Abida Haque

Pulmonary capillary hemangiomatosis lesion is seen in association with pulmonary veno-occlusive disease and pulmonary hypertension.

Histologic Features:

- Capillary hemangiomatosis is characterized by the presence of proliferating alveolar capillaries with presence of double capillaries on both sides of the alveolar walls, back-to-back capillaries, and capillary invasion of airways and blood vessels.
- Often, there is a distinct transition of the abnormal capillaries to normal areas.

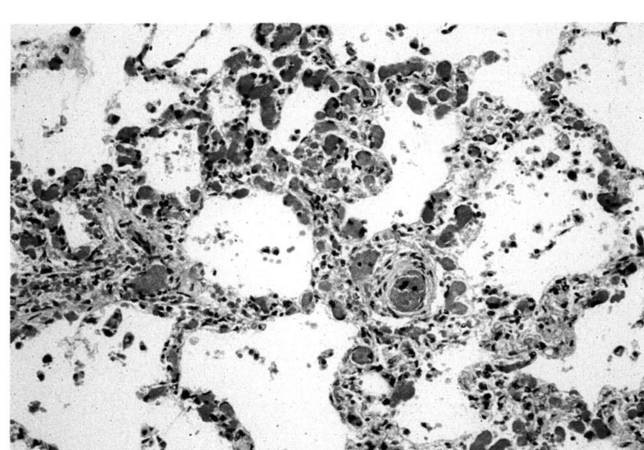

Figure 54.1 Proliferating alveolar capillaries with marked congestion and dilation.

Pulmonary Thrombi and Emboli

55

Emboli to the lungs include thrombi (usually from deep leg veins) and a variety of other materials and tissues. The latter are often clues to underlying medical conditions or injuries.

Part 1

Thromboemboli

▶ Abida Haque

Pulmonary thromboemboli may be massive, resulting in sudden death, or they may be smaller, with symptoms of mild respiratory distress. Large thromboemboli often originate in the deep leg veins and impact at the pulmonary artery bifurcation with complete occlusion, forming a "saddle embolus."

Histologic Features:

- Thrombi show a laminated appearance, and the lines of Zahn are firm and granular.
- Postmortem clots are soft and have two distinct components resembling red currant jelly and chicken fat.
- Once lodged in the pulmonary artery, the thrombi show evidence of organization, with an initial neutrophilic response in the vessel wall, followed by neutrophil infiltration of the thromboembolus and then fibroblast ingrowth within approximately 1 week.
- Thrombus is ultimately fibrosed and may be recanalized.

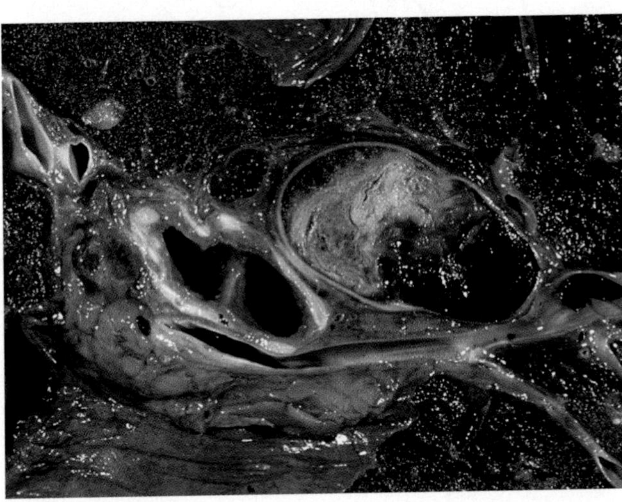

Figure 55.1 Gross figure showing a pulmonary artery distended with an endoluminal thromboembolus.

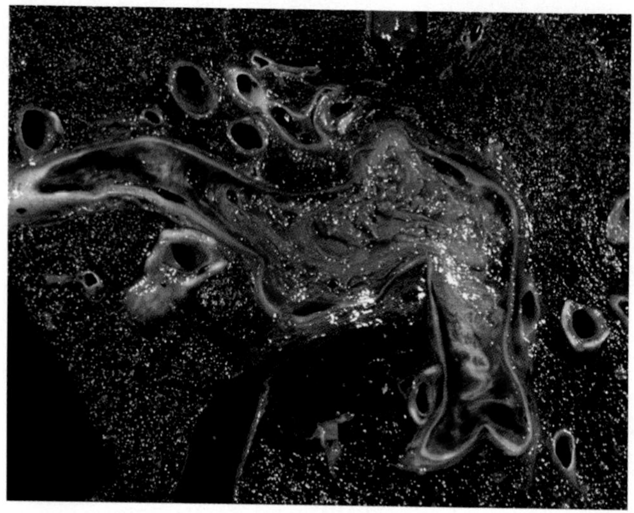

Figure 55.2 Gross figure showing a pulmonary artery with a laminated, firm, granular thromboembolus.

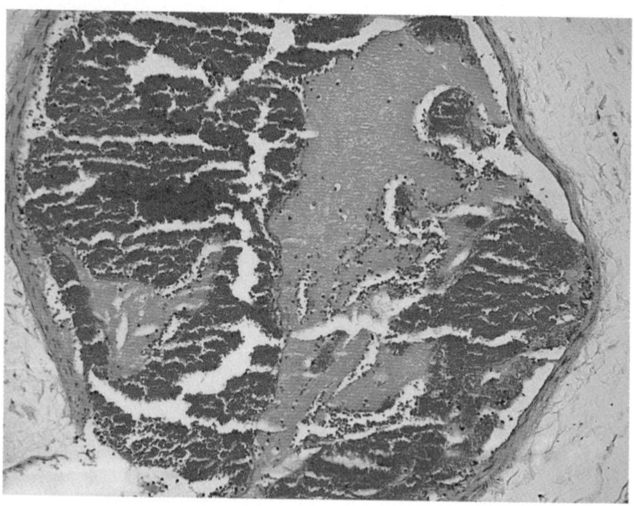

Figure 55.3 Small pulmonary artery distended with a recent thromboembolus, consisting mostly of fibrin and red blood cells.

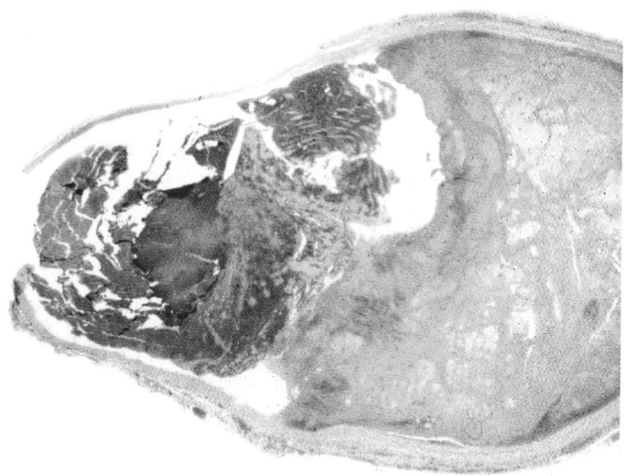

Figure 55.4 Organizing thromboembolus with lysed red blood cells suggesting a slightly less recent event.

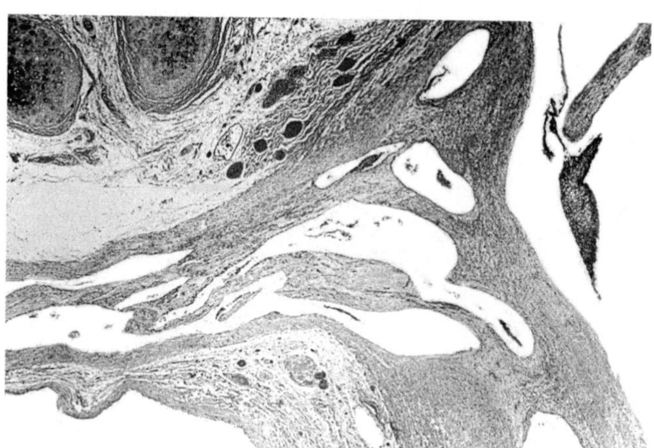

Figure 55.5 Large pulmonary artery branch with old organized thrombus replaced by pulmonary webs.

Part 2

Disseminated Intravascular Coagulation

▶ Dani S. Zander

Disseminated intravascular coagulation (DIC) is characterized by activation of the coagulation sequence with formation of microthrombi in multiple sites throughout the body. There is consumption of platelets, fibrin, and coagulation factors with concurrent activation of fibrinolytic pathways. Manifestations of DIC may stem from ischemic consequences of the thrombi and/or hemorrhagic consequences resulting from depletion of elements needed for coagulation with activation of fibrinolysis. DIC that develops acutely, such as in the setting of major trauma, tends to lead to hemorrhagic manifestations, whereas chronic

DIC, such as may be associated with a carcinoma, tends to reveal itself by thrombotic complications. DIC can complicate a wide variety of processes. Some of the more common associated disorders are obstetric complications (placental abruption, retained dead fetus, toxemia), infections (Gram-negative sepsis, meningococcemia, Rocky Mountain spotted fever, aspergillosis), neoplasms (carcinomas of the pancreas, lung, stomach, prostate, and acute promyelocytic leukemia), severe trauma, burns, and acute intravascular hemolysis.

Histologic Features:

- Fibrin thrombi in alveolar capillaries; a stain for fibrin (Carstairs stain, Lendrum stain, phosphotungstic acid-hematoxylin stain) is useful for highlighting microthrombi.
- Variably present:
  - Fibrin thromboemboli in larger blood vessels.
  - Infarction.
  - Alveolar hemorrhage.
  - Diffuse alveolar damage.

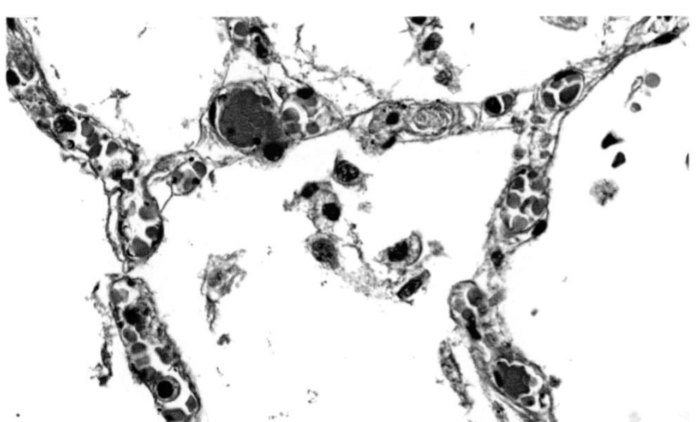

Figure 55.6 Histology showing microthrombi filling the lumens of the alveolar capillaries.

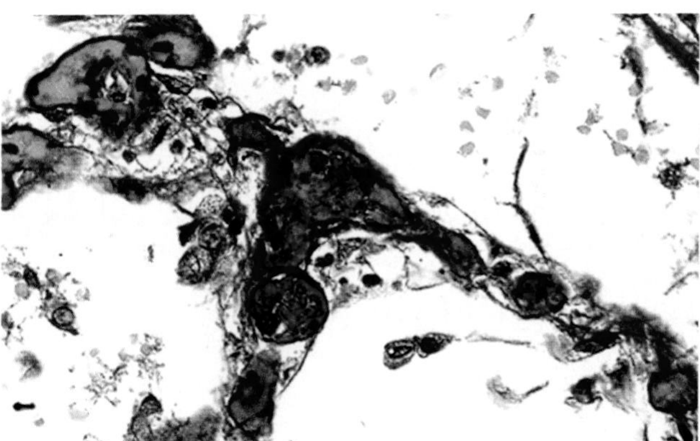

Figure 55.7 Histology showing fibrin-platelet Carstairs stain highlighting the fibrin microthrombus (red) occluding the capillary lumen.

Part 3

Foreign Body Emboli

▶ Abida Haque

Intravenous entries of fragments of plastic catheters and tubings, cotton fibers, and rarely bullets have been reported. Diagnosis is based on gross observation and clinical history.

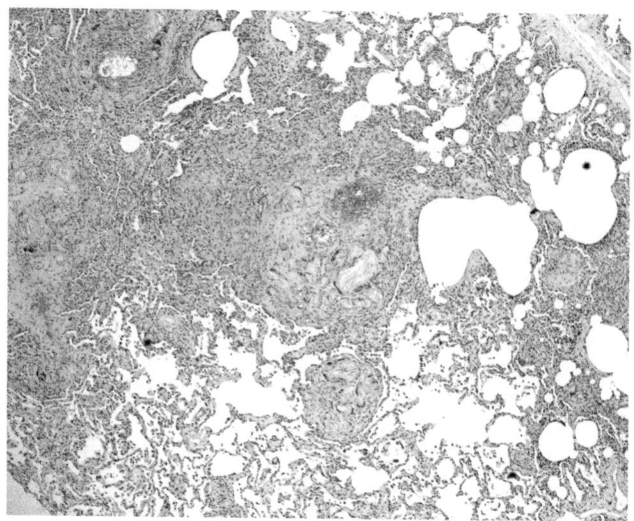

Figure 55.8 Multiple foreign body giant cell granulomas with multiple refractile platelike crystals.

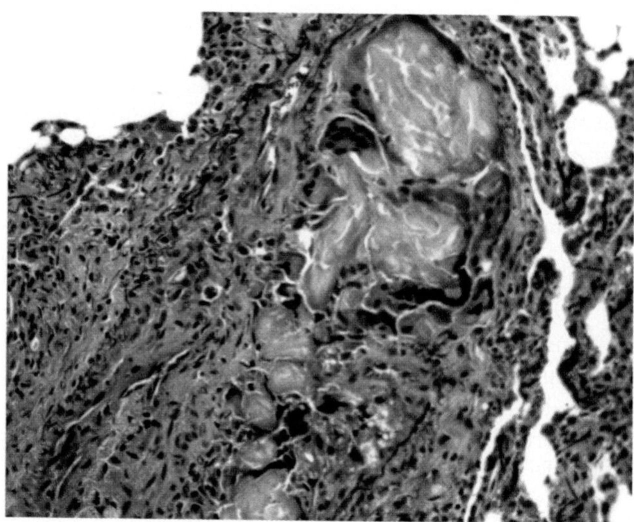

Figure 55.9 Movat stain of a muscular pulmonary artery with multiple refractile crystals (orange) surrounded by giant cells and focal destruction of the arterial wall.

Part 4

Bone Marrow Emboli

▶ Abida Haque

Bone marrow emboli can occur after bone fractures, vigorous cardiopulmonary resuscitation, and bone marrow infarction due to sickle cell disease or steroid therapy.

Histologic Features:

- Small to medium pulmonary arteries are distended with one or more of the hematopoietic elements with vacuolated and oval to round adipose cells.
- If the emboli are small, only myeloid precursors or erythroid precursors may be seen.
- Larger emboli may contain megakaryocytes.

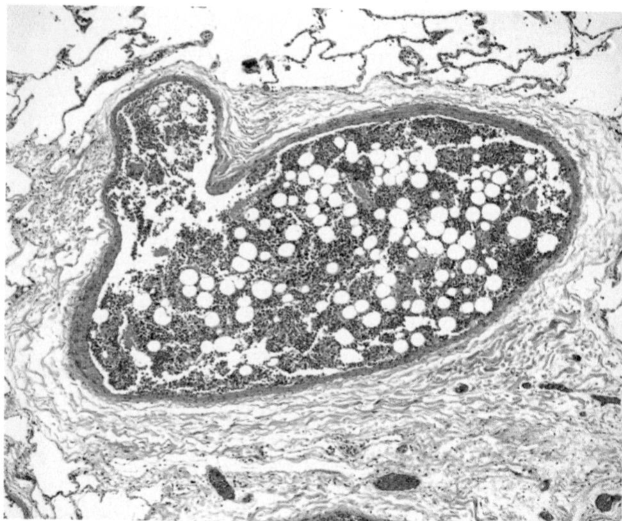

Figure 55.10 Low power of bone marrow embolus showing fat cells and erythropoietic marrow elements.

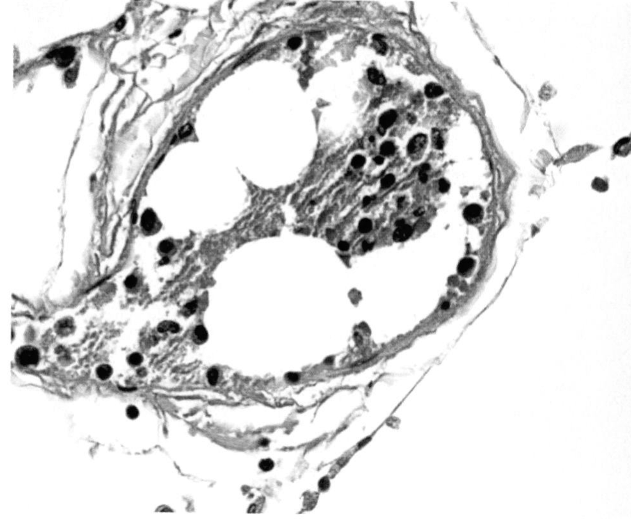

Figure 55.11 Higher power of bone marrow embolus showing a small vessel containing fat cells and erythropoietic marrow elements.

Part 5

Amniotic Fluid Embolism

▶ Abida Haque

Pulmonary amniotic fluid embolism is often associated with difficult labor or caesarean section; if massive, it can be fatal.

Histologic Features:

- Pulmonary artery branches contain squamous epithelial cells, lanugo hair, fat, meconium, and mucin.
- Rarely, trophoblast and decidua may be also found.

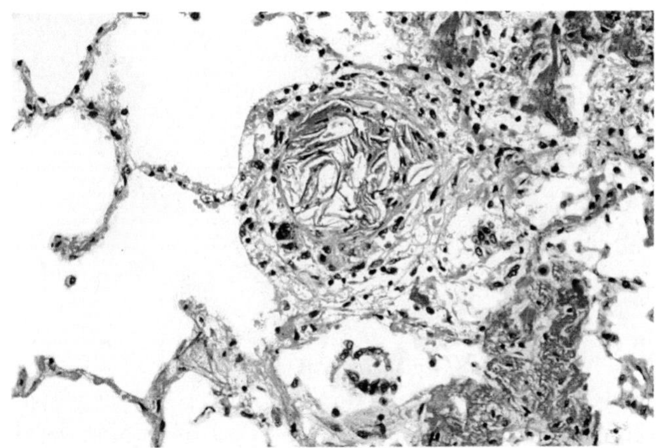

Figure 55.12 Compact clusters of squamous cells distending a small pulmonary vessel lumen.

Part 6

Body Tissues Emboli

▶ Abida Haque

Tissue emboli to the lungs may originate from any organ or tissues; however, bone, skin, brain, and liver are the most commonly reported sites. Liver and brain emboli are often associated with trauma and laceration of the brain or liver. Rarely, newborns with central nervous system malformations or severe head trauma during delivery have been reported to have brain tissue emboli in lungs. Severe hepatic necrosis has been reported to cause liver emboli in lungs.

Histologic Features:

- Fragments of various body tissues identified in vascular lumens.

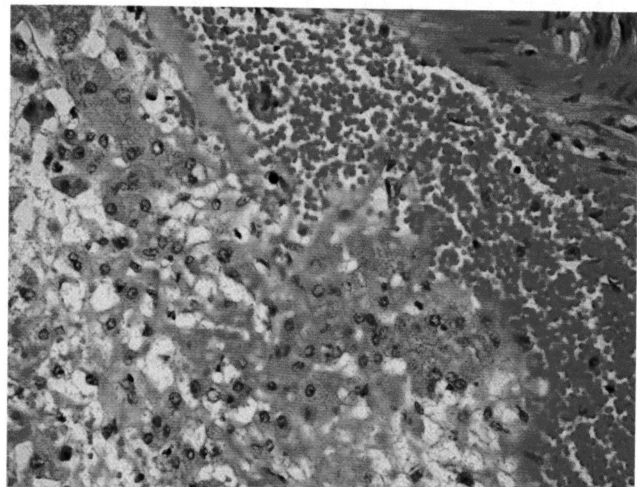

Figure 55.13 Lung section from a patient who died with severe trauma demonstrates a medium-size pulmonary artery with an embolus composed of hepatocytes.

Part 7

Tumor Emboli

▶ Abida Haque

Embolism of tumors from different sites is a fairly common occurrence. If extensive, the process may be referred to as embolic carcinamatosis and may cause pulmonary hypertension.

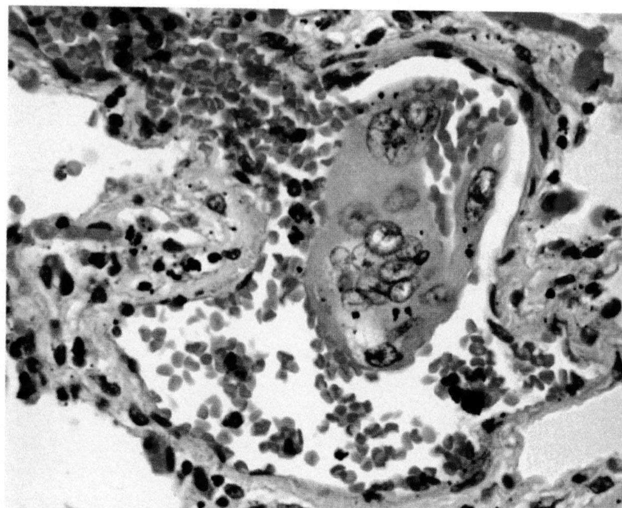

Figure 55.14 Tumor embolus within pulmonary vessel.

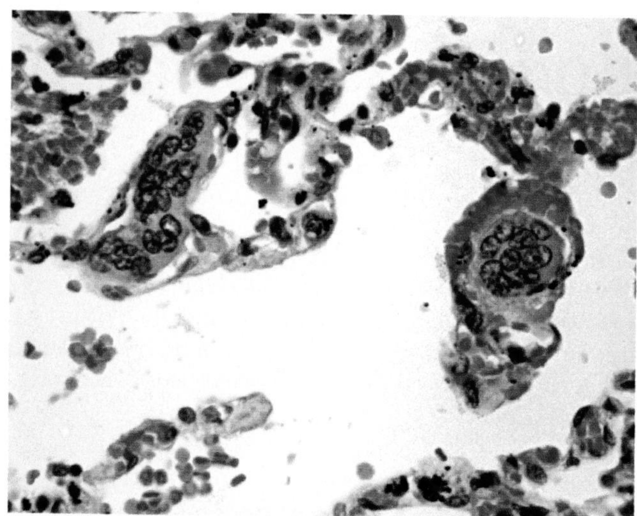

Figure 55.15 Higher power showing tumor emboli in capillaries.

Part 8

Parasitic Emboli

▶ Abida Haque

Dirofilaria immitis, filarial parasites (e.g., *Wuchereria*), *Strongyloides,* and *Ascaris* migrate through the lung during their developmental stages and may be found in the pulmonary vessels.

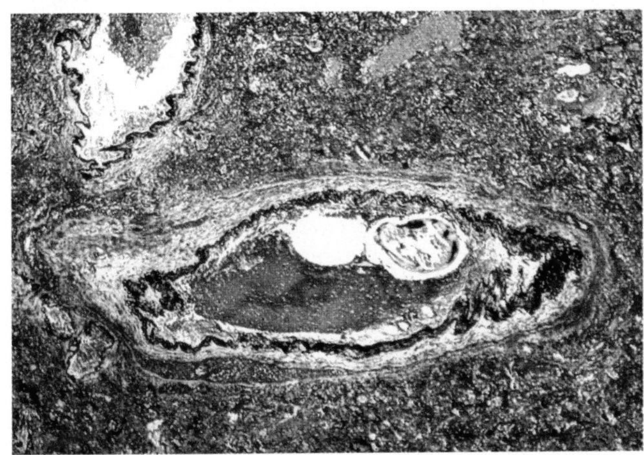

Figure 55.16 Verhoeff elastic stain of a pulmonary artery with fibrin thrombus and a cross section of a parasite confirmed to be *Dirofilaria immitis* on deeper sections.

Part 9

Air Emboli

▶ Abida Haque

Air can enter circulation during surgery, trauma with laceration of veins, intravenous injection, therapeutic insufflation of fallopian tubes, ventilation therapy, and hyperbaric decompression. Large amounts of air can produce obstruction to pulmonary blood flow, pulmonary edema, and death.

Histologic Features:

- Frothy blood in the pulmonary vessels.
- Dilation of right heart and contracted left heart.
- Pulmonary arteries show empty circular spaces within the column of blood.

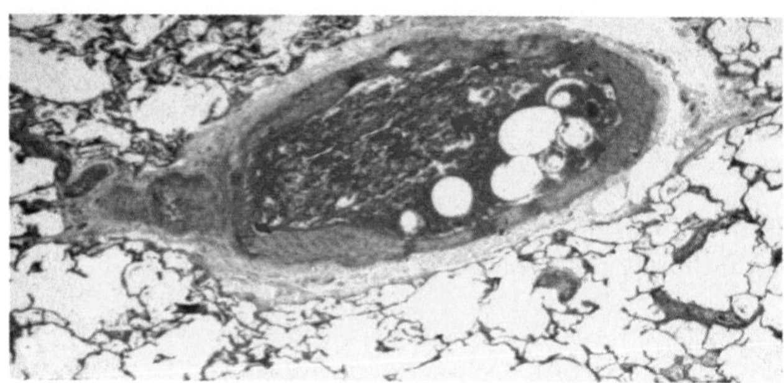

Figure 55.17 Pulmonary artery with distinct clear circular spaces within its lumen.

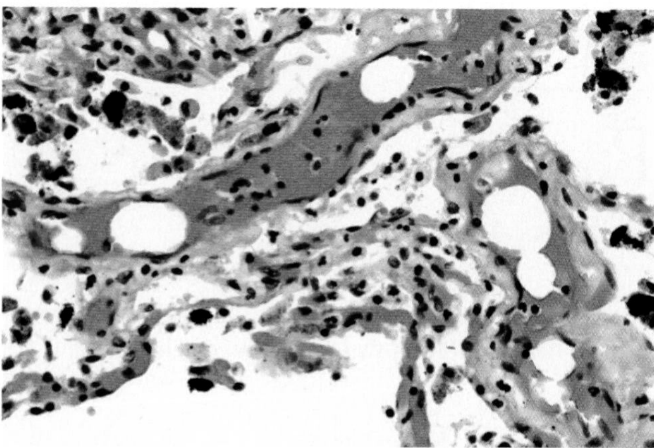

Figure 55.18 Changes consistent with air embolism. The alveoli also contain multiple hemosiderin-laden macrophages.

56

Pulmonary Infarct

▶ Abida Haque

Pulmonary infarcts resulting from occlusion of pulmonary artery branches are hemorrhagic, wedge shaped, and often pleural based.

Histologic Features:

- In early infarcts, there is edema and hemorrhage, followed by loss of cellular detail (coagulative necrosis) and neutrophilic infiltrate starting at the margin of the infarct at 24 to 48 hours.
- This is followed by macrophage response, hemosiderin deposition, and removal of necrotic debris.
- Infarct continues to organize with fibroblast proliferation, collagen deposition, and scar formation.
- Evolution and organization depends on the size of the infarct, with large infarcts taking several months to even one year for complete collagenization.

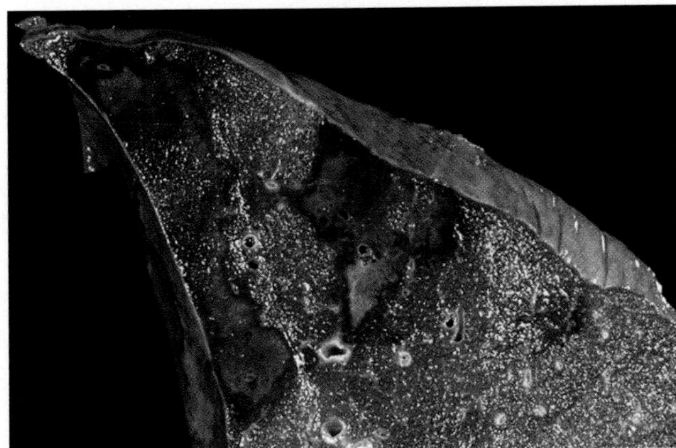

Figure 56.1 Gross figure showing an organizing infarct with a roughly triangular shape, central tan color and peripheral red-brown color.

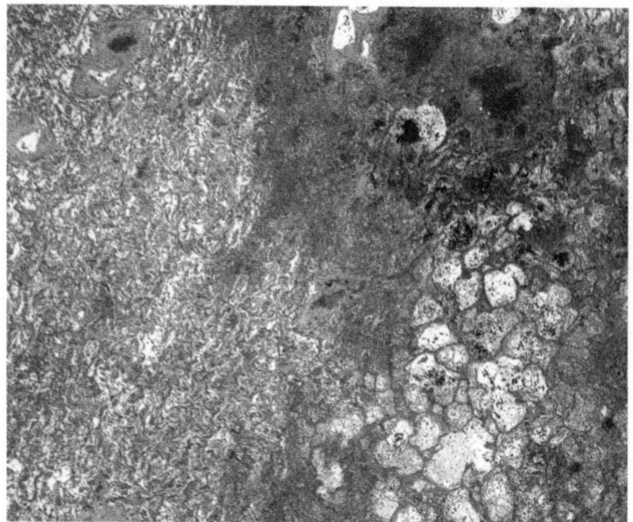

Figure 56.2 Ischemic necrosis of the lung parenchyma associated with hemorrhage, with centrally located ghostlike outlines of the alveolar septa and a blood vessel.

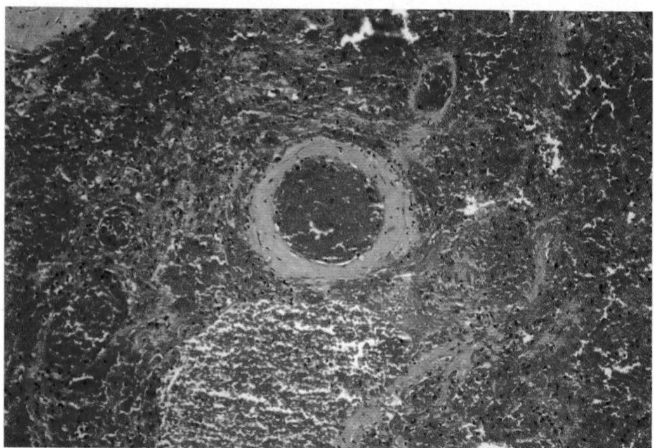

Figure 56.3 Higher power showing ischemic necrosis of pulmonary structures and severe hemorrhage.

Section 11

Large Airways

57

Bronchiectasis

▶ Alvaro C. Laga
▶ Timothy Allen
▶ Philip T. Cagle

Bronchiectasis refers to the irreversible pathologic dilation of bronchi due to inflammation and fibrosis, most often associated with chronic infection. There are many underlying predisposing conditions, including airway obstruction (tumors, foreign bodies, mucous plugs), cystic fibrosis, Kartagener syndrome, and immune deficiency. The lower lobes are more commonly involved.

Histologic Features:

- Varying degrees of inflammation, ulceration, and squamous metaplasia may be present within dilated bronchi.
- Lymphoid follicles are frequently observed in the bronchial walls.
- Extensive destruction of the bronchial wall including cartilage, muscle, and submucosal glands.
- Fibrosis and inflammation of the bronchial wall and peribronchial tissues.
- Associated acute and chronic pneumonias, organizing pneumonia, and postobstructive fibrosis and inflammation.

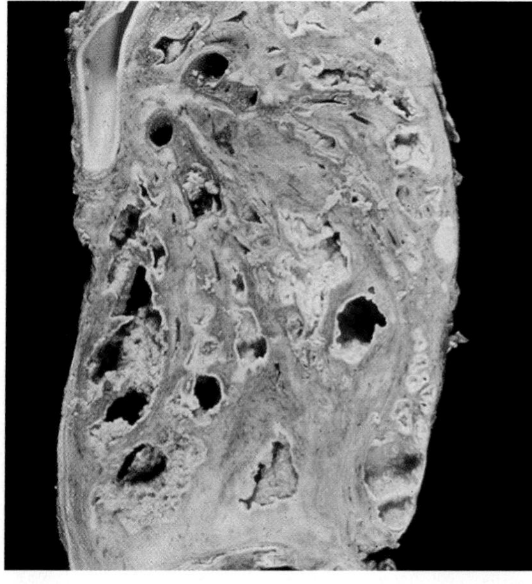

Figure 57.1 Gross figure of bronchiectasis showing dilated infected segmental bronchi and fibrosis of surrounding lung parenchyma.

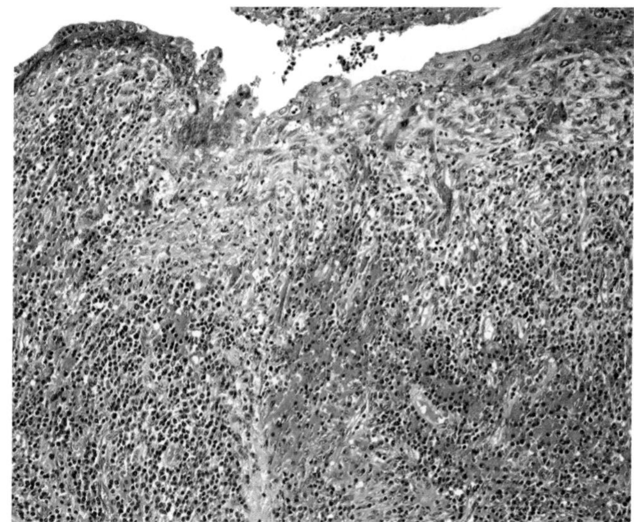

Figure 57.2 Bronchus with squamous metaplasia, mucosal erosion, granulation tissue, chronic inflammation, and fibrosis.

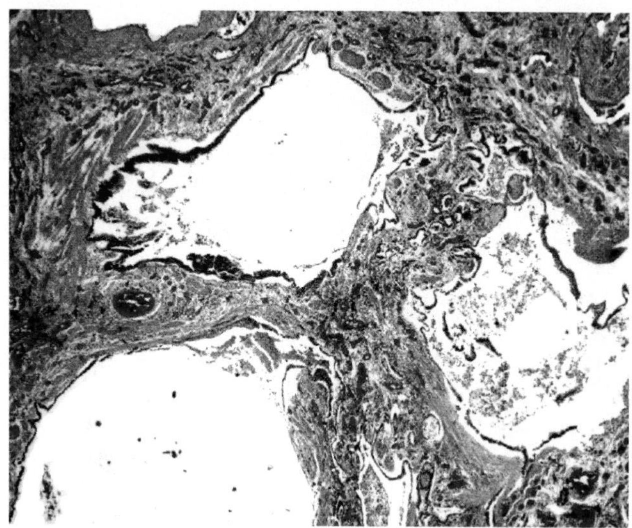

Figure 57.3 Honeycomb lung due to bronchiectasis consists of residual spaces lined by metaplastic columnar epithelium within severe fibrosis with smooth muscle hyperplasia.

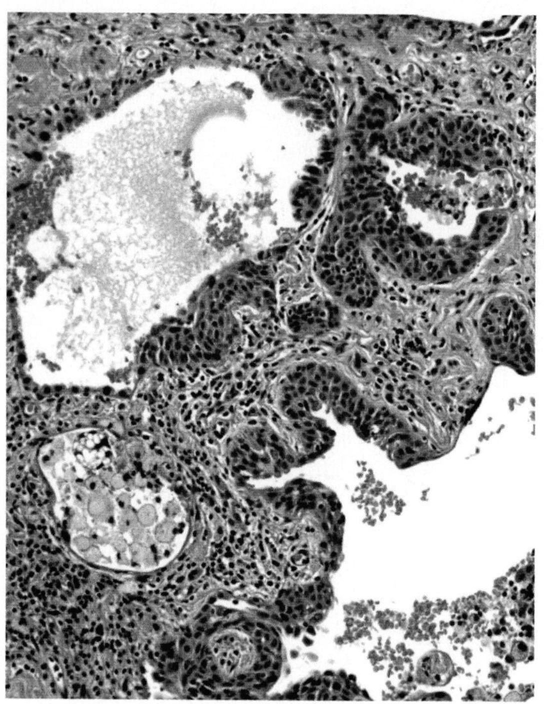

Figure 57.4 Severe fibrosis due to bronchiectasis with residual spaces lined by metaplastic squamous epithelium with lipid-laden macrophages within a residual space.

Part 1

Middle Lobe Syndrome

▶ Dani S. Zander

Middle lobe syndrome is an uncommon process in which there is chronic or recurrent atelectasis or radiographic opacification of the right middle lobe, lingula, or both. It can develop in adults and children. A cause of bronchial obstruction can be identified in some patients. Benign and malignant neoplasms have been associated with this disorder, as well as a wide variety of nonneoplastic conditions causing extrinsic or intrinsic airway obstruction. In other patients, no obstructing process can be defined. Chronic right middle lobe or lingular infection by *Mycobacterium avium-intracellulare,* developing predominantly in older women, has been termed *Lady Windemere's syndrome.*

Histologic Features:

Various combinations of the following features may be present:

- Bronchiectasis.
- Chronic airway inflammation.
- Atelectasis.
- Lymphoid hyperplasia.
- Organizing pneumonia.
- Abscesses.
- Granulomatous inflammation should prompt performance of stains for mycobacteria and fungi.

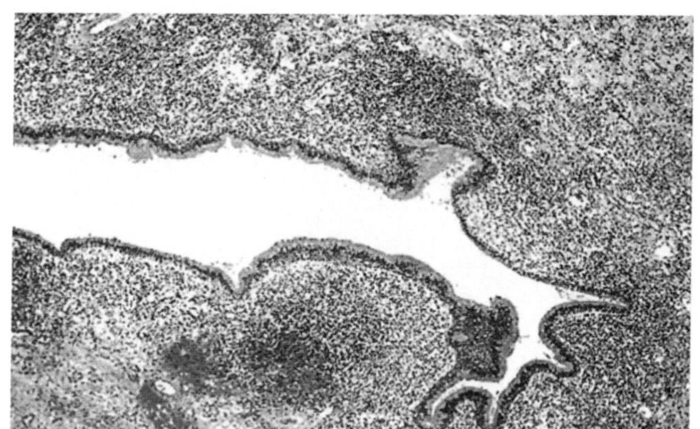

Figure 57.5 Bronchiectasis with active chronic inflammation and alveolar collapse in upper right.

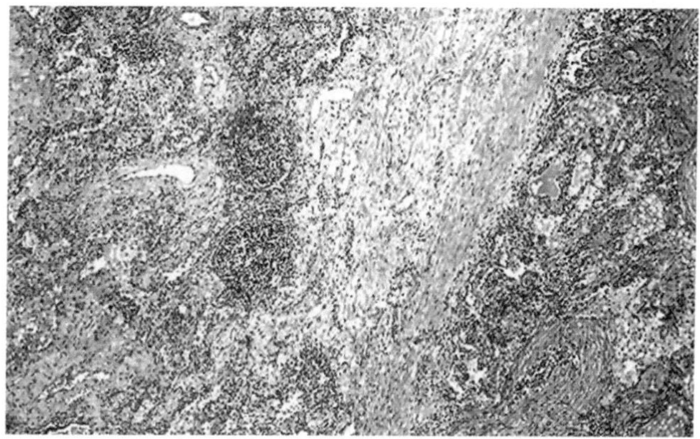

Figure 57.6 Fibrotic, thickened interlobular septum lies in the center. The lung parenchyma on the **left** of the septum is collapsed and fibrotic, and the parenchyma on the **right** demonstrates organizing pneumonia and edema. Lymphoid aggregates are also present.

Chronic Bronchitis

58

▶ Alvaro C. Laga
▶ Timothy Allen
▶ Philip T. Cagle

Chronic bronchitis is defined clinically as persistent cough with sputum production for at least 3 months in at least 2 consecutive years. Two factors are important in the pathogenesis of chronic bronchitis: 1) chronic irritation by inhaled substances, and 2) microbiologic infections. Cigarette smoking remains the primary cause. Other causes include heavy exposures to certain fumes and dusts.

Histologic Features:

- Enlargement of the mucus-secreting glands of the trachea and bronchi.
- Goblet cell metaplasia.
- Increase in inflammatory cells, particularly lymphocytes.
- Squamous metaplasia and dysplasia may be seen in the bronchial epithelium.
- Increased bronchial smooth muscle.
- Goblet cell metaplasia, mucous plugging, inflammation, and fibrosis in the bronchioles.

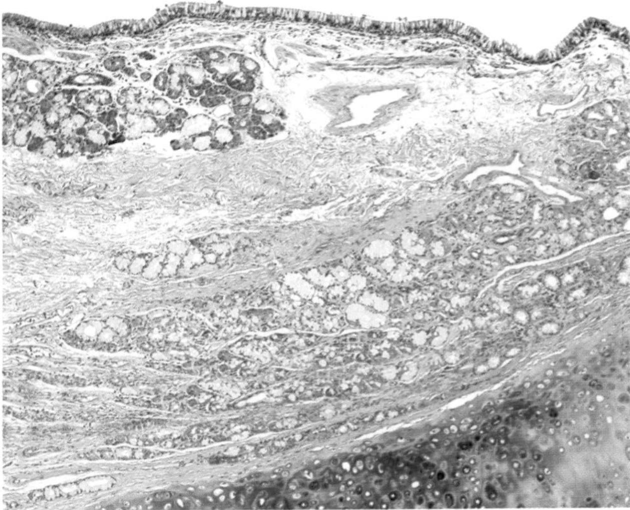

Figure 58.1 Bronchial wall shows increased numbers of bronchial glands characteristic of chronic bronchitis.

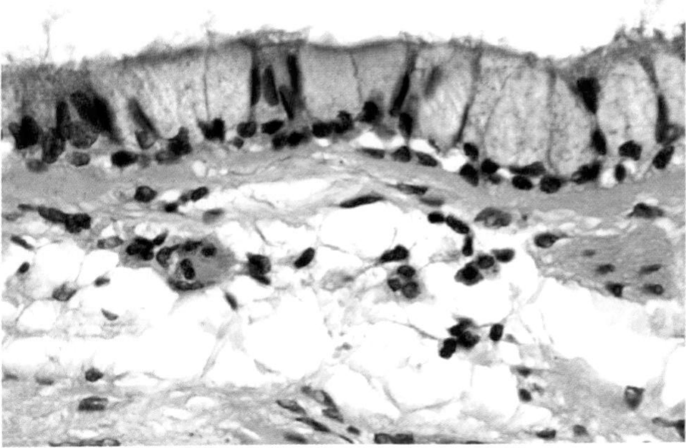

Figure 58.2 Chronic bronchitis shows bronchial surface epithelium with goblet cell metaplasia.

Part 1

Mucoid Impaction

▶ Alvaro C. Laga, Timothy Allen, and Philip T. Cagle

In obstructive airways diseases, including asthma, mucus may become impacted in airways, creating further airway obstruction due to impaction of mucus plugs. Patients may expectorate the rubbery mucous plugs that may form "casts" of the airways.

Histologic Features:

- Mucus casts containing laminated material with a variable number of degenerating inflammatory cells.
- Thinned bronchial wall.
- Bronchial mucosa may be ulcerated, stretched thin, or show focal squamous metaplasia.

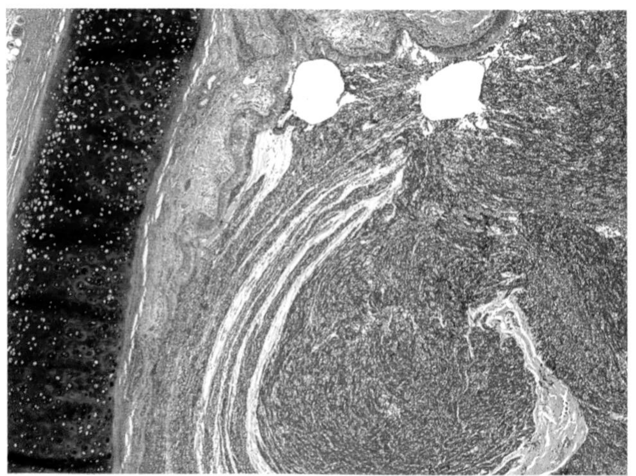

Figure 59.3 Dilated bronchus with compressed mucosa containing laminated mucoid material.

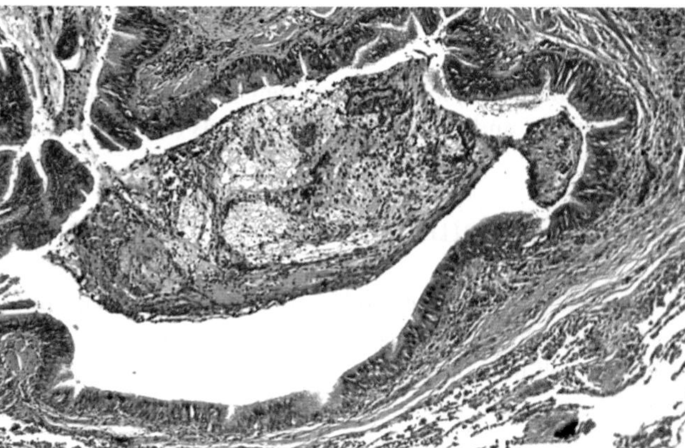

Figure 59.4 Low power shows a dilated small bronchus containing a mucus cast and inflammation.

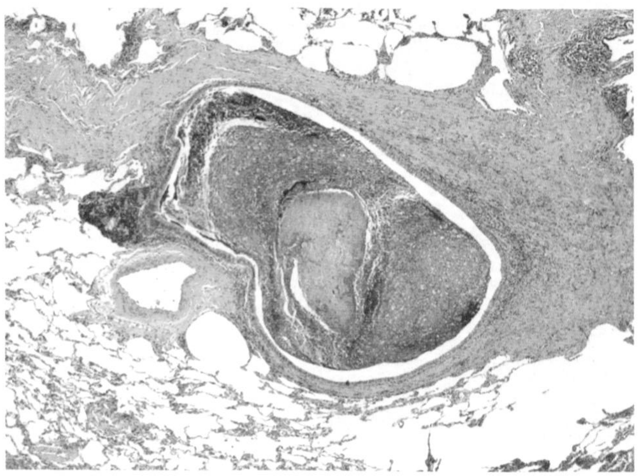

Figure 59.5 Higher power shows a bronchiole with flattened mucosa overlying a mucus cast.

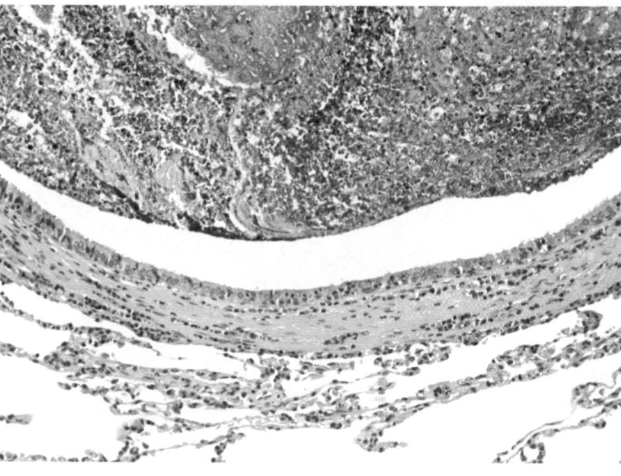

Figure 59.6 Thinned bronchial mucosa with mucus cast and degenerating inflammatory cells.

Part 2

Allergic Bronchopulmonary Aspergillosis

▶ Alvaro C. Laga, Timothy Allen, and Philip T. Cagle

Allergic bronchopulmonary aspergillosis (ABPA) is a hypersensitivity disorder caused by colonization of the bronchial tree with *Aspergillus fumigatus.* Patients have asthma and generally will fulfill serologic and radiologic criteria for ABPA. Severe forms are associated with bronchiectasis. Underlying conditions such as cystic fibrosis may be present.

Histologic Features:

- Proximal bronchi show the changes of asthma.
- Small numbers of *A. fumigatus* hyphae can be seen in the bronchial mucus.
- Large numbers of eosinophils, some of which may be shrunken (mummified), can be seen within the mucus.
- Desquamated epithelium, neutrophils, and macrophages may be seen in the mucus.

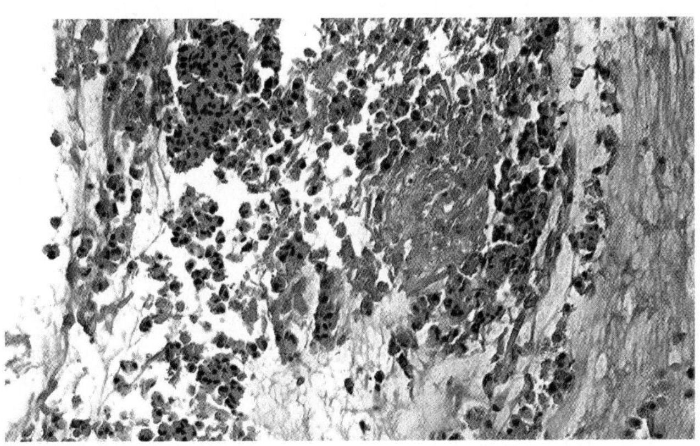

Figure 59.7 Allergic bronchopulmonary aspergillosis shows mucus containing a dense eosinophilic infiltrate and occasional fungal hyphae.

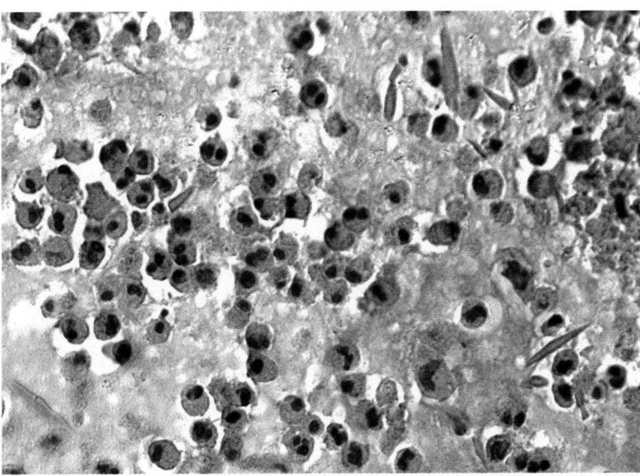

Figure 59.8 Higher power showing eosinophils and scattered Charcot-Leyden crystals within a background of mucus.

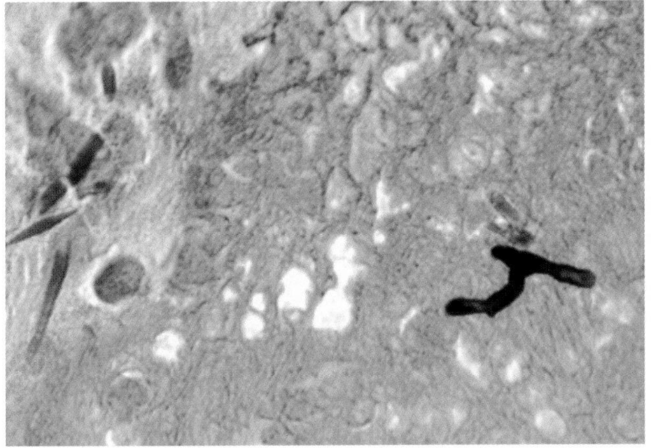

Figure 59.9 Gomori methenamine silver stain showing acute branching hyphae consistent with *Aspergillus* sp and a Charcot-Leyden crystal.

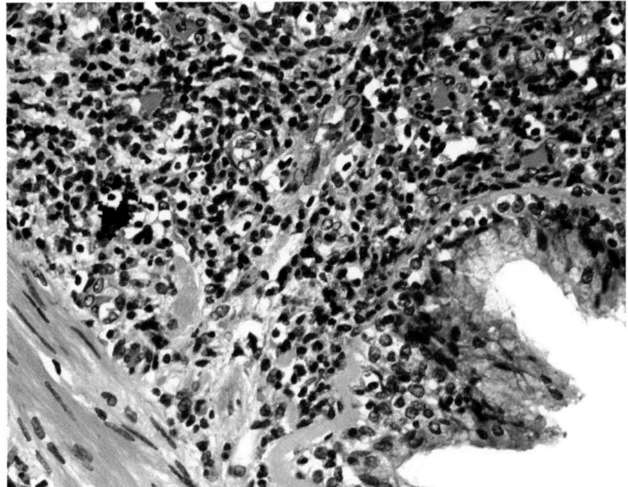

Figure 59.10 Underlying bronchiolar mucosa showing features of asthma, including a dense chronic inflammatory infiltrate rich in eosinophils, a thickened basement membrane, and smooth muscle hyperplasia.

Section 12

Small Airways

Bronchiolar and Peribronchiolar Inflammation, Fibrosis, and Metaplasia

60

▸ Philip T. Cagle

Bronchioles may be involved by inflammation and scarring as either an isolated or focal condition (e.g., a scarred bronchiole from a prior focal infection) or as a widespread or diffuse process. Inflammation and scarring of bronchiolar walls and the adjacent alveolar septa may be accompanied by metaplasia of the bronchiolar or alveolar epithelium. The bronchiolar epithelium may undergo goblet cell metaplasia or squamous metaplasia. The metaplasia on the surface of adjacent fibrotic alveoli may take the form of bronchiolar epithelium, goblet cell metaplasia, or squamous metaplasia. The appearance of bronchiolar-type epithelium on the surface of fibrotic alveoli next to a scarred bronchiole is sometimes called *lambertosis,* which refers to an older concept that this epithelium grew onto the alveolar surface from the bronchiolar lumen via the canals of Lambert.

Some of the diseases that may involve bronchioles with inflammation and possibly scarring include bronchopneumonia (see Chapter 61), organizing pneumonia (formerly known as *bronchiolitis obliterans organizing pneumonia,* see Chapter 62), constrictive bronchiolitis (see Chapter 63), respiratory and membranous bronchiolitis due to tobacco smoke (see Chapter 64), follicular bronchiolitis (see Chapter 65), diffuse panbronchiolitis (see Chapter 66), and small airway reactions to inorganic dust exposures (see Chapter 67). Histopathologic clues to the cause of bronchiolar scarring may be found in some cases (e.g., pigment-laden macrophages in respiratory bronchiolitis or foreign body giant cells in chronic aspiration).

Histologic Features:

- Scarred or inflamed bronchioles may be isolated focal lesions, perhaps purely incidental findings from an old focal infection, or may represent a widespread or diffuse process associated with functional changes in airflow.
- Inflammation and scarring in the walls of bronchioles and in the alveolar septa adjacent to the bronchioles.
- Goblet cell metaplasia or squamous metaplasia of the bronchiolar epithelium.
- Bronchiolar metaplasia, goblet cell metaplasia, or squamous metaplasia of the surface lining of adjacent scarred alveolar septa (lambertosis).
- In some cases, histopathologic findings may provide clues to the cause of the airway fibrosis and inflammation.

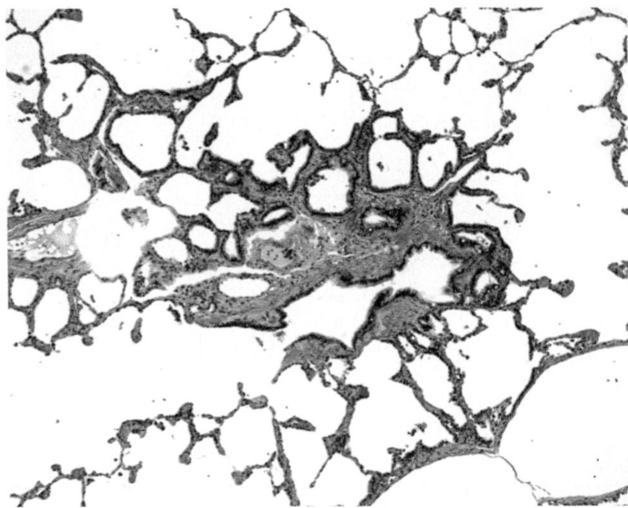

Figure 60.1 Fibrosis of the wall of the bronchiole and the first tiers of adjacent alveoli with metaplastic bronchiolar-type epithelium lining the surfaces of the fibrotic alveolar septa (lambertosis).

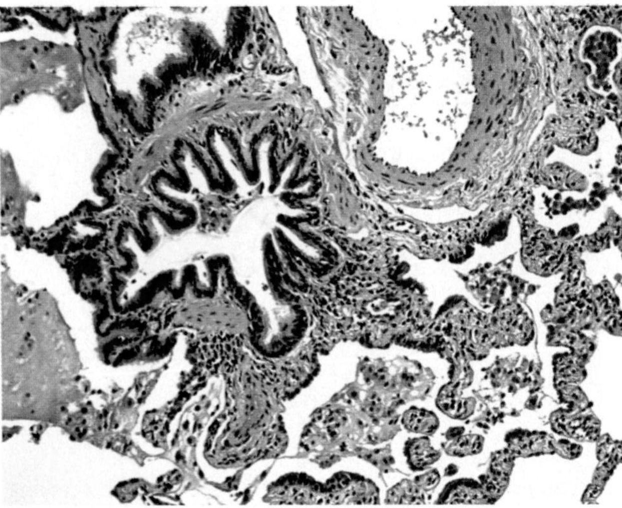

Figure 60.2 Bronchiole shows fibrosis and chronic inflammation of its wall and the walls of adjacent alveoli, which are lined on their surfaces by metaplastic bronchiolar-type epithelium.

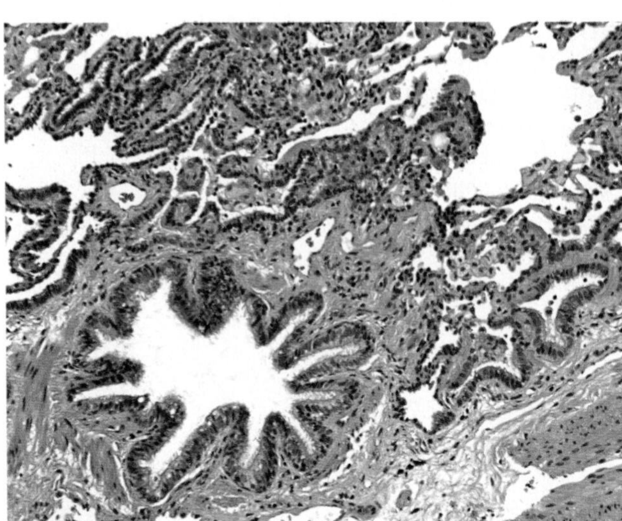

Figure 60.3 Lambertosis (metaplastic bronchiolar-type epithelium) of the fibrotic alveolar walls adjacent to this scarred bronchiole.

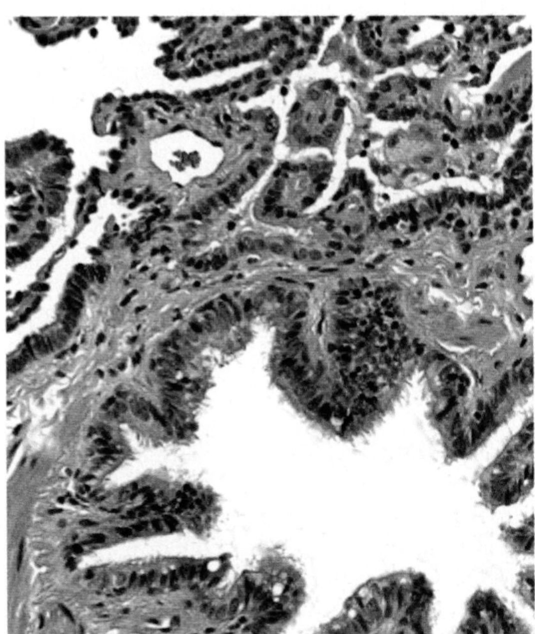

Figure 60.4 Higher power of lambertosis of the lining of fibrotic alveolar septa around a scarred bronchiole.

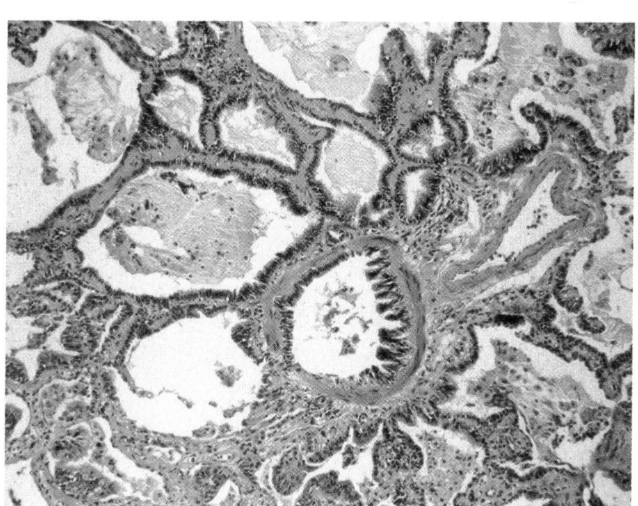

Figure 60.5 Extensive fibrosis and metaplastic lining of alveolar septa around a scarred bronchiole.

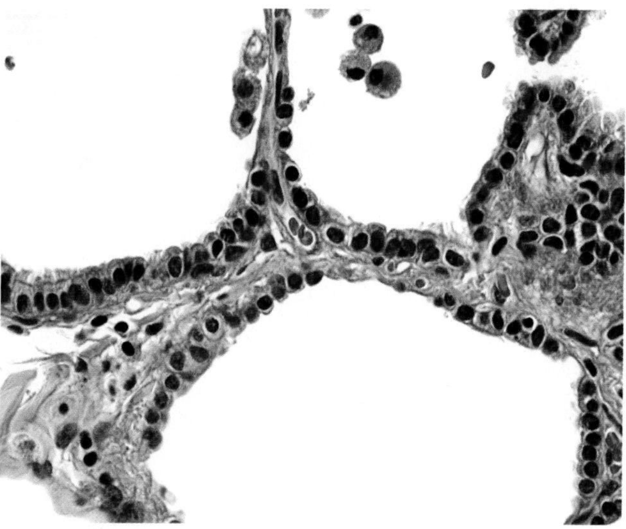

Figure 60.6 High power of metaplastic bronchiolar-type epithelium lining the surfaces of fibrotic alveolar walls.

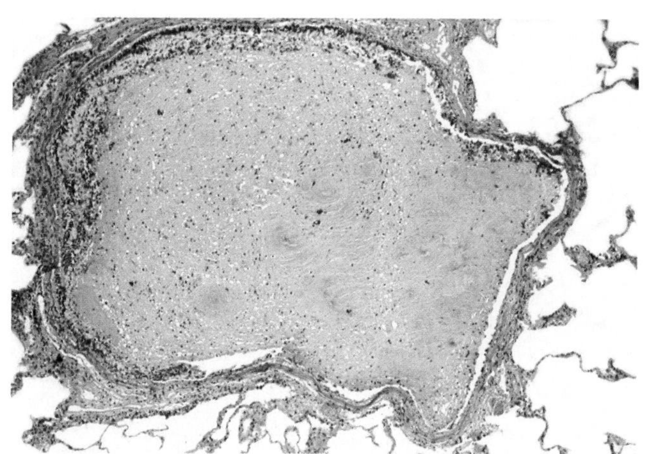

Figure 60.7 Goblet cell metaplasia of a bronchiole, with the lumen filled with mucus plug.

61 Bronchopneumonia

▶ Philip T. Cagle

Bronchopneumonia is also called *focal pneumonia* or *lobular pneumonia.* Bronchopneumonia is discussed here because the acute inflammation involves the respiratory bronchioles and adjacent alveolar ducts and alveoli (involves the center of the lobule). This is in contrast to lobar pneumonia, which involves an entire lobe. Pneumonias are discussed further in Chapters 68 and 69, and specific organisms that can cause pneumonias are discussed in Chapters 95 through 100.

Histologic Features:

- Acute inflammation composed of neutrophils fills respiratory bronchioles and spills into adjacent alveolar ducts and alveoli.

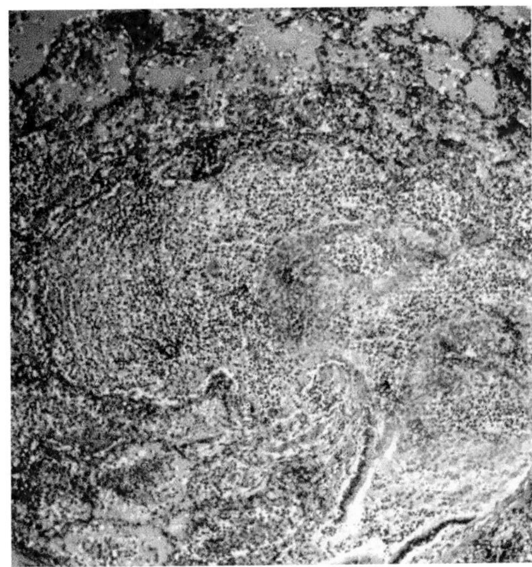

Figure 61.1 Low power shows neutrophils filling a bronchiole *(lower right)* and expanding into the adjacent alveoli. Other nearby alveoli are filled with pink edema fluid.

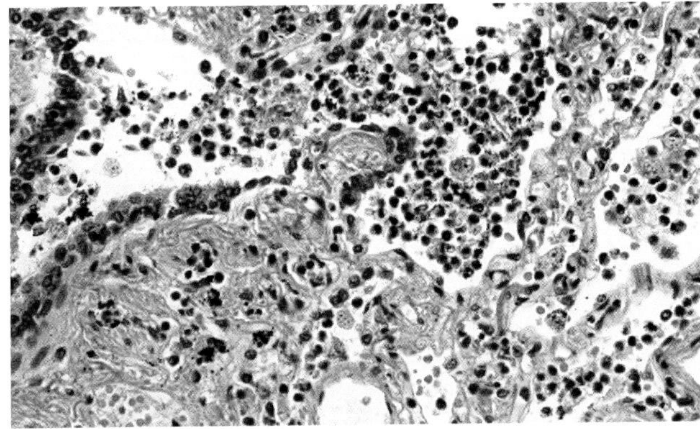

Figure 61.2 Higher power shows bronchiole and adjacent alveoli filled with neutrophils.

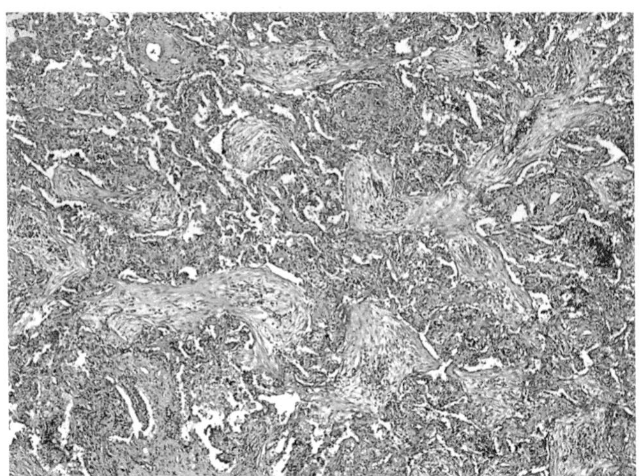

Figure 62.1 Low power shows branching plugs of granulation tissue in bronchioles, alveolar ducts, and alveoli.

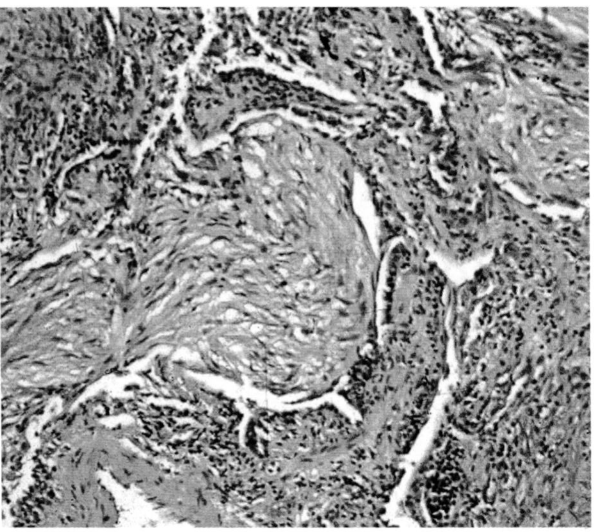

Figure 62.2 Granulation tissue plug in the lumen of a bronchiole.

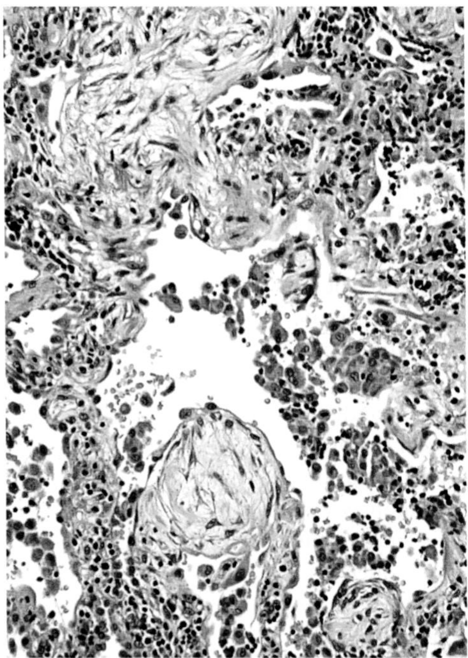

Figure 62.3 Masson bodies are rounded nodules of granulation tissue in alveolar spaces.

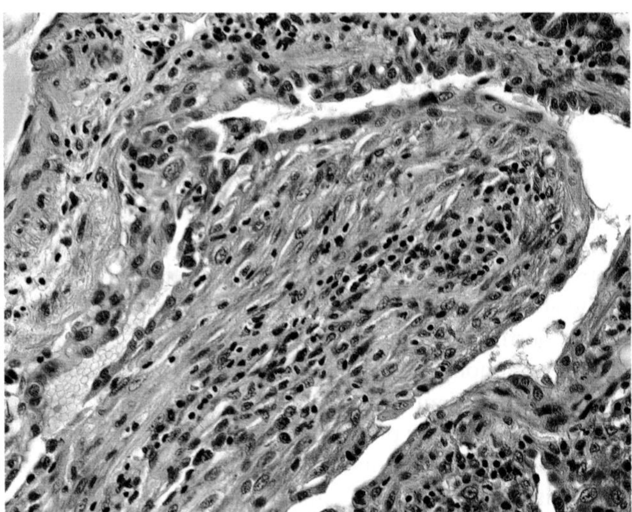

Figure 62.4 Higher power of granulation tissue plug in the lumen of a bronchiole. Lymphocytes can be seen in the granulation tissue.

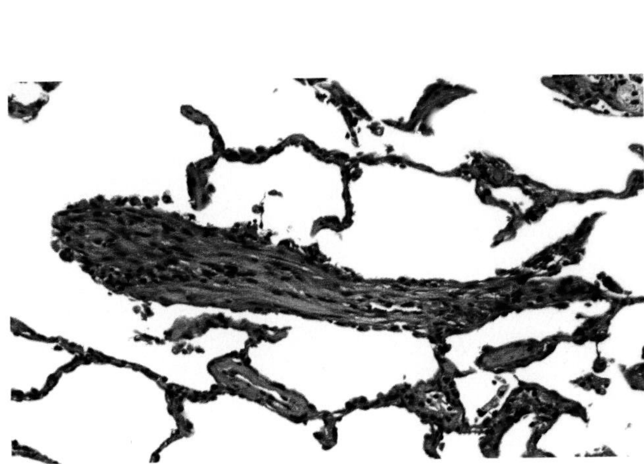

Figure 62.5 Plug of granulation tissue in the lumen of an alveolar duct.

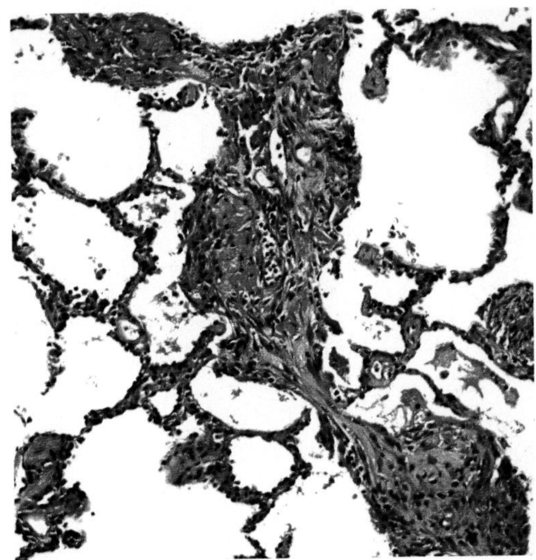

Figure 62.6 Granulation tissue fills an alveolar duct and extends through a pore of Kohn from one alveolus into another.

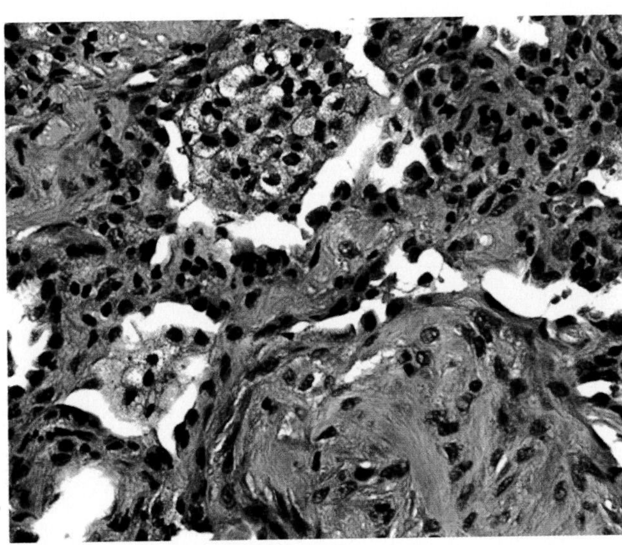

Figure 62.7 Intraalveolar foamy macrophages indicate small airways obstruction.

63

Constrictive Bronchiolitis

▶ Philip T. Cagle

Constrictive bronchiolitis is a condition in which the bronchiolar lumens are severely narrowed or obliterated by submucosal scarring. Constrictive bronchiolitis is also called *bronchiolitis obliterans* and *obliterative bronchiolitis.* Constrictive bronchiolitis results from scarring caused by infections (especially viral infections that affect the bronchioles), collagen vascular diseases involving the lungs (particularly rheumatoid arthritis), drug reactions, exposures to fumes and toxins, and bone marrow transplant. Constrictive bronchiolitis is a major histopathologic finding in chronic lung transplant rejection (see Chapter 104). It may be a component of bronchiectasis, cystic fibrosis, or asthma. It is also seen in some rare conditions, as in inflammatory bowel disease with lung involvement (see Chapter 90) and diffuse idiopathic pulmonary neuroendocrine cell hyperplasia (see Chapter 14, Part 4). Idiopathic cases also occur.

In constrictive bronchiolitis there is narrowing of the bronchiolar lumen by submucosal fibrous tissue. The narrowing may be subtle, and the clinical symptoms and findings may be disproportionate to the histologic narrowing. In other cases, some of the bronchiolar lumens may be completely obliterated, leaving only a scarred remnant of the airway. However, in contrast to cryptogenic organizing pneumonia (formerly known as *bronchiolitis obliterans organizing pneumonia*), there is concentric constriction of the lumen without intraluminal granulation tissue plugs and, in contrast to granulation tissue plugs, the mature submucosal fibrosis does not potentially resolve and disappear. There also may be adventitial scarring and smooth muscle hypertrophy. Inflammation may be present, or it may be minimal or absent. Trichrome stain may assist in identifying bronchioles by highlighting their muscle when their lumens have been replaced by scar.

Histologic Features:

- Bronchiolar lumen is narrowed by submucosal fibrous tissue.
- Luminal narrowing may be subtle, and airflow obstruction may be disproportionate to the amount of histologic narrowing.
- Bronchiolar lumens may be completely obliterated leaving only a scar; trichrome stain may help identify obliterated bronchioles by highlighting their smooth muscle.
- There may also be adventitial scarring and smooth muscle hypertrophy.
- Inflammation may be present, or it may be minimal or absent.

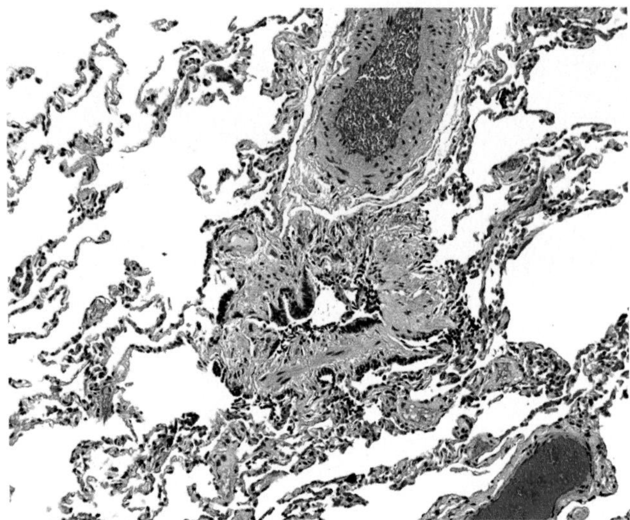

Figure 63.1 Terminal (membranous) bronchiolar lumen is narrowed by submucosal fibrosis in a case of fume exposure.

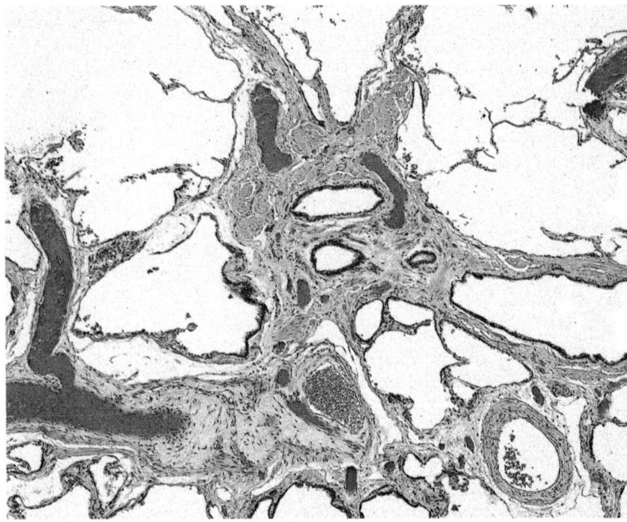

Figure 63.2 Scarring of the terminal (membranous) bronchiolar lumen and surrounding alveolar septa in a case of healed viral infection.

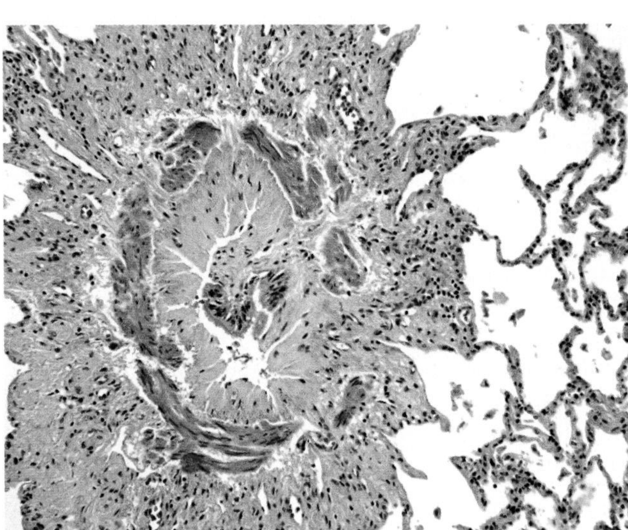

Figure 63.3 Nearly complete obliteration of a terminal (membranous) bronchiolar lumen by submucosal fibrosis in chronic rejection of a transplanted lung.

Respiratory Bronchiolitis and Membranous Bronchiolitis

64

▶ Philip T. Cagle

Tobacco smoking results in inflammatory, sometimes fibrotic, lesions of the membranous (terminal) bronchioles and respiratory bronchioles, referred to as *membranous bronchiolitis* and *respiratory bronchiolitis,* respectively. The extent and severity of these lesions vary widely, and they may be accompanied by emphysema, chronic bronchitis, or interstitial lung disease in the form of respiratory bronchiolitis-associated interstitial lung disease or desquamative interstitial pneumonia. More often, the lesions are unaccompanied by clinically significant findings, although, physiologically, measurements of FEV_1, $FEF_{25\%-75\%}$, or $FEF_{75\%}$ in smokers may indicate small airways obstruction.

Clinically significant small airway obstruction is often referred to as *small airways disease,* but FEV_1, $FEF_{25\%-75\%}$, and $FEF_{75\%}$ measurement cannot distinguish between proximal (membranous or terminal bronchiole) and distal (respiratory bronchiole) obstruction. In patients with clinical chronic obstructive pulmonary disease, the severity of disease and obstruction appears to correlate with the severity of bronchiolitis.

Histologic Features: Respiratory Bronchiolitis

- Lesions may be seen involving occasional respiratory bronchioles of smokers or may be more extensive and accompanied by clinical changes called *respiratory bronchiolitis-associated interstitial lung* disease.
- Collections of macrophages containing a finely granular brown cytoplasmic pigment within lumens of respiratory bronchioles and adjacent alveolar ducts and alveoli and connecting membranous (terminal) bronchioles.
- Mild to moderate infiltrates of lymphocytes and/or histiocytes in the bronchiolar wall; histiocytes may contain black anthracotic pigment or the same finely granular brown cytoplasmic pigment as the macrophages.
- Minimal to mild fibrosis in the bronchiolar wall and first tiers of adjacent alveolar septa, which may be lined by hyperplastic type II pneumocytes or metaplastic bronchiolar epithelium.

Membranous Bronchiolitis

- Lesions may be seen involving occasional membranous bronchioles of smokers or may be more extensive and accompanied by respiratory bronchiolitis or other smoking-related changes, such as emphysema and/or desquamative interstitial pneumonia.
- Collections of macrophages containing a finely granular brown cytoplasmic pigment within lumens of membranous bronchioles and often in lumens of respiratory bronchioles, alveolar ducts, and alveoli.
- Mild to moderate infiltrates of lymphocytes and/or histiocytes in the bronchiolar wall, smooth muscle hyperplasia, adventitial fibrosis, and/or hyperplasia or metaplasia of the bronchiolar epithelium.

- Histiocytes in the bronchiolar wall may contain coarse black anthracotic pigment or the same finely granular brown cytoplasmic pigment as the intraluminal macrophages.
- Mucus plugs may accompany goblet cell metaplasia of the bronchiolar epithelium.

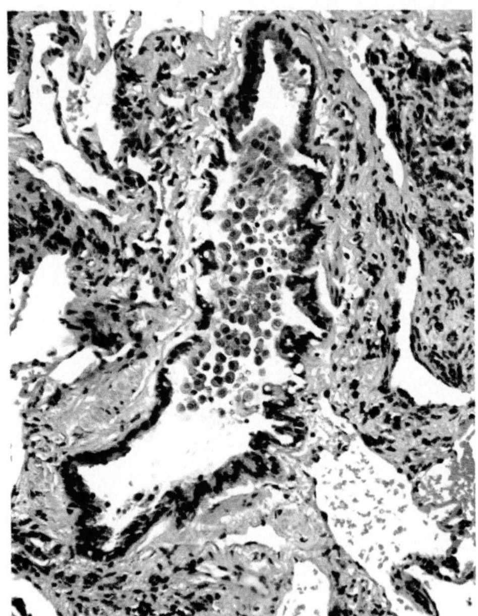

Figure 64.1 Membranous bronchiolitis consists of peribronchiolar fibrosis with mild inflammation and macrophages containing anthracotic pigment and lumen filled with macrophages containing finely granular brown cytoplasmic pigment.

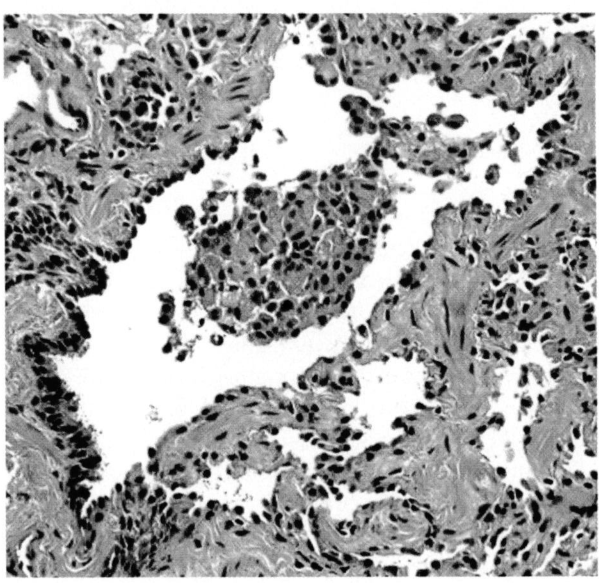

Figure 64.2 Membranous bronchiole from a smoker shows peribronchiolar fibrosis and focal inflammation and macrophages containing finely granular brown pigment within the lumen.

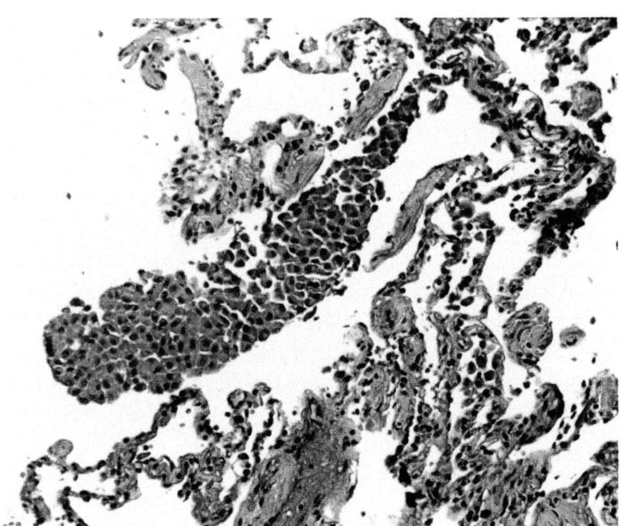

Figure 64.3 Collections of macrophages containing finely granular brown pigment are present within the lumen of an alveolar duct.

65 Follicular Bronchiolitis

▸ Timothy Allen
▸ Philip T. Cagle

Follicular bronchiolitis consists of hyperplasia of the bronchus-associated lymphoid tissue so that airways have prominent lymphoid tissue with follicles and germinal centers. Follicular bronchiolitis can occur in collagen vascular diseases involving the lungs (particularly rheumatoid arthritis and Sjögren syndrome), in bronchiectasis, in immunodeficiency states of various types, and in hypersensitivity reactions. Some cases are idiopathic. It may also be seen in association with lymphoma of the bronchus-associated lymphoid tissue.

Histologic Features:

- Prominent lymphoid tissue with follicles and germinal centers along airways.

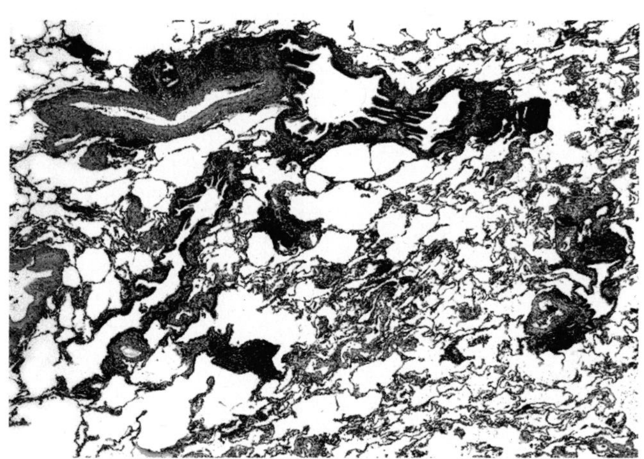

Figure 65.1 Low power of follicular bronchiolitis shows prominent lymphoid tissue along airways.

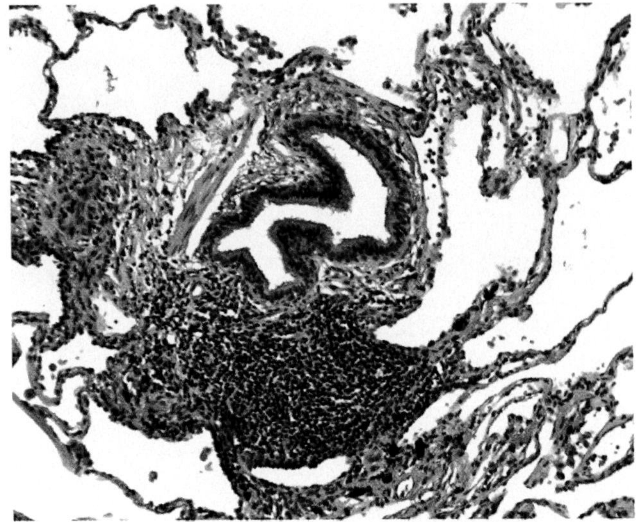

Figure 65.2 Prominent lymphoid tissue adjacent to a bronchiole.

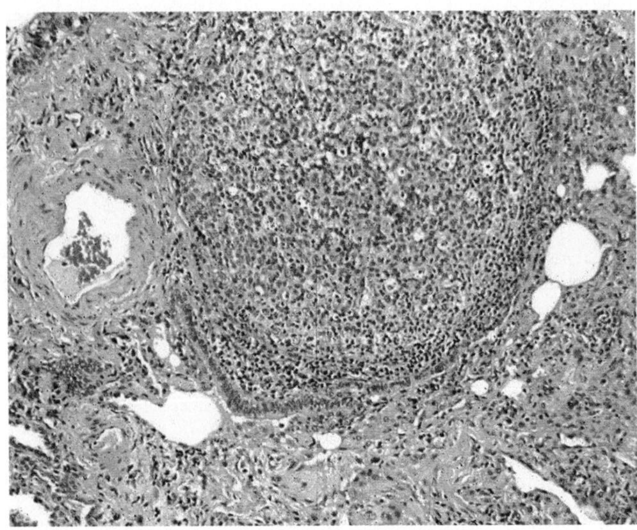

Figure 65.3 Lymphoid follicle with germinal center adjacent to a bronchiole in follicular bronchiolitis.

66 Diffuse Panbronchiolitis

▶ Philip T. Cagle

Diffuse panbronchiolitis is a progressive obstructive small airway disease associated with sinusitis that occurs primarily in adults of Japanese heritage. The disease is typically complicated by infections and, when untreated, leads to bronchiectasis and eventually death. An association with rheumatoid arthritis in Japan has been reported.

Grossly, bronchiolocentric yellow 1- to 3-mm nodules are present. Histologically, the bronchiolar interstitium in diffuse panbronchiolitis is infiltrated by foamy macrophages, lymphocytes, and plasma cells. Follicular bronchiolitis may be present, and there may be histopathologic findings of superimposed acute or organizing pneumonia.

Histologic Features:

- Respiratory bronchioles, terminal (membranous) bronchioles, and alveolar ducts may be involved; membranous (terminal) bronchioles may be ectatic.
- Transmural infiltration of bronchiolar interstitium and peribronchiolar tissue by foamy macrophages, lymphocytes, and plasma cells.
- Follicular bronchiolitis may be present.
- Acute inflammation may be present in bronchiolar lumens.
- Histopathologic findings of superimposed acute or organizing pneumonia and bronchiectasis may be present.

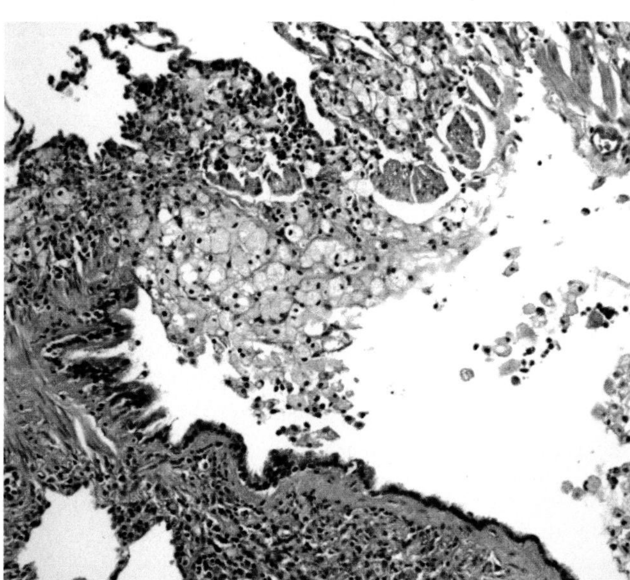

Figure 66.1 Bronchiolar wall is infiltrated by chronic inflammatory infiltrates and foamy macrophages that have spilled into the lumen in this section from a Japanese patient.

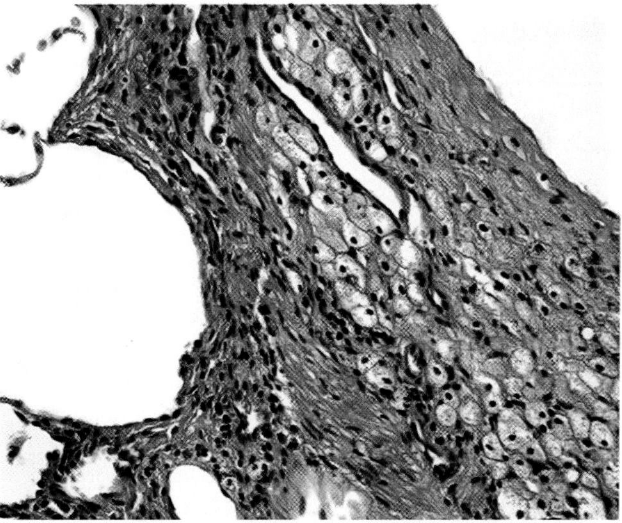

Figure 66.2 Foamy macrophages and lymphocytes in the interstitium in a Japanese patient.

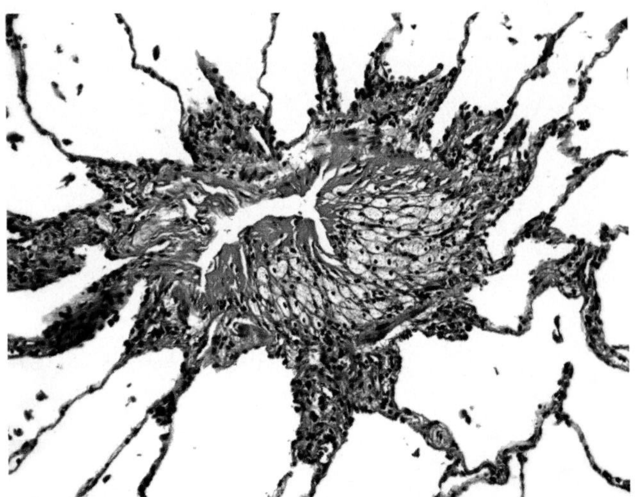

Figure 66.3 Lumen of small bronchiole is narrowed by foamy macrophages and lymphocytes in its wall in a North-American patient. This patient had a xanthomatous bronchiolitis obliterans with some features resembling diffuse panbronchiolitis in Japanese patients and required lung transplantation.

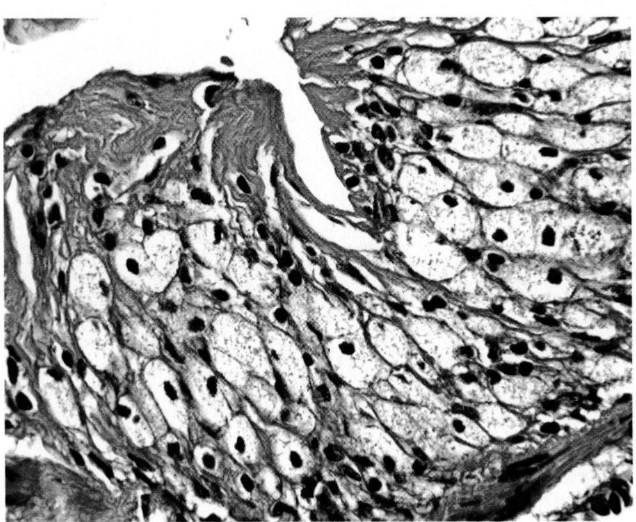

Figure 66.4 Higher power of Figure 66.3 shows foamy macrophages in the bronchiolar wall.

Small Airways and Inorganic Dusts

67

▶ Philip T. Cagle

Small airways (terminal or membranous bronchioles, respiratory bronchioles, and alveolar ducts) may be affected by exposure to both fibrous and nonfibrous mineral particles, including silica, silicates, coal dust, asbestos, iron, and mixed dusts. Small airways are often involved by macules and nodules of various dust exposures (see Chapter 85).

The term *mineral dust-associated small airways disease* has been coined to describe fibrosis of small airways that evolves from nonfibrotic dust macules. There is deposition of mineral dusts and minimal fibrosis in the walls of the membranous bronchioles, respiratory bronchioles, and alveolar ducts. With time, the lesions may progress, with fibrotic distortion of the airways and focal emphysema of the adjacent parenchyma.

Dust-related small airway fibrosis involves the same anatomic locations as tobacco smoke: terminal (membranous) bronchioles and respiratory bronchioles. In the past, it was suggested that mineral dusts caused more respiratory bronchiolitis and that tobacco smoke caused more membranous bronchiolitis, but in recent years, respiratory bronchiolitis and respiratory bronchiolitis-associated interstitial lung disease have emerged as important tobacco-related lesions (see Chapters 64, 78, 79, and 80).

Histologic Features:

- Small airways are often involved by macules and nodules of various dust exposures.
- In mineral dust-associated small airways disease, there are deposits of dust and dust-laden macrophages in the walls of terminal (membranous) bronchioles, respiratory bronchioles, and alveolar ducts associated initially with minimal fibrosis.
- With progression of mineral dust-associated small airways disease, there is increasing fibrosis of the walls of small airways, with distortion and potentially focal emphysema of parenchyma around the affected airways.

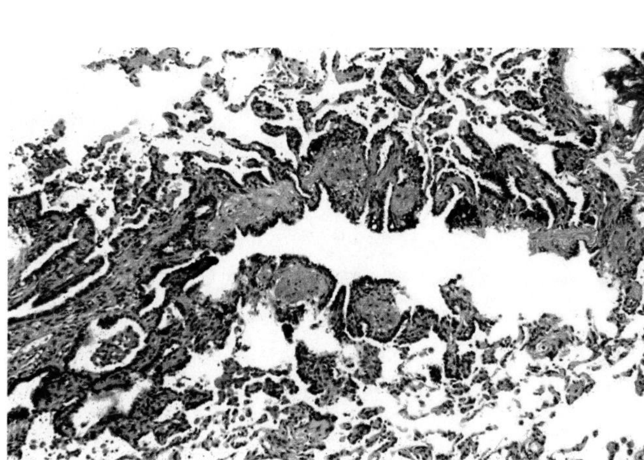

Figure 67.1 Low power of bronchiole with fibrotic wall and fragmentation of the adjacent alveolar septa in a patient with mineral dust exposure.

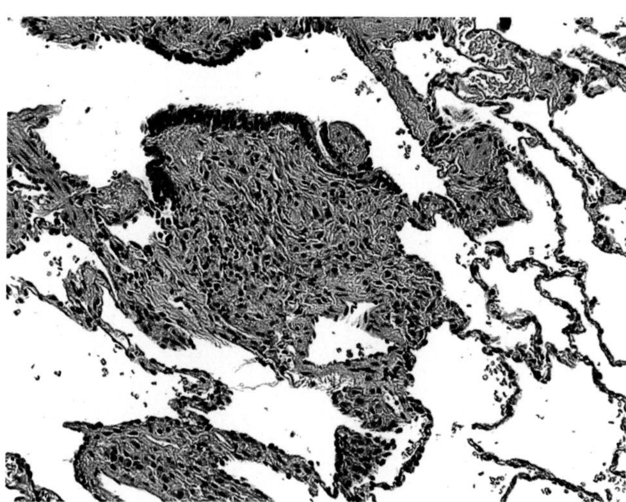

Figure 67.2 Early silicotic nodule consisting of pigmented macrophages and irregular collagen in the wall of a bronchiole.

Section 13

Alveolar Infiltrates

68

Acute Pneumonia

▶ Roberto Barrios

Acute pneumonia is characterized by acute inflammation of the lung involving distal air-spaces. Acute pneumonias can be classified in several different ways: according to epidemiology, pathogenesis, anatomic distribution, clinical presentation, and specific etiologic agent. The tissue response depends, to a certain extent, on the inflammatory response to specific etiologic agents. *Streptococcus pneumoniae* and *Haemophilus influenzae* often produce lobar consolidation, but tissue necrosis is rarely present. In contrast, staphylococci and many Gram-negative bacilli often produce necrosis and even abscess formation. Classic examples of acute pneumonia, such as pneumococcal pneumonia, are characterized by abundant polymorphonuclear leukocyte exudates. In patients with lobar pneumonia, the lesions progress over time from edema to red hepatization, gray hepatization, and resolution. These classic descriptions are now rarely seen because of antibiotic administration, which has modified the natural history of the disease and has sharply reduced the overall case-fatality rate (Table 68.1).

Table 68.1. Major Causes of Infectious Pneumonia

Gram-positive cocci	*Streptococcus pneumoniae, Streptococcus pyogenes,* other streptococci, staphylococci
Gram-positive bacilli	*Bacillus anthracis*
Gram-negative cocci	*Neisseria meningitidis, Moraxella catarrhalis*
Gram-negative coccobacilli	*Haemophilus influenzae;* Gram-negative bacilli: *Klebsiella pneumoniae, Pseudomonas* sp, *Escherichia coli, Proteus, Serratia* sp, *Acinetobacter, Yersinia pestis, Francisella tularensis, Enterobacter* sp, *Bacteroides, Legionella* sp
Mixed flora (frequently found in aspiration pneumonia)	
Mycobacteria	*Mycobacterium tuberculosis, Mycobacterium avium complex*
Fungi	*Histoplasma, Coccidioides, Blastomyces, Cryptococcus, Candida, Aspergillus, Mucoraceae*
Parasites	*Pneumocystis carinii, Toxoplasma gondii*
Mycoplasmas	*Mycoplasma pneumoniae*
Chlamydiae	*Chlamydia psittaci, Chlamydia trachomatis, Chlamydia pneumoniae*
Rickettsias	*Coxiella brunetti*
Viruses	Influenza virus, parainfluenza virus, adenovirus, respiratory syncytial virus, rhinovirus, measles virus, varicella zoster virus, cytomegalovirus

Modified from Simon HB. Pulmonary infections. In: Dale DC, ed. *Scientific American Medicine.* WebMD, 2003.

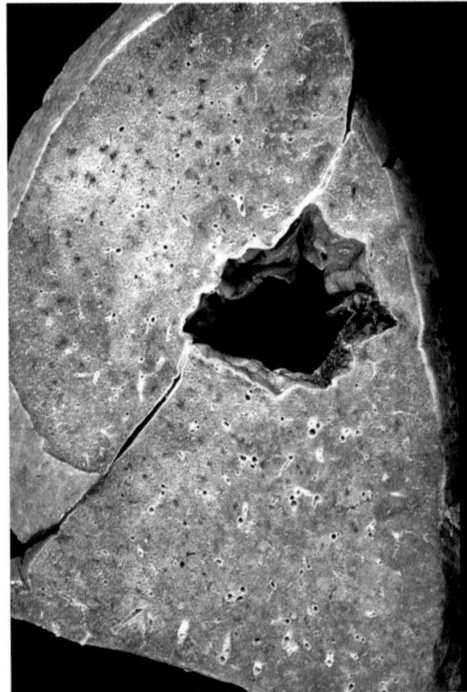

Figure 68.4 Gross figure shows an acute pulmonary abscess having a thin, irregular cavity wall in an alcoholic patient who died of sepsis.

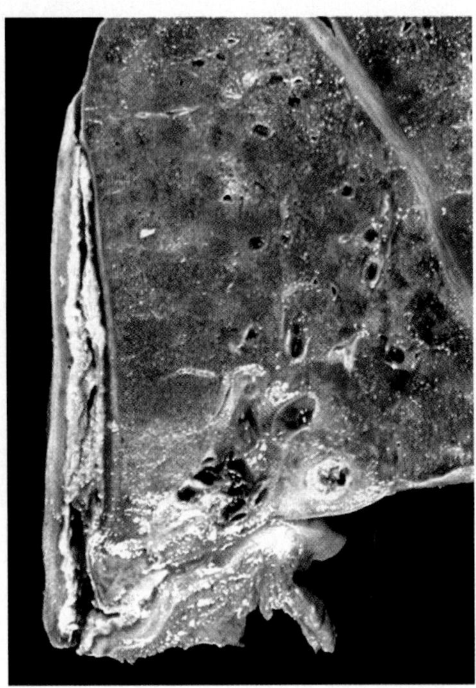

Figure 68.5 Gross figure of a chronic abscess shows pleural thickening and fibrosis secondary to pleural rupture and empyema in a patient with staphylococcal septicemia following abdominal surgery.

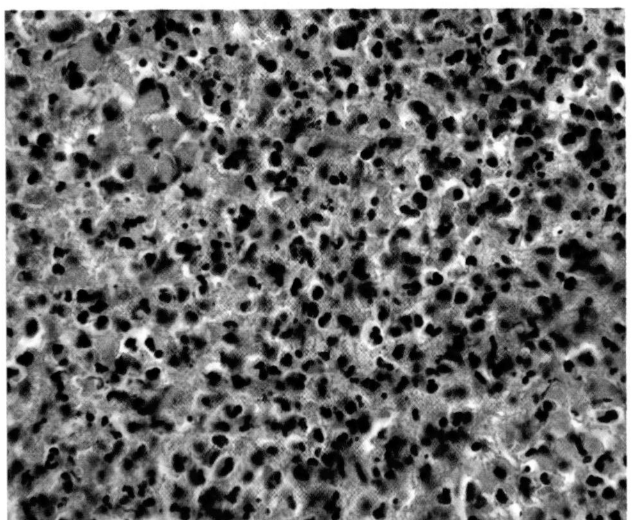

Figure 68.6 Acute abscess characterized by neutrophils, macrophages, and necrotic debris.

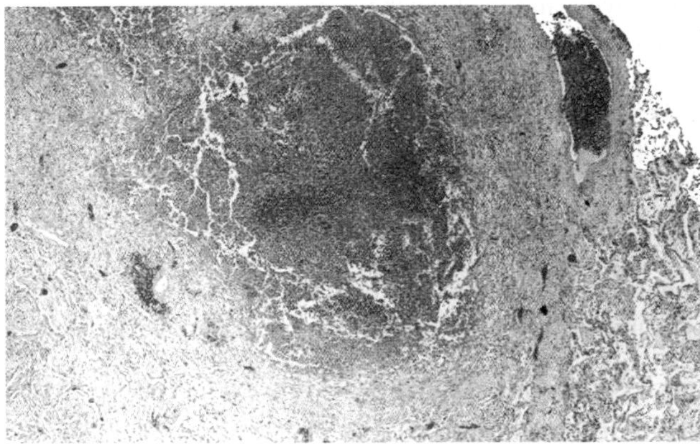

Figure 68.7 Small chronic abscess shows thick fibrous walls surrounding necrotic debris and remnants of fibrinous exudates. The central debris may be evident for several weeks or months.

Part 3

Aspiration Pneumonia

▶ Abida Haque

Aspiration of oropharyngeal or gastric contents produces an acute exudative response within minutes, followed by necrotizing pneumonia, abscess formation, and cavitation.

Chronic aspiration of lipid material, such as milk consumption by infants, mineral oil ingestion, or use of oily nasal drops by adults, can cause lipoid pneumonia. Aspiration of mineral oil may result in lipoid pneumonia. Aspiration of barium solution, charcoal, foreign bodies (in children), and polyurethane foam has been reported.

Histologic Features:

- Acute aspiration pneumonia shows diffuse pulmonary congestion, edema, alveolar epithelial necrosis, and atelectasis.
- Within 4 to 5 hours there is intense neutrophil infiltrate, followed by hyaline membrane formation in 24 to 48 hours.
- Resolution may start at 72 hours or later.
- Lipoid pneumonia is characterized by collections of foamy histiocytes within the alveoli and alveolar interstitium.
- Interstitial fibrosis may be seen in chronic cases.
- Chronic inflammation of bronchioles with foreign body granulomata has been recently reported and referred to as *diffuse aspiration bronchiolitis.*

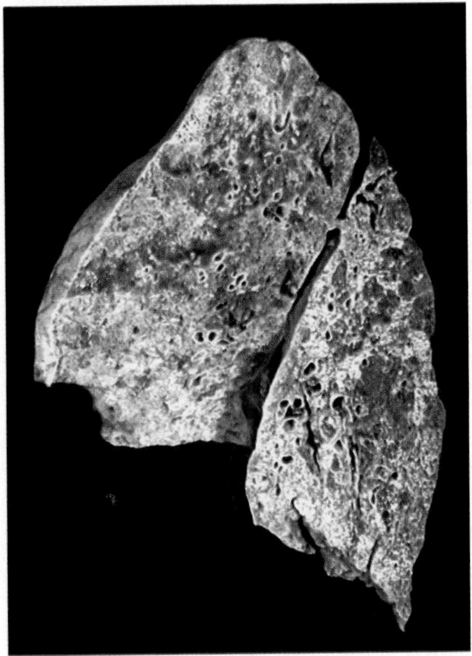

Figure 68.8 Gross figure showing chronic aspiration pneumonia with organizing bronchopneumonia and extensive bilateral fibrosis, characterized by grayish-white areas at the lung periphery, with the only normal lung tissue appearing dark brown.

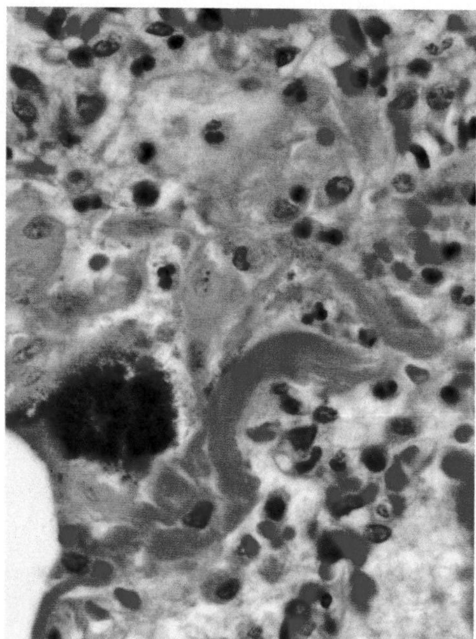

Figure 68.9 Alveolus filled with fibrinous exudates, neutrophils, degenerated muscle fibers, and bacterial colonies consistent with acute aspiration pneumonia.

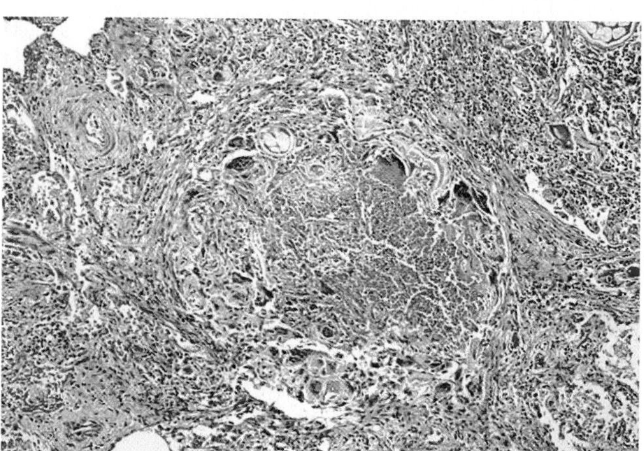

Figure 68.10 Chronic aspiration pneumonia showing granulomatous lesion with central necrosis surrounded by macrophages, neutrophils, multinucleated giant cells, and aspirated starch particle.

Organizing Acute Pneumonia

69

▶ Roberto Barrios

When an acute pneumonia does not resolve, it progresses to a subacute and chronic stage, with organization of the acute fibrinous exudates by fibroblast ingrowth. An organized acute pneumonia consists of consolidation of the lung, with fibroblastic proliferation (granulation tissue) filling the airspaces. This early fibrosis may be admixed with inflammatory cells, residual acute pneumonia, and aggregates of macrophages in a patchy pattern.

A pattern of lung injury previously referred to as *bronchiolitis obliterans organizing pneumonia* consists of plugs of granulation tissue with bronchiolar lumens and in adjoining airspaces. This particular pattern is now more often designated *organizing pneumonia* and, when idiopathic, *cryptogenic organizing pneumonia.* These patterns are discussed in Chapters 62 and 94, respectively.

Histologic Features:

- Aggregates of macrophages, mostly intraalveolar.
- Fibroblastic proliferation that passes through alveolar pores in some areas.
- Chronic inflammation in varying degrees.

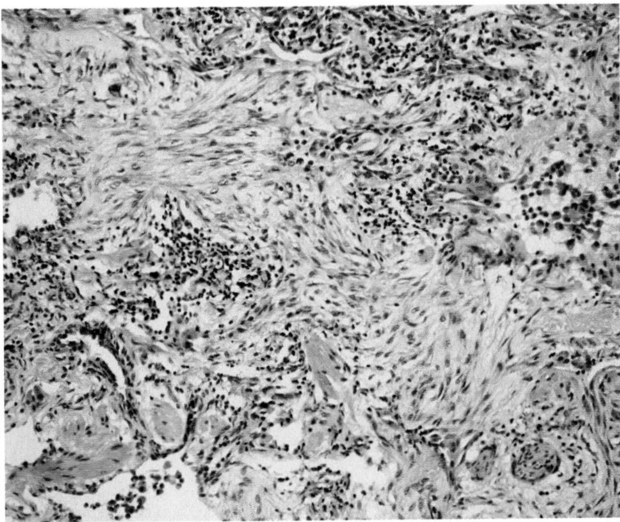

Figure 69.1 Organizing acute pneumonia with fibroblastic proliferation filling airspaces and a mild lymphocytic infiltrate.

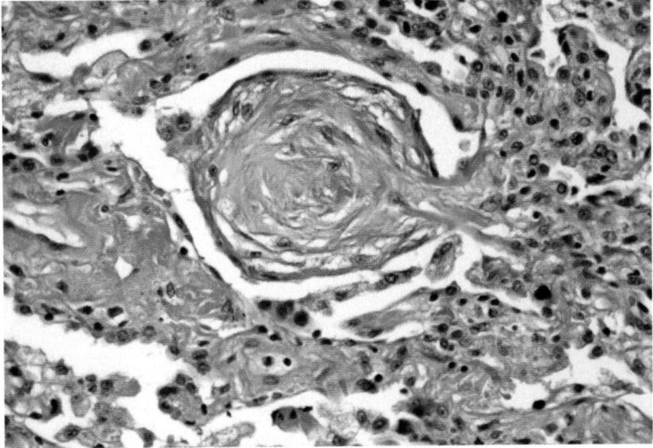

Figure 69.2 Well-defined fibroblastic proliferation within an alveolar space and mildly thickened alveolar septa.

70

Pulmonary Edema

▶ Roberto Barrios

The buildup of extravascular fluid in the lungs is called *pulmonary edema.* Pulmonary edema is a common complication of cardiac and noncardiac disorders. Cardiogenic pulmonary edema results from left heart failure, valvular heart disease, and obstruction in the left chambers of the heart (pulmonary edema can be the first sign of coronary heart disease). Noncardiogenic causes include fluid overload, renal failure, acute respiratory distress syndrome, drug reactions, narcotics (heroin), toxic inhalation, and near drowning. The actual mechanism may be due to increased hydrostatic pressure in the capillaries and venules and/or changes in vessel permeability. Pulmonary edema can be a chronic condition, or it can develop suddenly and quickly become life threatening. The life-threatening type of pulmonary edema occurs when a large amount of fluid suddenly shifts from the pulmonary blood vessels into the interstitium and/or alveoli.

The sequence of events for the development of pulmonary edema is always the same, regardless of the etiology. It consists of an early interstitial phase, where fluid accumulates in the alveolar interstitium, and a second stage, where fluid is present in the alveoli. The pathologist depends on the staining of protein within the edema fluid to make a histologic diagnosis of edema. If there is edema fluid with a minimal amount of protein, it may be difficult to make the diagnosis of pulmonary edema even when clinical, radiologic, and physiologic methods detect the presence of edema in the patient. The protein that accompanies edema fluid is seen as intraalveolar eosinophilic material filling the airspaces. Other conditions in which eosinophilic material occupies alveoli are pulmonary alveolar proteinosis and *Pneumocystis carinii* pneumonia. Pulmonary edema lacks the granularity, coarse granules, cholesterol clefts, and macrophages of alveolar proteinosis. *Pneumocystis* pneumonia also shows intraalveolar eosinophilic material, but the intraalveolar material displays a foamy appearance that corresponds to the cysts.

Histologic Features:

- Microscopic changes are identical, regardless of the cause.
- In sections stained with hematoxylin and eosin, protein that leaks with the fluid is stained as a pink homogeneous eosinophilic material.
- Differential diagnosis includes pulmonary alveolar proteinosis and *P. carinii* pneumonia.

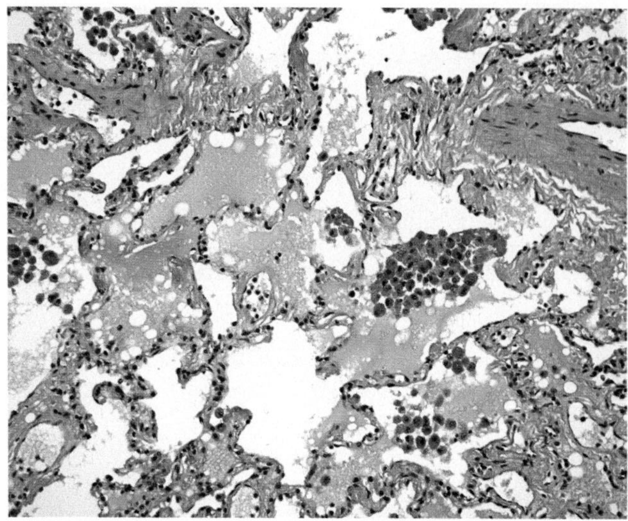

Figure 70.1 Pulmonary edema with some alveolar spaces occupied by an eosinophilic proteinaceous material and some hemosiderin-laden macrophages associated with chronic passive congestion.

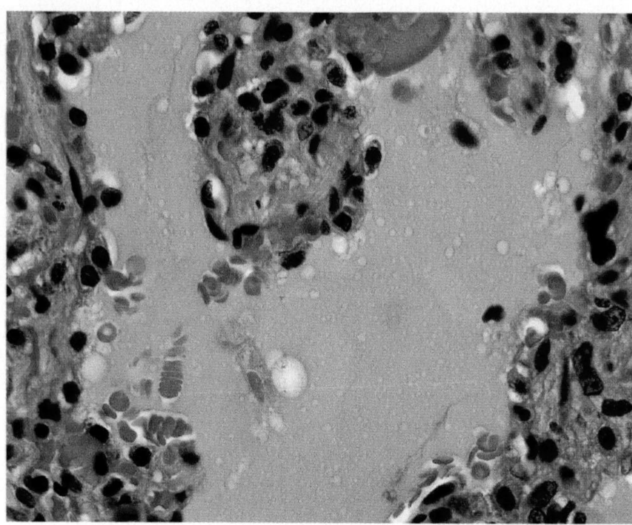

Figure 70.2 Higher power shows intraalveolar edema and engorgement of alveolar capillaries.

71 Diffuse Alveolar Damage

▸ Roberto Barrios

Diffuse alveolar damage (DAD) is a term that describes a tissue response to a wide variety of acute lung injuries. The lung has limited ways to respond to injury; therefore, the pathologic findings present in this entity are similar regardless of the causal agent. The clinical expression of this tissue reaction is acute respiratory distress syndrome (ARDS), also known in the literature as acute lung injury, traumatic wet lung, Da Nang lung, noncardiogenic pulmonary edema, congestive atelectasis, and adult hyaline membrane disease. Causes of DAD include infections, trauma including neurotrauma, burns, shock, inhalation of fumes and toxins, drug reactions, chemotherapy and radiation, aspiration, oxygen and ventilation, and other insults. Many patients with ARDS/DAD have a combination of several possible causes superimposed on one another, such as trauma followed by oxygen therapy and infection. Approximately 50% of cases resolve. In some cases, there is progression to a fibrotic phase with end-stage fibrosis. From clinical and experimental observations it is known that DAD progresses through several histologic and clinical stages. Most authors recognize an early exudative, a proliferative, and a late resolving phase.

During early stages, grossly the lungs are heavy due to congestion and edema. The histologic findings depend on the stage of the disease. The early exudative phase shows edema and necrosis of alveolar epithelium. After 72 hours, fibrin and hyaline membranes appear. During the proliferative phase, there is fibroblastic and myofibroblastic interstitial proliferation, as well as type II cell hyperplasia. Finally, the fibrotic phase is characterized by areas of interstitial fibrosis with occasional cystic spaces and occasionally changes that resemble the bronchopulmonary dysplasia seen in infants. Acute interstitial pneumonia has histopathologic features similar to organizing DAD and is a pathologic correlate of the idiopathic clinical syndrome Hamman-Rich (see Chapter 91).

Histologic Features: Exudative (Acute) Phase

- Congestion of alveolar capillaries.
- Interstitial and intraalveolar edema.
- Focal intraalveolar hemorrhage.
- Hyaline membranes.
- Intracapillary neutrophil margination.
- Interstitial inflammation.
- Microvascular thromboemboli (capillaries and arterioles).

Proliferative (Organizing) Phase (Starting at End of First Week)

- Type 2 pneumocyte proliferation ("cuboidalization" of alveolar epithelium).
- Fibroblastic proliferation.

- Squamous metaplasia (occasionally).
- Thromboemboli and small peripheral infarcts.

Fibrotic (Chronic) Phase (3–4 Weeks After Onset)

- Lung architecture remodeled by dense fibrous tissue.
- Alveolar spaces and bronchioles surrounded by dense fibrosis.
- Honeycomb cystic changes may occur.

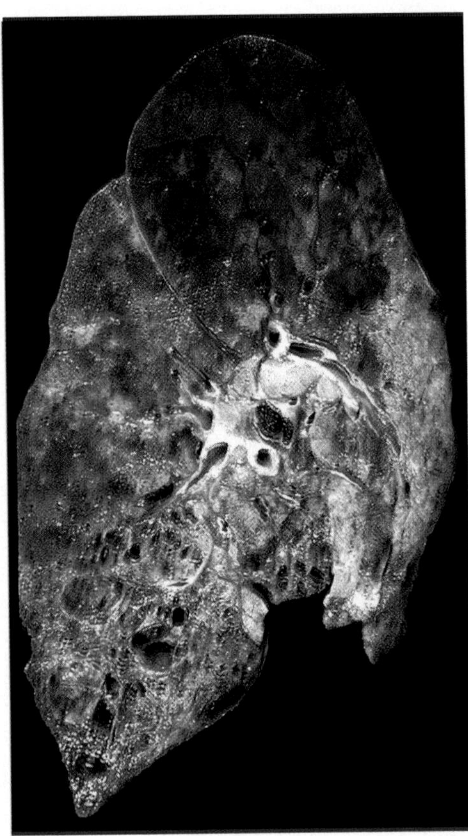

Figure 71.1 Gross figure of diffuse alveolar damage shows diffuse congestion.

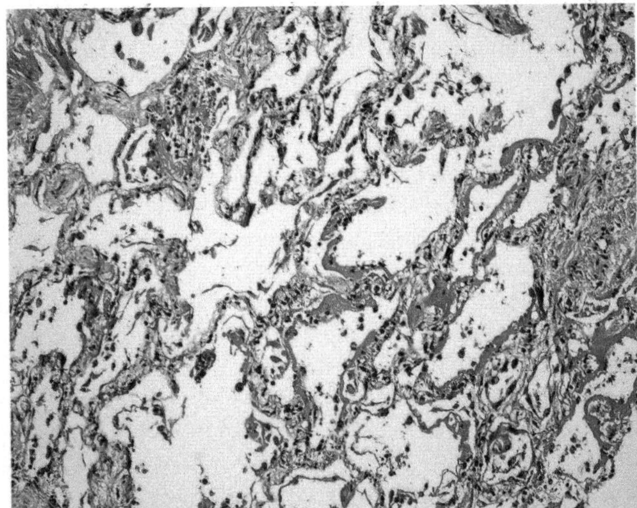

Figure 71.2 Diffuse alveolar damage characterized by edema, hyaline membranes, and scattered inflammatory cells. The architecture is preserved but inflammatory changes are diffuse.

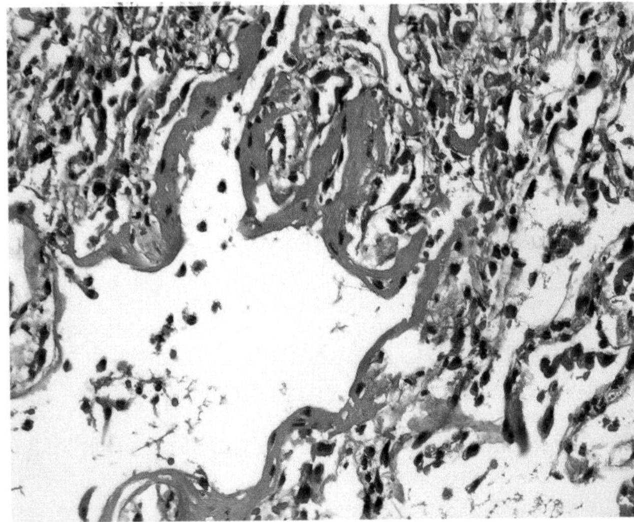

Figure 71.3 Higher power shows hyaline membranes admixed with scattered inflammatory cells.

Acute Fibrinous and Organizing Pneumonia

72

▶ Mary Beth Beasley

Acute fibrinous and organizing pneumonia (AFOP) is a recently described pattern of lung injury that has a mortality rate similar to that of diffuse alveolar damage (DAD) and likely represents a variant histology. The pattern lacks classic histologic features seen in other histologic patterns of lung injury associated with an acute or subacute clinical presentation, namely, DAD, eosinophilic pneumonia, and organizing pneumonia.

AFOP may have an acute or subacute clinical presentation and is associated with a variety of underlying conditions (infection, collagen vascular disease, environmental exposure) or may be idiopathic. The mortality rate is approximately 50%, although some patients present with a more indolent clinical course with good recovery. AFOP likely represents a variant histology of DAD, but further investigation is needed.

Histologic Features:

- Intraalveolar fibrin balls without hyaline membrane formation or significant numbers of eosinophils.
- Relatively patchy distribution with average 50% airspace involvement; not exclusively bronchiolocentric.
- Variable amounts of organizing pneumonia.
- Interstitium with scant inflammation, typically lymphocytic.
- Small degree of myxoid interstitial connective tissue, similar to that seen in DAD.
- Small numbers of interstitial neutrophils may be present.
- Neutrophilic capillaritis absent.
- Absent or very rare eosinophils.
- No granulomas.
- Lung parenchyma not involved by intraalveolar fibrin relatively normal in appearance.
- Does not meet classic criteria of DAD, eosinophilic pneumonia, or organizing pneumonia (formerly known as bronchiolitis obliterans organizing pneumonia).
- No histologic feature correlated with outcome.

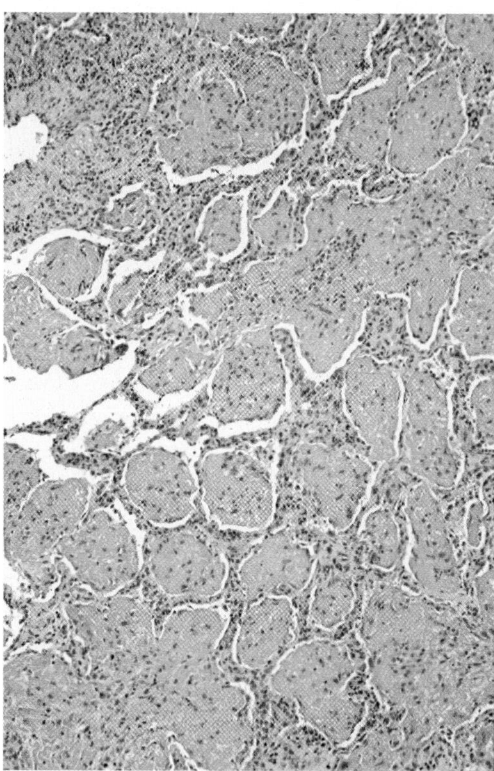

Figure 72.1 Low power of AFOP shows filling of airspaces with intraalveolar fibrin balls.

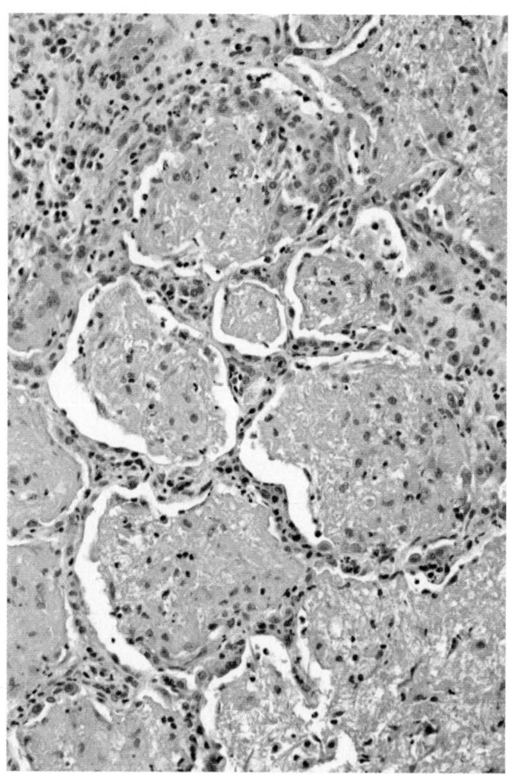

Figure 72.2 Higher power shows intraalveolar fibrin and mild associated interstitial inflammation.

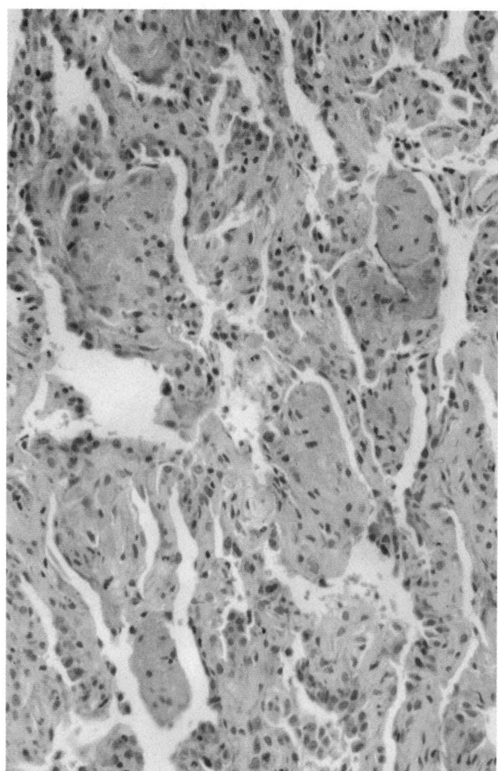

Figure 72.3 Higher power demonstrates interstitial myxoid connective tissue and intraalveolar fibrin balls.

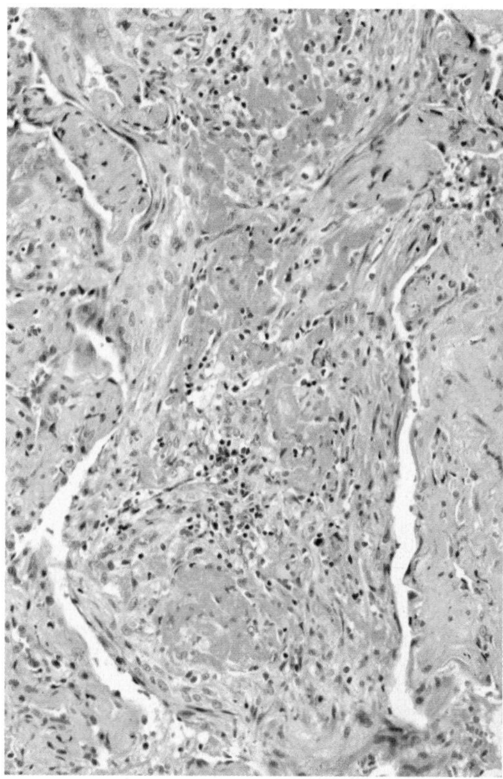

Figure 72.4 Organizing intraalveolar focus of fibroblastic tissue with central core of residual fibrin.

73

Lipoid Pneumonia

▶ Roberto Barrios

Lipoid pneumonia can be subdivided into exogenous and endogenous lipoid pneumonia, depending on the origin of the lipid products associated with this lesion.

Exogenous lipoid pneumonia is produced by inhalation of mineral oil or similar product. It usually occurs due to chronic inhalation of small quantities of these products, which reach the distal lung. Most cases are seen in individuals who use mineral oil as a laxative or use oily nose drops, or who are exposed to industrial inhalation of oily substances or conditions predisposing to chronic aspiration. Over time, fibrosis develops in the areas of pneumonia. Differential diagnosis includes nontuberculous mycobacterial infection (special stains for mycobacteria should always be obtained).

Endogenous lipoid pneumonia is much more common than exogenous lipoid pneumonia. It is also known as *postobstructive pneumonia* or *golden pneumonia* (because of the yellow color produced by the lipids). It is characterized by accumulation of foamy macrophages in the alveolar spaces and interstitium. Their cytoplasm is finely vacuolated (in contrast to the large vacuoles seen in exogenous lipoid pneumonia). Endogenous lipoid pneumonia is frequently seen distal to areas of obstruction (due to malignancy, inflammation, foreign bodies, etc.) where there is accumulation of endogenous lipids and cholesterol from cellular debris and blood due to the obstruction.

Histologic Features:

Exogenous Lipoid Pneumonia

- Numerous macrophages in alveoli and interstitium.
- Macrophages containing large clear vacuoles.
- Multinucleated foreign body giant cells.
- Chronic interstitial inflammation.
- Demonstration of oil by fat stains on frozen sections.
- Bronchoalveolar lavage (BAL) specimens may suggest the diagnosis.

Endogenous Lipoid Pneumonia

- Foci of finely vacuolated foamy macrophages in alveoli.
- Occasional interstitial foamy macrophages may be seen.
- Associated mild chronic inflammation.
- Cholesterol crystals.

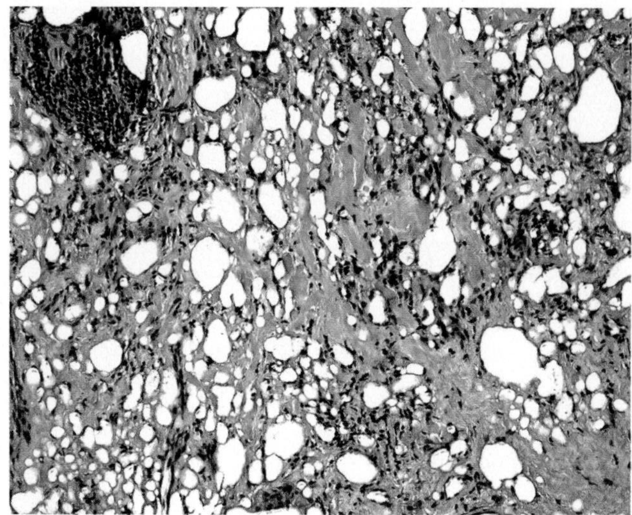

Figure 73.1 Exogenous lipoid pneumonia characterized by large spaces of lipid surrounded by fibrosis and inflammation.

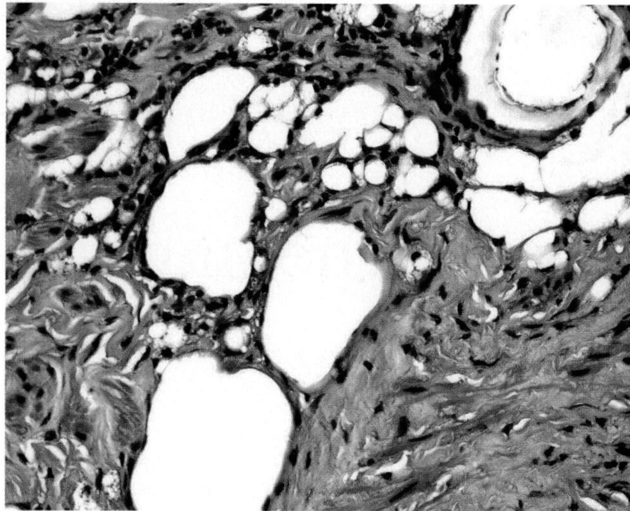

Figure 73.2 Higher power illustrates tissue reaction around the lipid deposits.

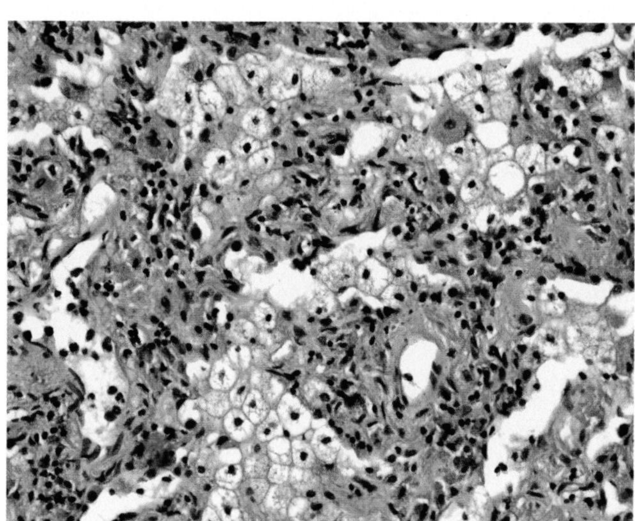

Figure 73.3 Endogenous lipoid pneumonia with alveolar spaces occupied by foamy macrophages.

Eosinophilic Pneumonia

74

▶ Dani S. Zander
▶ Roberto Barrios

The eosinophilic pneumonias are a group of diseases characterized histologically by the accumulation of numerous eosinophils in alveolar spaces and often by peripheral blood eosinophilia. Recognized triggers of eosinophilic pneumonia include infections (especially parasitic and fungal) and drugs. The process can be a component of a variety of immunologic or systemic diseases, including asthma, allergic bronchopulmonary mycoses, collagen vascular diseases, hypereosinophilic syndrome, and Churg-Strauss syndrome. Eosinophilic pneumonia can also be associated with human immunodeficiency virus infection and malignancies. Many examples, however, are idiopathic.

Chronic eosinophilic pneumonia presents with cough, dyspnea, and low-grade fevers that occur over months to years. The condition is commonly associated with asthma and peripheral blood eosinophilia, produces peripheral airspace consolidation on chest radiograph, usually shows a rapid response to corticosteroids, and frequently relapses with withdrawal of corticosteroids. With acute eosinophilic pneumonia, patients develop hypoxemia and respiratory failure over a period of days, chest radiograph demonstrates diffuse infiltrates, and the process resolves rapidly with corticosteroid therapy, without relapses.

Histologic Features:

- Numerous eosinophils filling alveoli and in the interstitium, sometimes forming eosinophil abscesses surrounded by palisaded histiocytes.
- Variable accompaniment of macrophages, fibrin, and necrotic debris in alveoli.
- Organizing pneumonia is commonly present in chronic eosinophilic pneumonia.
- Diffuse alveolar damage is present in acute eosinophilic pneumonia.
- Charcot-Leyden crystals may be present.
- Vascular infiltration by eosinophils may be present.
- In patients treated with steroids, eosinophils may not be prominent, but increased numbers of alveolar macrophages may persist.

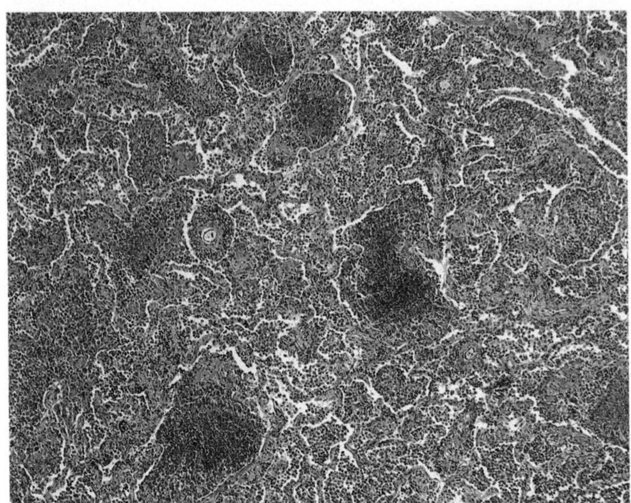

Figure 74.1 Eosinophilic pneumonia with multiple eosinophil abscesses in alveoli.

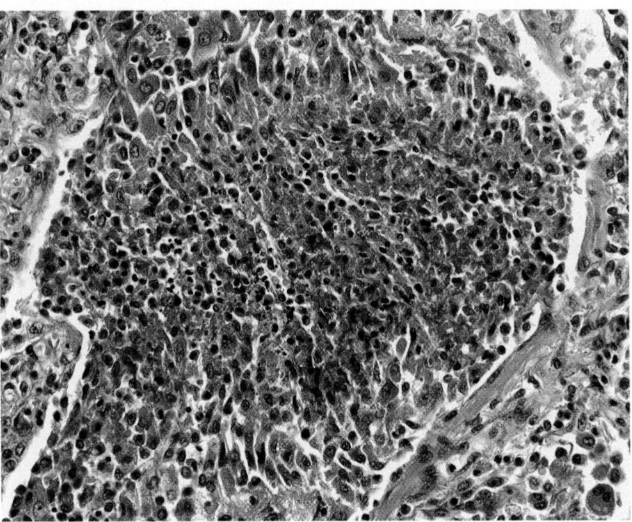

Figure 74.2 Higher power of an eosinophil abscess showing a central zone of necrotic and intact eosinophils surrounded by palisaded histiocytes.

Desquamative Interstitial Pneumonialike Pattern

75

▶ Alvaro C. Laga
▶ Robert Barrios

The term *desquamative interstitial pneumonia (DIP)-like pattern* describes the accumulation of macrophages in the alveoli that can take place as a nonspecific reaction adjacent to a variety of lesions, the most classic example being pulmonary Langerhans cell histiocytosis (see Chapter 29). Many of these cases of DIP-like reaction represent respiratory bronchiolitis-associated interstitial lung disease (see Chapter 80). However, a DIP-like reaction can be seen in and around localized parenchymal masses and interstitial fibrosis in the lung. DIP-like reactions can be seen with usual interstitial pneumonia, nonspecific interstitial pneumonia, asbestosis, human immunodeficiency virus infection, drug reactions, scars, tumors, and infarcts.

Histologic Features:

- Intraalveolar accumulation of macrophages in and around interstitial fibrosis and localized parenchymal masses.
- In smokers, the macrophages may contain cytoplasmic finely granular brown pigment.

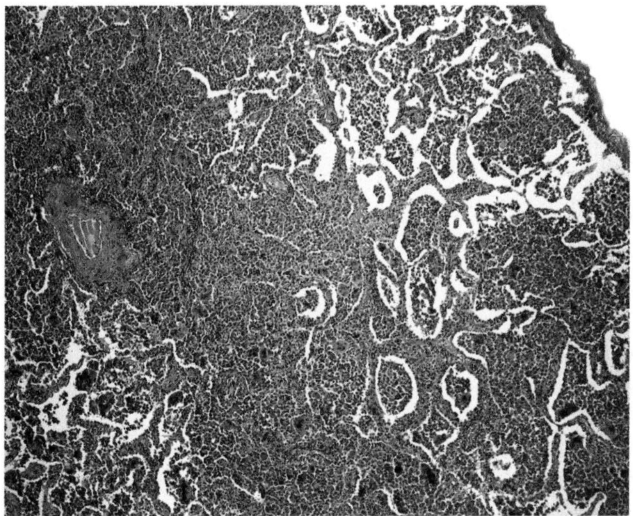

Figure 75.1 Low power shows a localized lesion with interstitial pneumonia and filling of alveolar spaces by numerous macrophages.

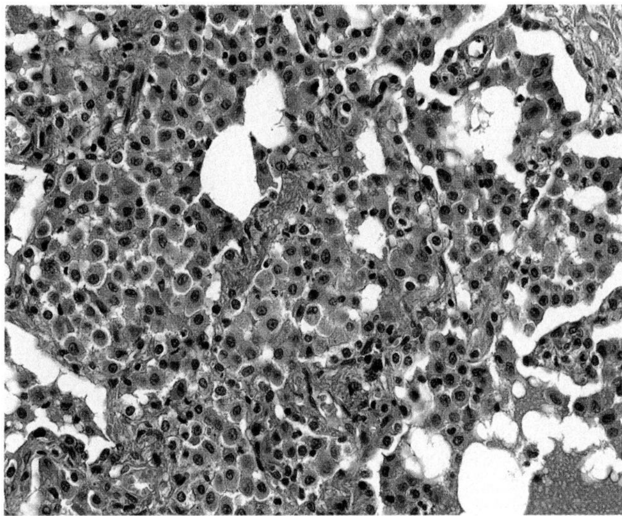

Figure 75.2 Higher power of alveolar spaces filled with abundant macrophages in a DIP-like reaction.

76

Pulmonary Alveolar Proteinosis

▶ Roberto Barrios
▶ Carlos Bedrossian

Pulmonary alveolar proteinosis is a rare lesion characterized by accumulation of a granular eosinophilic material in the alveoli. It can be seen as a primary "idiopathic" disease or associated with other conditions, such as infections, massive inhalation of inorganic dusts, malignancy, immune deficiency, lysinuric protein intolerance, and in lung transplants. Overproduction of surfactant by type 2 pneumocytes or its impaired clearance by alveolar macrophages have been proposed as mechanisms for this entity. Microscopic examination reveals that the alveoli and alveolar ducts are occupied by an eosinophilic material with a superficial resemblance to pulmonary edema; however, the material seen in proteinosis is finely granular, is periodic acid–Schiff (PAS) positive, and contains occasional cholesterol crystals and foamy macrophages.

Differential diagnosis includes pulmonary edema, *Pneumocystis carinii* pneumonia, and alveolar mucinosis. Pulmonary edema is generally homogeneous and lacks the granularity, cholesterol clefts, and foamy macrophages seen in proteinosis. The intraalveolar eosinophilic material seen in *Pneumocystis* pneumonia is foamy and corresponds to the cysts of the microorganism. The diagnosis can sometimes be made by bronchoalveolar lavage (BAL). Examination of sputum may suggest the diagnosis by identification of PAS-positive macrophages.

Cytologic Features:

- Amorphous proteinaceous eosinophilic granular material and alveolar macrophages.

Histologic Features:

- Accumulation of eosinophilic proteinaceous granular material in alveoli, alveolar ducts, and occasional bronchioles.
- In addition, cholesterol clefts and small, dense, globular clumps of eosinophilic material are characteristic.
- Accumulated material is PAS positive.
- Inflammation or interstitial fibrosis is inconspicuous or mild, but interstitial fibrosis or inflammation may occur in patients with longstanding disease.
- Occasional foamy macrophages and type 2 pneumocytes are seen within the alveoli.
- Intraalveolar material stains with an antibody to surfactant apoprotein.
- Electron microscopy reveals concentrically laminated myelin figures and lamellar bodies identical to the cytoplasmic inclusions of type 2 pneumocytes.
- Infection with *Nocardia,* mycobacterial, fungal, and viral agents can be associated with pulmonary alveolar proteinosis.

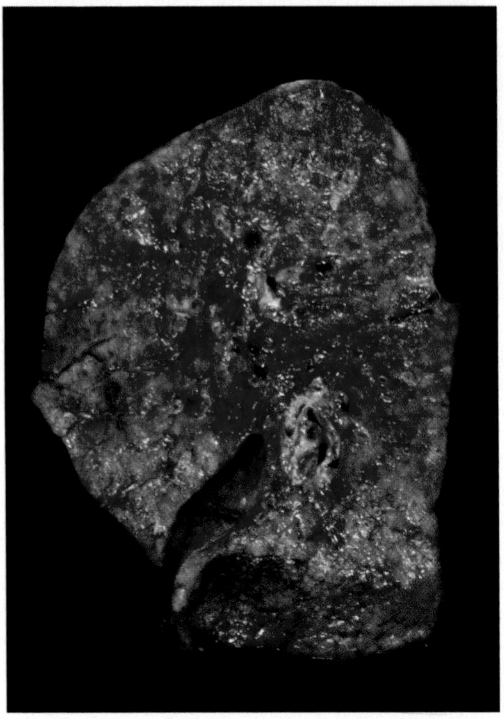

Figure 76.1 Gross figure of pulmonary alveolar proteinosis shows a heavy lung with red-gray areas of consolidation throughout.

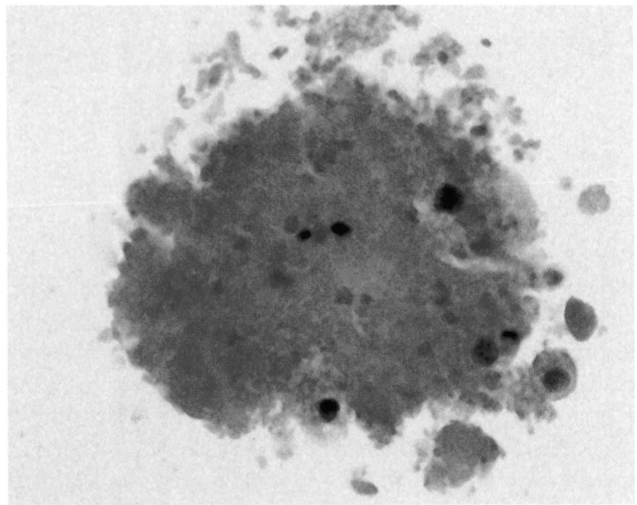

Figure 76.2 Cytology figure shows proteinaceous granular material and alveolar macrophages from a bronchoalveolar lavage (Papanicolaou stain).

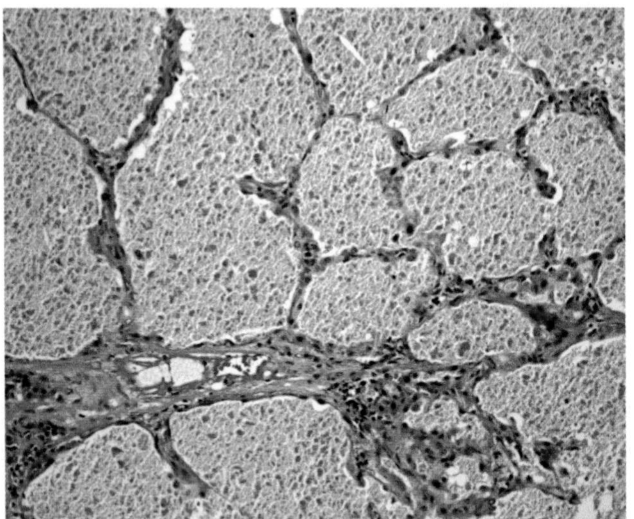

Figure 76.3 Parenchyma shows alveoli filled with an eosinophilic finely granular material. Alveolar septa are unremarkable.

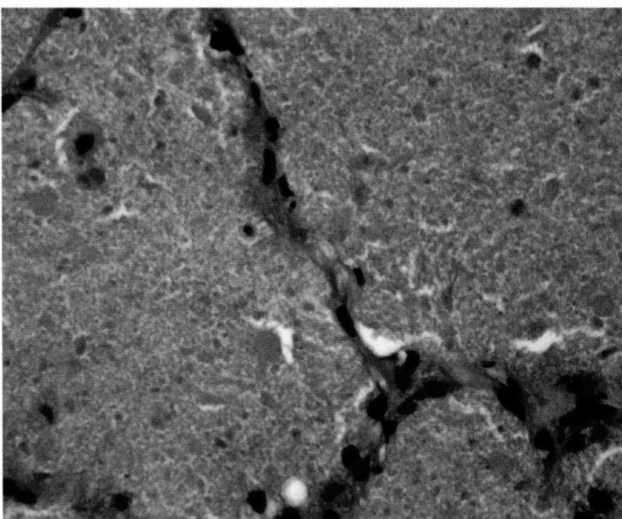

Figure 76.4 Higher power of alveolar proteinosis shows minimal interstitial reaction.

Section 14

Tobacco-Related Diseases

Emphysema

77

▶ Timothy Allen
▶ Philip T. Cagle

Emphysema is characterized by destruction of respiratory bronchioles, alveolar ducts, and alveoli leaving enlarged airspaces. There are several types of emphysema, but the most common type is centrilobular (also known as *centriacinar* or *proximal acinar*) emphysema caused by tobacco smoking that involves primarily the respiratory bronchioles. It is most prominent in the upper lung zones. Panacinar emphysema, like that seen with α_1-antitrypsin deficiency, involves alveolar ducts as well as the respiratory bronchioles.

The destruction of lung parenchyma in emphysema leaves residual fragments of tissue, including islands of fibrovascular tissue. Although it has been emphasized that emphysema is not the same as diffuse interstitial fibrosis, remodeling of lung tissue also appears to have a role in emphysema, and there may be mild fibrosis. Additional histopathologic changes related to tobacco smoking, including respiratory and membranous bronchiolitis, respiratory bronchiolitis-associated interstitial lung disease, and desquamative and related findings, may be seen in association with emphysema from tobacco smoking. Anthracotic pigment and/or macrophages containing smoker's pigment may be present. Bullae are cystic spaces that are found in the lung apices, subpleurally, and elsewhere in emphysematous lungs.

Histologic Features:

- Fragmentation and loss of respiratory bronchioles and septal tissue creating enlarged spaces.
- Bullae are typically subpleural and have residual islands of fibrovascular tissue within grossly evident enlarged spaces.
- Other findings related to tobacco smoking may be observed, including anthracotic pigment, smoker's pigment, respiratory bronchiolitis, membranous bronchiolitis, respiratory bronchiolitis-associated interstitial lung disease, and related conditions.
- Tissue sections may show mild fibrosis and secondary changes, including focal scars and focal acute or organizing pneumonia.

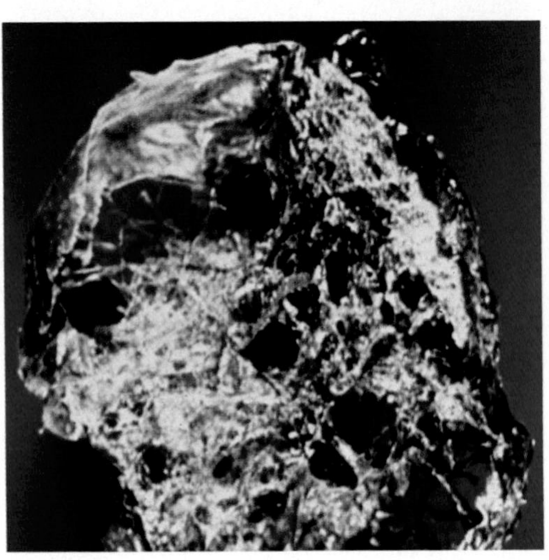

Figure 77.1 Lung with severe emphysema showing extensive destruction of lung parenchyma.

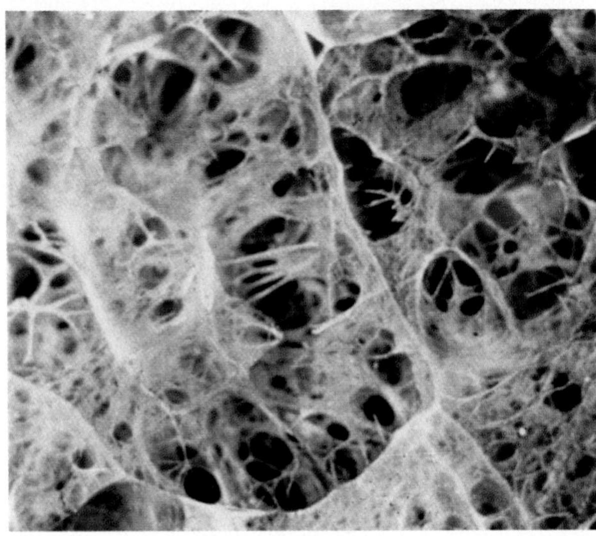

Figure 77.2 Residual strands of fibrovascular tissue in severe emphysema cross spaces created by destruction of lung parenchyma.

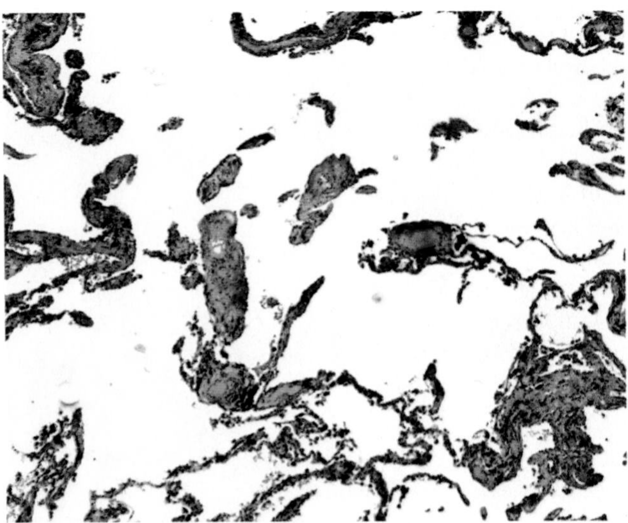

Figure 77.3 Destruction by emphysema leaves enlarged spaces with "floating" parenchymal fragments.

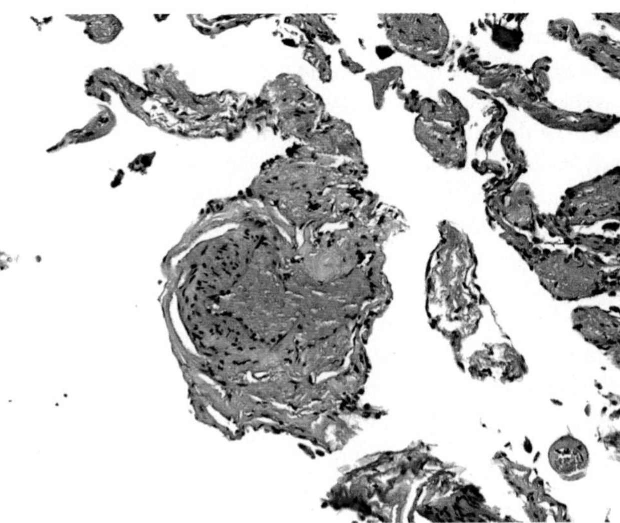

Figure 77.4 Higher power shows residual fibrovascular tissue fragment "floating" in an enlarged space.

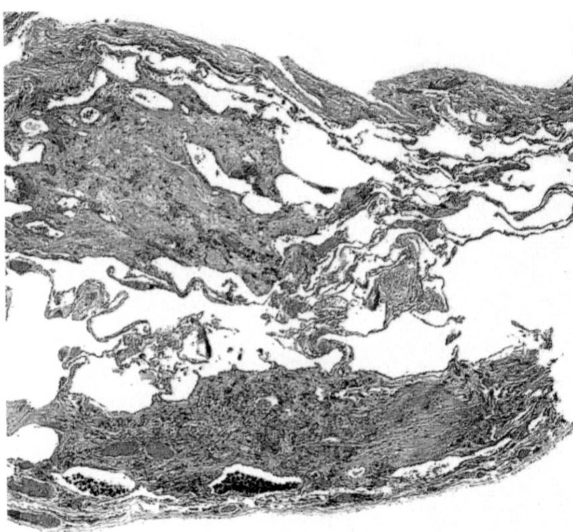

Figure 77.5 Focal subpleural scars in association with emphysema.

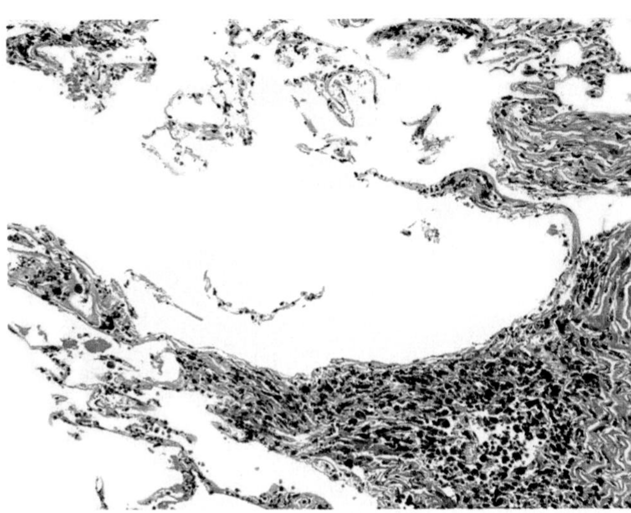

Figure 77.6 Space created by destruction of lung parenchyma with anthracotic pigment in associated focal scar.

78 Membranous Bronchiolitis

▸ Philip T. Cagle

Tobacco smoke effects on the small airways can often be measured physiologically as an obstructive change in FEV_1, more specifically in $FEF_{25\%-75\%}$ or $FEF_{75\%}$. When clinically significant, these changes are referred to as *small airways disease.* However, FEV_1, $FEF_{25\%-75\%}$, and $FEF_{75\%}$ do not distinguish between proximal (membranous or terminal) and distal (respiratory) bronchioles.

Tobacco smoke causes morphologic changes in both the respiratory bronchioles and the membranous (terminal) bronchioles. These changes may be observed together or in combination with other tobacco-related changes such as emphysema. Bronchiolitis of little or no clinical significance can frequently be observed in lung tissue from many smokers. In patients with clinical chronic obstructive pulmonary disease, physiologic obstruction and severity of clinical disease appear to correlate with the severity of histologic bronchiolitis.

Membranous (terminal) bronchiolitis may be seen in occasional membranous bronchioles of smokers or may be more extensive and accompanied by other smoking-related changes, including emphysema, respiratory bronchiolitis, and/or desquamative interstitial pneumonia. The histopathologic changes of membranous (terminal) bronchiolitis include lymphocytic infiltrates of the bronchiolar wall, smooth muscle hyperplasia, adventitial fibrosis, and hyperplasia and metaplasia of bronchiolar epithelium. Goblet cell metaplasia of the membranous bronchiolar epithelium (normally goblet cells are not found in the bronchiolar epithelium) may be accompanied by mucus plugs. Macrophages containing finely granular brown pigment (smoker's pigment), such as those seen in respiratory bronchiolitis and desquamative interstitial pneumonia, are often seen in the lumens of the membranous bronchioles, as well as in the lumens of adjacent respiratory bronchioles, alveolar ducts, and alveoli. Histiocytes containing the same finely granular brown pigment and/or macrophages containing coarse black anthracotic pigment may also be seen in the fibrotic walls of membranous bronchioles.

Histologic Features:

- Lesions may be seen involving occasional membranous bronchioles of smokers or may be more extensive and accompanied by respiratory bronchiolitis or other smoking-related changes such as emphysema and/or desquamative interstitial pneumonia.
- Collections of macrophages containing a finely granular brown cytoplasmic pigment within lumens of membranous bronchioles and often in lumens of respiratory bronchioles, alveolar ducts, and alveoli.
- Infiltrates of lymphocytes and/or histiocytes in the bronchiolar wall, smooth muscle hyperplasia, adventitial fibrosis, and/or hyperplasia or metaplasia of the bronchiolar epithelium.
- Histiocytes in the bronchiolar wall may contain coarse black anthracotic pigment or the same finely granular brown cytoplasmic pigment as the intraluminal macrophages.
- Mucus plugs may accompany goblet cell metaplasia of the bronchiolar epithelium.

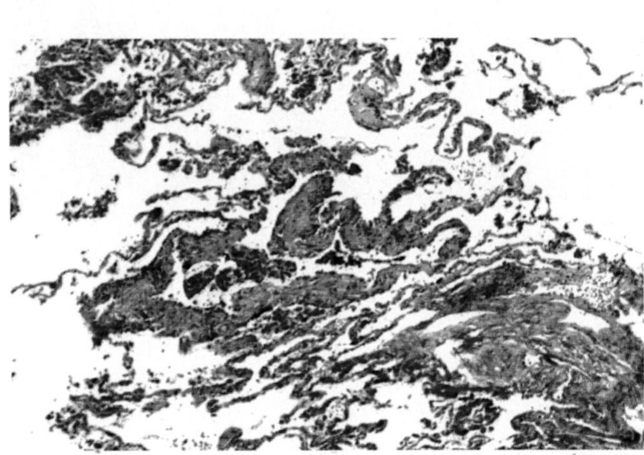

Figure 78.1 At low power, aggregates of macrophages containing finely granular brown pigment can be seen in the bronchiolar lumen and in adjacent airspaces in a tobacco smoker.

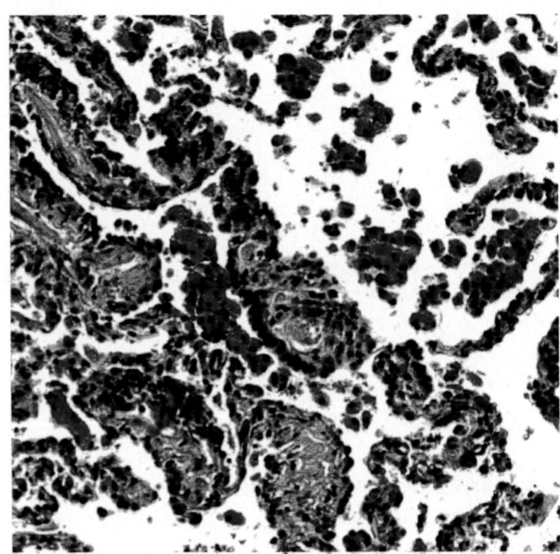

Figure 78.2 Higher power shows macrophages containing finely granular brown pigment in the lumen of a bronchiole and in adjacent alveolar spaces.

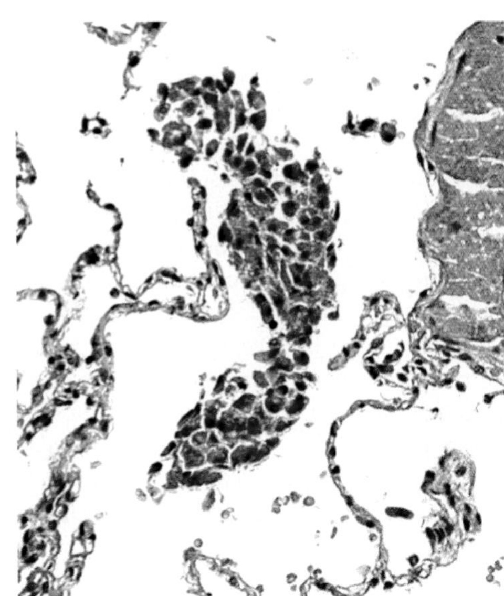

Figure 78.3 Macrophages containing finely granular brown pigment fill the lumen of an alveolar duct in a tobacco smoker.

Respiratory Bronchiolitis

79

▸ Philip T. Cagle

Lesions of respiratory bronchiolitis may be observed involving occasional respiratory bronchioles in lung specimens from cigarette smokers unaccompanied by clinically significant findings. Less frequently, respiratory bronchiolitis may be more extensive and accompanied by clinical and morphologic changes called *respiratory bronchiolitis-associated interstitial lung disease* (see Chapter 80). Respiratory bronchiolitis consists of collections of lightly pigmented macrophages within the lumens of respiratory bronchioles. The cytoplasm of the macrophages contains finely granular particles that are brown on hematoxylin and eosin and stain faintly with iron stain. This material has been referred to as *smoker's pigment.* Collections of similar pigmented macrophages are typically found in the lumens of adjacent alveolar ducts and alveoli and may be seen in the lumens of membranous (terminal) bronchioles as well. The walls of the bronchioles exhibit variable infiltrates of lymphocytes and histiocytes containing the same finely granular pigment as the macrophages and/or coarse black anthracotic pigment. Variable peribronchiolar fibrosis may also be present involving the bronchiolar walls and first tiers of adjacent alveolar septa. The fibrotic alveolar septa may exhibit type 2 pneumocyte hyperplasia or metaplastic bronchiolar epithelium (lambertosis). In some individuals, the respiratory bronchiolitis may be extensive or severe enough to result clinically in diffuse interstitial lung disease called *respiratory bronchiolitis-associated interstitial lung disease* (see Chapter 80).

Histologic Features:

- Lesions may be seen involving occasional respiratory bronchioles of smokers or may be more extensive and accompanied by clinical changes called *respiratory bronchiolitis-associated interstitial lung disease.*
- Collections of macrophages containing a finely granular brown cytoplasmic pigment within lumens of respiratory bronchioles and adjacent alveolar ducts and alveoli; collections of pigmented macrophages may also be seen in lumens of adjacent membranous (terminal) bronchioles.
- Infiltrates of lymphocytes and/or histiocytes in the bronchiolar wall; the histiocytes may contain coarse black anthracotic pigment and/or the same finely granular brown cytoplasmic pigment as the macrophages.
- Minimal to mild fibrosis in the bronchiolar wall and first tiers of adjacent alveolar septa, which may be lined by hyperplastic type 2 pneumocytes or metaplastic bronchiolar epithelium (lambertosis).

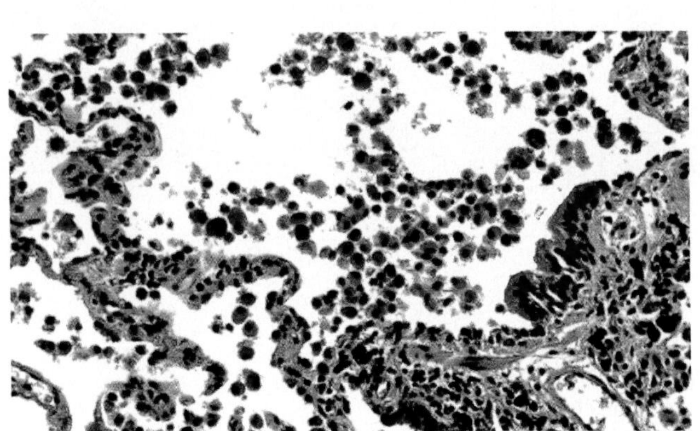

Figure 79.1 Macrophages containing finely granular brown pigment fill the lumen of a respiratory bronchiole and adjacent alveolar spaces in a tobacco smoker.

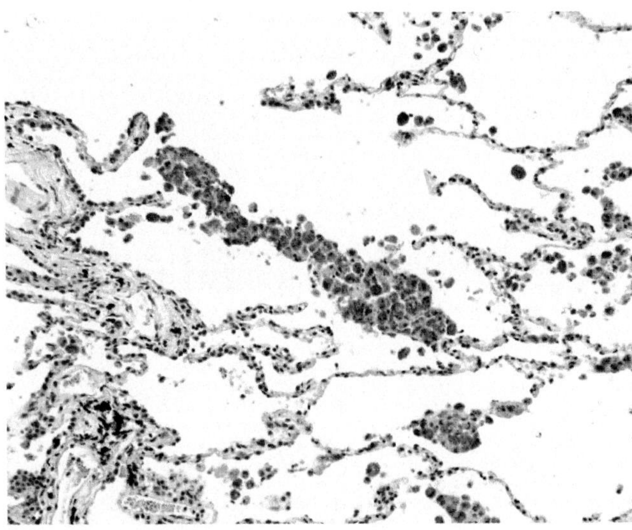

Figure 79.2 Alveolar duct contains aggregate of macrophages with cytoplasmic finely granular brown pigment within its lumen in a tobacco smoker.

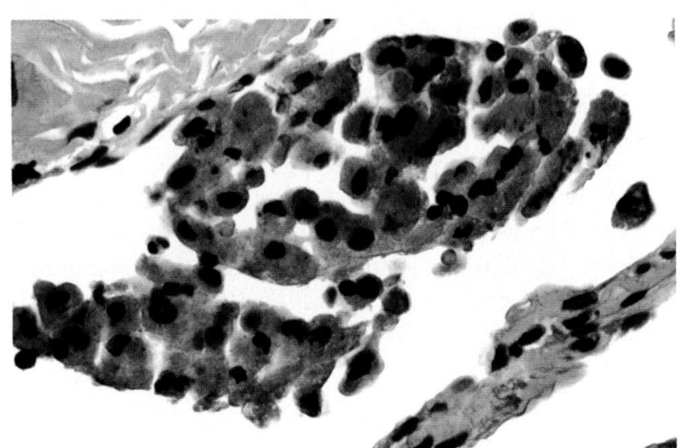

Figure 79.3 High power shows characteristic macrophages of respiratory bronchiolitis containing finely granular brown pigment within their cytoplasm.

Respiratory Bronchiolitis-Associated Interstitial Lung Disease/Desquamative Interstitial Pneumonia

80

▸ Philip T. Cagle

Respiratory bronchiolitis may uncommonly be associated with a generally mild and generally nonprogressive interstitial lung disease characterized by dyspnea, cough, and radiographic abnormalities referred to as *respiratory bronchiolitis-associated interstitial lung disease* (RBILD). The histopathologic findings of respiratory bronchiolitis are discussed in Chapter 79. In desquamative interstitial pneumonia (DIP), the alveolar spaces are filled with collections of macrophages containing the same finely granular brown cytoplasmic pigment seen in respiratory bronchiolitis and RBILD. Like respiratory bronchiolitis and RBILD, DIP occurs primarily in smokers. The primary difference between DIP and RBILD is that in DIP the alveolar spaces, alveolar ducts, and respiratory bronchioles are much more diffusely and uniformly involved, whereas in RBILD the lesions are patchy and bronchiolocentric. It seems likely that respiratory bronchiolitis and RBILD are less extensive forms of DIP, either mild forms of the same disease or "precursor" lesions, and increasingly these entities are considered together. Histopathologically, a spectrum of varying degrees of lung involvement between patchy airway-centered respiratory bronchiolitis and diffusely distributed DIP can be observed in different cases.

In DIP the diffuse filling of alveoli, alveolar ducts, and respiratory bronchioles with pigmented macrophages is accompanied by a relatively uniform thickening of alveolar septa by lymphocytes with lesser numbers of plasma cells and occasionally eosinophils. The thickened alveolar septa are lined by prominent cuboidal type 2 pneumocytes.

When originally described, consideration was given to the possibility that the pigmented macrophages in DIP might be pneumocytes shed into the alveolar spaces, although the correct interpretation that these were macrophages was given preference. Focal DIP-like histopathologic patterns and collections of intraalveolar macrophages are seen adjacent to lung fibrosis and lung nodules of many types, including focal scars, cancers, Langerhans cell histiocytosis, and usual interstitial pneumonia (UIP) (see Chapter 75). Respiratory bronchiolitis and focal DIP-like areas are relatively common in lung tissue from smokers. Therefore, diagnosis of RBILD and DIP should take into account limitations of biopsy sampling and clinical context. The frequent association of focal DIP-like macrophage aggregates in and around areas of UIP probably contributed to earlier speculation that DIP progresses to UIP, a concept that has not been supported by studies over the past decade.

Histologic Features:

- In RBILD and DIP, the respiratory bronchioles, alveolar ducts, and/or alveolar spaces contain collections of macrophages containing finely granular brown cytoplasmic pigment.
- In DIP the alveolar spaces, alveolar ducts, and respiratory bronchioles are much more diffusely and uniformly involved, whereas in RBILD the lesions are patchy and bronchiolocentric.
- In DIP the alveolar septa are relatively uniformly thickened by lymphocytes with lesser numbers of plasma cells and occasionally eosinophils and are lined by prominent cuboidal-type 2 pneumocytes.
- Lungs from smokers may show varying extents of involvement by collections of pigmented macrophages and interstitial pneumonia within a spectrum from RBILD to DIP.

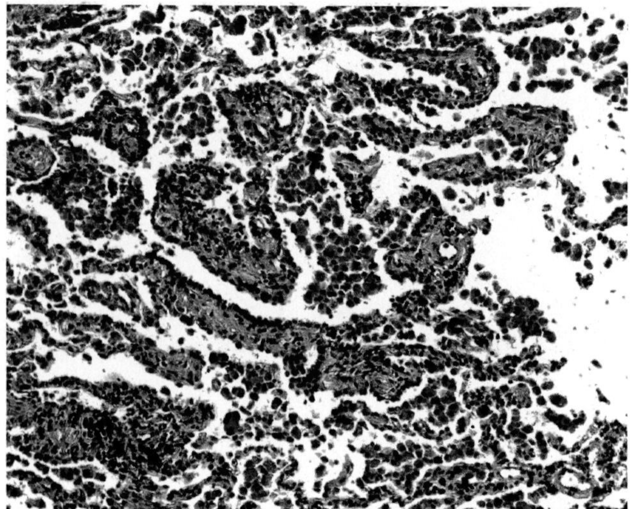

Figure 80.1 Low power of RBILD shows mild fibrosis of a respiratory bronchiole and collections of pigmented macrophages in the bronchiolar lumen and surrounding alveolar spaces.

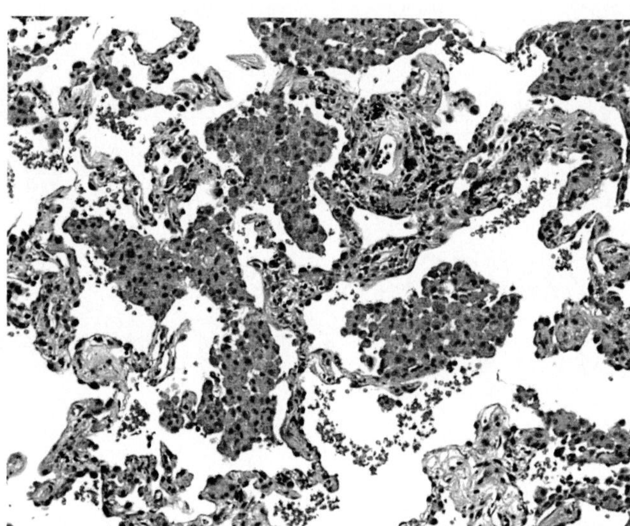

Figure 80.2 Patchy collections of pigmented macrophages are present in alveolar spaces associated with mild interstitial pneumonia and reactive type 2 pneumocytes in the lungs of smokers, apparently signifying a spectrum from RBILD to DIP.

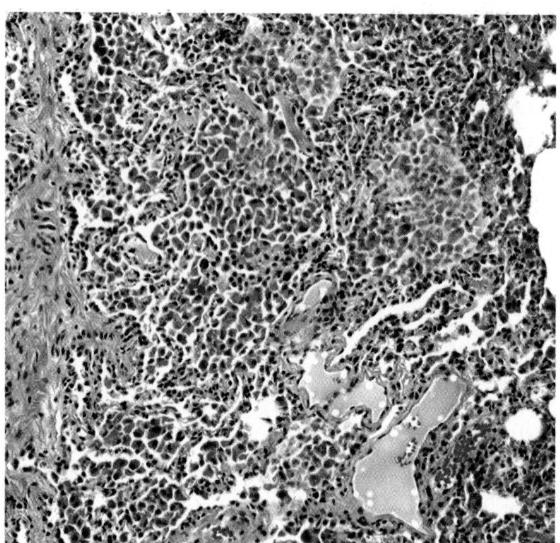

Figure 80.3 Low power of DIP shows collections of pigmented macrophages filling alveolar spaces with mild interstitial fibrosis and lymphocytic infiltrates in the alveolar septa.

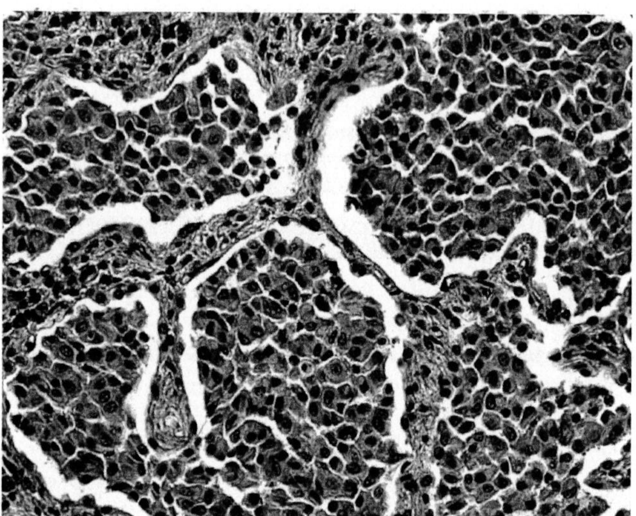

Figure 80.4 Medium power shows collections of pigmented macrophages filling alveolar spaces and mild fibrosis of alveolar septa in DIP.

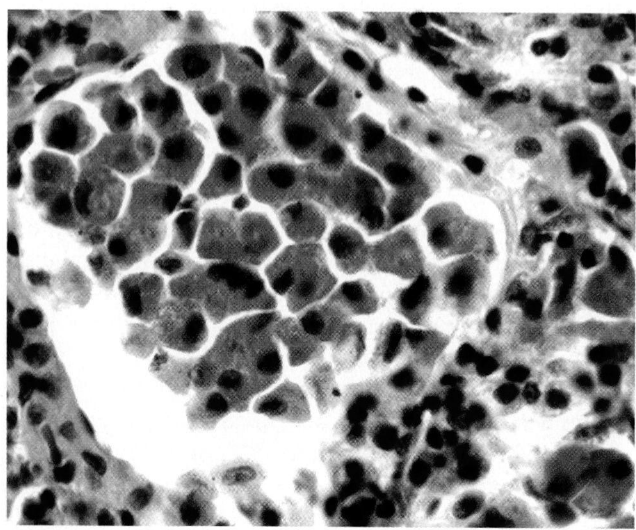

Figure 80.5 Higher power of DIP shows the finely granular brown pigment in the cytoplasm of macrophages that is observed in respiratory bronchiolitis, RBILD, and DIP.

Section 15

Diffuse Interstitial Lung Diseases

81 Infectious Interstitial Pneumonias

▸ Abida Haque

Interstitial pneumonia is most often the result of viral infection. Several viruses produce this pattern, in addition to causing airway inflammation and necrosis, and in severe cases result in diffuse alveolar damage. The overall pattern of injury and the presence of characteristic viral inclusions often provide clues to the etiologic agent in most cases. The most common viruses that produce interstitial inflammation are influenza and parainfluenza virus, measles, respiratory syncytial virus, *Cytomegalovirus,* herpes simplex virus, and adenovirus. Chronic Epstein-Barr virus also produces an interstitial pneumonia. Other less common causes include congenital listeriosis, toxoplasmosis, rubella, and congenital varicella zoster infection.

Histologic Features:

- Alveolar septa are infiltrated with mononuclear cells, predominantly lymphocytes, macrophages, and plasma cells.
- Mild edema and capillary congestion may also be present.
- The small airways may have mononuclear infiltrates in the walls and may show hyperplasia of the bronchus-associated lymphoid tissue.
- Presence of viral inclusions can provide clues to the etiology of the interstitial infection.
- If there are no inclusions, use of immunoperoxidase stains or immunofluorescence is often helpful to identify the virus.

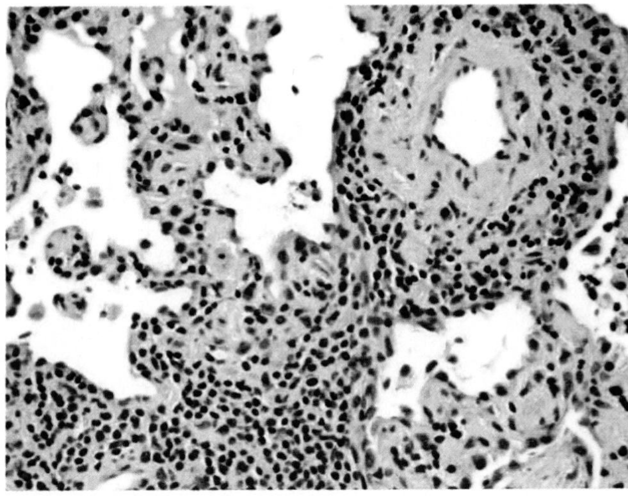

Figure 81.1 Expansion of the alveolar septa with inflammatory cell infiltrate and hyperplastic lymphoid nodules in a patient with chronic Epstein-Barr virus infection.

Hypersensitivity Pneumonitis

82

Roberto Barrios

Hypersensitivity pneumonitis, also known as *hypersensitivity pneumonia* and *extrinsic allergic alveolitis,* is a diffuse interstitial granulomatous pneumonia secondary to inhalation of organic antigens. Other synonyms used for this disease represent the causative antigen, and terms such as *farmer's lung, bagassosis, bird fancier's lung,* and *pigeon breeder's disease* have been used. Hypersensitivity pneumonitis most likely represents a combination of an immune complex-mediated (type III) and T-cell–mediated, delayed (type IV) immunologic mechanisms. In advanced lesions, a picture of nonspecific interstitial pneumonia (NSIP) fibrotic pattern or of end-stage fibrosis may be found. Differential diagnosis includes sarcoidosis, NSIP, usual interstitial pneumonia, lymphoid interstitial pneumonia, and infections. The granulomas seen in hypersensitivity pneumonitis are loose and "poorly formed" and consist of aggregates of lymphocytes, plasma cells, and occasional multinucleated cells. They are usually bronchiolocentric and show extension into adjacent alveolar septa. In contrast, the sarcoidal granuloma is well developed and usually well circumscribed and tends to follow the lymphatic routes (pleura, interlobular septa, and bronchovascular bundles).

Lymphoid interstitial pneumonia is a rare entity characterized by a much more prominent interstitial lymphoid infiltrate than hypersensitivity pneumonia, but sometimes the differential diagnosis between these entities is difficult and history of exposure should be correlated. The cellular pattern of NSIP resembles the changes seen in hypersensitivity pneumonitis, and it is well recognized that some cases diagnosed as NSIP are found to be hypersensitivity pneumonitis. The presence of granulomas and an exposure history help distinguish between the two conditions. The final diagnosis depends on good clinical, radiologic, and histopathologic correlation.

Histologic Features:

- The acute phase is not well characterized; a neutrophilic infiltrate in the alveoli and respiratory bronchioles (acute bronchiolitis) and a pattern of diffuse alveolar damage has been reported.
- The chronic phase is characterized by the triad of: interstitial pneumonitis predominantly around airways (including a "cellular bronchiolitis"), noncaseating "poorly formed" granulomas (75% of cases), and intraluminal budding fibrosis or organizing pneumonia.
- Small foci of organizing pneumonia, bronchiolitis, and scant or absent eosinophils may also be present.

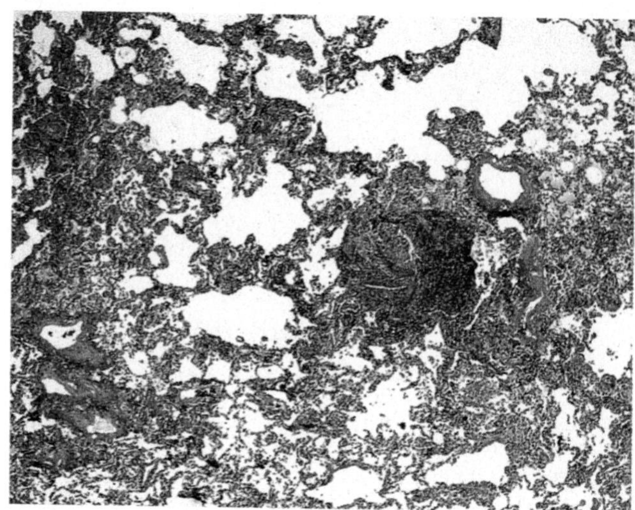

Figure 82.1 Low power shows a bronchiolocentric interstitial lymphoplasmacytic infiltrate with no significant fibrosis.

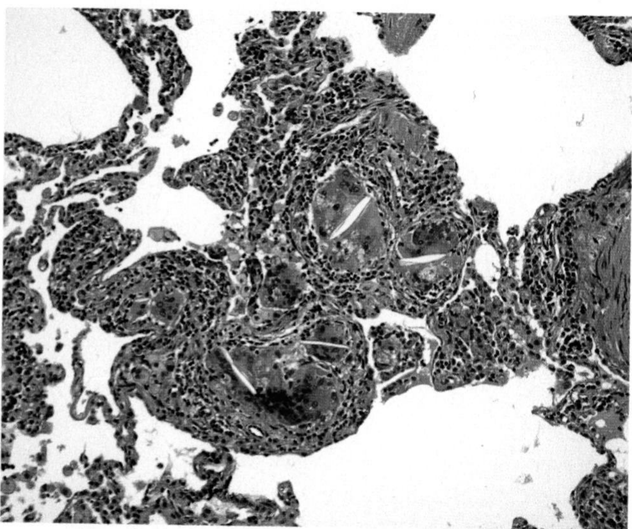

Figure 82.2 Higher power shows a "loose" poorly defined granuloma. Cholesterol clefts are associated with multinucleated giant cells.

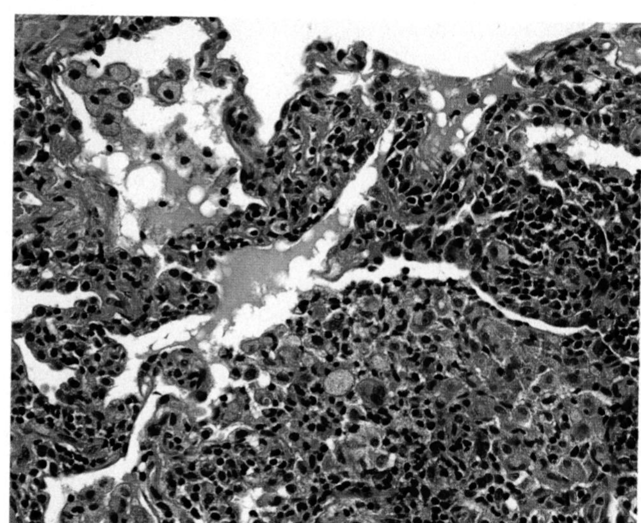

Figure 82.3 Focus of intraalveolar foamy macrophages, which occasionally form small foci of endogenous lipoid pneumonia.

83

Hot Tub Lung

▶ Andras Khoor

Hot tub lung is a diffuse granulomatous interstitial lung disease that develops in immunocompetent individuals caused by inhalation of aerosolized nontuberculous mycobacteria (usually *Mycobacterium avium* complex), which can occur if a contaminated hot tub is used. It may represent hypersensitivity reaction, infection, or both. Diagnostic criteria include detection of nontuberculous mycobacteria in sputum, bronchoalveolar lavage, or lung biopsy specimen, usually by cultures.

Histologic Features:

- Well-formed nonnecrotizing granulomas are present in every case; the granulomas are better formed than those seen in typical cases of hypersensitivity pneumonia.
- Necrotizing granulomas occur rarely.
- The granulomas show random or, less often, bronchiolocentric distribution.
- Organizing pneumonia pattern or patchy chronic interstitial pneumonia may be seen.
- Acid-fast bacilli are rarely detected by special stains.

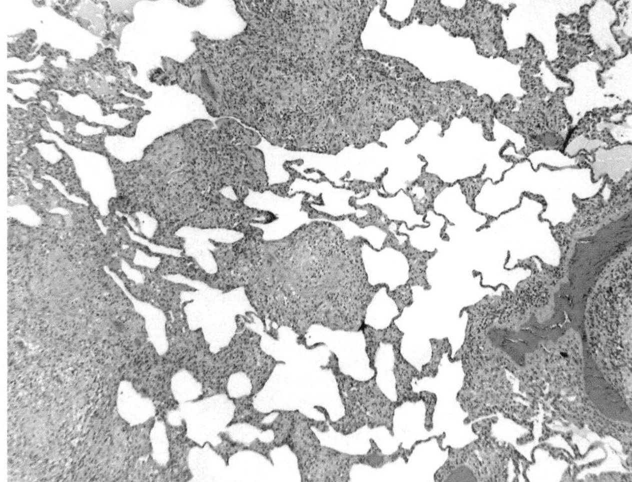

Figure 83.1 Low power shows randomly distributed granulomas.

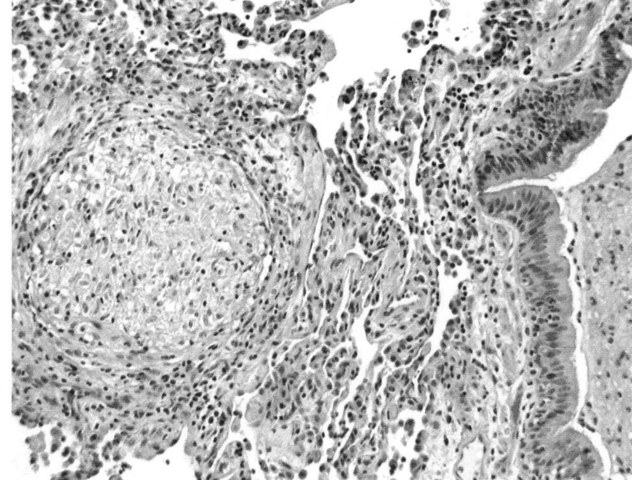

Figure 83.2 Medium power shows a bronchiolocentric granuloma.

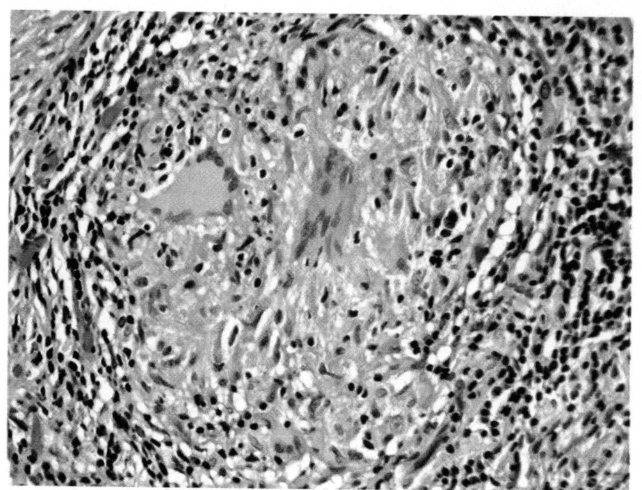

Figure 83.3 High power shows a well-formed nonnecrotizing granuloma.

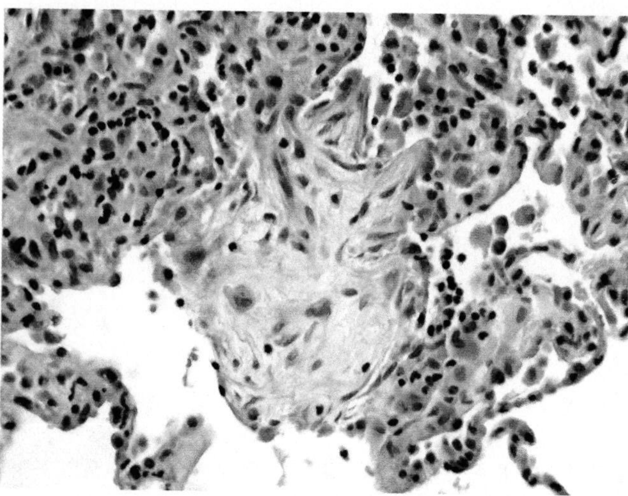

Figure 83.4 High power shows focal organizing pneumonia pattern.

84

Flock Lung

▸ Armando Fraire

Flocking is a widely used industrial process in which short segments of nylon or similar synthetic fibers are applied to backing fabric materials to produce plush material. Flock lung refers to a clinicopathologic syndrome that can be observed in workers in the flocking industry who are exposed to respirable microfibers. Clinically, the process closely resembles a hypersensitivity pneumonitis. Pathologically, the process also mimics hypersensitivity pneumonitis, but other lung injury patterns such as bronchiolitis obliterans organizing pneumonia and nonspecific interstitial pneumonitis may be present.

Histologic Features:

- Peribronchiolar lymphocytic interstitial inflammation.
- Peribronchial or parenchymal lymphoid hyperplasia.
- Bronchiolar mural lymphocytic infiltration.
- Peribronchiolar accumulation of alveolar macrophages.
- Focal organizing pneumonia.
- Absence of granulomas.

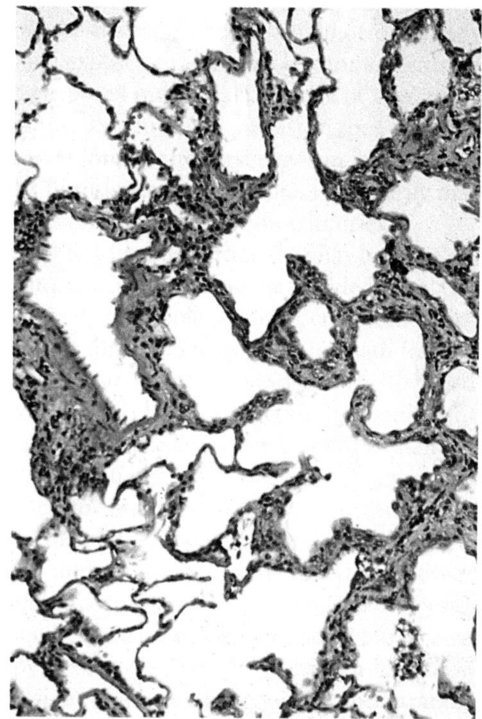

Figure 84.1 Low power shows nonspecific interstitial pneumonitis pattern.

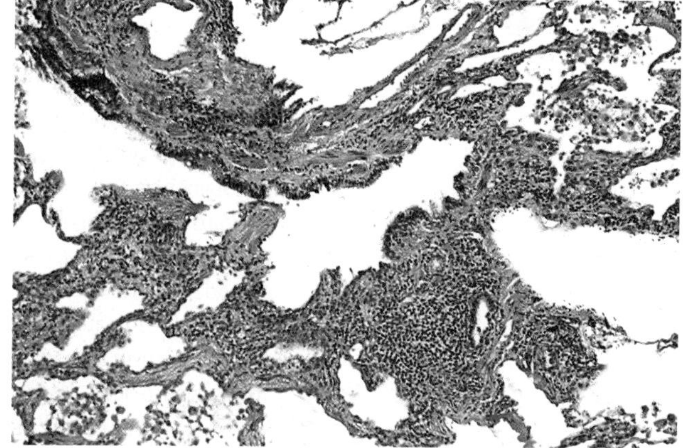

Figure 84.2 Low power shows mural bronchiolar lymphocytic infiltration.

It is important to distinguish between history of exposure to asbestos and asbestosis. By themselves, asbestos bodies or asbestos fibers indicate exposure but do not indicate whether a person has the disease asbestosis, which requires evaluation of the lung tissue for characteristic fibrosis in addition to asbestos exposure. Asbestos bodies may be observed in lung tissue of occupationally exposed individuals who do not have any resulting fibrosis. Studies have also shown that virtually all individuals in the general population who have not had occupational exposure have asbestos fibers and bodies in their lungs that they have inhaled from the background levels of asbestos present in the ambient air, primarily in urban environments. Therefore, it is possible to observe asbestos bodies in any person in the general population who has not had occupational or bystander exposure to asbestos, but, if observed, these bodies would not be in quantities sufficient to produce asbestosis. In actual practice, it is uncommon to come across asbestos bodies in routine tissue sections or cytology specimens from persons without some exposure to asbestos above background levels.

Asbestosis is a specific type of fibrosis related to asbestos exposure and begins in the first tiers of alveolar septa in respiratory bronchioles (see Chapter 67). Asbestosis may progress and the amount of interstitial fibrosis increase until there is end-stage honeycomb lung. The radiologic and gross distribution of asbestosis mimics that of usual interstitial pneumonia in that it is worse in the lower lung zones and periphery. Therefore, the clinical and radiologic presentation of asbestosis may mimic other interstitial lung diseases and *vice versa.* Gross examination of lungs from autopsies of patients with asbestosis reveals fibrosis and honeycombing that is more severe in the lower zones and peripheral lung parenchyma.

Although asbestosis may be accompanied by pleural changes, including pleural plaques and pleural thickening, these pleural changes can also be present without parenchymal fibrosis; therefore, they should not be called asbestosis. The term *asbestosis* should be reserved only for the parenchymal disease.

Cytologic Features:

- Asbestos fibers may be found in sputum and lavage specimens of persons with asbestos exposure, with or without asbestosis (asbestosis cannot be diagnosed from cytology specimens).
- The asbestos fiber is clear on Papanicolaou stain, but its iron-containing proteinaceous coat stains golden yellow to brown.
- Occasionally asbestos bodies may be partially encased by macrophages.

Histologic Features:

- Diagnosis of asbestosis requires (i) a characteristic pattern of diffuse interstitial fibrosis, as discussed later, and (ii) the presence of asbestos bodies, as discussed later.
- Interstitial fibrosis in asbestosis consists of mature collagen from the chronic course of the disease; young fibrosis consisting of granulation tissue (such as that seen with organizing pneumonia or organizing diffuse alveolar damage) is not asbestosis.
- Interstitial fibrosis of asbestosis generally begins around the respiratory bronchioles where the earliest or minimal changes is fibrosis of the first tier(s) of alveolar septa of the respiratory bronchioles; this should be distinguished from respiratory bronchiolitis caused by smoking or other etiologies.
- Fibrosis of asbestosis may progress to involve more alveolar septa between bronchioles and eventually progress to end-stage honeycomb lung.
- The severity of asbestosis is worse in the lower lung zones and at the peripheries; fibrosis that is worse in the upper lung zones, that is focal, or that is not bilateral does not fulfill criteria of asbestosis.

- Limited biopsies such as transbronchial biopsies or needle biopsies do not permit evaluation of enough lung tissue to exclude or confirm a diagnosis of asbestosis; peribronchiolar fibrosis may not be sampled and focal scars cannot be ruled out; a wedge biopsy is required as a minimum to evaluate for asbestosis.
- In addition to a characteristic pattern of fibrosis, a minimum of two asbestos bodies is required to diagnose asbestosis (this rule is used to eliminate the chance of occasionally finding an asbestos body in persons without sufficient asbestos exposure as the cause of any observed fibrosis); generally, as the observed severity of the fibrosis of asbestosis increases, the number of asbestos bodies observed in the tissue sections increases.
- There may be ancillary changes associated with asbestosis, such as multinucleated giant cells (which may contain asbestos bodies), presence of blue bodies, pseudo-desquamative interstitial pneumonia reaction to the fibrosis and superimposed infections, tobacco-related changes, or mixed dust pneumoconioses; confirmation or exclusion of asbestosis requires careful evaluation of at least a wedge biopsy of lung tissue.
- Asbestos bodies, by themselves, are only markers of asbestos exposure and do not represent the interstitial lung disease asbestosis unless the characteristic interstitial fibrosis is also present.
- Pleural plaques due to asbestos exposure by themselves are only markers of asbestos exposure and do not represent the interstitial lung disease asbestosis; unlike asbestos bodies, pleural plaques are not required for a diagnosis of asbestosis.

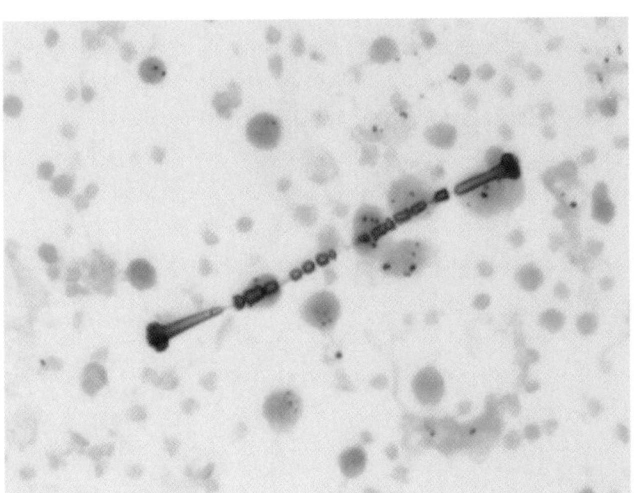

Figure 85.1 Papanicolaou stain of a bronchoalveolar lavage shows an asbestos body with a clear fibrous core coated with golden brown iron forming a barbell-shaped structure.

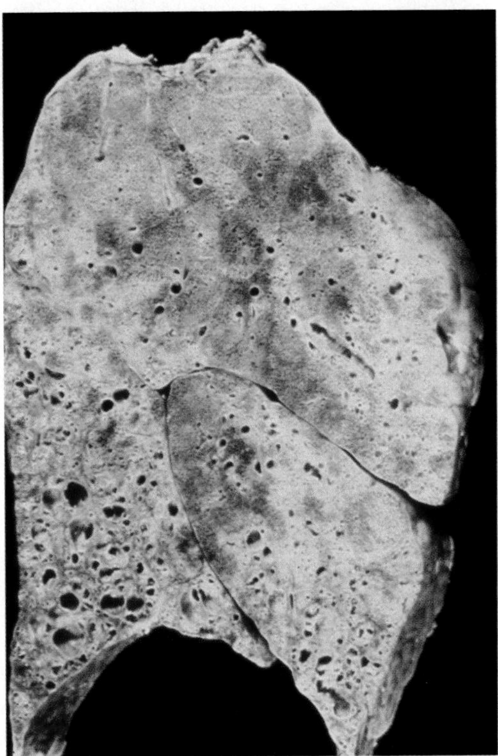

Figure 85.2 Gross lung figure from autopsy of patient with severe asbestosis shows peripheral fibrosis and end-stage honeycomb lung in the lower zones.

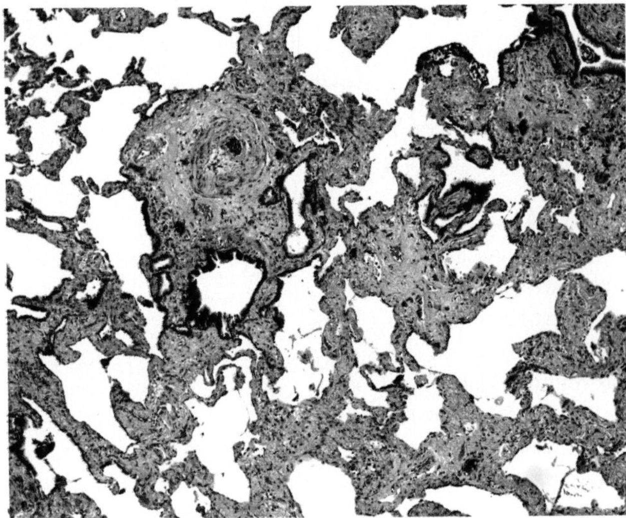

Figure 85.3 Asbestosis shows mature interstitial fibrosis of the alveolar septa.

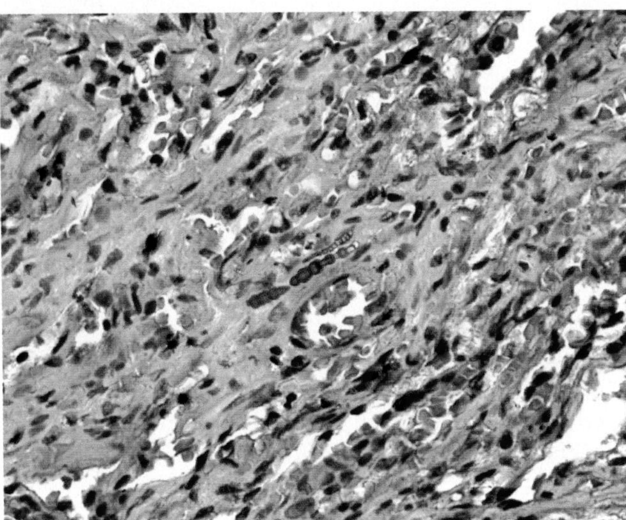

Figure 85.4 Interstitial scarring of asbestosis with asbestos bodies in the mature collagen. They are composed of clear cores coated with refractile golden brown beads of iron.

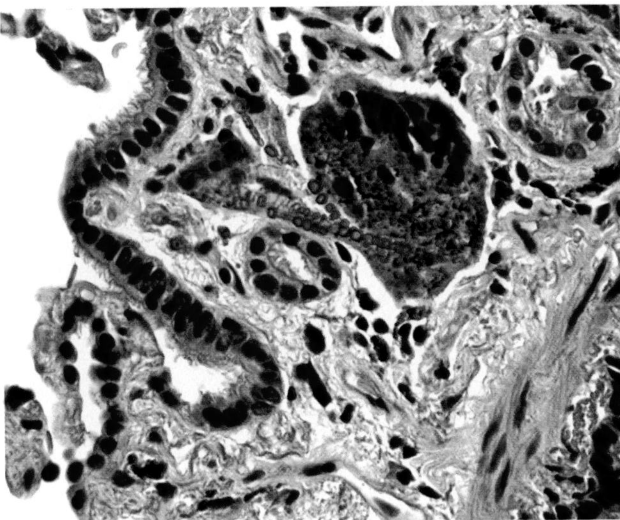

Figure 85.5 Submucosal multinucleated giant cell partially engulfing asbestos bodies with clear cores coated with refractile golden brown beads of iron.

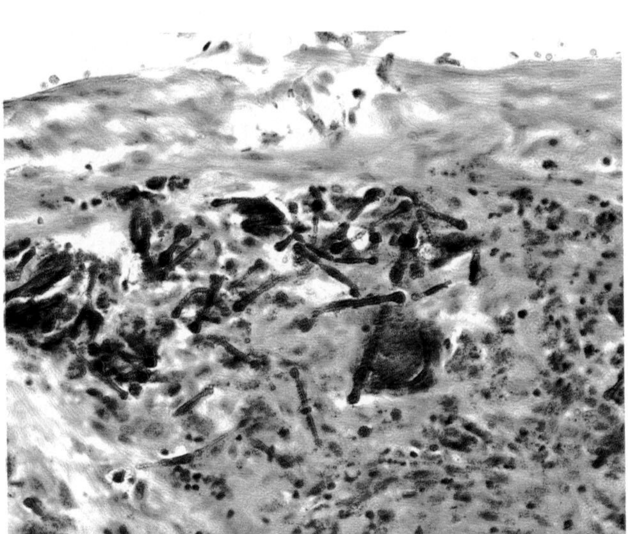

Figure 85.6 Large numbers of golden brown barbell-shaped asbestos bodies are within a large interstitial scar of severe asbestosis.

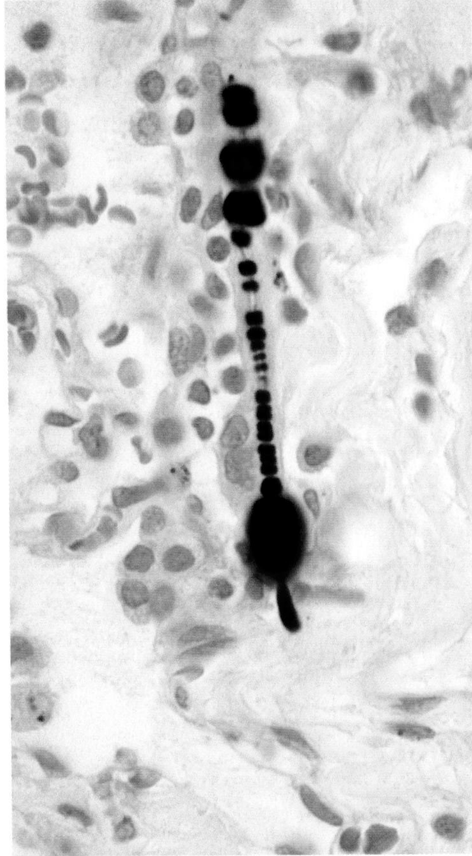

Figure 85.7 Iron stain stains the beaded iron coat of an asbestos body bright blue around a clear asbestos fiber core, highlighting the asbestos body against a pale pink background.

Part 2

Silicosis

▶ Alvaro C. Laga, Timothy Allen, and Philip T. Cagle

Silicosis is the pulmonary disease that results from exposure to large amounts of crystalline silica (quartz). High levels of silica exposure potentially occur in coal and other miners, sandblasters, glass manufacturers, quarry workers, and stone dressers. The lesions found in silicosis are referred to as *silicotic nodules.*

The classic nodular or chronic silicosis has a latency period averaging 20 to 40 years after initial exposure. Development and progression of silicosis may occur after cessation of exposure to silica. Rarely, accelerated silicosis may develop in 3 to 10 years. Acute silicosis is the result of a massive, overwhelming exposure and produces a pulmonary alveolar proteinosis (see Chapter 76).

In contrast to asbestosis, silicosis is more severe in the upper lung zones. The number and extent of silicotic nodules that can be observed range widely. Silicotic nodules may be found in the hilar lymph nodes without involvement of lung parenchyma, and this should not be called silicosis. It is not unusual to find an occasional small, clinically irrelevant silicotic nodule as an incidental finding in lung specimens. The presence of multiple silicotic nodules smaller than 1 cm in size is called *simple silicosis.* A minority of patients with simple silicosis progress to complicated silicosis or progressive massive fibrosis (PMF). PMF consists of silicotic nodules measuring greater than 1 cm in diameter, and there is confluence of silicotic nodules involving large areas of lung parenchyma. These large conglomerates of silicotic nodules may be cavitated. Patients with PMF may die of respiratory failure. In accelerated silicosis the silicotic nodules tend to be less well formed, and there is more accompanying interstitial fibrosis.

Grossly, the nodules are whorled, round, well-circumscribed, hard, slate gray, and sometimes calcified. Grossly, the visceral pleural nodules have been referred to as candle-wax lesions and consist of gray waxy nodules with an anthracotic rim.

Silica creates nodules in a lymphangitic distribution, including along the bronchovascular bundles, interlobular septa, and pleura, but nodules can be seen elsewhere in the lung parenchyma. Bronchial and hilar lymph nodes also often have similar nodules. Early nodules begin as collections of dust-laden macrophages typically containing anthracotic pigment mixed with minimal reticulin and collagen fibers. Gradually, the center of the nodule becomes increasingly more collagenized and fibrotic but retains the surrounding rim of dust-laden macrophages. Eventually, the nodule matures into a round to oval nodule composed primarily of whorls of hyalinized collagen with a peripheral rim of dust-laden macrophages. There may be so-called focal emphysema surrounding the silicotic nodule with fragmentation of the lung parenchyma adjacent to the fibrotic nodule.

In polarized light, silica particles are tiny 2-μm crystals that are typically only weakly birefringent. The silica particles are less conspicuous than the larger and more brightly birefringent silicate particles that often accompany them in the inhaled dust. It is important to distinguish silica particles as well from endogenous calcium oxalate crystals, "dirt" on the slide, or other endogenous or incidental particles that may be birefringent in polarized light (see Chapters 7, 8, and 9). In addition, tobacco smokers may have small collections of macrophages containing anthracotic pigment and birefringent particles that are a result of tobacco smoke and do not represent silicosis.

Patients with silicosis have an increased susceptibility to infection with Mycobacterium tuberculosis, atypical Mycobacteria, and fungus. Laboratory findings in simple silicosis include increased sedimentation rate, antinuclear antibodies, and immune complexes. Scleroderma has been found to be prevalent in silicotics.

Histologic Features:

- Early silicotic nodules consist of aggregates of dust-laden macrophages containing anthracotic pigment mixed with minimal reticulin and collagen fibers.
- With progression, collagen begins to accumulate centrally within the nodule.
- Mature silicotic nodules are characterized histologically by concentric, acellular, whorled bundles of dense hyalinized collagen with a rim of dust-laden macrophages.
- Calcification may be present, and variable amounts of anthracotic pigment may be present centrally or at the periphery.
- Parenchymal nodules may result in focal emphysema of the adjacent lung tissue.
- The nodules often occur in a subpleural location or in a perivascular or peribronchiolar location, but they may occur anywhere within the lung parenchyma; silicotic nodules also typically occur in the bronchial and hilar lymph nodes, where they show similar histologic features; silicotic nodules limited to the lymph nodes without parenchymal involvement should not be diagnosed as silicosis.
- Examination of sections under polarized light generally shows a mixture of very small weakly birefringent silica particles and larger more brightly birefringent silicate particles inhaled with the silica particles.

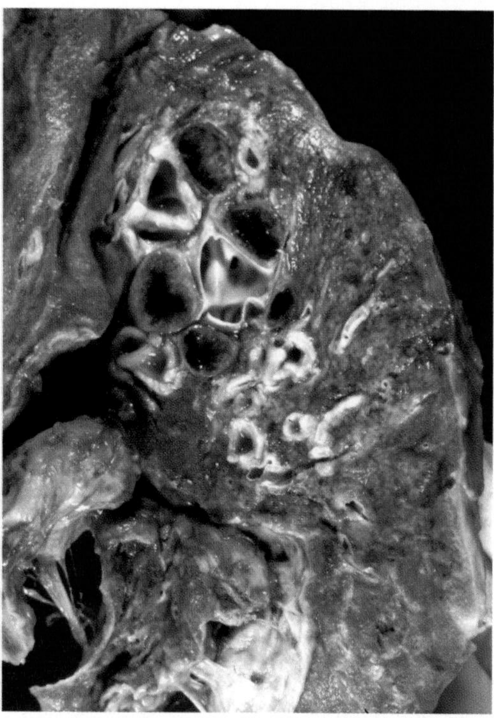

Figure 85.8 Gross figure of complicated silicosis or progressive massive fibrosis shows slate gray confluent nodules, predominantly in the upper lobe, with hilar node involvement.

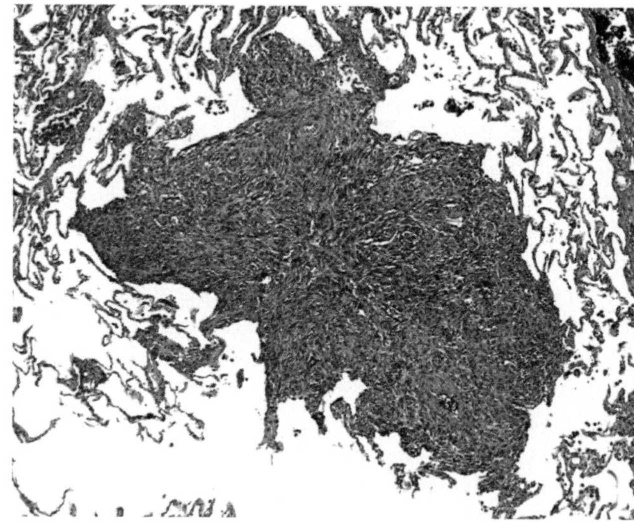

Figure 85.9 Early silicotic nodule in lung parenchyma consists of an aggregate of dust-laden macrophages with irregularly arranged collagen and focal emphysema of the adjacent alveolar septa.

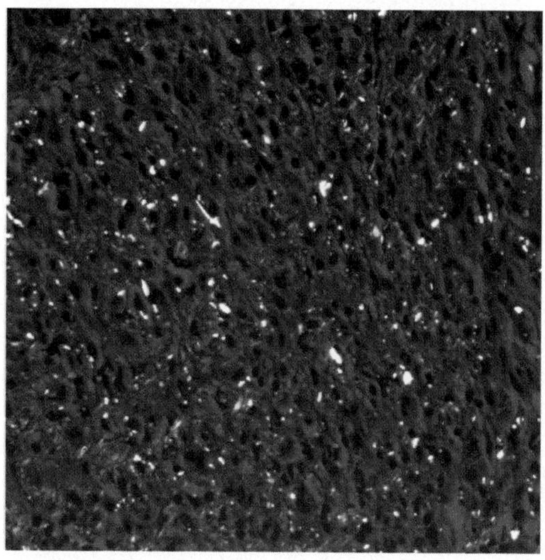

Figure 85.10 Polarized light examination of dust-laden macrophages in an early silicotic nodule shows abundant tiny, weakly birefringent silica particles mixed with larger brightly birefringent silicate particles.

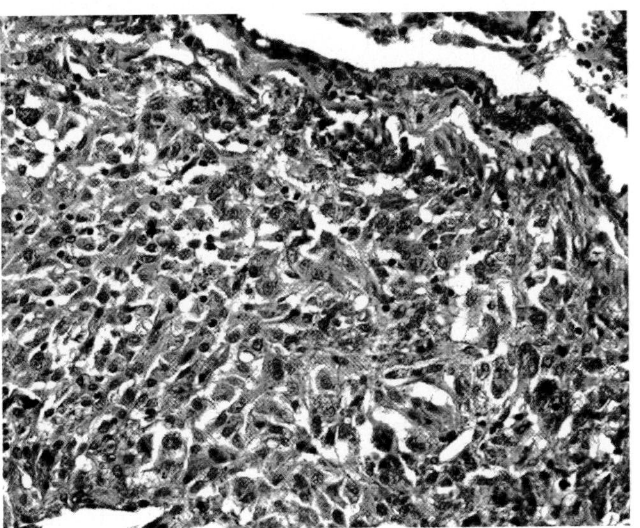

Figure 85.11 Early silicotic nodule beneath airway mucosa consists of an aggregate of dust-laden macrophages.

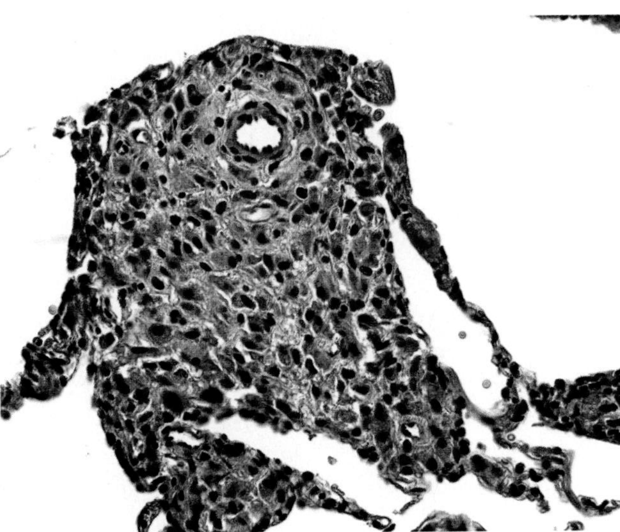

Figure 85.12 Early silicotic nodule in a perivascular location consists of aggregates of dust-laden macrophages and irregularly arranged collagen.

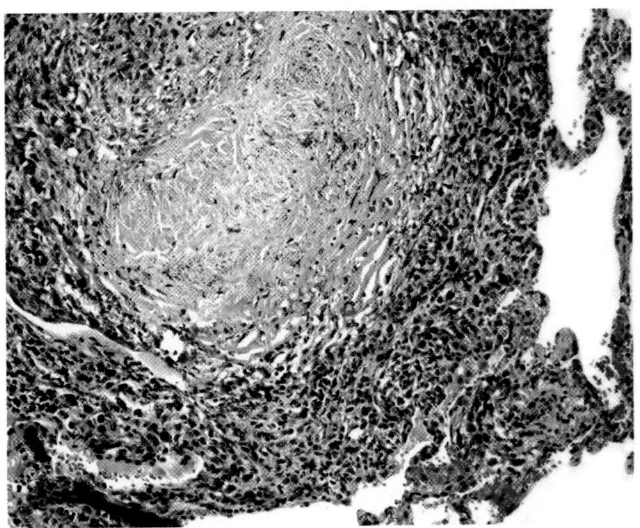

Figure 85.13 Maturing silicotic nodule exhibits central whorls of virtually acellular, hyalinized collagen and anthracotic pigment and peripheral dust-laden macrophages, many of which also contain anthracotic pigment.

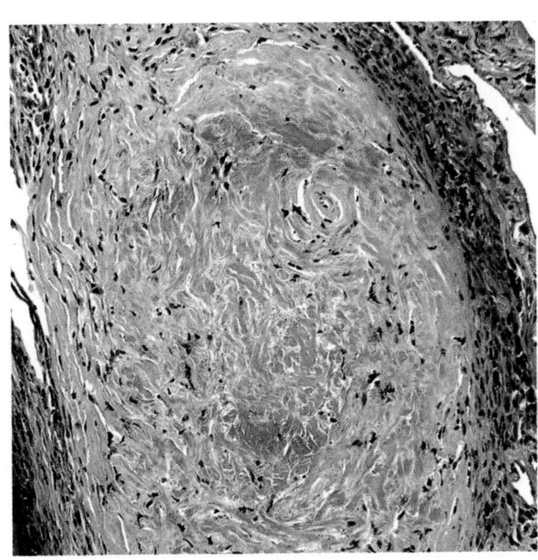

Figure 85.14 More advanced silicotic nodule shows mostly whorls of dense, virtually acellular, hyalinized collagen with a thin rim of dust-laden macrophages.

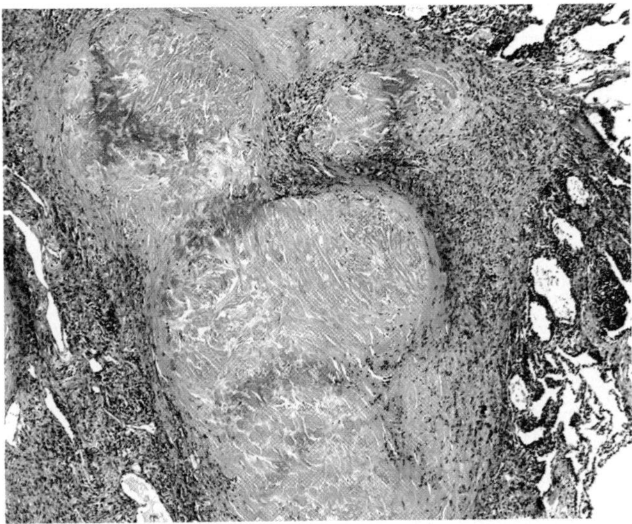

Figure 85.15 Multiple large confluent advanced silicotic nodules in complicated silicosis (progressive massive fibrosis).

Part 3

Silicatosis

▶ Alvaro C. Laga, Timothy Allen, and Philip T. Cagle

The nonasbestos silicates include talc, mica, kaolin, and clays. Individuals are exposed in mining, in foundries, and in the manufacturing of building materials, ceramics, cosmetics, and other products. Compared with asbestos or silica, pneumoconiosis caused by the nonasbestos silicates is relatively uncommon. Silicates may be contaminated with silica or asbestos in certain settings, and these contaminating materials are often responsible for greater contribution to the lung disease than the nonasbestos silicates in these circumstances (see Chapter 85, Part 4).

Silicates produce several types of lesions. (i) *Macules* are nonpalpable collections of dust-laden macrophages around respiratory bronchioles with minimal fibrosis. (ii) *Nodules* (2-10 mm) are hard fibrotic lesions containing dust, dust-laden macrophages and collagen. Nodules may have central hyalinized collagen probably reflecting silica contamination and reaction to the silica. Nodules may also contain multinucleated giant cells. Nodules are most prominent in the upper and mid lung zones. (iii) *Fibrosis* and *dust deposits* in the walls of terminal (membranous) bronchioles, respiratory bronchioles, and alveolar ducts is a type of mineral dust–induced small airway disease. (iv) *Foreign body granulomas* may occur. (v) *Interstitial fibrosis* consisting of interstitial pneumonia and fibrosis with abundant dust particles, and giant cells may be present. (vi) *Massive fibrosis* consisting of severe extensive fibrosis and numerous dust particles, probably arising from coalescence of numerous nodules, may be seen.

Histologic Features:

- Silicate macules consist of dust-laden macrophages associated with minimal fibrosis within the walls of respiratory bronchioles.
- Silicate nodules are composed of haphazardly arranged bundles of collagen interspersed with dust and dust-laden macrophages; they are predominantly found in the upper and mid lung zones.
- Nodules may have central hyalinization, probably as a result of silica contamination.
- Giant cells may be seen in silicate nodules.
- Mineral dust-induced small airway disease consists of fibrosis and dust deposits in the walls of terminal (membranous) bronchioles, respiratory bronchioles, and alveolar ducts.
- Silicates may produce interstitial fibrosis with fibrotic interstitial pneumonia in association with numerous dust particles and sometimes foreign body giant cells.
- Massive fibrosis consists of expansive fibrosis associated with copious dust deposits.
- Pleural thickening may be present.

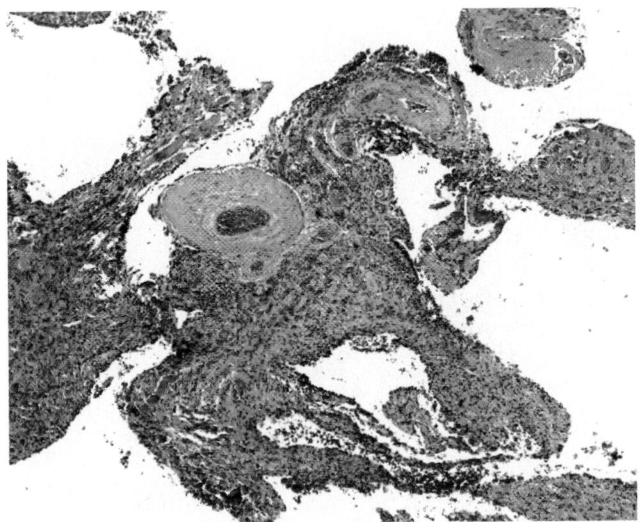

Figure 85.16 Kaolinosis shows fibrotic nodule and interstitial fibrosis with numerous dust-laden macrophages.

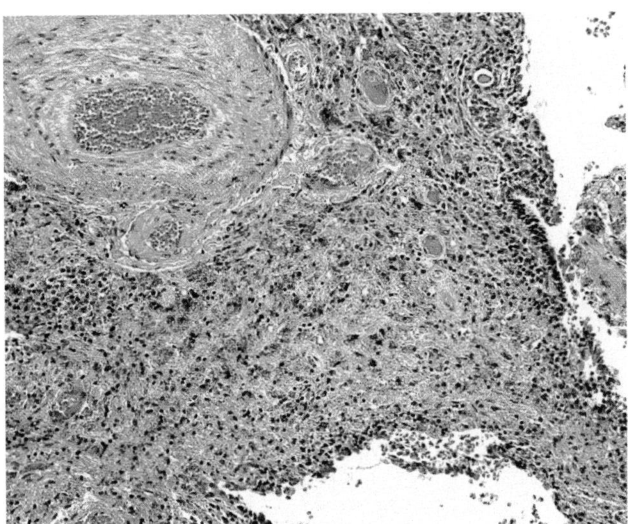

Figure 85.17 Perivascular nodule in kaolinosis consists of irregular collagen and multiple dust-laden macrophages.

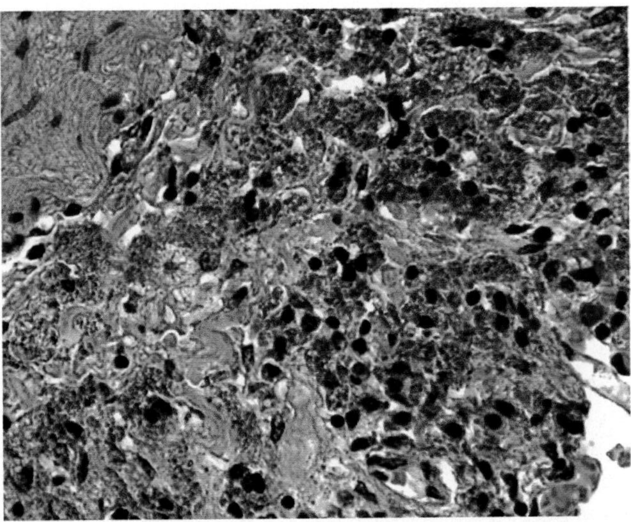

Figure 85.18 High power of dust-laden macrophages within kaolinosis nodule.

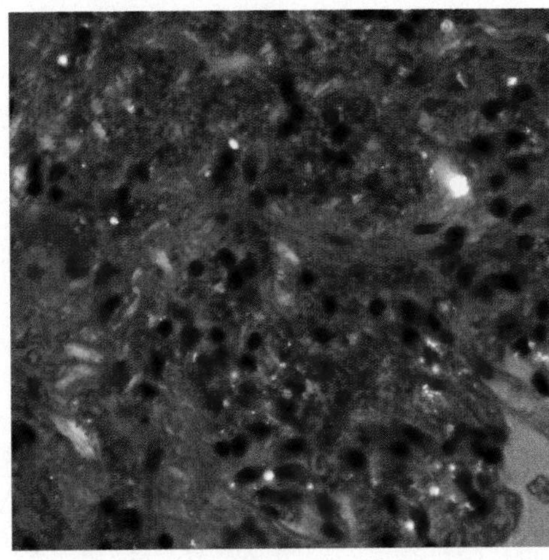

Figure 85.19 Polarization of kaolinosis nodule in Figure 85.18 shows brightly birefringent silicate particles.

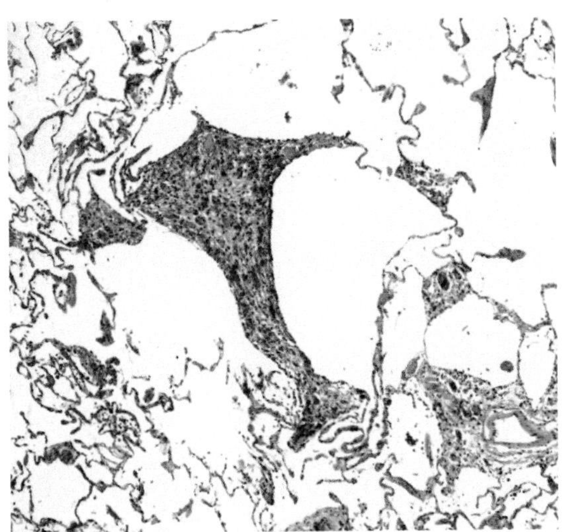

Figure 85.20 Talcosis shows fibrotic nodule containing dust-laden macrophages with focal emphysema of the adjacent lung parenchyma.

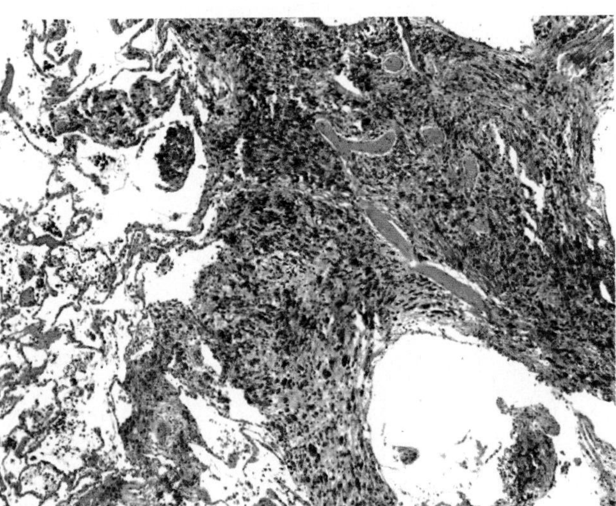

Figure 85.21 Talcosis shows fibrotic nodule and interstitial fibrosis with abundant dust-laden macrophages.

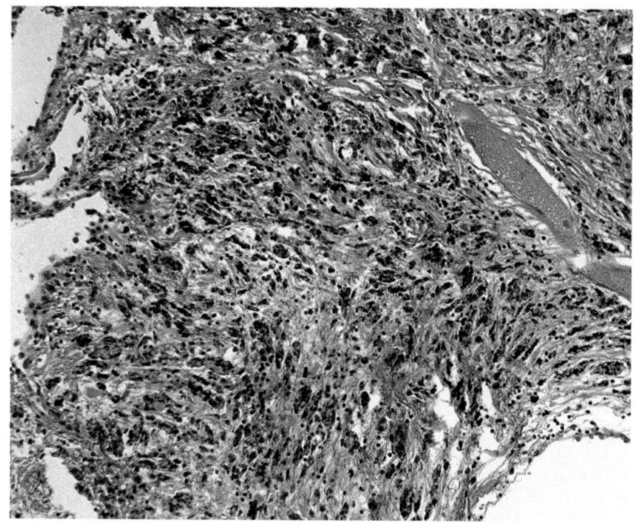

Figure 85.22 Talcosis nodule consists of irregular collagen interspersed dust-laden macrophages.

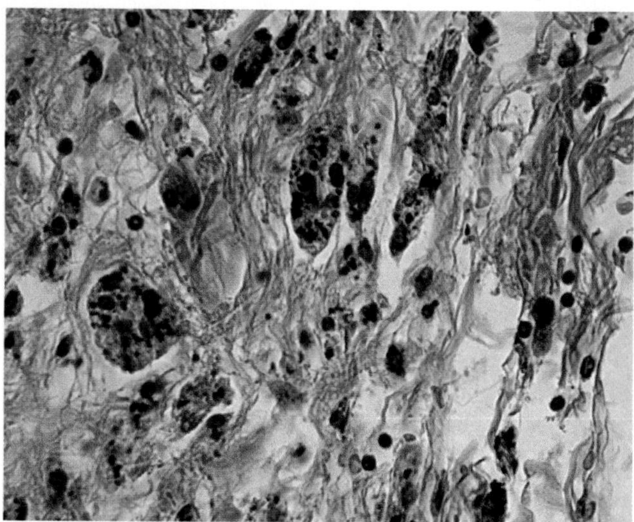

Figure 85.23 High power of dust-laden macrophages within talcosis nodule.

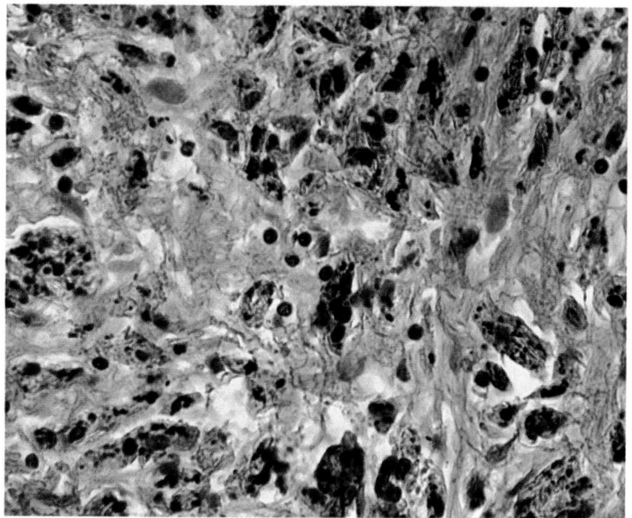

Figure 85.24 Macrophages contain dust particles within their cytoplasm in this talcosis nodule.

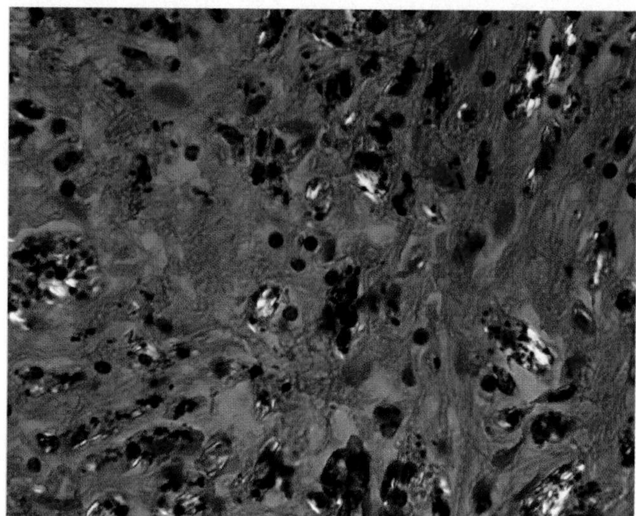

Figure 85.25 Polarization of talcosis nodule in Figure 85.24 shows brightly birefringent silicate particles.

Part 4

Mixed Pneumoconiosis and Mixed Dust Pneumoconiosis

▶ Alvaro C. Laga, Timothy Allen, and Philip T. Cagle

Some workers may have exposures to more than one inorganic dust, either simultaneously in one setting or at different times in different settings. The terms *mixed pneumoconiosis* and *mixed dust pneumoconiosis* have been used for pneumoconioses from exposures to more than one type of inorganic dust. These terms are often used loosely or interchangeably, and strict definitions of these terms may not be necessary or universally accepted. However, in a stricter sense, *mixed pneumoconiosis* has been defined as having recognizably distinctive pathologic features of more than one pneumoconiosis in the same patient. For example, an individual might have both asbestosis (characteristic pattern of fibrosis and asbestos bodies) and silicosis (silicotic nodules) in the lung tissue essentially as two separate but simultaneous diseases. The term *mixed dust pneumoconiosis* has been used for exposures to dusts containing more than one component, often producing hybrid lesions that are not classic for either dust alone. For example, exposure to silicates contaminated with silica may produce lesions that are neither classic silicotic nodules nor classic pure silicate nodules but rather a variable hybrid of the two. The resulting nodules will have more collagen than the pure silicate nodule but will not have the large central whorls of collagen expected of a silicotic nodule, with the amount of collagen apparently depending on the amount of silica content in the mixed dust (see Chapter 85, Part 2). Nonspecific interstitial fibrosis is also a frequent component of mixed dust pneumoconiosis.

Histologic Features:

- Distinct pathologic features of two or more separate dust exposures are present and recognizable (mixed pneumoconiosis).
- Hybrid lesions that have combined pathologic features of two different dust exposures; for example, silicate nodules with central hyalinization because of silica contamination.

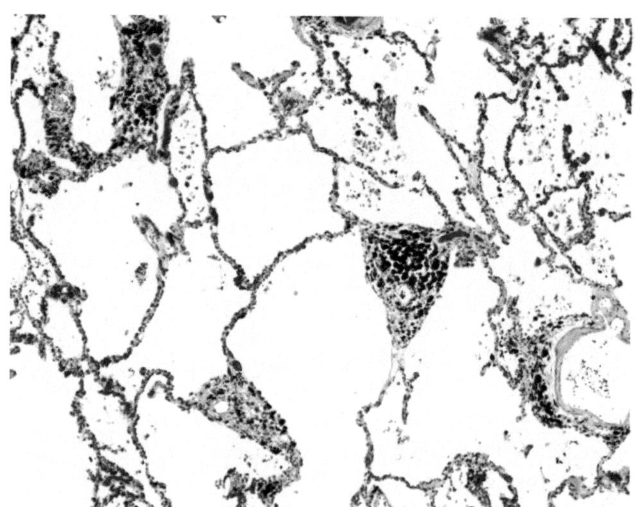

Figure 85.26 Small perivascular nodules containing dust-laden macrophages, anthracotic pigment, and increased collagen in a patient with mixed dust pneumoconiosis with silicate and silica exposure.

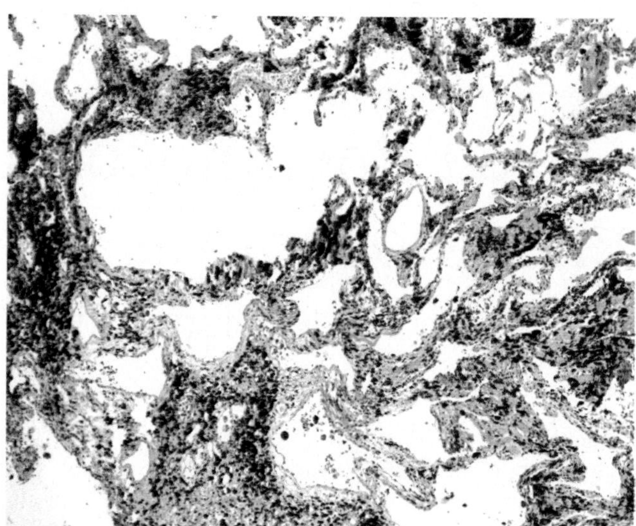

Figure 85.27 Fibrotic nodules with dust-laden macrophages, anthracotic pigment, and focal hyalinization mixed with irregular interstitial fibrosis with dust-laden macrophages and anthracotic pigment in a patient with mixed dust pneumoconiosis.

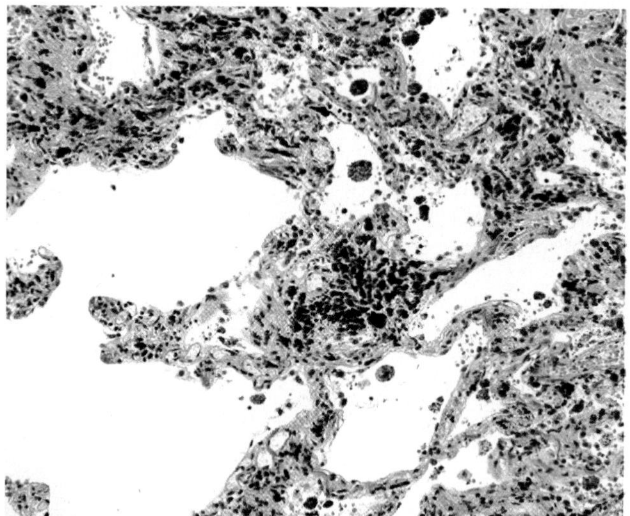

Figure 85.28 Nonspecific pattern of interstitial fibrosis with multiple dust-laden macrophages and anthracotic pigment mixed with irregular nodules in mixed dust pneumoconiosis.

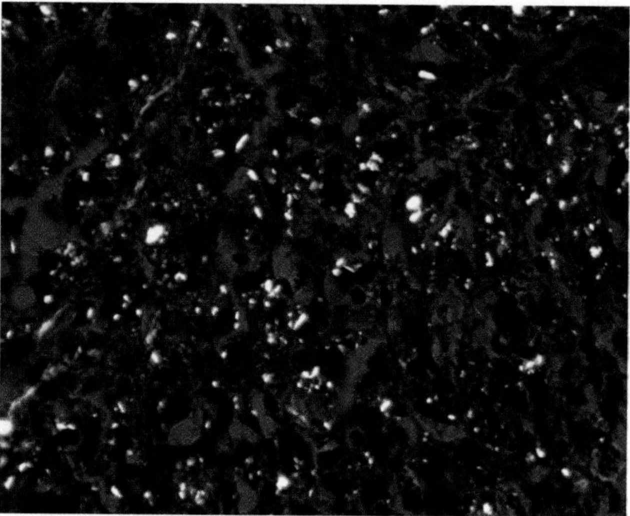

Figure 85.29 Polarized light in mixed dust pneumoconiosis shows tiny weakly birefringent particles of silica and larger strongly birefringent silicates.

Part 5

Coal Worker's Pneumoconiosis

▶ Alvaro C. Laga, Timothy Allen, and Philip T. Cagle

Coal worker's pneumoconiosis (CWP) results from exposure to coal dust in coal miners. Coal dust is composed of noncrystalline carbon and varying amounts of crystalline silica (quartz), kaolin, mica, and other silicates. The quartz content of the coal dust is a major determinant of the pulmonary pathologic response, and it varies among different types of coal (e.g., anthracite vs. soft coal). The most common radiologic abnormality in simple CWP consists of multiple, small, rounded opacities in the upper zones of both lungs.

The coal dust macule is characteristic of CWP and is accompanied by focal emphysema, an integral component of the diagnosis. Macules consist of aggregates of coal dust-laden macrophages with minimal fibrosis. The focal emphysema is seen even in miners who have never smoked, but it is typically more severe in heavy smokers. Coal dust nodules are fibrotic nodules containing dust-laden macrophages that are seen in the respiratory bronchioles (where they may evolve from macules), bronchovascular bundles, and pleura. They result primarily from the silica (quartz) mixed with the coal dust, although less fibrogenic silicates also may contribute. Thus, a coal dust nodule is a lesion of mixed dust pneumoconiosis composed of various combinations of coal dust, silica, and silicates (see Chapter 85, Part 4). The amount of whorled hyalinized collagen in the coal dust nodule reflects the amount of contaminating silica in the dust. Coal dust nodules are typically seen in association with macules, and both macules and nodules are more common in the upper lobes. Coal dust nodules are divided into micronodules (≤7 mm) and macronodules (7-20 mm) based on size.

Simple CWP consists of macules and/or nodules. Nodules may coalesce, causing complicated CWP or progressive massive fibrosis (PMF). The nodules in PMF are at least 2 cm in diameter. Cavitation may occur in PMF.

Histologic Features:

- Coal dust macules are composed of coal dust-laden macrophages in a reticulin stroma within the walls of respiratory bronchioles, alveolar ducts, and adjacent alveoli.
- Focal emphysema around the macule is an integral criterion for the diagnosis of CWP.
- Coal dust nodules consist of dust-laden macrophages in a fibrotic stroma; they are more common in the upper zones of the lung but also may be seen in the interlobular septa and in subpleural and peribronchial connective tissue.
- Coal dust nodules are arbitrarily classified into micronodules (≤0.7 cm), macronodules (0.7–2 cm), and progressive massive fibrosis (≥2 cm).
- Progressive massive fibrosis lesions consist of extensive fibrosis and abundant dust-laden macrophages; necrosis with cavitation and cholesterol clefts may be seen.

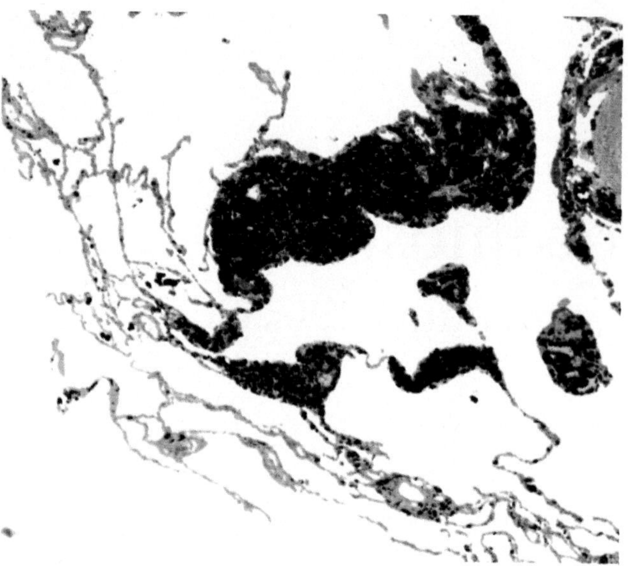

Figures 85.30 Low power of a coal dust macule consisting of abundant coal dust-laden macrophages in the wall of an alveolar duct and focal emphysema.

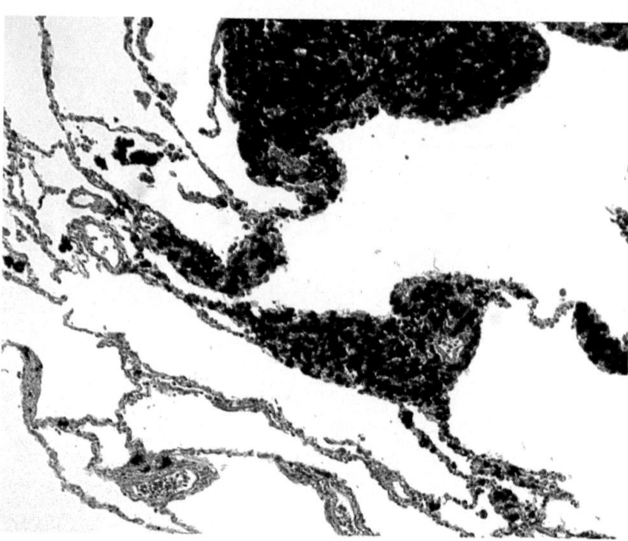

Figure 85.31 Higher power of coal dust macule showing deposits of coal dust-laden macrophages with minimal fibrosis in an alveolar duct wall.

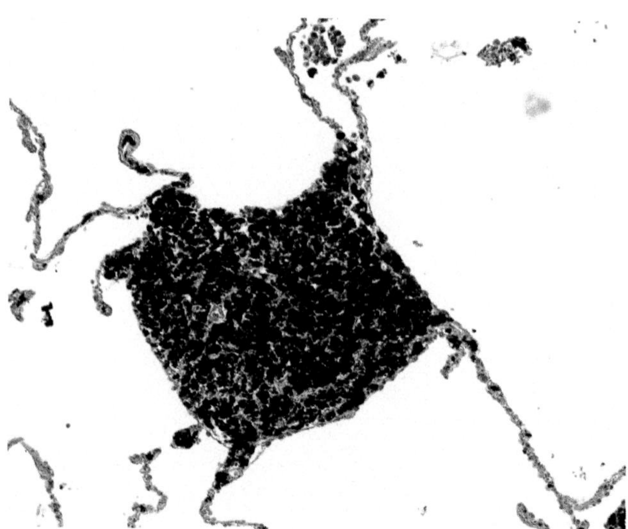

Figure 85.32 Coal dust macule shows only minimal fibrosis but numerous macrophages containing coal dust.

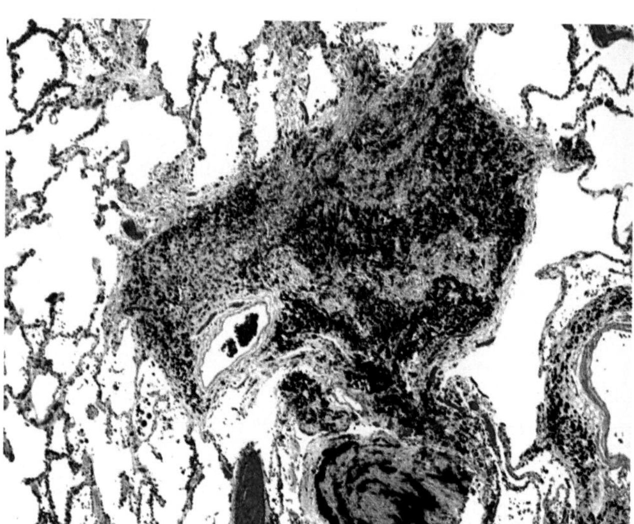

Figure 85.33 Coal dust nodule shows fibrosis with dust-laden macrophages with focal whorls of denser hyalinized collagen seen in the *lower part* of the figure.

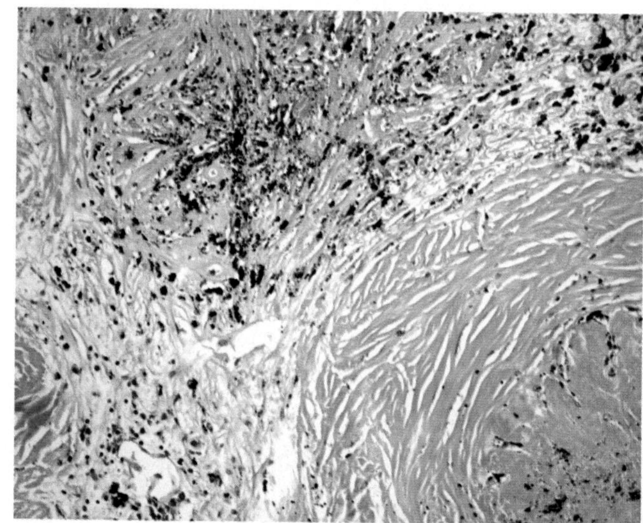

Figure 85.34 Higher power of coal dust nodules shows fibrosis and dust-laden macrophages with area of whorled hyalinized collagen indicating exposure to coal dust containing silica.

Part **6**

Giant Cell Interstitial Pneumonia/ Hard Metal Pneumoconiosis

▶ Alvaro C. Laga, Timothy Allen, and Philip T. Cagle

Most cases of giant interstitial pneumonia are hard metal pneumoconiosis resulting from inhalation of hard metal particles. Hard metal is a mixture primarily of tungsten carbide and cobalt, although other metals may be present. It is a very hard substance used for grinding, polishing, cutting, and bearings in tools, drills, and high-temperature conditions. Cobalt, rather than tungsten carbide, is thought to be the primary cause of the lung disease, but tungsten carbide and other metals usually are identified in tissue samples because of the solubility of cobalt.

The histologic features consist of an interstitial pneumonia with interstitial fibrosis and lymphocytic infiltrates and filling of alveolar spaces with macrophages and numerous multinucleated giant cells. The multinucleated giant cells are characterized by their unusually large number of nuclei and by emperipolesis in which intact lymphocytes, neutrophils, or mast cells are seen in the cytoplasm of the giant cells.

Not all cases of giant cell interstitial pneumonia are caused by hard metal exposure. Therefore, hard metal pneumoconiosis needs to be confirmed by work history and analysis of lung tissue for metals by energy-dispersive x-ray elemental analysis or other techniques. Exposure to hard metals may also produce reactions other than giant cell interstitial pneumonia, including asthma and hypersensitivity pneumonitis.

Histologic Features:

- Interstitial pneumonia with interstitial fibrosis and lymphocytic infiltrates plus macrophages and numerous multinucleated giant cells in the alveolar spaces.
- Large multinucleated giant cells often have tremendous numbers of nuclei, as many as 20 to 30 nuclei.
- Asteroid bodies and abundant dust may be present in the cytoplasm of the giant cells.
- Emperipolesis or presence of intact lymphocytes, neutrophils, or mast cells in the cytoplasm of multinucleated giant cells.

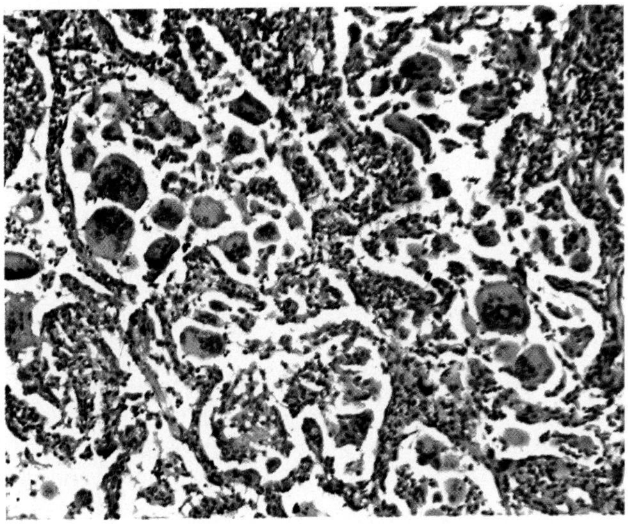

Figure 85.35 Low power of giant cell interstitial pneumonia shows interstitial fibrosis and lymphocytic infiltrates and macrophages and multinucleated giant cells within the alveolar spaces.

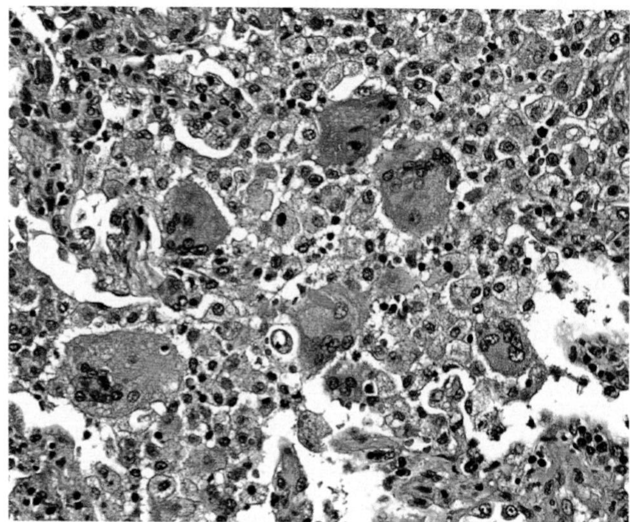

Figures 85.36 Alveolar spaces are filled with macrophages and multinucleated giant cells, some of which exhibit emperipolesis.

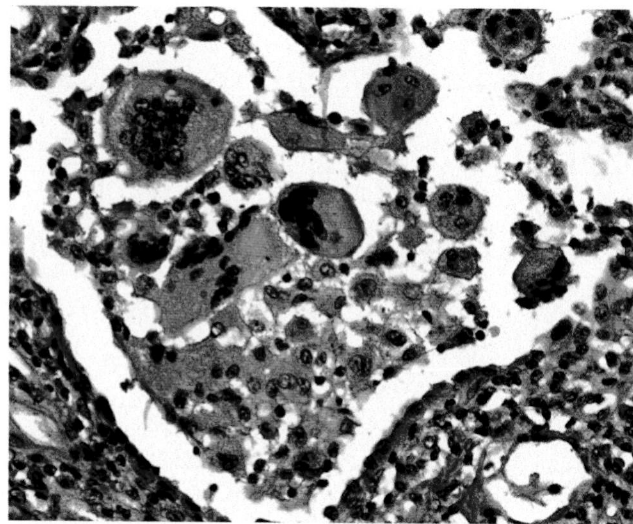

Figure 85.37 Higher power shows multinucleated giant cells and alveolar macrophages filling the alveolar spaces. Some of the giant cells show unusually numerous nuclei.

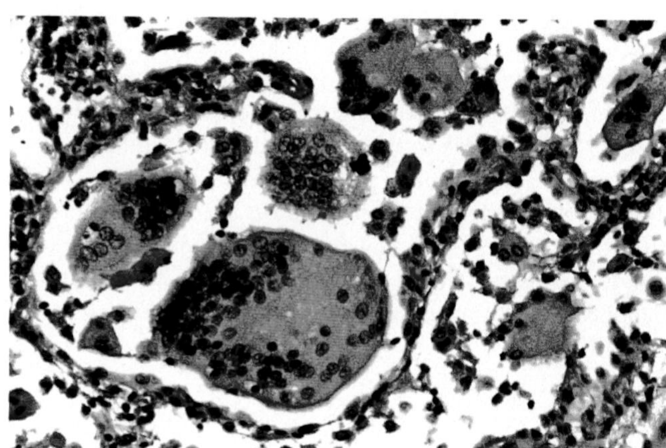

Figure 85.38 High power of alveolar space containing large multinucleated giant cells with tremendous numbers of nuclei.

Part 7

Siderosis

▶ Alvaro C. Laga, Timothy Allen, and Philip T. Cagle

Siderosis is pneumoconiosis caused by inhalation of iron particles. Mixed dust pneumoconioses such as silicosiderosis are caused by combined exposure to iron and other dusts (see Chapter 85, Part 4). Siderosis can occur in miners, steel mill workers, foundry workers, and welders, as well as workers in other occupations. Siderosis is usually a pneumoconiosis that produces radiologic abnormalities but no clinical disease. For this reason, iron is often referred to as an *inert* mineral. In many occupations, individuals exposed to iron are also exposed to silica and may be exposed to other dusts such as asbestos. This results in mixed dust pneumoconioses in which the iron may contribute little or not at all to the clinical lung disease. However, with very heavy exposures to iron, iron alone may produce macules, fibrotic nodules, and small airways fibrosis.

Ferruginous bodies of inhaled iron particles are often round to oval with golden brown endogenous iron deposited around oval to round black exogenous iron cores. The endogenous iron is Prussian blue positive but the inhaled iron is not.

Histologic Features:

- Iron appears as brown to black free dust, as ferruginous bodies with black cores (typically round ferruginous bodies with round black cores), and in macrophages.
- Macules consist of deposits of iron, ferruginous bodies, and iron-laden macrophages with minimal fibrosis around bronchioles and blood vessels.
- Fibrosis in walls of respiratory bronchioles with free iron dust, ferruginous bodies, and iron-laden macrophages.
- Nodules consist of nodular fibrosis with collagen and free iron dust, ferruginous bodies, and iron-laden macrophages.
- Modifications of these lesions may be seen in silicosiderosis with denser hyalinized collagen due to the silica.

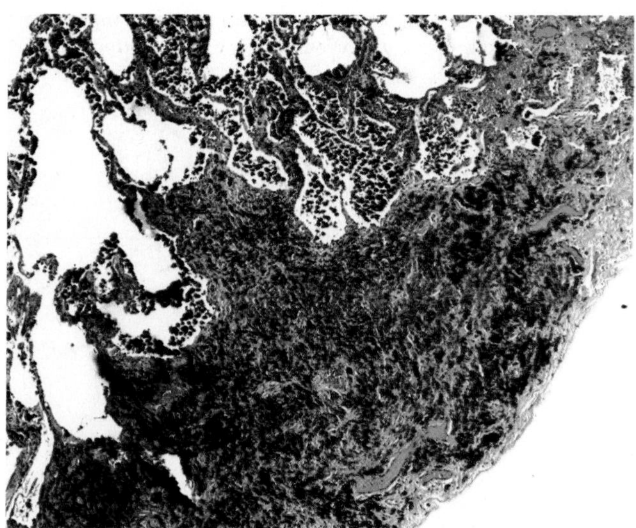

Figure 85.39 Subpleural fibrotic nodule consists of collagen, iron dust, ferruginous bodies, and iron-laden macrophages with iron dust and iron-laden macrophages in the adjacent alveolar spaces.

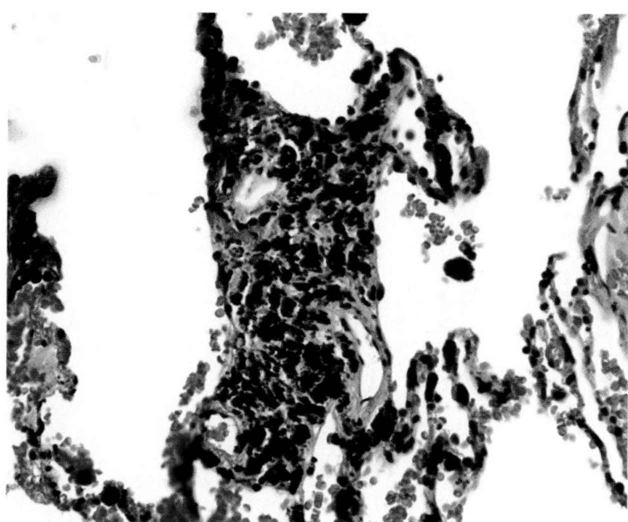

Figure 85.40 Perivascular macule contains iron dust, ferruginous bodies, and iron-laden macrophages with minimal fibrosis.

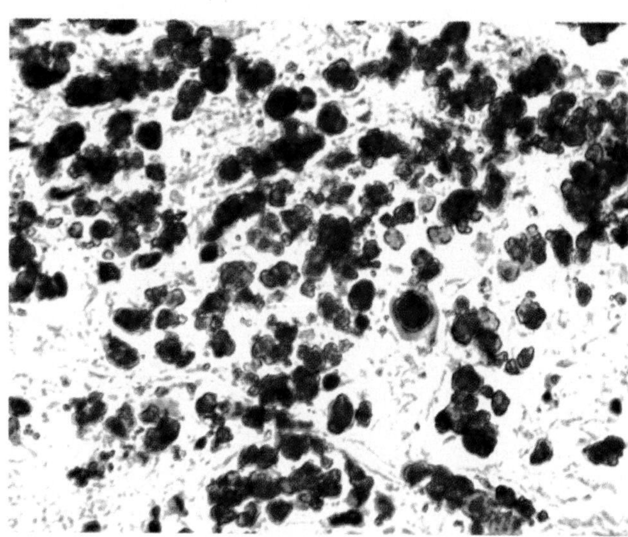

Figure 85.41 High power shows golden brown iron particles and ferruginous bodies with round black cores.

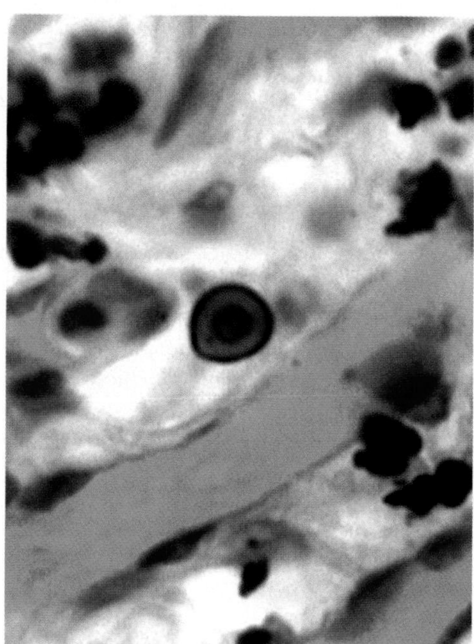

Figure 85.42 High power of a round ferruginous body with a round black core of exogenous iron surrounded by a rim of brown endogenous iron.

Part 8

Aluminosis

▶ Philip T. Cagle

Although millions of workers are exposed to aluminum, aluminum pneumoconiosis or aluminosis is very rare. The rare fibrotic reaction to aluminum appears to depend in part on the industrial setting when nonpolar lubricants are substituted for stearin in the manufacturing of aluminum powders. In this setting, protection against formation of aluminum hydroxide is not provided, and the resultant aluminum hydroxide is believed to cause the pulmonary fibrosis.

Aluminosis consists of interstitial fibrosis associated with macrophages containing aluminum particles or small black jagged particles. Fibrotic nodules containing macrophages with intracytoplasmic material may be found in a predominantly lymphangitic distribution in the bronchovascular bundles and in the pleura. The intracytoplasmic material within the macrophages is brown-gray and refractile, but it is not birefringent on polarized light and is negative for iron stain.

Other very rare reactions to aluminum exposure, including pulmonary alveolar proteinosis, have been reported.

Histologic Features:

- Interstitial fibrosis including fibrotic nodules in a lymphangitic distribution in the bronchovascular bundles and pleura.

- Macrophages containing brown-gray refractile material or small black jagged particles are present in the interstitial fibrosis and fibrotic nodules.
- Macrophage cytoplasmic material is not birefringent on polarized light and is negative on iron stain.

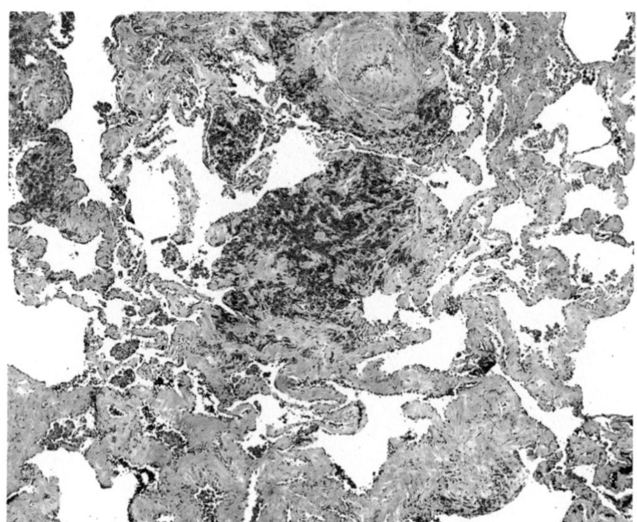

Figure 85.43 Low power shows interstitial fibrosis with dust-laden macrophages containing a brown-gray refractile material.

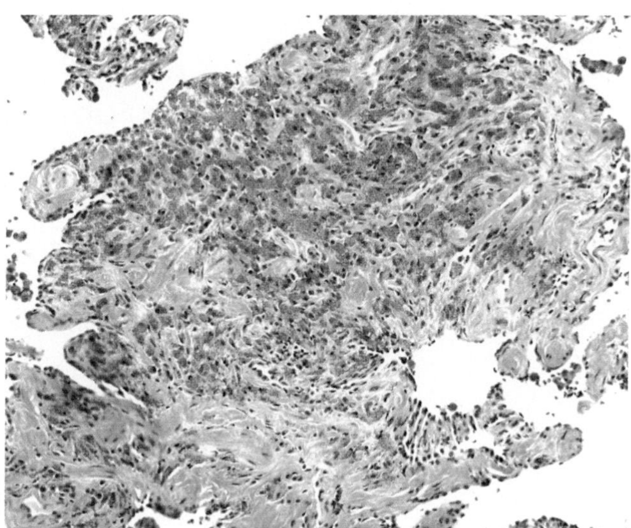

Figure 85.44 Higher power of fibrotic nodule shows macrophages with cytoplasmic brown-gray refractile dust.

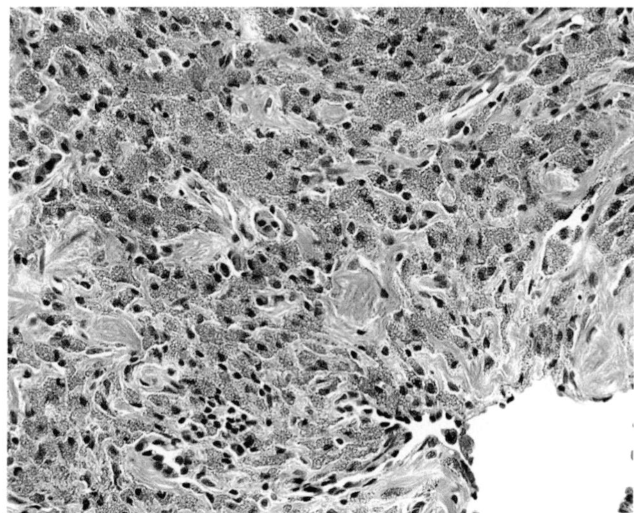

Figure 85.45 Higher power shows refractile brown-gray dust particles in the cytoplasm of numerous macrophages within a fibrotic nodule.

Interstitial Disease in Collagen Vascular Diseases

86

▶ Abida Haque

Collagen vascular diseases represent a group of chronic inflammatory conditions that are immunologically mediated. They are associated with both localized and diffuse pulmonary lesions, and the latter account for a significant part of the diffuse interstitial lung disease spectrum. The pulmonary changes of rheumatoid arthritis and systemic lupus erythematosus are the most widely recognized. However, other collagen vascular diseases may also present with pulmonary involvement. Collagen vascular disease should be considered in the differential diagnosis of interstitial lung disease (see Chapter 113).

Histologic Features:

- Interstitial pneumonias with lymphocytes and/or plasma cells may be seen.
- Nonspecific inflammatory cell infiltrates are common around the airways.
- Usual interstitial pneumonia (UIP)-like pattern may be seen, and some cases are inseparable from examples of idiopathic UIP on histopathology.
- Nonspecific interstitial pneumonia pattern may be observed in some cases.

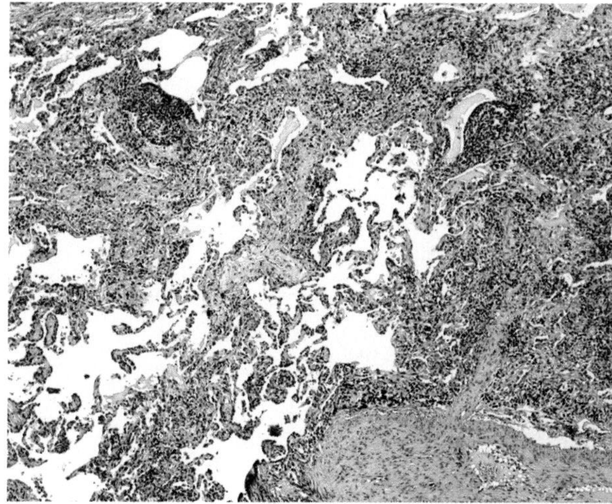

Figure 86.1 Rheumatoid lung shows septal thickening and infiltration by chronic inflammatory cells. Follicular bronchiolitis is also present.

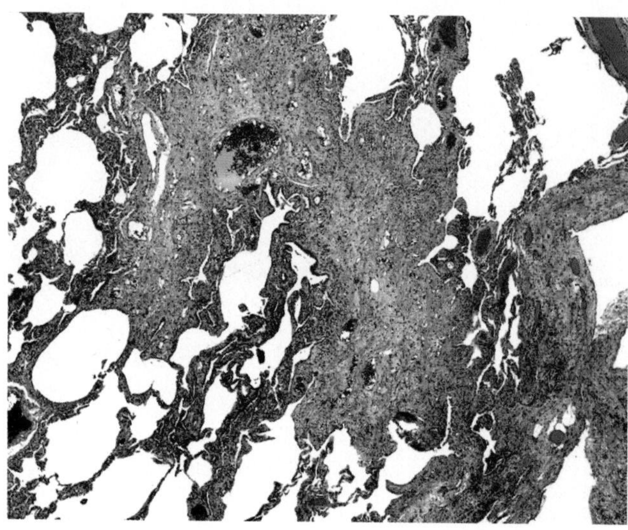

Figure 86.2 Patchy interstitial fibrosis consistent with UIP-like pattern in rheumatoid lung.

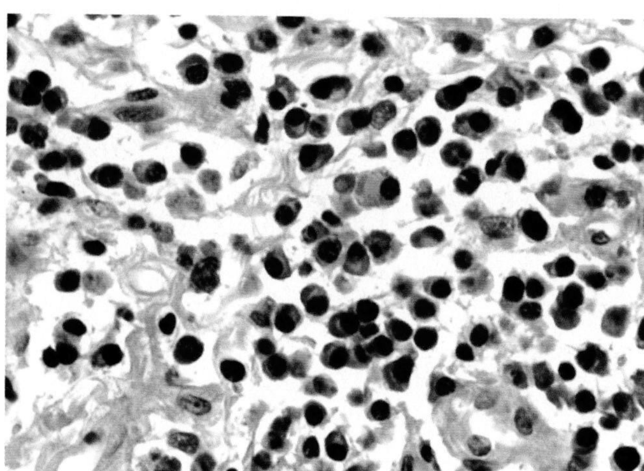

Figure 86.3 Plasma cell-rich inflammatory infiltrate is frequently seen in interstitial lung disease associated with rheumatoid arthritis.

87

Organized Diffuse Alveolar Damage

▶ Alvaro C. Laga
▶ Abida Haque

The organizing phase of diffuse alveolar damage (DAD) generally begins approximately 7 days after a lung insult and is characterized by dramatic proliferation of interstitial fibroblasts associated with marked hyperplasia of type 2 pneumocytes. Organized DAD may grossly show firm smooth areas of consolidated lung parenchyma and small cysts. Organized DAD must be distinguished from other forms of fibrosis, including usual interstitial pneumonia (UIP). In the early stages of organization of DAD, the fibrosis is predominantly immature. In rare cases, the fibrosis may progress to mature fibrosis and result in honeycomb change. Whereas UIP has a slow progressing course, DAD has a rapid onset, often arising in the setting of severe inflammatory or traumatic events (see Chapter 71).

Histologic Features:

- Septal thickening.
- Fibroblastic proliferation.
- Type 2 pneumocyte hyperplasia.
- Squamous metaplasia may be seen in some cases.
- Dense fibrosis and honeycomb change may occur.

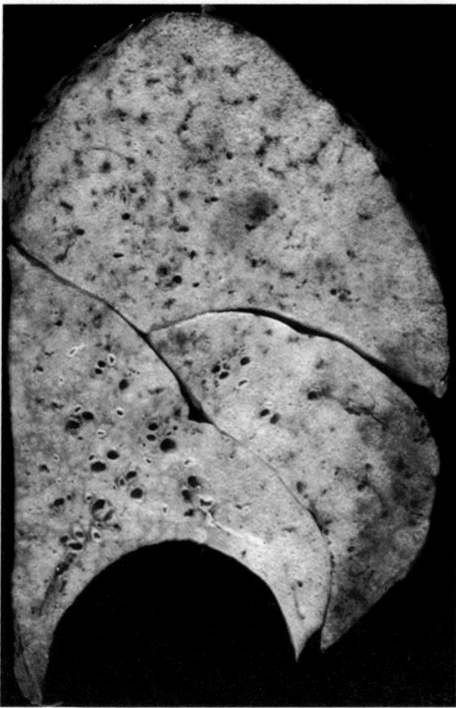

Figure 87.1 Gross figure shows organized DAD with consolidated lung parenchyma and small cysts.

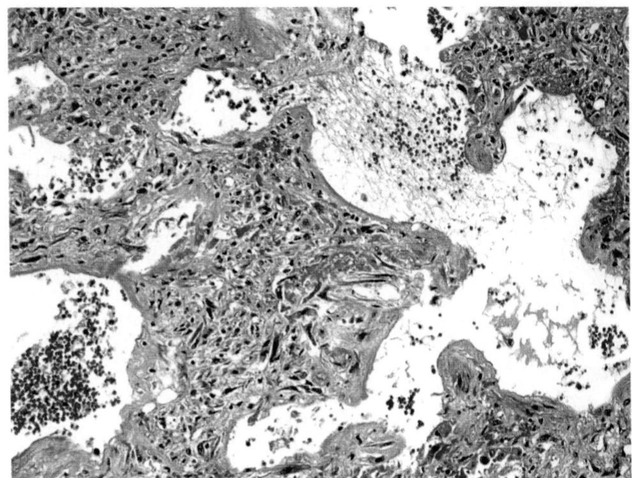

Figure 87.2 Organizing DAD with florid interstitial fibroblastic proliferation distorting the lung architecture.

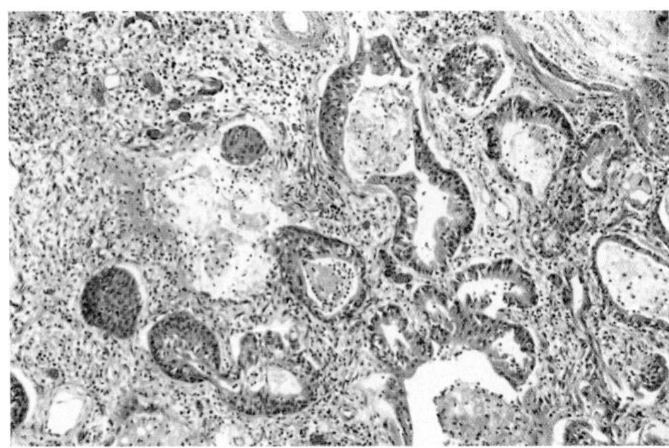

Figure 87.3 Distorted lung parenchyma with alveolar septal thickening and extensive squamous metaplasia.

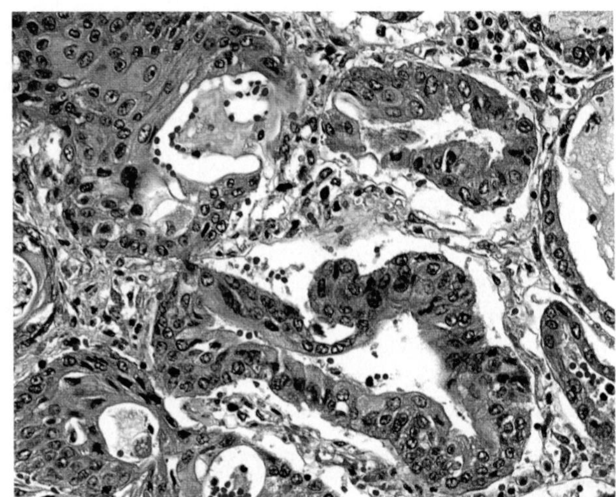

Figure 87.4 Higher power of organizing DAD shows squamous metaplasia.

Diffuse Alveolar-Septal Amyloidosis

88

▶ Alvaro C. Laga
▶ Timothy Allen
▶ Philip T. Cagle

Lung involvement as diffuse alveolar-septal amyloidosis occurs in most cases of systemic primary amyloidosis. Involvement limited to the lungs and lung involvement by secondary amyloidosis are both very rare. Diffuse alveolar-septal amyloidosis produces bilateral reticulonodular interstitial infiltrates that may be mistaken for pulmonary fibrosis radiographically. Patients may die of progressive respiratory insufficiency. Grossly, the lungs are bulky and the cut surfaces have a diffuse rubber-sponge appearance and texture. Histologically, the lung architecture is generally preserved with thickening of alveolar septa by amorphous eosinophilic amyloid diffusely or as multiple interstitial nodules.

Histologic Features:

- Diffuse uniform deposition of amyloid in the alveolar septa, interstitium, and tracheobronchial tree or multiple small interstitial nodules.
- Giant cell reaction and a chronic inflammatory infiltrate may occasionally occur.
- Apple green birefringence with Congo red stain.

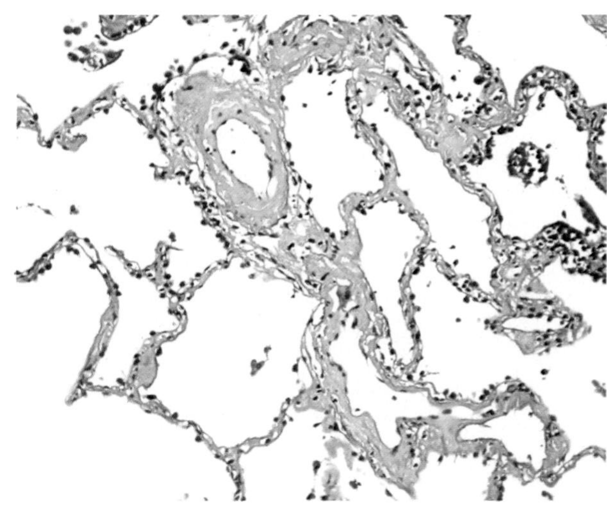

Figure 88.1 Septal amyloidosis with septa thickened by eosinophilic waxy material.

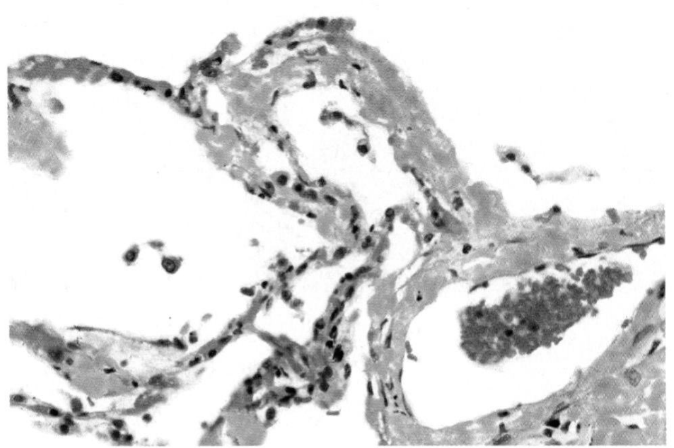

Figure 88.2 Higher power shows deposition of amorphous waxy eosinophilic material within alveolar septa.

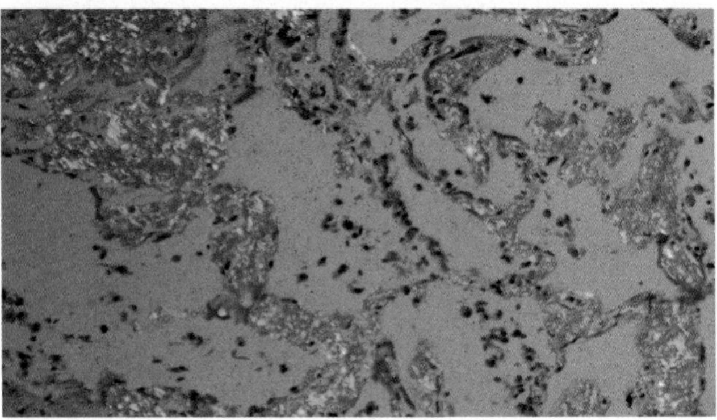

Figure 88.3 Septal amyloidosis shows characteristic apple green birefringence of amyloid on Congo red stain.

89

Honeycomb Lung

- Roberto Barrios
- Timothy Allen
- Hakan Cermik
- Dani S. Zander

Honeycomb lung represents an end-stage common pathway for a number of lung diseases; however, the gross and microscopic appearance is the same regardless of the initial lung disease. The radiologic and gross pathologic appearance of end-stage fibrosis of the lungs consists of cystic spaces separated by bands of fibrous tissue that give the appearance of a honeycomb. Honeycomb lung may result from idiopathic interstitial pneumonias (it is an integral part of the definition of usual interstitial pneumonia; see Chapter 92), sarcoidosis, chronic hypersensitivity pneumonitis, drug reactions, chronic aspiration, chronic infections, bronchiectasis, pneumoconioses, organized diffuse alveolar damage, and other chronic lung injuries.

The lungs are small and firm with a nodular ("cobblestone") pleural surface, which resembles the surface of a cirrhotic liver. This external appearance is due to irregular fibrosis of the underlying parenchyma, which shows fibrosis and smooth muscle proliferation (hence the term *muscular cirrhosis of the lungs*). On section, there is obliteration of the normal architecture with replacement by cystic spaces and grayish-white to yellow fibrous tissue that, as noted, resembles a honeycomb.

Histologic Features:

- Distortion of the normal architecture by severe fibrosis with cysts separated by broad bands of fibrous tissue.
- Fibrosis may show focal chronic inflammatory infiltrates, focal lymphoid aggregates, and/or focal smooth muscle hyperplasia.
- Cysts may accumulate mucus, debris, macrophages, and acute inflammation.
- Cysts may have metaplasia of their lining, including bronchiolar metaplasia ("bronchioloectasis"), cuboidal epithelium ("cuboidalization"), and squamous metaplasia.

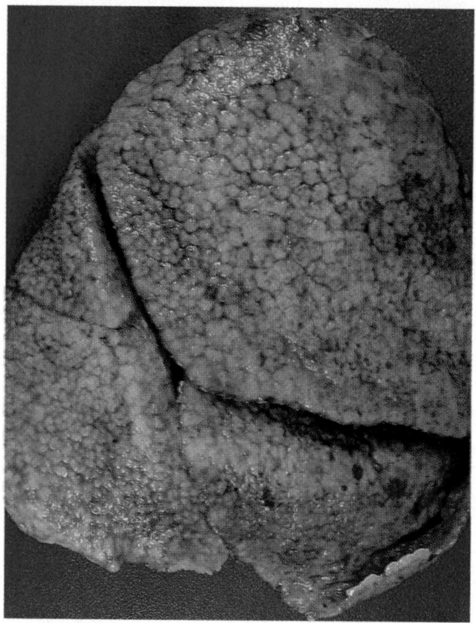

Figure 89.1 Gross figure of pleural surface of honeycomb lung shows nodularity ("cobblestoning") due to underlying parenchymal fibrosis with retraction.

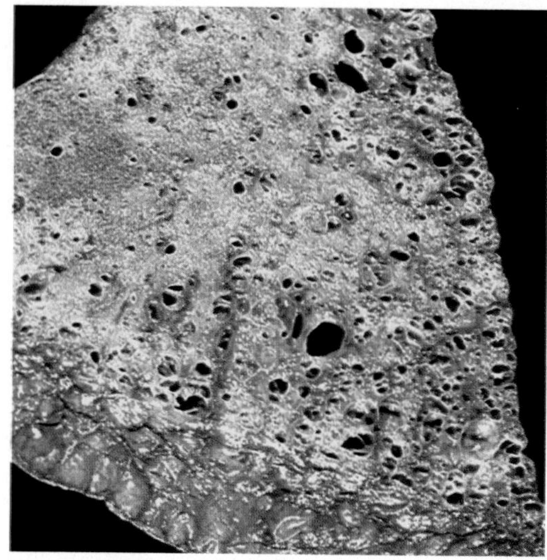

Figure 89.2 Gross figure of cut section of honeycomb lung shows severe fibrosis with cystic spaces.

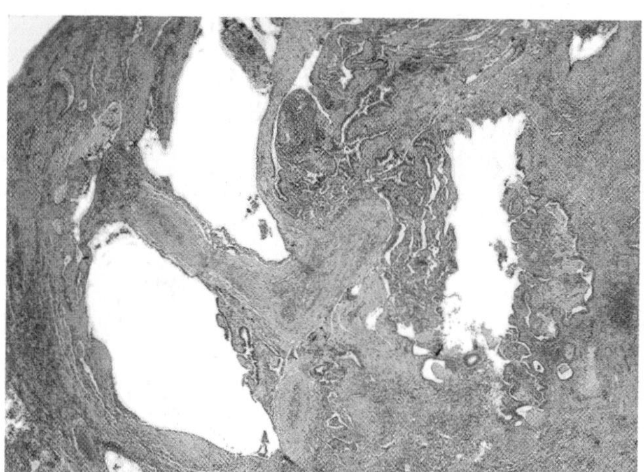

Figure 89.3 Distortion of normal architecture by severe fibrosis and cyst formation.

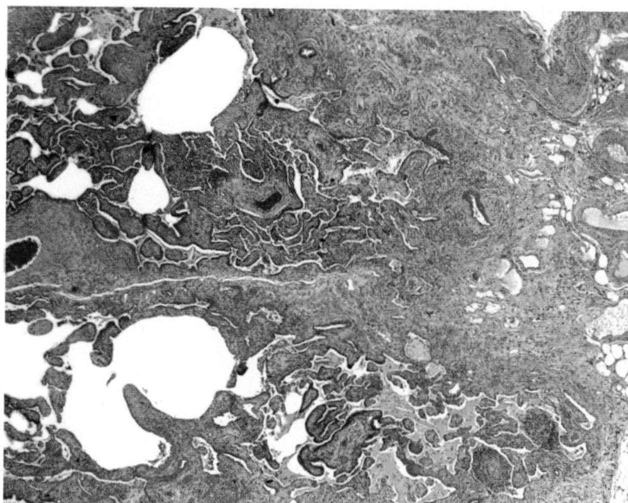

Figure 89.4 Honeycomb lung with fibrosis, distortion of normal architecture, cyst formation, and bronchiolar metaplasia of the cyst epithelium.

Lung Disease in Inflammatory Bowel Disease

90

▶ Alvaro C. Laga
▶ Philip T. Cagle

Pulmonary involvement in inflammatory bowel disease is rare and can present as airway, interstitial, or pleural lesions. Lung symptoms usually develop after the onset of bowel disease but occasionally may be the initial manifestation. Pulmonary complications of inflammatory bowel disease include chronic bronchitis, bronchiectasis, bronchiolitis, serositis, necrobiotic nodules, and interstitial lung disease. Radiologic findings include multiple bilateral nodular opacities and thickening of the trachea and bronchial walls.

Histologic Features:

- Large airway involvement characterized by inflammation, ulceration, and narrowing of the trachea and/or bronchi.
- Necrotic parenchymal nodules with numerous neutrophils.
- Organizing pneumonia.
- Interstitial lung disease with patterns of interstitial inflammation and/or fibrosis.

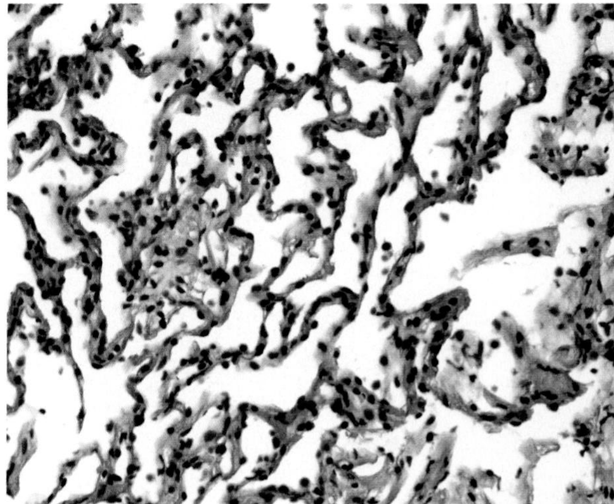

Figure 90.1 Minimal lymphocytic inflammatory infiltrate in a lung biopsy of a patient with inflammatory bowel disease.

Section 16

Idiopathic Interstitial Pneumonias

91 Acute Interstitial Pneumonia

▸ Abida Haque

Acute interstitial pneumonia (AIP) is the pathologic correlate of Hamman-Rich syndrome, a rapidly progressive interstitial fibrosis of unknown etiology. The onset of shortness of breath is typically preceded by a prodrome of viral-like illness with cough and fever, and respiratory failure within days or weeks. AIP has many pathologic features of organizing diffuse alveolar damage (see Chapters 71 and 87). There is no known precipitating factor for AIP as opposed to adult respiratory distress syndrome. Mortality is high, up to 60%. Cultures for viruses, bacteria, and fungal organisms are negative in the early stages; however, nosocomial infections may occur during hospitalization.

Histologic Features:

- There is diffuse interstitial fibroblast proliferation associated with abundant edematous, myxomatous stroma.
- Marked alveolar type 2 pneumocyte hyperplasia with large atypical cells lining the alveolar septa.
- Hyaline membranes and alveolar fibrinous exudates may be absent or minimal.
- Pulmonary vessels may have organizing and recent thrombi.
- The temporal heterogeneity of usual interstitial pneumonia is not seen.
- Immunostains for viral antigens have been consistently negative in several studies.

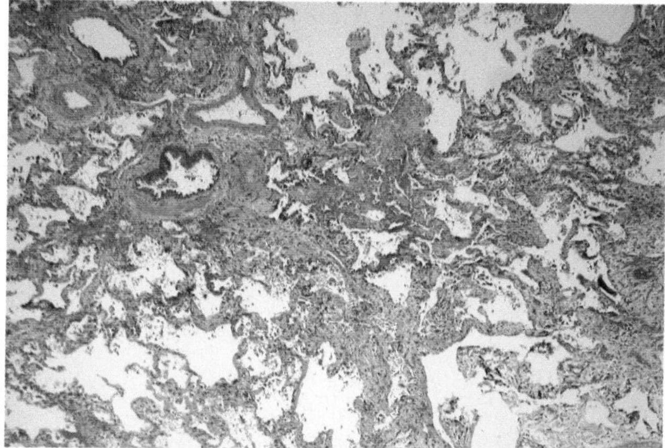

Figure 91.1 Low power shows expansion of interstitium with light blue myxomatous edematous stroma, characteristic of AIP.

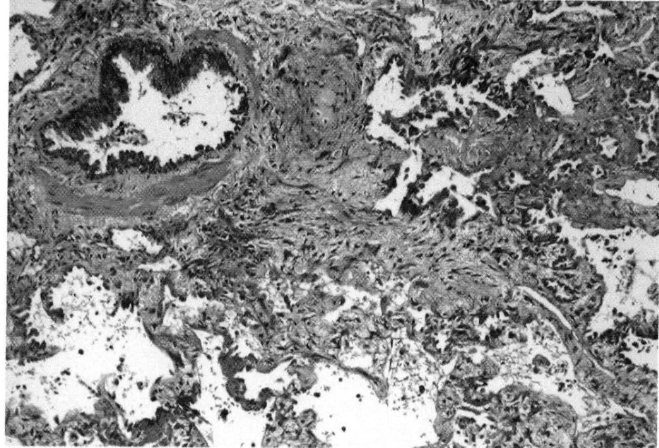

Figure 91.2 Higher power shows details of the fibrous tissue.

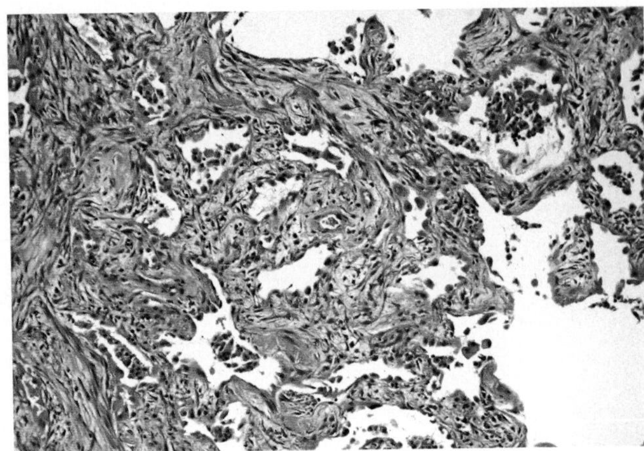

Figure 91.3 Interstitial fibroblastic proliferation surrounded by minimal stroma may be present in other areas. Type 2 pneumocyte hyperplasia may also be present.

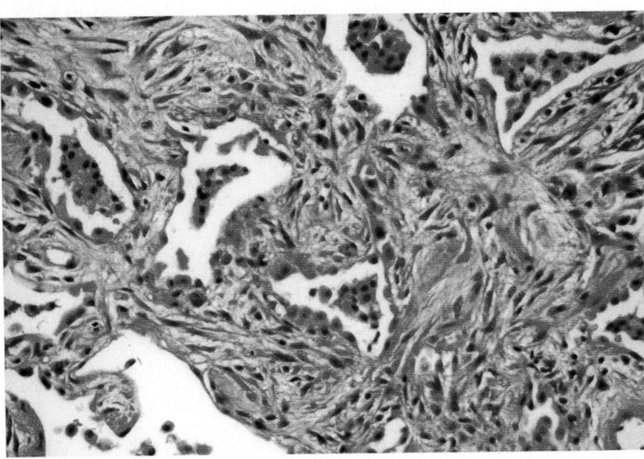

Figure 91.4 Higher power of interstitial fibroblastic proliferation.

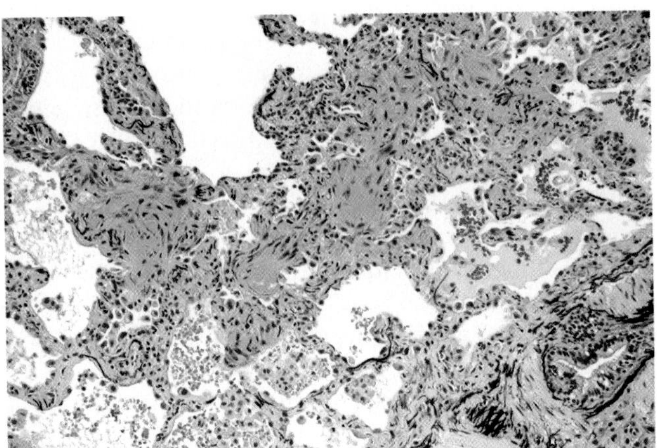

Figure 91.5 Movat stain highlighting the interstitial myxomatous stroma associated with fibroblastic proliferation.

Usual Interstitial Pneumonia 92

▸ Alvaro C. Laga
▸ Timothy Allen
▸ Philip T. Cagle

The American Thoracic Society and the European Respiratory Society define *usual interstitial pneumonia* (UIP) as the pathologic abnormality essential to the diagnosis of the distinct clinical disorder *idiopathic pulmonary fibrosis* (IPF), also known as *cryptogenic fibrosing alveolitis.* IPF is a chronic progressive form of interstitial pulmonary fibrosis that occurs in middle-aged to elderly patients and does not respond to immunosuppressive therapy, unlike many other interstitial lung diseases. The patient classically presents with insidious onset of shortness of breath. Over months or years, as increasingly more lung tissue is gradually replaced by scar, large areas (especially in the lower zones and subpleurally) become end-stage honeycomb lung, and the disease becomes progressively more clinically severe, eventually resulting in respiratory failure. The great majority of patients with IPF are smokers, and it is probable that smoking has a causative role in IPF. In comparison to many other forms of interstitial pneumonia, including most other idiopathic interstitial pneumonias, the prognosis of UIP is poor, and, as noted, UIP does not respond to steroids. Therefore, it is important to correctly diagnose UIP versus other interstitial pneumonias.

UIP is characterized histologically by a patchy pattern of chronic interstitial fibrosis (mature collagen) with relatively minimal to mild interstitial chronic inflammation. This patchy pattern results in areas of variable interstitial fibrosis mixed with areas of normal or nearly normal lung parenchyma and areas of architectural distortion consisting of honeycomb lung or solid scars. Radiologically, grossly, and microscopically, the fibrosis and honeycombing of UIP are more prominent in lower lung zones and in the periphery of the lung. Microscopically, the fibrosis is also worse in the periphery of the lobule. Essential to the concept and diagnosis of UIP is temporal heterogeneity (the process is ongoing and not of the "same age" or same duration throughout the biopsy). The temporal heterogeneity is demonstrated by the presence of active fibroblast foci representing "younger" foci of active ongoing disease compared to the more abundant "older" mature scarring. Fibroblast foci consist of small tufts of granulation tissue (fibroblasts in a myxoid or edematous stroma), typically on the fibrotic walls at the interface between fibrotic and normal lung.

Honeycomb areas may show lymphoid aggregates, smooth muscle hyperplasia, bronchiolar or squamous metaplasia of cyst linings and neutrophils, macrophages, or debris in the cystic spaces (see Chapter 89). Desquamative interstitial pneumonialike reactions with collections of macrophages containing granular brown cytoplasmic material may be seen in the honeycomb areas (see Chapter 75). Infections or other superimposed pathologies are possible. There is an increased risk of lung cancer in patients with UIP. Whether or not this is due to the UIP itself or to smoking as an etiologic agent common to both diseases is not known.

Lung involvement in collagen vascular diseases, particularly rheumatoid arthritis and scleroderma, can produce a UIP pattern of fibrosis. It has been proposed that fibroblast foci are less prevalent in UIP associated with collagen vascular disease and that these patients have better survival than patients with IPF. Other diseases that may produce a pattern of fibrosis mimicking UIP include drug reactions, chronic aspiration, radiation fibrosis and "burnt out" chronic infections, sarcoidosis, chronic hypersensitivity pneumonitis, Langerhans histiocytosis, and other conditions that may lead to widespread fibrosis and honeycomb lung in some cases. A more uniform pattern of mature interstitial fibrosis without fibroblast foci may represent organized diffuse alveolar damage (see Chapter 87) or acute interstitial pneumonia (see Chapter 91). The fibrotic form of nonspecific interstitial pneumonia (NSIP) enters into the differential diagnosis, and it is likely that some biopsies interpreted as NSIP represent untypical areas of UIP (see Chapter 93). Although some pneumoconioses may mimic UIP radiologically and/or clinically, asbestos bodies or other specific clues to diagnosis are apparent on histologic examination (see Chapter 85). Histologic observation of granulomas, hyaline membranes, extensive areas of organizing pneumonia, foreign body giant cells, bronchiolocentric fibrosis, and other specific findings suggest that the fibrosis has another etiology that should be investigated.

Histologic Features:

- Chronic interstitial fibrosis composed predominantly of mature collagen with relatively minimal to mild interstitial chronic inflammation.
- Patchy pattern of interstitial fibrosis with areas of normal or nearly normal lung parenchyma mixed with areas of minimal to mild interstitial fibrosis and areas of architectural distortion consisting of honeycomb lung or solid scars.
- Fibrosis and honeycombing of UIP are more prominent in the lower lung zones, in the peripheral (subpleural) areas, and in the periphery of the lobule.
- Fibroblast foci consisting of small tufts of granulation tissue (fibroblasts in a myxoid or edematous stroma), typically on the fibrotic walls at the interface between fibrotic and normal lung.
- Most of the fibrosis observed in UIP is mature collagen, including areas of honeycomb lung and solid scars, but the scattered small fibroblast foci represent the active areas of ongoing disease (temporal heterogeneity).
- Granulomas, hyaline membranes, extensive areas of organizing pneumonia, foreign body giant cells, bronchiolocentric fibrosis, and other specific findings suggest that the fibrosis has another cause.

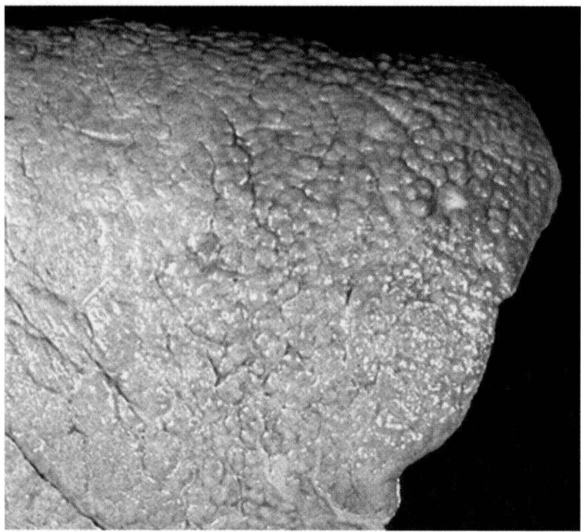

Figure 92.1 "Cobblestoning" of the pleural surface in UIP caused by retraction of interlobular septa due to subpleural fibrosis.

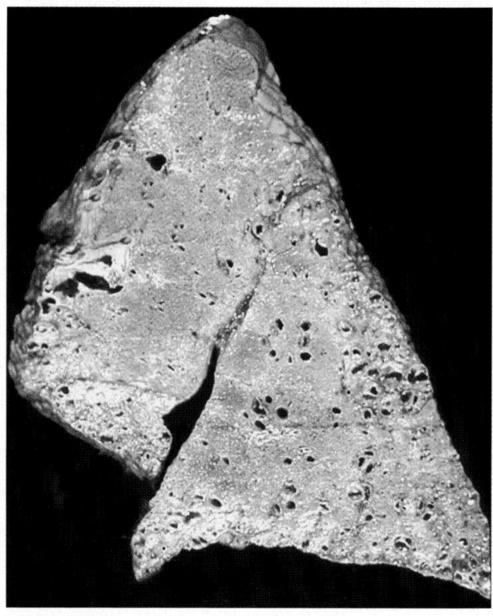

Figure 92.2 Cut surface shows more severe fibrosis subpleurally and in the lower lung zones.

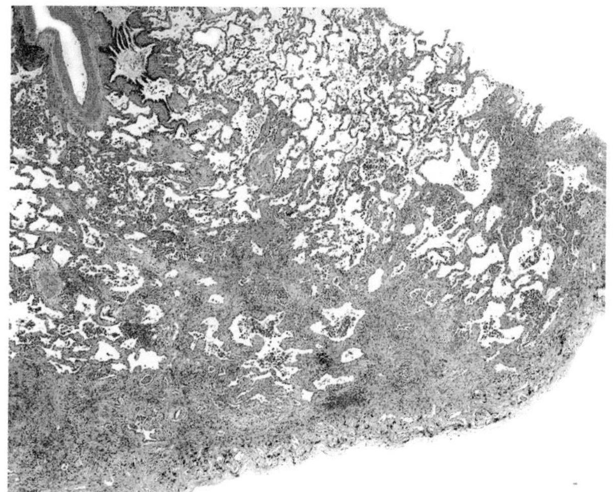

Figure 92.3 Low power of a wedge biopsy shows a patchy pattern of predominantly mature interstitial fibrosis with areas of normal or near normal alveolar septa mixed with areas of minimal to mild interstitial fibrosis and denser subpleural scar and honeycombing.

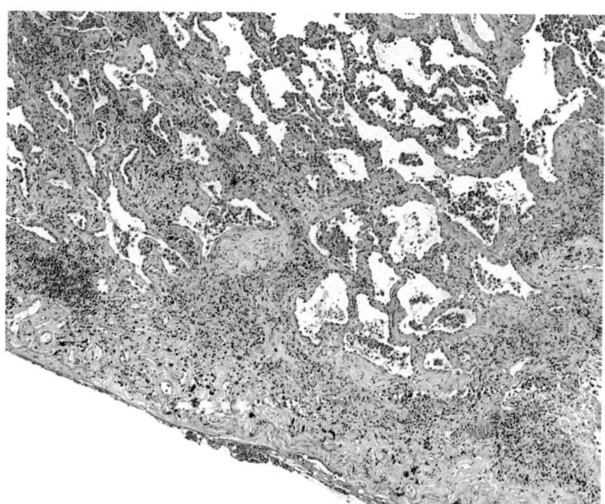

Figure 92.4 Medium power shows subpleural architectural distortion by solid scar, as well as adjacent areas of mild interstitial fibrosis where alveolar septa are thickened but retain regular architecture.

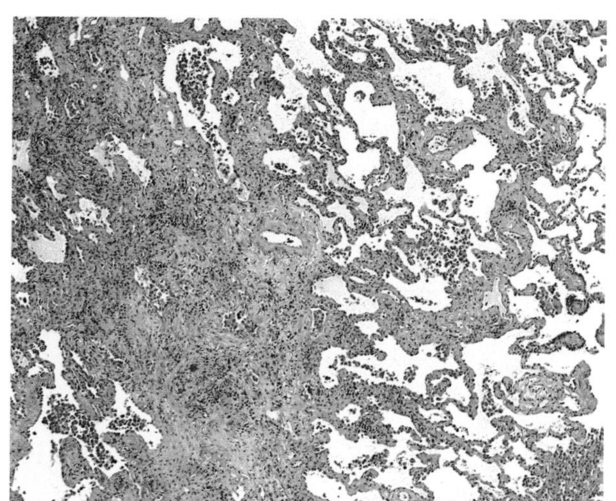

Figure 92.5 Medium power shows area of dense scar with adjacent alveolar septa with mild fibrosis and alveolar septa of normal thickness.

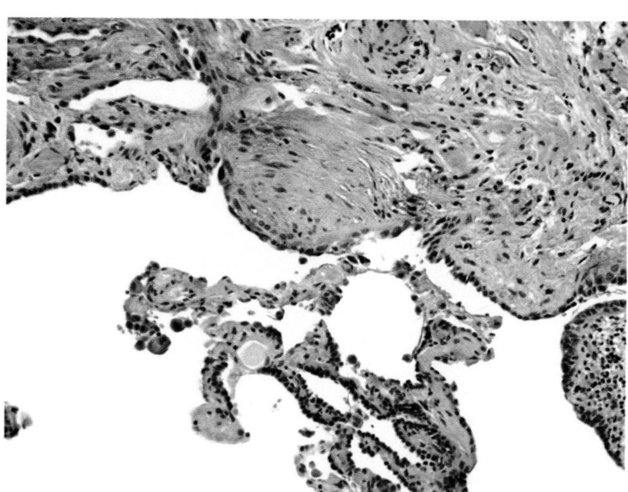

Figure 92.6 High power shows a fibroblast focus consisting of a clump of fibroblasts in a myxoid stroma located at the interface of fibrotic lung.

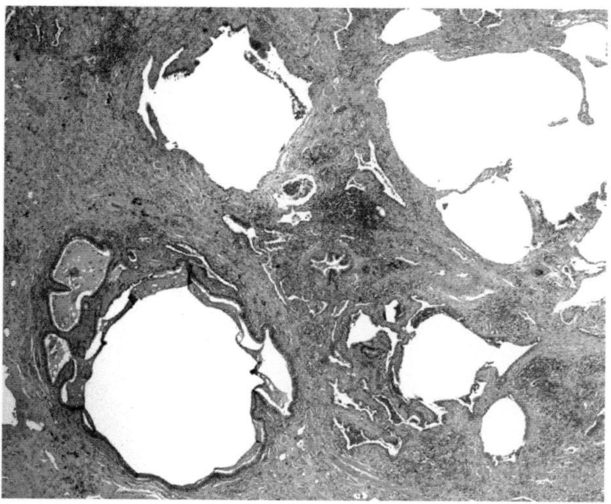

Figure 92.7 Normal lung architecture is replaced by broad bands of dense fibrous tissue containing cystic spaces in an area of honeycomb lung.

Nonspecific Interstitial Pneumonia

93

▶ Alvaro C. Laga
▶ Timothy Allen
▶ Philip T. Cagle

Nonspecific interstitial pneumonia (NSIP) is defined as a chronic idiopathic interstitial pneumonia that is temporally "uniform" (the process is of the "same age" or same duration throughout the biopsy). Biopsies of several specific entities can also show features that meet the criteria for NSIP, as discussed further later. NSIP occurs most often in middle-aged adults and usually presents as shortness of breath. Histologically, NSIP is divided into cellular and fibrotic forms. Most cases of NSIP show cellular interstitial infiltrates composed of lymphocytes and plasma cells arranged in a homogeneous "linear" pattern in which the lung architecture is preserved (cellular type of NSIP). Less often, cases show predominantly interstitial fibrosis arranged in a homogenous "linear" pattern in which the lung architecture is largely preserved (fibrotic type of NSIP). Some cases may show varying amounts of both cellular interstitial infiltrates and interstitial fibrosis. In contrast to usual interstitial pneumonia (UIP; see Chapter 92), NSIP has minimal or absent honeycombing. NSIP lacks the fibroblast foci that represent the temporal heterogeneity of UIP. In contrast to UIP, cellular NSIP has a good response to steroids and a good prognosis. Fibrotic NSIP may respond to steroids, although generally fibrotic NSIP has a much worse prognosis than cellular NSIP and, therefore, is more similar to UIP in prognosis and response to steroids.

NSIP is a common histologic pattern in collagen vascular diseases involving the lung (see Chapters 86 and 113). Some cases of NSIP are hypersensitivity pneumonitis (extrinsic allergic alveolitis; see Chapter 82). In particular, some biopsies of hypersensitivity pneumonitis have temporally homogeneous interstitial lymphoplasmacytic infiltrates consistent with NSIP but lack the poorly formed granulomas characteristic of hypersensitivity pneumonitis. Areas with histopathologic features of NSIP may sometimes be present in cases of UIP and may be the only areas sampled on a biopsy. Other types of interstitial fibrosis or inflammation that may have an NSIP-like pattern include drug reactions and organized diffuse alveolar damage (see Chapter 87) or acute interstitial pneumonia (see Chapter 91).

Histologic Features:

- NSIP is temporally homogeneous and lacks the fibroblast foci that are the hallmark of temporal heterogeneity in UIP.
- NSIP may be patchy in distribution.
- In cellular NSIP, the alveolar septa have lymphoplasmacytic infiltrates that may vary from minimal to severe and may be accompanied by lymphoid nodules, but the underlying alveolar architecture is relatively preserved and recognizable.
- In fibrotic NSIP, the alveolar septa have fibrosis that may vary from minimal to severe, but the underlying alveolar architecture is relatively preserved and recognizable.
- Mixed patterns with varying amounts of cellular lymphoplasmacytic infiltrates and interstitial fibrosis may be observed.
- Honeycombing is minimal or absent.
- Organizing pneumonia may be present.

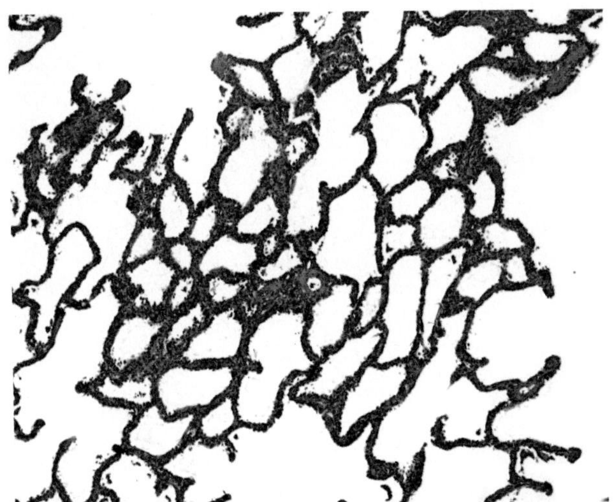

Figure 93.1 Low power of cellular NSIP with homogeneous "linear" pattern of lymphoplasmacytic infiltrates in preserved alveolar septa.

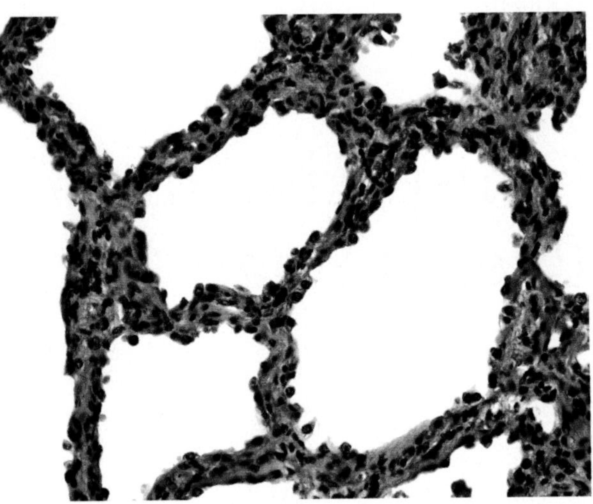

Figure 93.2 Higher power shows homogeneous "linear" pattern of lymphoplasmacytic infiltrates in alveolar septa in cellular NSIP.

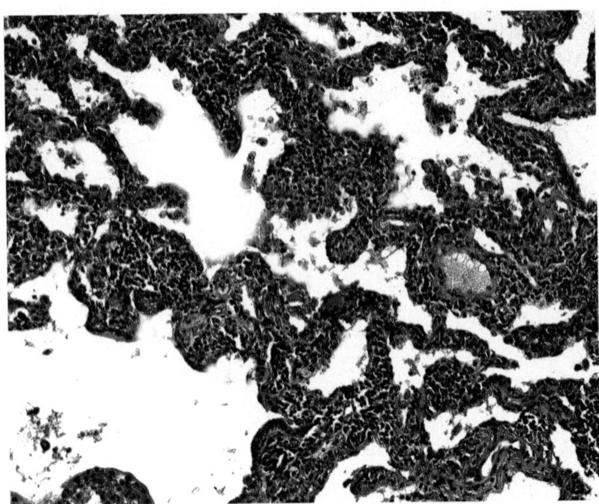

Figure 93.3 In this case of cellular NSIP, the alveolar septa are more distended by the lymphoplasmacytic infiltrates, but the underlying alveolar architecture is still recognizable.

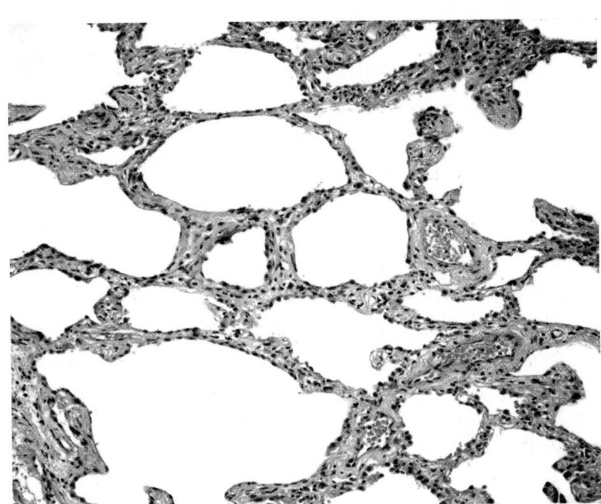

Figure 93.4 Low power of fibrotic NSIP shows a homogeneous "linear" pattern of alveolar septal fibrosis with preservation of the alveolar architecture.

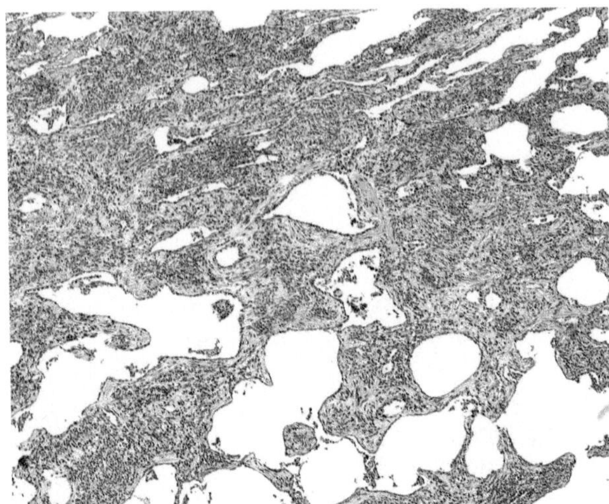

Figure 93.5 Medium power shows a mixed cellular and fibrotic pattern of NSIP with thickening of the alveolar septa by both lymphoplasmacytic infiltrates and fibrosis and focal remodeling of the lung architecture without fibroblast foci.

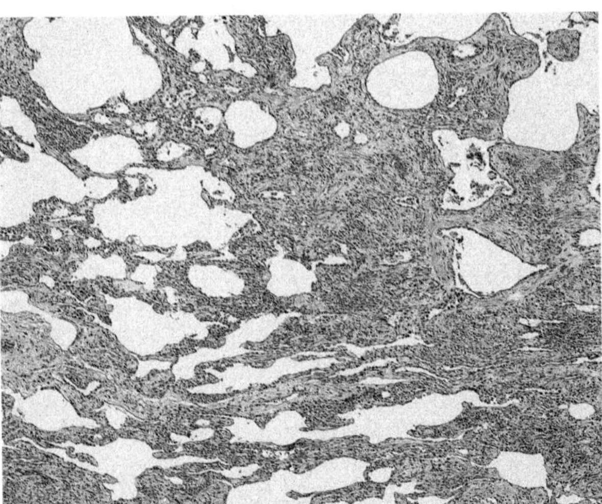

Figure 93.6 Mixed cellular and fibrotic pattern of NSIP showing both lymphoplasmacytic infiltrates and fibrosis. The architecture is relatively preserved but shows focal remodeling without fibroblast foci.

Cryptogenic Organizing Pneumonia (Idiopathic Bronchiolitis Obliterans Organizing Pneumonia)

94

▸ Alvaro C. Laga
▸ Timothy Allen
▸ Philip T. Cagle

Cryptogenic organizing pneumonia (COP), formerly termed *idiopathic bronchiolitis obliterans organizing pneumonia* (idiopathic BOOP), consists of proliferation of granulation tissue within small airways, alveolar ducts, and alveoli. The clinical syndrome occurs most often in middle-aged to older adults and is often preceded by a flulike illness. Persistent nonproductive cough and shortness of breath are the usual presenting symptoms. Most, but not all, patients respond rapidly to steroids, and in most cases prognosis is excellent.

COP is an idiopathic clinical syndrome, but similar lesions can be seen in various specific pulmonary injuries (see Chapter 62). These identifiable causes of organizing pneumonia must be excluded clinically and pathologically before a diagnosis of COP can be made. When an organizing pneumonia pattern is present, the pathologist should examine the tissue for viral inclusions, poorly formed granulomas or isolated giant cells (hypersensitivity pneumonitis), and foreign body giant cells (aspiration).

At low power, COP consists of a patchy pattern of nodules of granulation tissue that typically center on a small airway surrounded by normal or near normal lung. At higher power there are arborizing branches of granulation tissue (fibroblasts in an edematous or myxoid stroma) that fill the lumens of bronchioles, alveolar ducts, and adjacent alveoli. Rounded plugs of granulation tissue in the alveolar spaces are referred to as *Masson bodies.* The general architecture of the lung is preserved, with no significant interstitial fibrosis or honeycombing. There may be small foci of lymphocytes, plasma cells, and macrophages in some bronchioles, and interstitial inflammation is usually minimal to moderate. Transbronchial biopsies may fail to sample bronchioles and sample only alveoli with organizing pneumonia. Intraalveolar collections of foamy macrophages may result from the bronchiolar obstruction.

Histologic Features:

- Nodules of granulation tissue in and around small airways consist of polypoid plugs of granulation tissue (fibroblasts in an edematous or myxoid stroma) in the lumens of bronchioles branching into lumens of adjacent alveolar ducts and alveoli.
- Rounded nodules of granulation tissue within alveolar spaces (Masson bodies).
- Cellular bronchiolitis may be present.
- Normal alveolar parenchyma adjacent to the organizing pneumonia.
- Interstitial inflammation is minimal to moderate.
- No significant architectural distortion.
- Only alveoli with organizing pneumonia may be sampled with transbronchial biopsies.
- Intraalveolar collections of foamy macrophages may result from bronchiolar obstruction.

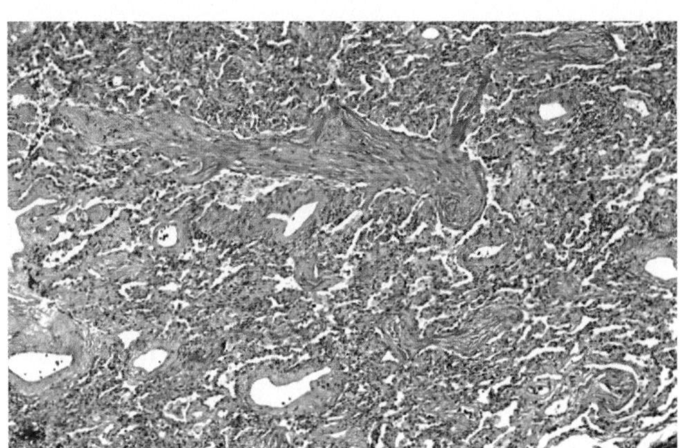

Figure 94.1 Granulation tissue fills lumens of alveolar ducts.

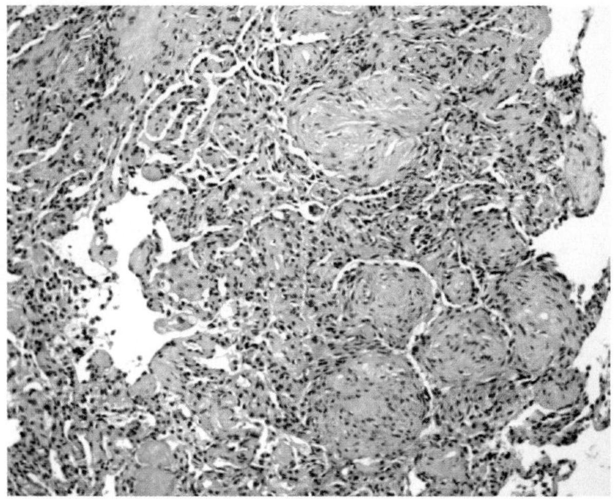

Figure 94.2 Rounded nodules of granulation tissue (Masson bodies) in alveolar spaces.

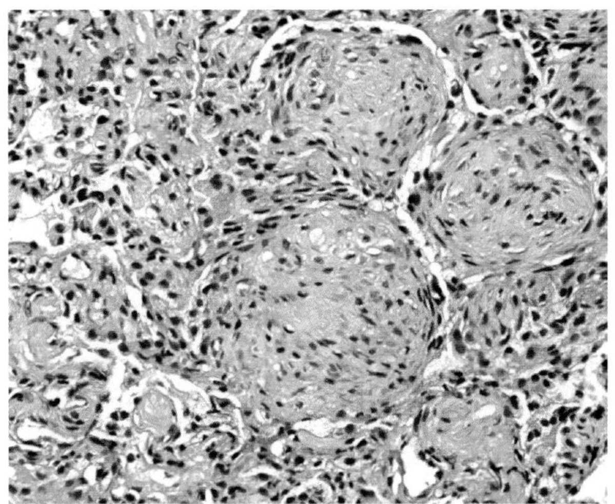

Figure 94.3 Higher power of rounded Masson bodies shows that they are composed of fibroblasts in an edematous or myxoid stroma.

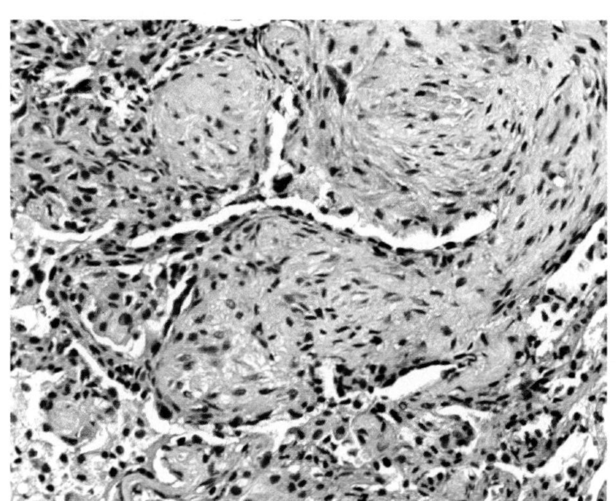

Figure 94.4 Plugs of intraluminal granulation tissue in COP.

Section 17

Specific Infectious Agents

- The infected cell shows enlarged nucleus with a single, round to oval inclusion surrounded by a clear halo (Cowdry type A) with margination of chromatin on the inner aspect of the nuclear membrane.
- Fully developed inclusions are easily seen at low power, permitting quick diagnosis; however, in the early stages, the inclusions resemble those seen in other Herpesviridae families (HSV, VZV).
- Masson trichrome stain highlights the inclusions.
- Cytoplasmic inclusions are valuable in the diagnosis of CMV; these are small, granular, and basophilic in early stages but later become larger (up to 3 μm) and aggregate near the cell membrane.
- Inclusions are periodic acid–Schiff (PAS) and Gomori methenamine silver positive.

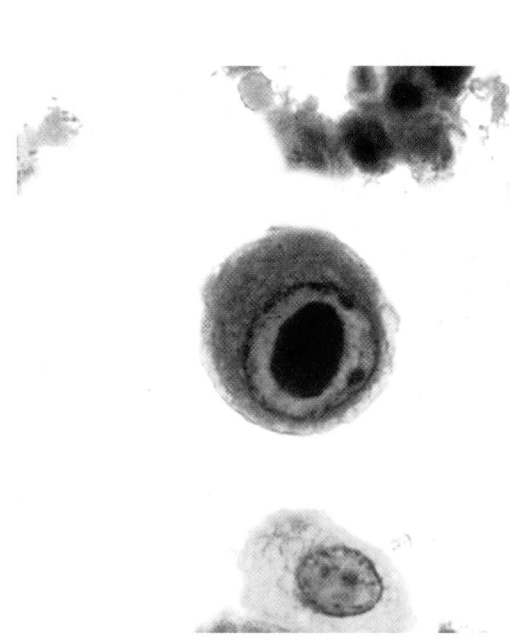

Figure 95.1 Cytology figure showing alveolar cell containing a large oval intranuclear inclusion (owl eye nucleus).

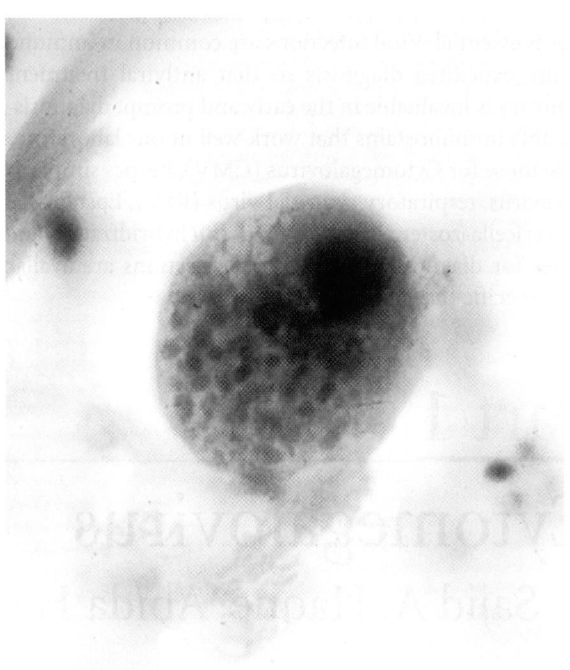

Figure 95.2 Cytology figure showing alveolar cell containing cytoplasmic inclusions consisting of small multiple round bodies.

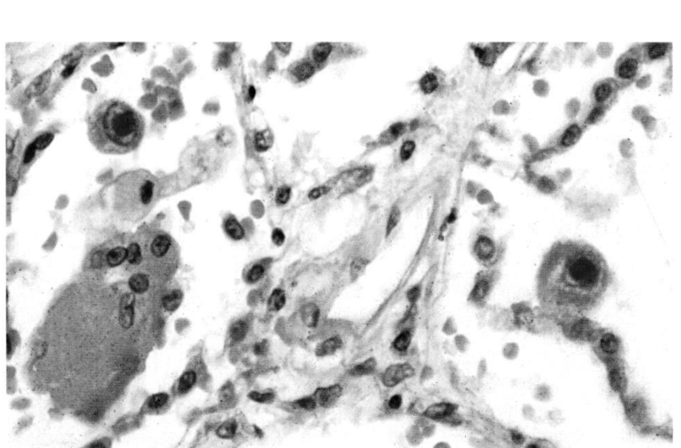

Figure 95.3 Two large alveolar cells with intranuclear Cowdry type A inclusions.

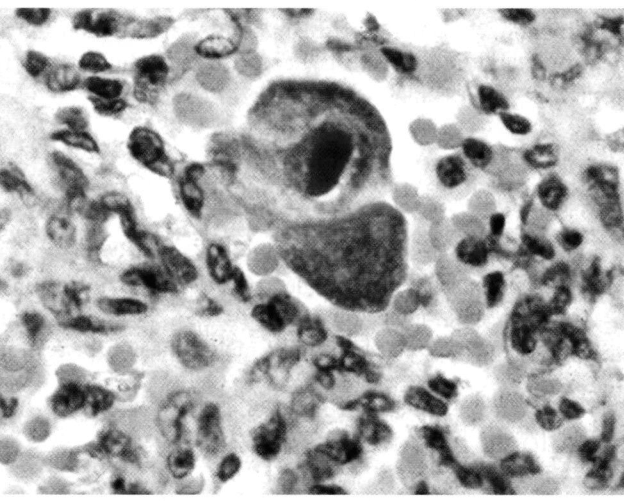

Figure 95.4 Higher power of a type 2 pneumocyte with intranuclear and cytoplasmic inclusions.

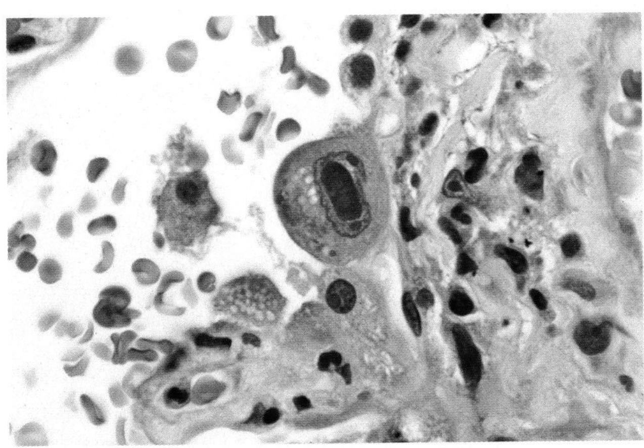

Figure 95.5 Type 2 pneumocyte with both intranuclear and cytoplasmic inclusions.

Part 2

Herpes Simplex Virus

▶ Sajid A. Haque, Abida Haque, and Mary Ostrowski

HSV infections are usually asymptomatic in immunocompetent individuals. In immunocompromised adults, the infection is associated with necrotizing tracheobronchitis and bronchopneumonia. The airway mucosa and/or the lung parenchyma may show acute inflammation with necrosis, fibrinous exudates, and DAD in severe infection. The viral inclusions occur early in the course of infection but may be obscured by the inflammation. Both HSV I and II infections have been identified in the lungs of infants and immunocompromised adults.

Cytologic Features:

- Multinucleated cells with nuclear molding.
- Chromatin pattern with opaque or ground-glass smudged appearance.
- Eosinophilic nuclear inclusions.

Histologic Features:

- Infected cells are enlarged, often multinucleated, and may show two types of nuclear inclusions.
- Characteristic amphophilic, homogenous, or "glassy" nuclear inclusions (3 to 8 μm in size) bordered by clumped chromatin (Cowdry type B), or deeply eosinophilic, homogenous, centrally placed, and surrounded by a clear halo (Cowdry type A).
- No cytoplasmic inclusions.

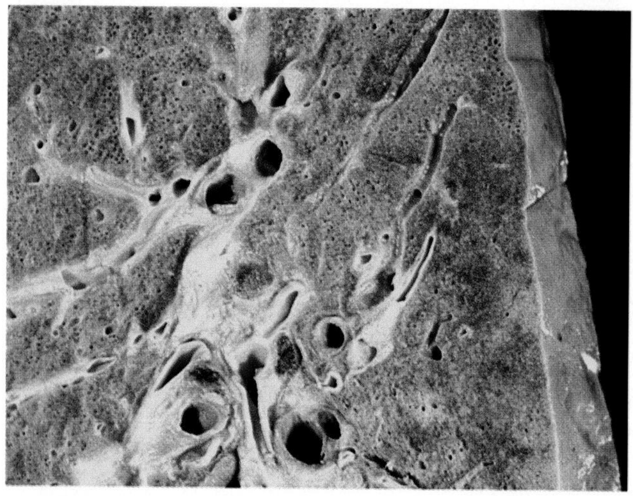

Figure 95.6 Gross figure showing small pale areas of consolidation.

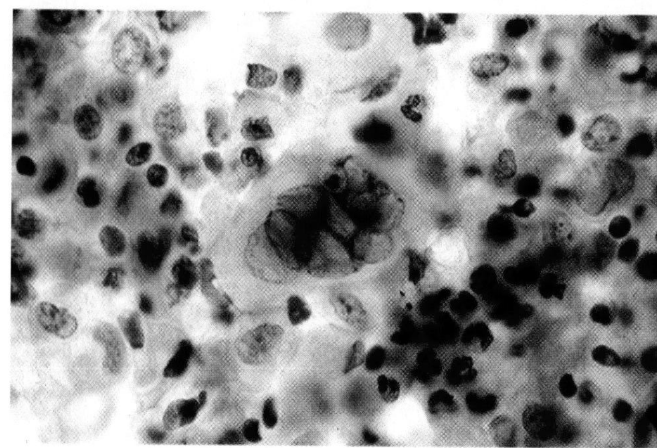

Figure 95.7 Cytologic figure showing a multinucleated giant cell with ground-glass nuclei diagnostic of HSV infection, surrounded by inflammatory cells.

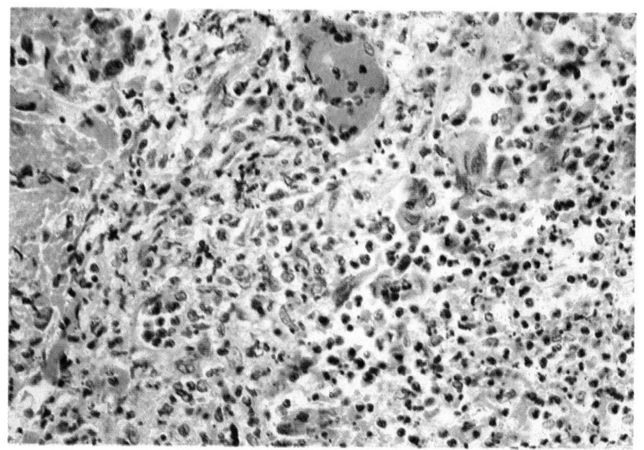

Figure 95.8 Low power showing an inflammatory infiltrate and a few multinucleated giant cells. Diagnosis of HSV pneumonia cannot be made at this magnification.

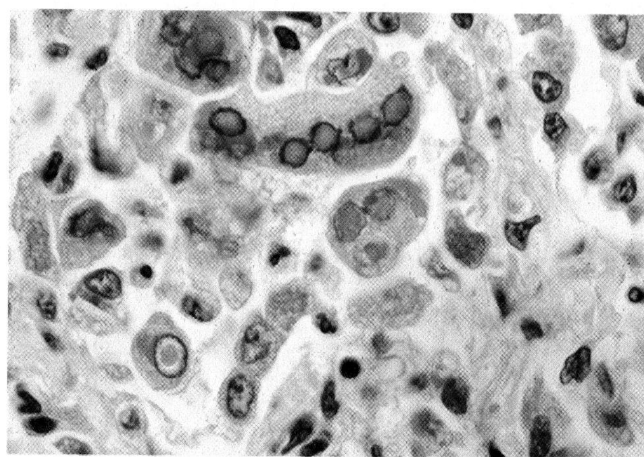

Figure 95.9 Higher power showing multinucleated giant cells with characteristic eosinophilic ground glass nuclei (Cowdry type B) and a single cell with early eosinophilic inclusion surrounded by a clear halo in the *bottom left corner* (Cowdry type A).

Part 3

Influenza and Parainfluenza Virus Pneumonia

▶ Sajid A. Haque and Abida Haque

The influenza and parainfluenza viruses primarily infect the respiratory epithelium. Infection in immunocompromised subjects and children may be severe, resulting in DAD. Secondary bacterial infection causes acute necrotizing tracheobronchitis and bronchopneumonia. Influenza virus A and B infections produce the influenza syndrome, whereas parainfluenza infection predominantly causes upper respiratory infection. Squamous metaplasia of airway epithelium is often present in the healing phase. Diagnosis of influenza virus pneumonia requires viral culture.

Histologic Features:

- Classic pathologic finding in severe influenza infection is alveolar epithelial damage, either focal or diffuse, and associated with hyaline membranes.
- Healing phase is characterized by interstitial lymphocytic infiltrate and bronchial epithelial squamous metaplasia.
- No viral inclusions are seen with influenza virus infection.
- Parainfluenza infection is characterized by formation of syncytial giant cells.
- No intranuclear inclusions are present, but small cytoplasmic inclusions may occur.

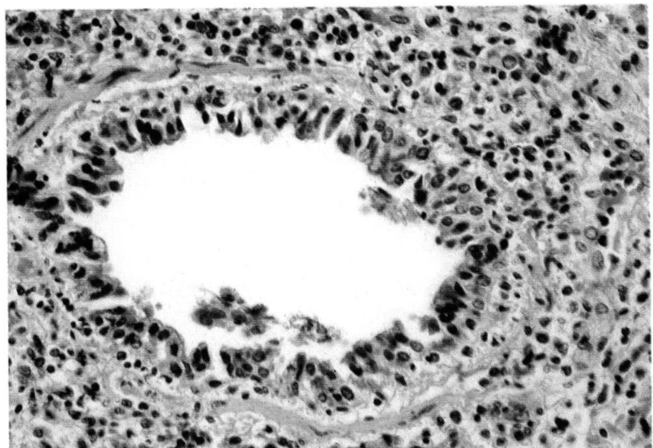

Figure 95.10 Small airway with characteristic pathologic changes of acute inflammation and damage to the lining epithelial cells.

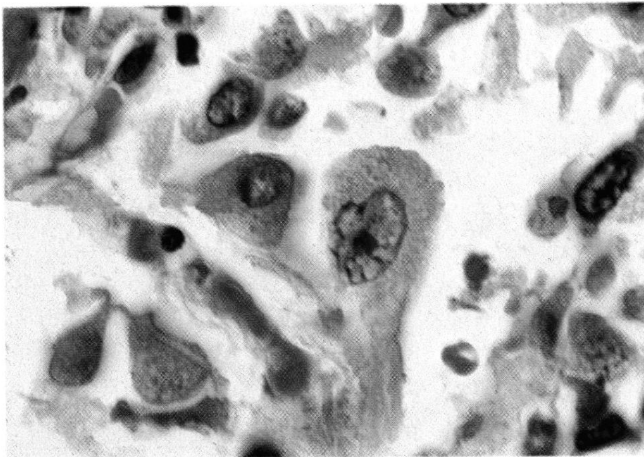

Figure 95.11 Small cytoplasmic inclusions are present in the centrally located large cell, probably a type 2 pneumocyte.

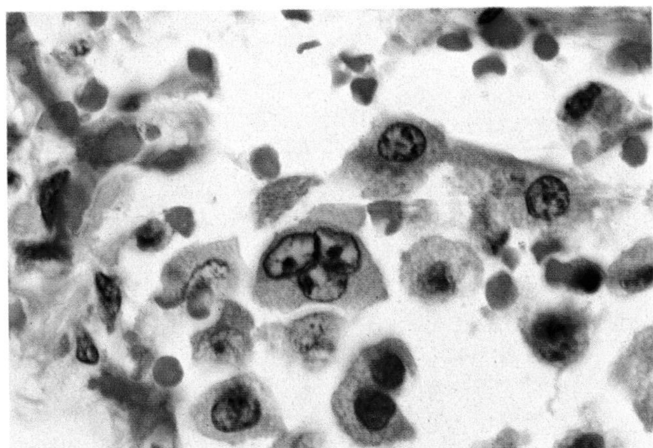

Figure 95.12 Centrally located multinucleated cell with viral cytopathic effect but no clear cytoplasmic inclusions.

Part 4

Adenovirus

▶ Sajid A. Haque and Abida Haque

Adenovirus infection may be seen in both immunocompromised and healthy subjects, particularly in children; however, life-threatening infections are only seen in the former. Two patterns of infection are seen in the lungs. The first pattern shows DAD, with interstitial and alveolar edema, inflammation, and hyaline membranes. The second pattern is a necrotizing bronchopneumonia, with extensive ulceration of the small airways and alveolar neutrophil and macrophage infiltrate associated with fibrinous exudates and necrosis.

Cytologic Features:

- Normal-sized bronchial epithelial cells with ground-glass appearing nucleus.
- Deeply basophilic intranuclear inclusions.

Histologic Features:

- The diagnostic lesion is the characteristic intranuclear viral inclusions, the so-called smudge cells in the airway and alveolar epithelial cells.
- These cells contain large deeply basophilic inclusions with blurring of nuclear membrane.
- Early inclusions are small and amphophilic, surrounded by artifactual halo and peripheralization of chromatin, progressing to larger basophilic inclusions, thus resembling HSV and VZV inclusions.
- Cytomegaly, multinucleated giant cells, and cytoplasmic inclusions are not present.

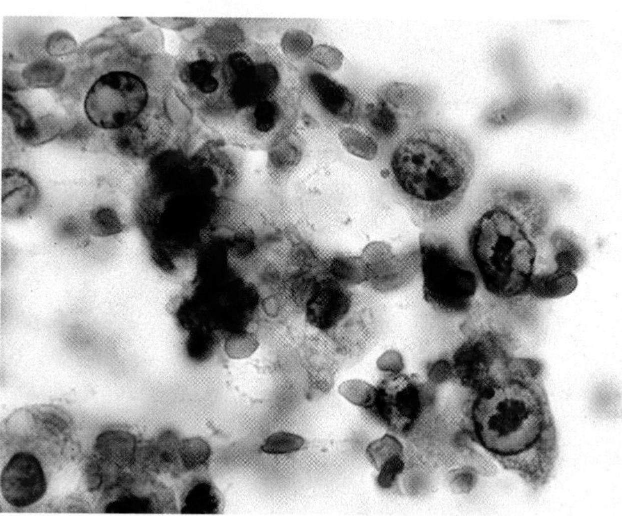

Figure 95.13 Cytology figure showing multiple cells with changes suggestive of early viral cytopathic effect.

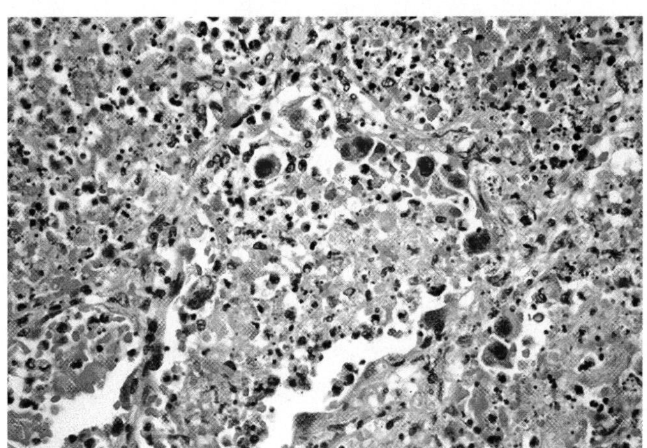

Figure 95.14 Necrotizing bronchopneumonia with several cells showing typical intranuclear inclusions of Adenovirus.

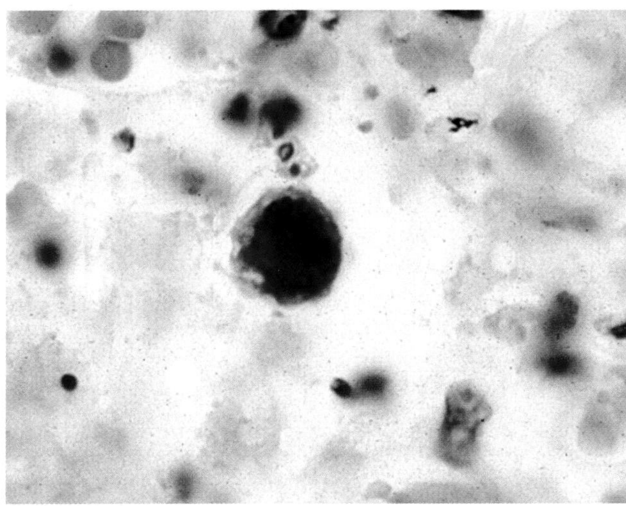

Figure 95.15 Higher power of a cell with deeply basophilic intranuclear inclusion (smudge cell) surrounded by necrotic debris.

Part 5

Respiratory Syncytial Virus

▶ Sajid A. Haque and Abida Haque

RSV infection is a common, self-limited infection in young children presenting as common cold, although almost half of the children develop bronchiolitis or pneumonia. Severe hypoxemia with respiratory failure may develop in children with underlying heart or lung disease. Grossly, the lungs show areas of hyperinflation alternating with areas of consolidation, and bronchial occlusion from mucus.

Histologic Features:

- Bronchi and bronchioles contain epithelial hyperplasia, squamous metaplasia, and obstruction of the lumen with mucus containing cellular debris and inflammatory cells.
- Large multinucleated syncytial cells line the alveolar spaces and, less commonly, the airways.
- Syncytial giant cells contain cytoplasmic inclusions, 1 to 20 μm in diameter, seen as homogenous eosinophilic globules, often in the perinuclear areas.
- Clear halos may surround the smaller inclusions.
- No intranuclear inclusions are seen.
- Mild to moderate mononuclear and neutrophil infiltrate may be seen in the interstitial and peribronchial areas.

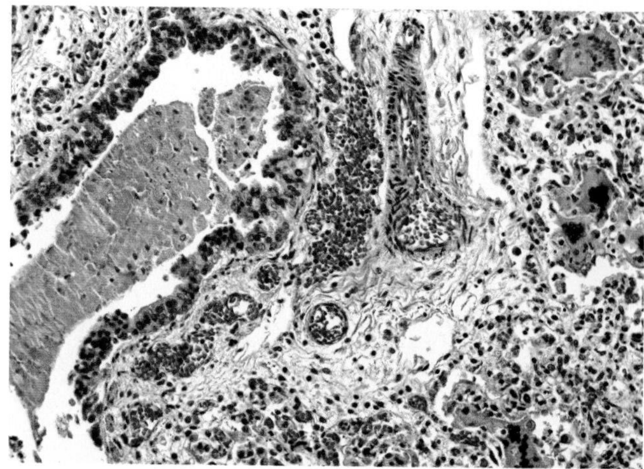

Figure 95.16 Small airway with epithelial inflammation, exudative infiltrate, and multinucleated syncytial giant cells in the surrounding lung parenchyma.

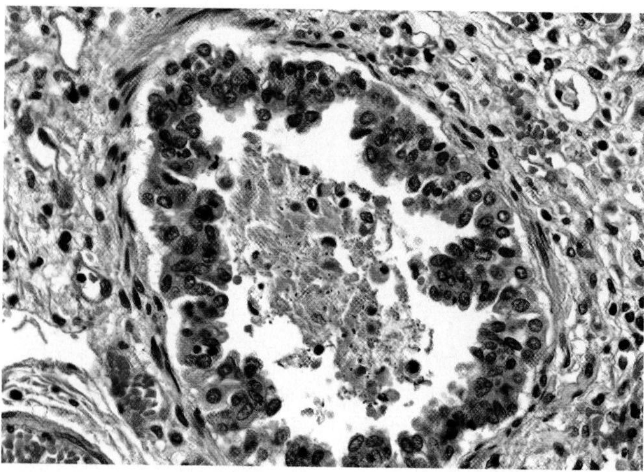

Figure 95.17 Higher power showing hyperplastic and focally necrotic epithelium and necrotic debris in the lumen.

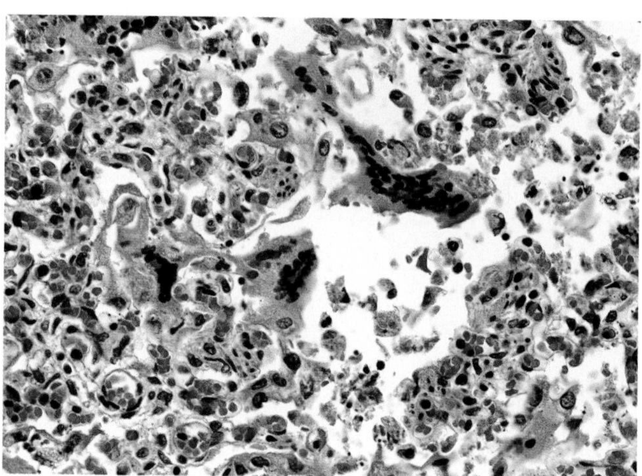

Figure 95.18 Multiple syncytial giant cells associated with exudative inflammation.

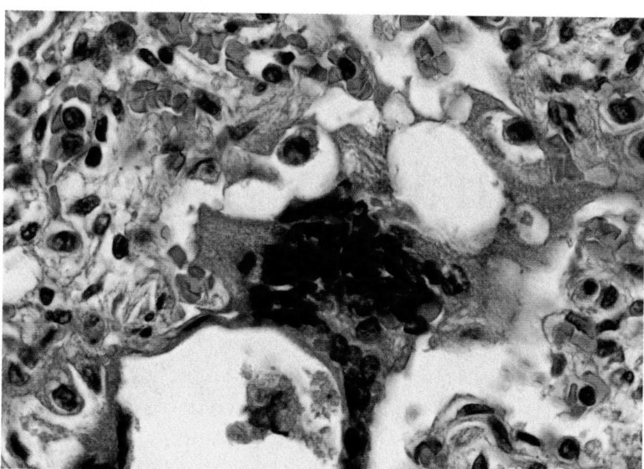

Figure 95.19 Syncytial cell containing many basophilic nuclei and multiple eosinophilic globular homogenous cytoplasmic inclusions; there are no intranuclear inclusions.

Part 6

Measles Virus

Sajid A. Haque and Abida Haque

Measles virus pneumonia may be seen in both healthy and immunocompromised subjects. Patients may show a focal or generalized interstitial pneumonia with interstitial and peribronchial mononuclear infiltrates, squamous metaplasia of airway epithelium, alveolar edema, and pneumocyte hyperplasia. In immunocompromised patients, extensive bronchopneumonia with hemorrhage may be seen. The hallmark of the infection is multinucleated giant cells formed by fusion of bronchiolar or alveolar epithelial cells. Another type of giant cell is seen in reticuloendothelial cells, the Warthin-Finkeldey cell; however, these cells do not have viral inclusions.

Histologic Features:

- Interstitial pneumonia is associated with abundant multinucleated giant cells lining the alveoli or lying free in alveolar spaces.
- Cells contain both intranuclear and cytoplasmic inclusions.
- Intranuclear inclusions are eosinophilic and separated from the surrounding marginated chromatin by indistinct haloes.
- Cytoplasmic inclusions are deeply eosinophilic and vary in size.

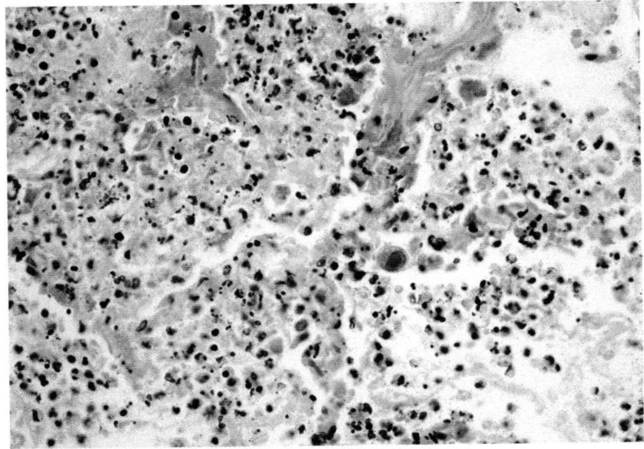

Figure 95.20 Acute necrotizing bronchopneumonia with a few larger cells suggestive of viral cytopathic effect.

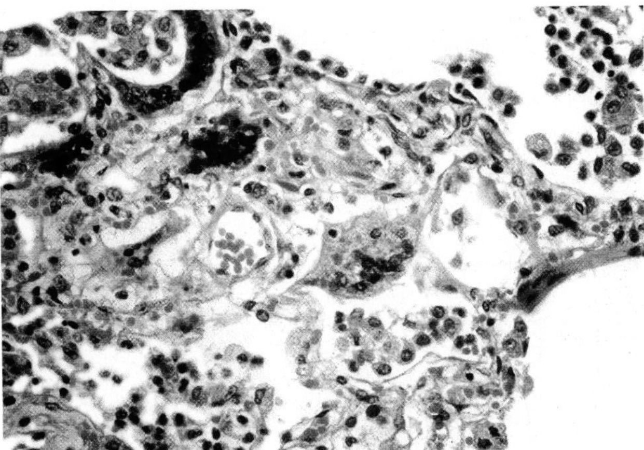

Figure 95.21 Multinucleated giant cells with eosinophilic cytoplasmic inclusions. Intranuclear inclusions also characteristic of measles pneumonia are not obvious. (From R. Tesh, University of Texas Medical Branch, Galveston, Texas, and R. Salas, Instituto Nacional de Higiene, Caracas, Venezuela.)

Part 7

Varicella-Zoster Virus

▶ Sajid A. Haque and Abida Haque

VZV is a ubiquitous virus that causes two distinct clinical infections: varicella (or chicken pox) and herpes zoster (shingles). Adults, immunodeficient patients, and pregnant women are susceptible to varicella pneumonia. VZV is morphologically similar to other herpesviruses.

Histologic Features:

- VZV pneumonia contains multinucleated giant cells and other findings similar to the findings in HSV pneumonia.

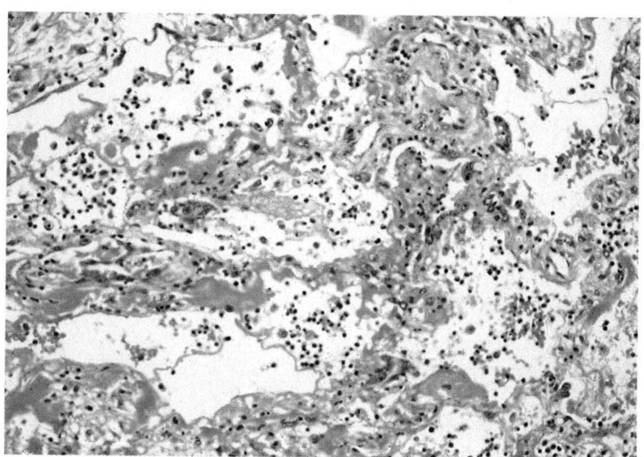

Figure 95.22 DAD with moderate inflammation and a few multinucleated giant cells. (From R. Tesh, University of Texas Medical Branch, Galveston, Texas, and R. Salas, Instituto Nacional de Higiene, Caracas, Venezuela.)

Part 8

Hantavirus

▶ Sajid A. Haque and Abida Haque

Hantaviruses are a group of closely related zoonotic viruses that cause pulmonary and renal infection syndromes. Hantavirus pulmonary syndrome (HPS) is characterized by rapidly progressive pulmonary edema, shock, and high mortality. The pathologic lesions of HPS are primarily vascular, with pulmonary capillary dilation and edema. Pulmonary hemorrhage is exceedingly rare. HPS should be suspected when previously healthy adults develop acute respiratory distress syndrome (ARDS), particularly if they have been exposed to rodents or have traveled to endemic areas.

Histologic Features:

- Mild to moderate interstitial pneumonitis with pulmonary congestion and edema.
- Alveolar mononuclear infiltrate of small and enlarged cells, the latter resembling immunoblasts.
- No inflammation of respiratory epithelium, no alveolar pneumocyte hyperplasia, and neutrophils are absent or scanty.
- In severe and fatal infections, exudative and fibrotic changes of DAD are seen.
- In patients who survive the illness, alveolar pneumocyte hyperplasia is prominent and associated with edema and fibrosis of alveolar septa.

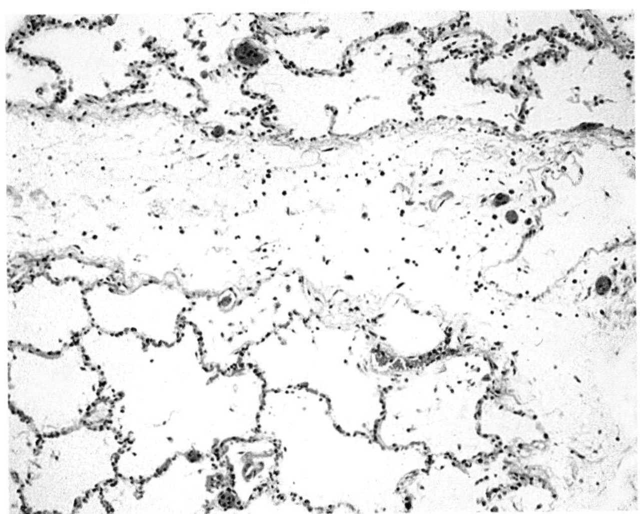

Figure 95.23 Low power showing marked septal edema associated with alveolar capillary congestion and mild alveolar edema. (From R. Tesh, University of Texas Medical Branch, Galveston, Texas, and R. Salas, Instituto Nacional de Higiene, Caracas, Venezuela.)

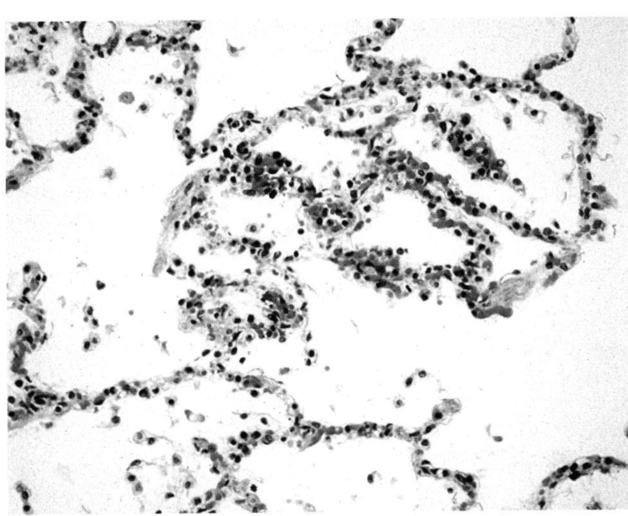

Figure 95.24 Higher power showing mononuclear cell infiltrate in the alveolar septa and capillary congestion, characteristic of HPS. (From R. Tesh, University of Texas Medical Branch, Galveston, Texas, and R. Salas, Instituto Nacional de Higiene, Caracas, Venezuela.)

Part 9

Severe Acute Respiratory Syndrome

▶ Armando Fraire, Daniel Libraty, Florencio Dizon, Remigo M. Olveda, and Bruce A. Woda

First recognized in China in the fall of 2002 as a lethal form of rapidly progressive pneumonia, severe acute respiratory syndrome (SARS) infected more than 8,000 individuals worldwide and killed nearly 800 before the initial outbreak waned in the spring of 2003. An outbreak of eight SARS cases occurred in the Philippine Islands in 2003. Two of the eight patients died early during the course of their disease. The causative agent, the SARS-associated coronavirus (SARS-RoV), is a new member of the family of viruses known as Coronaviridae. The Hong Kong criteria for clinical diagnosis includes contact with a known case, fever greater than 38° C, infiltrates seen on chest x-ray film, and two of the following symptoms: chills, new onset of cough, and malaise. Pathologic study of lungs from SARS patients shows a characteristic picture of DAD, closely resembling sequential time-related changes seen in non–SARS-associated DAD.

Histologic Features:

Major Histopathologic Features (Seen in Early Phases)

- Interstitial and intraalveolar edema.
- Eosinophilic hyaline membranes hugging alveolar wall, some containing neutrophils.
- Sparse mononuclear infiltrates in the interstitium.
- Bronchiolar epithelial denudation and fibrin deposition.

Other Histopathologic Features (Seen Later in the Organizational Phase)

- Loose fibroblastic proliferation.
- Type 2 pneumocyte hyperplasia.
- No evidence of nuclear or cytoplasmic inclusions.
- Multinucleated giant cells.

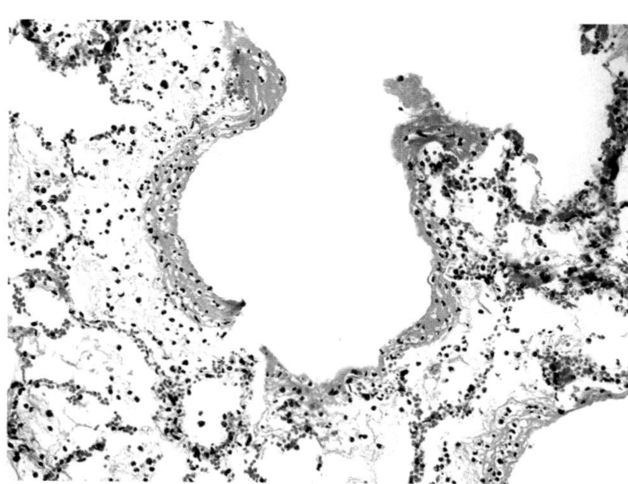

Figure 95.25 Eosinophilic membrane hugging the alveolar walls and acute inflammatory cells within the membrane. (From R. Tesh, University of Texas Medical Branch, Galveston, Texas, and R. Salas, Instituto Nacional de Higiene, Caracas, Venezuela.)

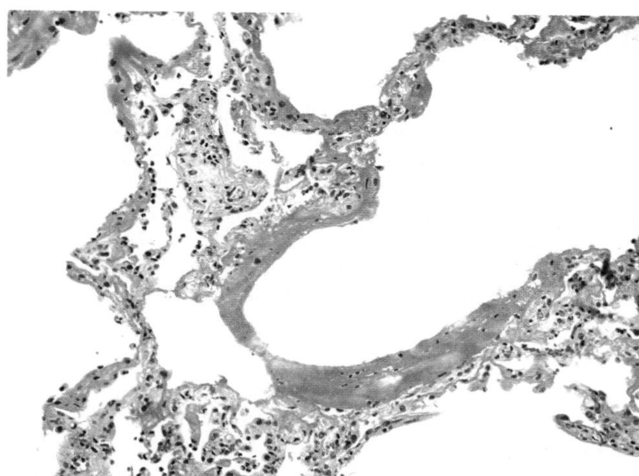

Figure 95.26 PAS stain showing a hyaline membrane with strong PAS positivity, indicating presence of glycoproteins. (From R. Tesh, University of Texas Medical Branch, Galveston, Texas, and R. Salas, Instituto Nacional de Higiene, Caracas, Venezuela.)

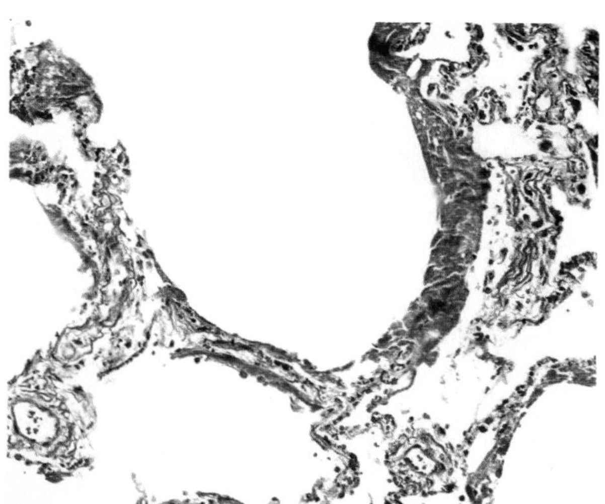

Figure 95.27 Masson trichrome stain of hyaline membrane showing a positive reaction in the membrane and loose collagenous material in the interstitium. (From R. Tesh, University of Texas Medical Branch, Galveston, Texas, and R. Salas, Instituto Nacional de Higiene, Caracas, Venezuela.)

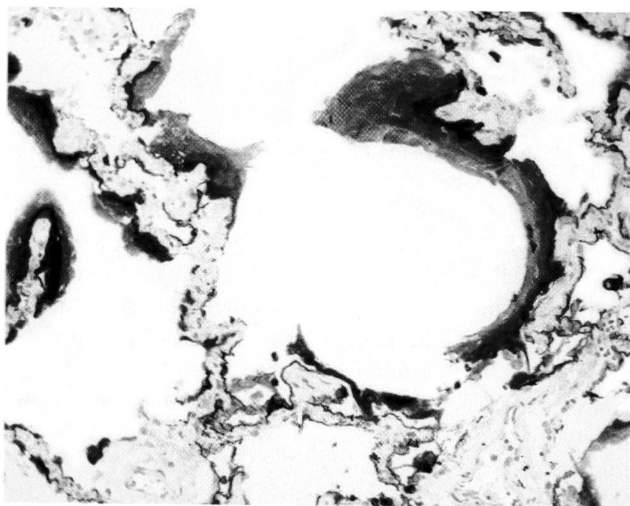

Figure 95.28 Immunohistochemical stain for pan-keratin showing a hyaline membrane with cytokeratin positivity in a membranous pattern and no formed cell elements, indicating that the membranes line bare alveolar walls. (From R. Tesh, University of Texas Medical Branch, Galveston, Texas, and R. Salas, Instituto Nacional de Higiene, Caracas, Venezuela.)

Part 10

Viral Hemorrhagic Fevers

Viral hemorrhagic fevers are acute febrile illnesses caused by a highly virulent group of viruses and associated with microvascular insufficiency and shock, with or without hemorrhage. Infection of macrophages with secretion of cytokines and other inflammatory agents probably plays a critical role in pathogenesis of the widespread vascular damage.

Viral hemorrhagic fevers are caused by at least 15 viruses in four viral families (Arenaviridae, Bunyaviridae, Flaviviridae, Filoviridae). The clinical diseases and pathologic findings vary among the viral hemorrhagic fevers. The Arenavirus hemorrhagic fevers include New World diseases (Argentine hemorrhagic fever, Bolivian hemorrhagic fever, Venezuelan hemorrhagic fever) and Old World diseases (Lassa fever). Examples illustrated here include Venezuelan hemorrhagic fever (Figs. 95.21–95.31) and a flavivirus disease, yellow fever (Figs. 95.32 and 95.33).

Subpart 10.1

Arenavirus Hemorrhagic Fevers

▶ Judith Aronson

The Arenaviridae are a family of viruses that are associated with rodent-transmitted disease in humans. Each of the viruses in this family is associated with a particular rodent species in which it is maintained. They are divided into two groups: the New World hemorrhagic fevers (Argentine, Bolivian, and Venezuelan hemorrhagic fevers) and the Old World hemorrhagic fever (Lassa fever). Human infection occurs when an individual comes into contact with the excretions of an infected rodent through ingestion, inhalation, or direct contact with abraded skin. They cause a syndrome recognized as viral hemorrhagic fever, which is characterized by fever, prostration, and generalized signs of increased vascular permeability.

Histologic Features:

- Fibrin microthrombi in capillaries are typical of New World hemorrhagic fevers.
- Hyaline membranes with DAD (present in one third of cases).
- Mononuclear interstitial pneumonitis may be seen.
- Pulmonary hemorrhage may be seen, particularly in New World Arenavirus hemorrhagic fevers; it is less common in Lassa fever.
- Bronchopneumonia is frequently seen, due to secondary bacterial infection.
- Immunohistochemistry demonstrates viral antigens in endothelial cells, pleural mesothelium, alveolar macrophages, and bronchial epithelium.

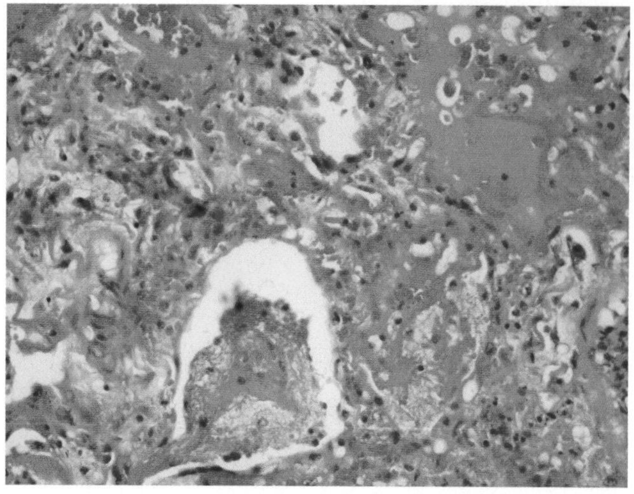

Figure 95.29 Venezuelan hemorrhagic fever with alveolar spaces filled with fibrin and hemorrhage and congested septal capillaries with fibrin microthrombi. (From R. Tesh, University of Texas Medical Branch, Galveston, Texas, and R. Salas, Instituto Nacional de Higiene, Caracas, Venezuela.)

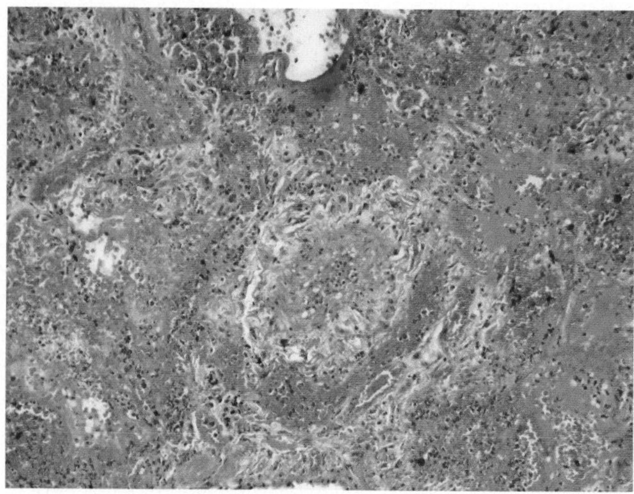

Figure 95.30 Venezuelan hemorrhagic fever with alveolar spaces filled with fibrin and hemorrhage with a thickened vessel. (From R. Tesh, University of Texas Medical Branch, Galveston, Texas, and R. Salas, Instituto Nacional de Higiene, Caracas, Venezuela.)

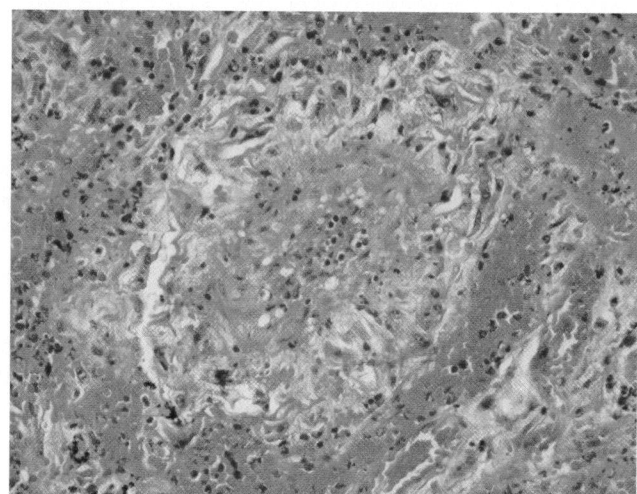

Figure 95.31 Higher power showing thrombosis and marginating neutrophils. (From R. Tesh, University of Texas Medical Branch, Galveston, Texas, and R. Salas, Instituto Nacional de Higiene, Caracas, Venezuela.)

Subpart 10.2

Yellow Fever

▶ Judith Aronson

A virus of the Flaviviridae family causes yellow fever. It is seen more frequently in tropical Africa and South America. The major pathology ascribed to yellow fever is in the liver and reticuloendothelial organs. It is associated with jaundice and hematemesis, and patients usually die of a syndrome comparable to hepatorenal syndrome. The lungs are not generally involved, but lung involvement has been described.

Histologic Features:

- Pulmonary hemorrhage is present, reflecting the severe hemorrhagic diathesis.
- DAD with hyaline membranes is often present.
- Bronchopneumonia may be present.

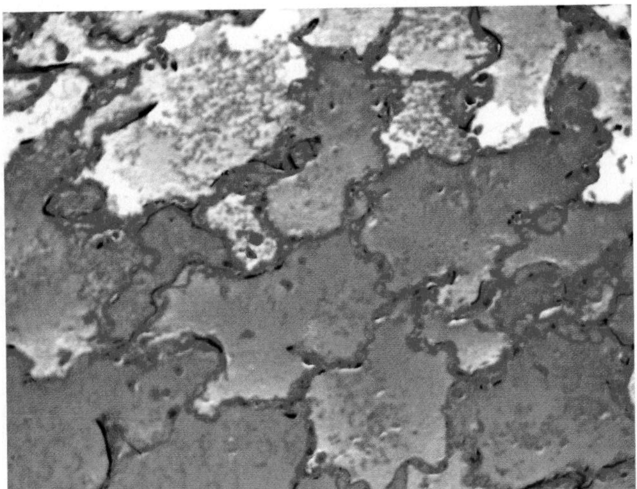

Figure 95.32 Yellow fever with diffuse alveolar edema and hemorrhage. (From D. Watts and R. Tesh, University of Texas Medical Branch, Galveston, Texas.)

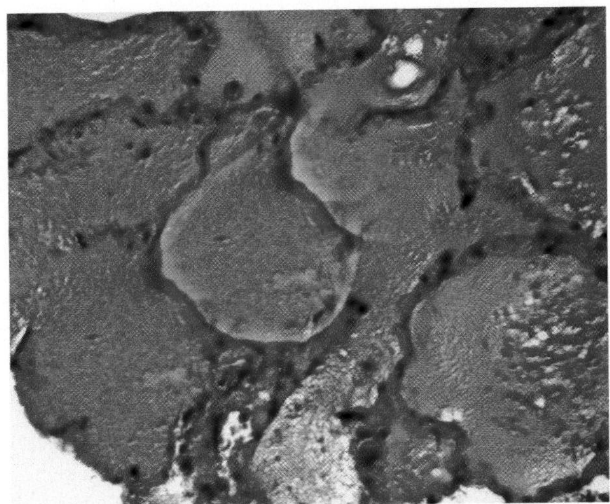

Figure 95.33 Higher power of yellow fever showing diffuse alveolar edema and hemorrhage. (From D. Watts and R. Tesh, University of Texas Medical Branch, Galveston, Texas.)

96 Mycoplasma

▸ Alvaro C. Laga
▸ Philip T. Cagle

Mycoplasma pneumoniae infection is typically a disease of otherwise healthy adolescents and adults and is a common pathogen in this population. Approximately 20% of infections are asymptomatic. The majority of symptomatic infections present as mild upper respiratory tract infections or tracheobronchitis. Only 5% of infections result in pneumonia. The usual clinical symptoms include fever, sore throat, cough, chills, headache, and malaise. The symptoms are often disproportionately compared to the radiologic findings. Few cases are biopsied. Acute bronchiolitis may be seen. Mycoplasma is in the differential diagnosis of organizing pneumonia formerly known as bronchiolitis obliterans organizing pneumonia (BOOP).

Histologic Features:

- Organizing pneumonia.
- Acute bronchiolitis.

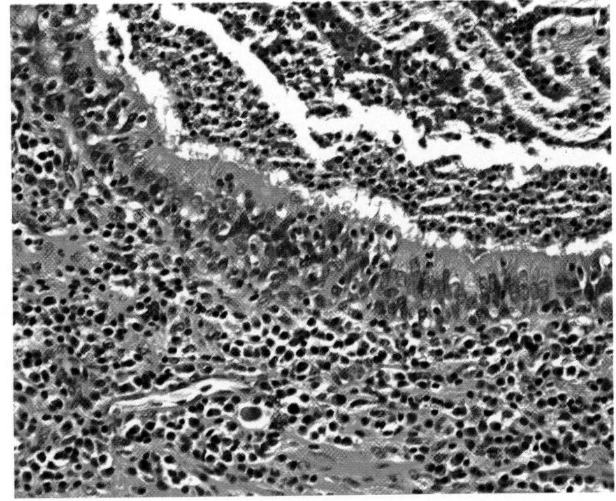

Figure 96.1 Mycoplasma infection with acute bronchiolitis showing a peribronchiolar infiltrate of lymphocytes and plasma cells.

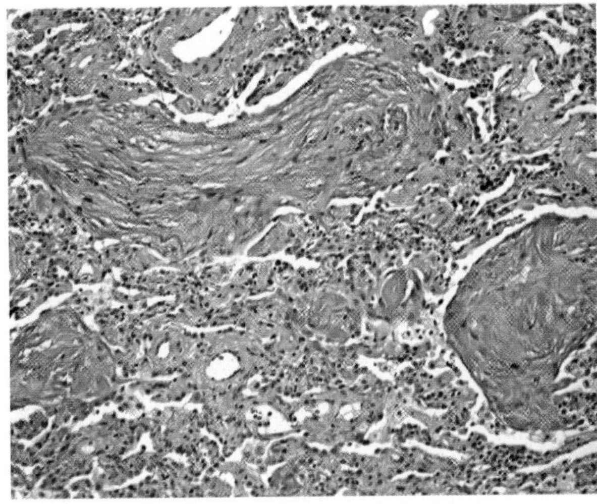

Figure 96.2 Organizing pneumonia associated with Mycoplasma infection.

97

Bacteria

Bacterial pneumonia may be primary within the lung or may be secondary to hematogenous dissemination from bacterial infection at another site. The virulence of the bacteria, host immunity, and other factors determine the pathology of bacterial pneumonias.

Part 1

Pseudomonas

▶ Alvaro C. Laga and Abida Haque

Pseudomonas sp. are Gram-negative bacilli. They tend to be thin and long compared to the shorter, fatter Enterobacteriaceae. *Pseudomonas aeruginosa* is the most virulent species of the genus and the predominant isolate in clinical laboratories. This microorganism produces powerful exoenzymes, including proteases and elastases that result in tissue destruction. Consequently, the hallmarks of *Pseudomonas* infection are hemorrhage, necrosis, and abscess formation. It may cause pneumonia by two different mechanisms: (i) aspiration of oral contents in the nosocomial setting, when patients change the oral flora to Gram-negative species, and (ii) secondary spread to the lungs from distant foci through the bloodstream. Macroscopic lesions may present as firm, yellow-brown or tan necrotic nodules, often sharply delimited from the surrounding tissue.

Histologic Features:

- Mixed inflammatory infiltrate composed of lymphocytes, macrophages, and neutrophils.
- Necrosis, vasculitis, and abscess formation can be often seen.
- Gram-negative bacilli may be observed on the adventitial surface of blood vessels.

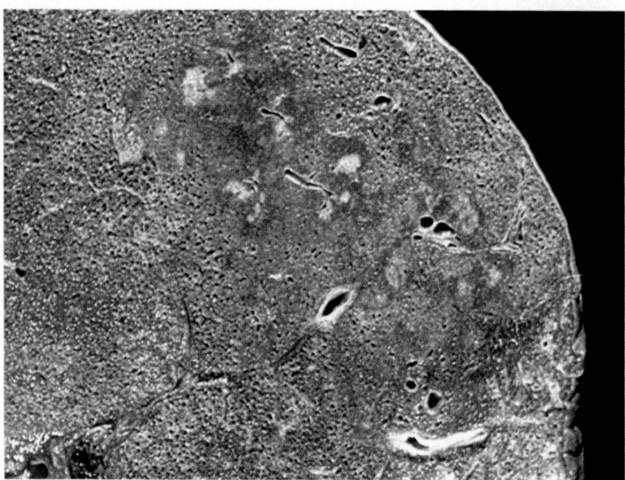

Figure 97.1 *Pseudomonas aeruginosa* pneumonia. Multiple well-defined yellow-brown nodules within the lung parenchyma are seen in this case.

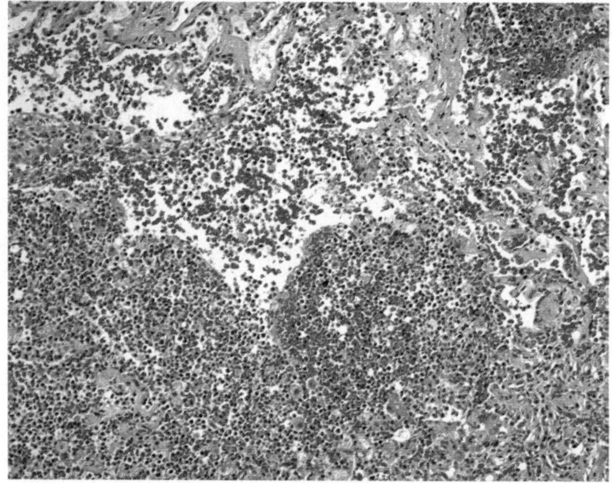

Figure 97.2 *Pseudomonas aeruginosa* pneumonia. Intense inflammatory infiltrate with destruction of alveolar septa and hemorrhage.

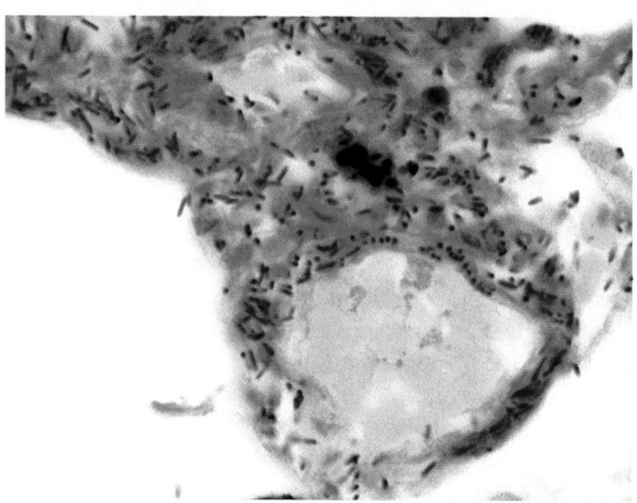

Figure 97.3 *Pseudomonas aeruginosa* pneumonia. Long and thin Gram-negative bacilli are seen surrounding blood vessels.

Part 2

Klebsiella Pneumonia

▶ Abida Haque

Klebsiella pneumoniae are Gram-negative, nonmotile bacilli, approximately 6 μm in length and 0.6 μm in width, and an important component of normal gastrointestinal flora. *K. pneumoniae* is also an important cause of community-acquired pneumonia, particularly in patients with diabetes mellitus, alcoholism, and chronic obstructive pulmonary disease.

Histologic Features:

- The acute pneumonia may be patchy or lobar; although there is consolidation in early stages, the later stages are associated with necrosis and abscess formation.

- Neutrophil infiltrates fill the alveoli in the acute stage, followed later by macrophages.
- Healing is often associated with formation of scars.
- The bacilli have a polysaccharide mucoid capsule, giving rise to mucoid colonies on agar, and a mucoid/gelatinous appearance to the consolidated areas.
- The bacilli are blackened and easily visible with silver stains [Gomori methenamine silver (GMS)].
- Pulmonary gangrene is a rare complication.

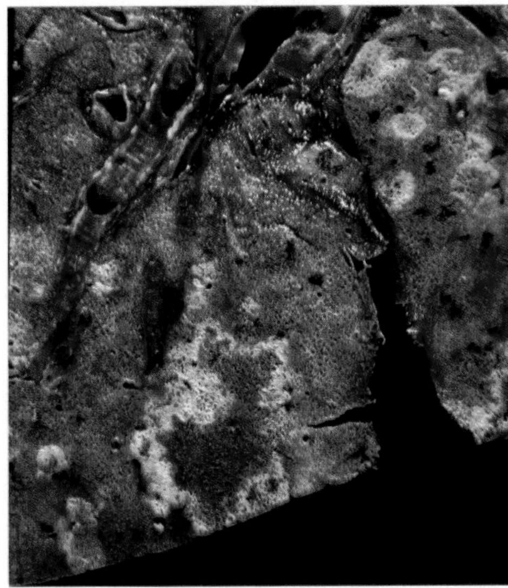

Figure 97.4 Gross figure shows areas of bronchopneumonia with a gelatinous center and pale tan borders due to the mucoid exudate produced by *K. pneumoniae* capsules.

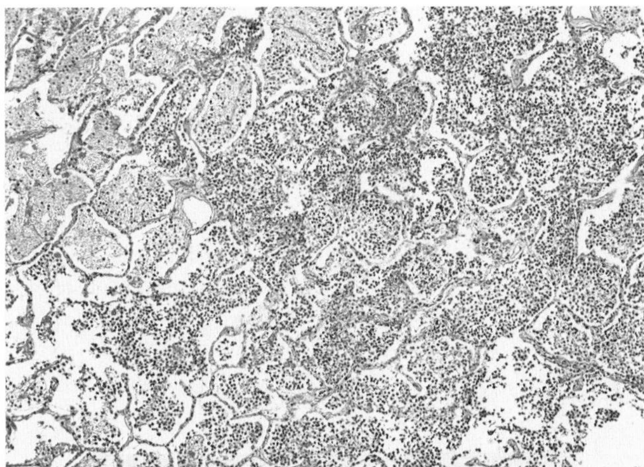

Figure 97.5 Bronchopneumonia with alveolar fibrinous exudates mixed with extensive inflammatory infiltrate. In the early stage of infection, neutrophils predominate in the infiltrate, mixed with a few macrophages and, later, a macrophage response may be seen.

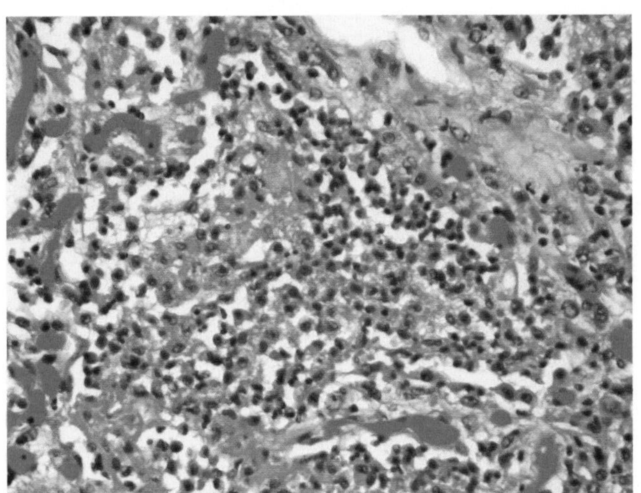

Figure 97.6 Higher power shows extensive inflammatory infiltrate and fibrin.

Part 3

Staphylococcus

▶ Abida Haque

Staphylococci colonize the skin, anterior nasal cavity, and sometimes the gastrointestinal tract of healthy individuals, resulting in 20% to 40% of the population becoming a carrier. Staphylococcal pneumonia may result from aspiration of oropharyngeal secretions or as a complication of viral pneumonia. The characteristic feature of infection is early necrosis and abscess formation, which may extend to the pleura, resulting in empyema.

Histologic Features:

- The abscess contains clusters of hematoxyphil-staining, Gram-positive bacteria, often in clusters.
- The bacterial colonies may be surrounded by an acellular eosinophilic matrix rich in immunoglobulins (Splendore-Hoeppli phenomena), also called a *botryomycotic abscess.*

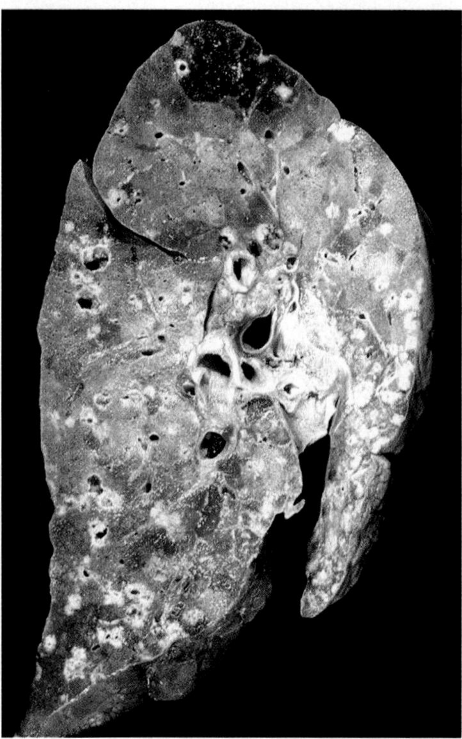

Figure 97.7 Gross figure shows extensive bronchopneumonia from hematogenous spread from an abdominal staphylococcus abscess. Central necrosis may be present in some of the areas of consolidation, a characteristic of staphylococcal infection.

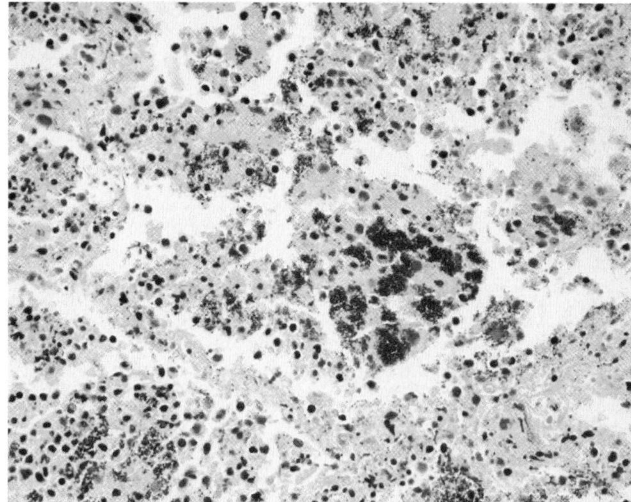

Figure 97.8 Clusters of hematoxyphil-staining bacteria within inflammatory infiltrate in alveolar spaces.

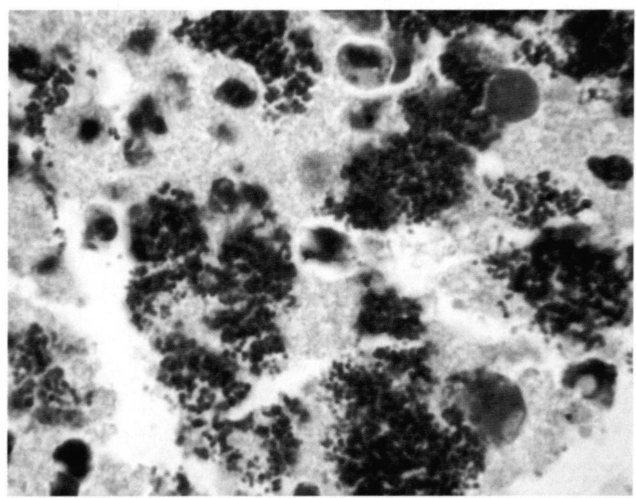

Figure 97.9 Higher power of bacteria mixed with necrotic debris and macrophages.

Part **4**

Nocardia

▶ Abida Haque

Nocardiosis of the lung is caused by infection with the bacteria *Nocardia* sp. Approximately 500 to 1,000 new cases of nocardiosis are diagnosed each year in the United States. *Nocardia* are aerobic, Gram-positive bacilli with a filamentous, beaded morphology. Pulmonary infection is usually acquired through inhalation of saprophytic organisms in the soil or decaying vegetable matter. Rarely, the organisms may reach the lungs via the bloodstream from indwelling catheters. Pneumonia is caused most often by *N. asteroids, N. brasiliensis,* and *N. otitidiscaviarum* (previously N. caviae). Rarely, *N. transvalensis, N. nova,* or *N. farcinica* causes pneumonia. The definitive diagnosis is established by culture of lung biopsy tissue or bronchoalveolar lavage fluid. Direct examination of respiratory specimens, including sputum, with the Gram or Fite stains is also useful.

Histologic Features:

- Multiple abscesses, which may be confluent with occasional cavitation.
- Extensive necrosis.
- Numerous neutrophils with microabscess formation.
- Chronic cases may contain multinucleated giant cells.
- Organisms are seen within the areas of necrosis and suppuration but are difficult to see on hematoxylin and eosin stains.
- Rarely, *Nocardia* sp. forms "fungus balls" (such as aspergillus) within preexisting cavities.
- Alveolar proteinosis may be associated with *Nocardia* pulmonary infection.
- *Nocardia* consists of long, thin, beaded, bacterial filaments measuring approximately 1 µm in thickness.
- Microorganisms branch at right angles in a manner referred to as a *Chinese character pattern.*
- Organisms can be demonstrated with GMS, Brown-Brenn, and Brown-Hopps stains; it is weakly acid fast.

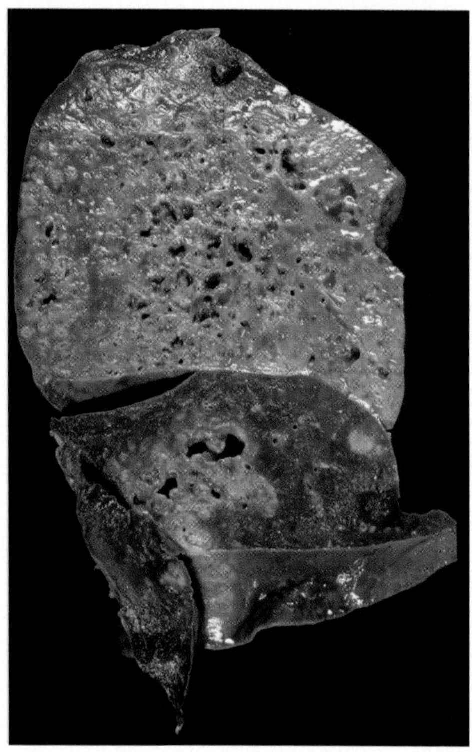

Figure 97.10 Gross figure of *Nocardia* infection showing consolidation and abscess formation.

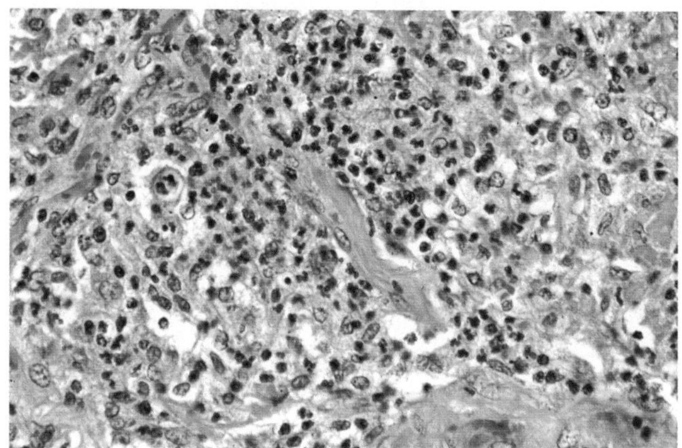

Figure 97.11 Numerous neutrophils forming a microabscess, characteristic of *Nocardia* infection.

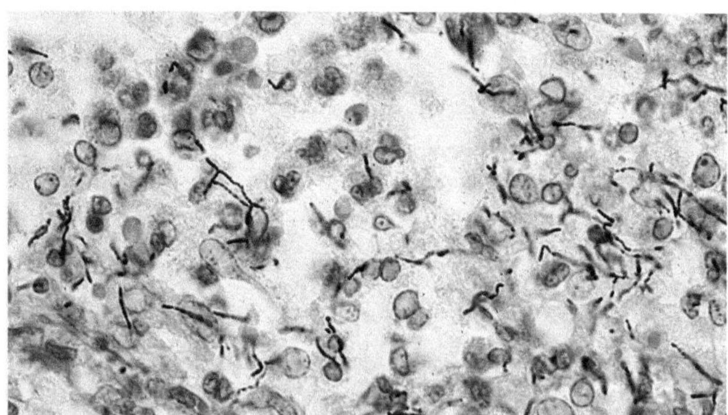

Figure 97.12 Higher power of *Nocardia* organisms showing typical branching Chinese character pattern.

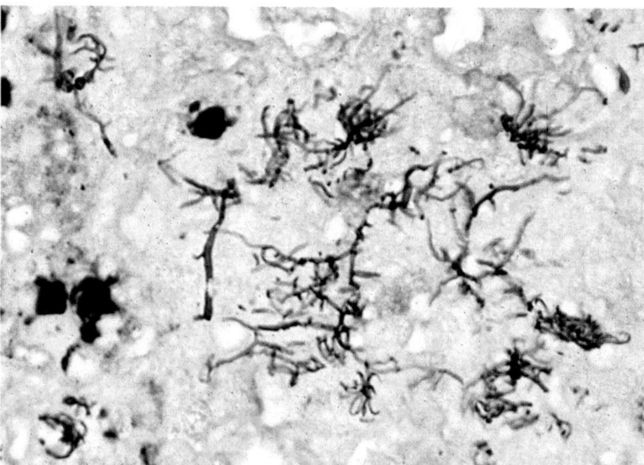

Figure 97.13 GMS stain shows *Nocardia* organisms with characteristic Chinese letter pattern.

Part 5

Actinomyces

▶ Abida Haque

Actinomyces are anaerobic or microaerophilic filamentous bacteria, commensal in the oropharynx, vagina, and gastrointestinal tract of healthy people, which cause endogenous infection. There is no increased incidence of infection in immunocompromised individuals. Thoracic actinomycosis is caused by aspiration of oropharyngeal contents.

Histologic Features:

- The characteristic histologic lesion is an abscess with one or more actinomycotic granules in the center of the abscess.
- The granules consist of aggregates of delicate, filamentous, branching, amphophilic, often beaded bacteria, measuring 1.0 μm in width.
- The filaments at the periphery of the granules are radially oriented and covered with fingerlike, deeply eosinophilic Splendore-Hoeppli material.
- The granules are surrounded by neutrophils and represent the "sulfur granules" seen in the draining actinomycotic sinuses.
- Actinomyces are Gram positive (Brown-Brenn) and acid-fast negative; they stain with silver stains.
- Gram-stained smears of the sulfur granules show the filamentous bacteria with right-angled branching pattern and beading.
- Culture and immunofluorescent antibody may be useful in confirming the diagnosis.

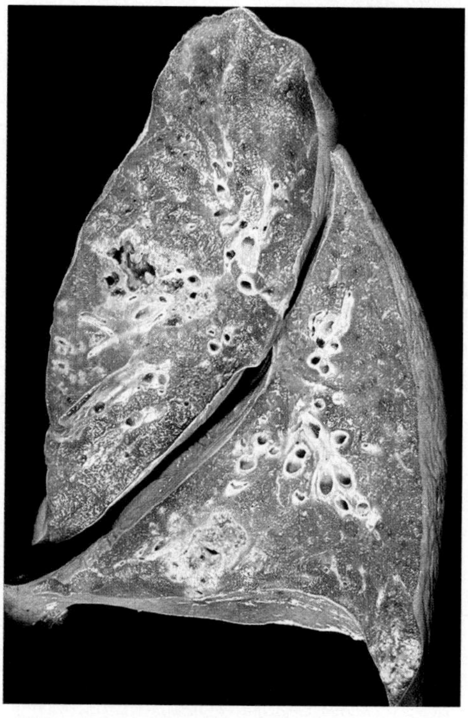

Figure 97.14 Gross figure showing multiple areas of confluent bronchopneumonia, some with central abscesses.

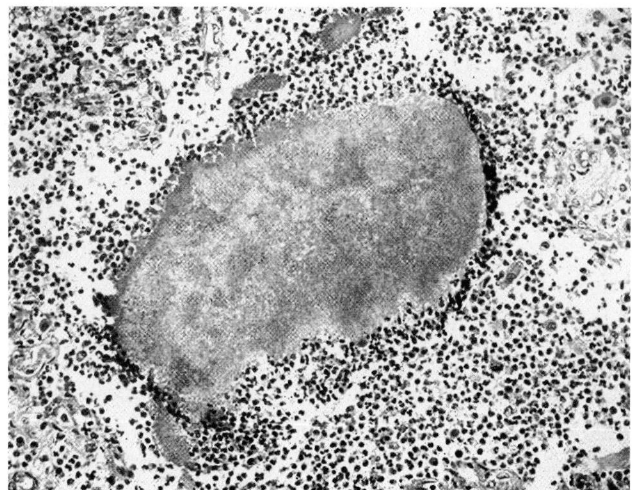

Figure 97.15 Characteristic granule with central aggregate of the bacteria surrounded by deeply eosinophilic Splendore-Hoeppli material.

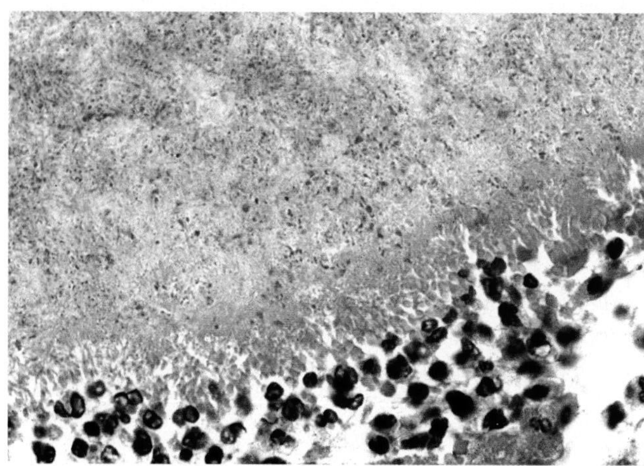

Figure 97.16 Higher magnification showing delicate, filamentous amphophilic, branching bacteria in the center and radially oriented filaments covered with deeply eosinophilic fingerlike material at the periphery.

Part 6

Legionella

▶ Abida Haque

Legionella pneumophila are aerobic, Gram-negative bacilli, with a ubiquitous aquatic distribution, particularly in water reservoirs. The pulmonary infection is often associated with symptoms of gastrointestinal and cerebral involvement and often serum electrolyte abnormalities. The bacilli are 0.3 to 1.0 μm wide and 2.5 μm long, and are facultative intracellular organisms that proliferate in phagocytic cells. The lungs are consolidated and firm and have focal necrosis.

Histologic Features:

- The alveoli are filled with fibrin and sheets of macrophages and neutrophils.
- Progression of disease may result in confluent and multilobar consolidation, followed by abscess formation.
- Silver stains, such as Steiner, Dieterle, or Warthin-Starry, are very useful for demonstration of the bacteria.
- Modified Brown-Hopps stain also may be used, although the organisms are weakly Gram negative and weakly acid fast.
- Immunoperoxidase and immunofluorescent stains are quite sensitive and may be used on paraffin blocks.
- Electron microscopy may be useful in some cases to identify the organism.

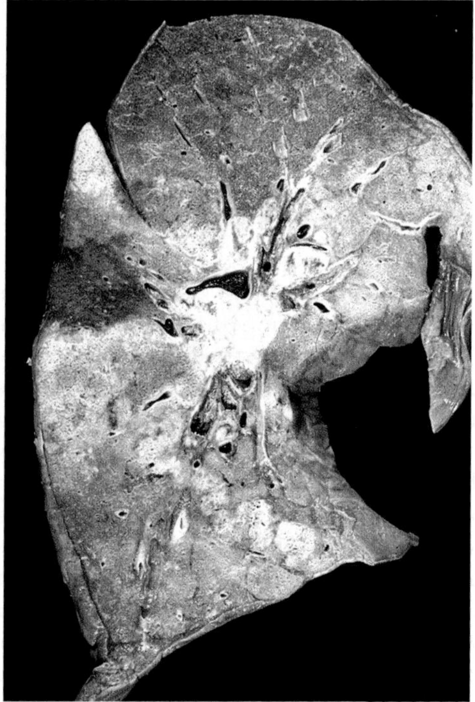

Figure 97.17 Gross figure shows multiple areas of confluent bronchopneumonia.

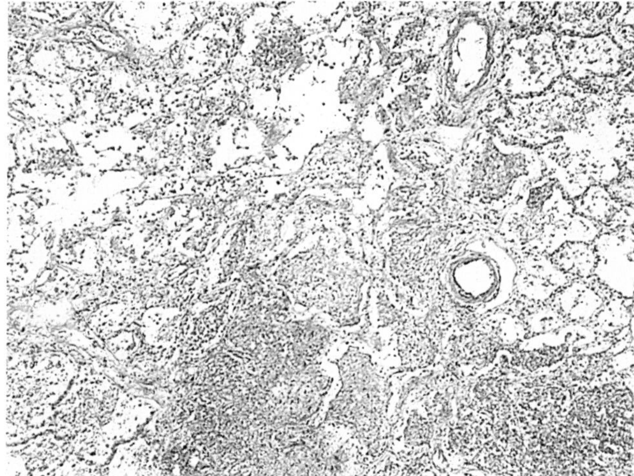

Figure 97.18 Extensive alveolar macrophage infiltrate with some neutrophils.

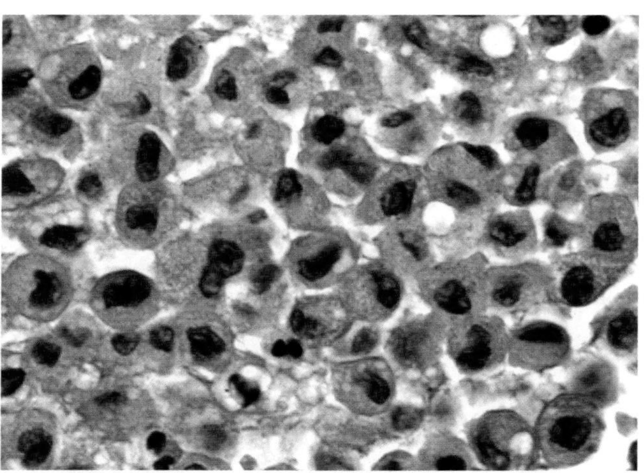

Figure 97.19 Higher power shows alveolar macrophage infiltrates.

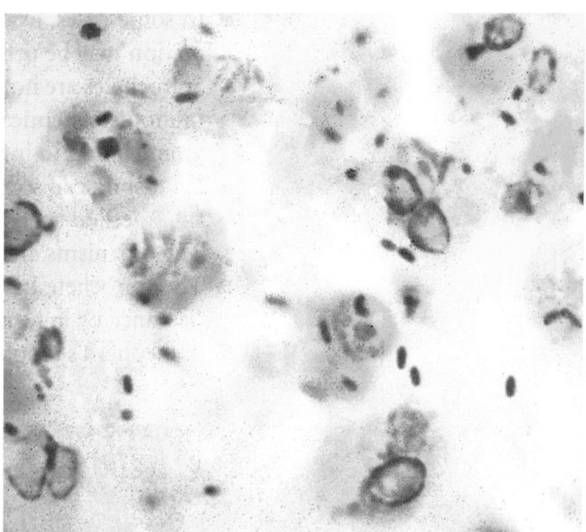

Figure 97.20 Silver (Dieterle) stain shows intracellular coccobacilli.

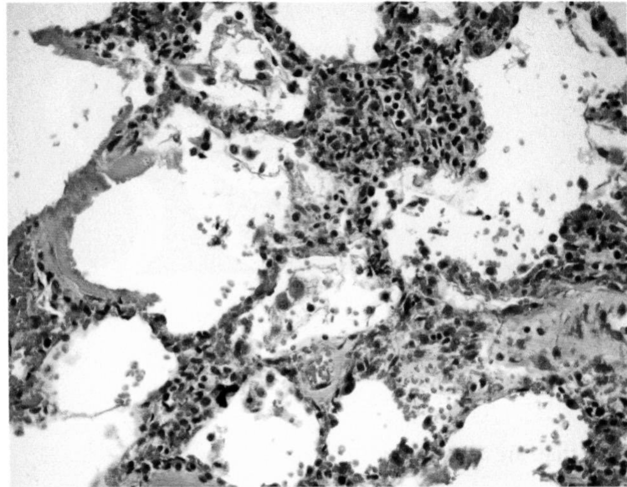

Figure 98.1 Abundant mononuclear cells in the interstitial compartment and hyaline membranes lining one alveolar septum, from a fatal case of Rocky Mountain spotted fever.

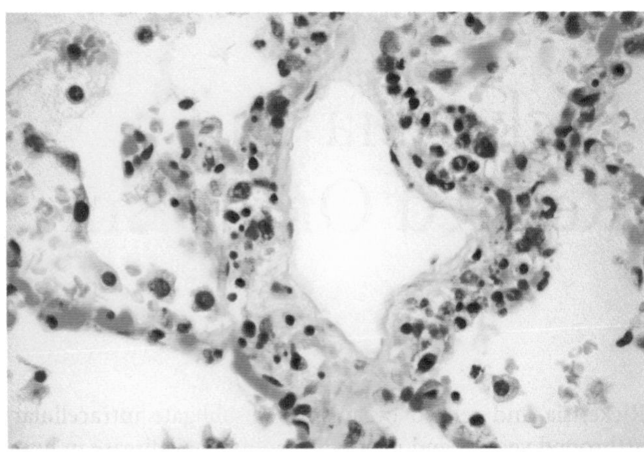

Figure 98.2 Higher power showing lymphocytes and macrophages in the interstitial compartment.

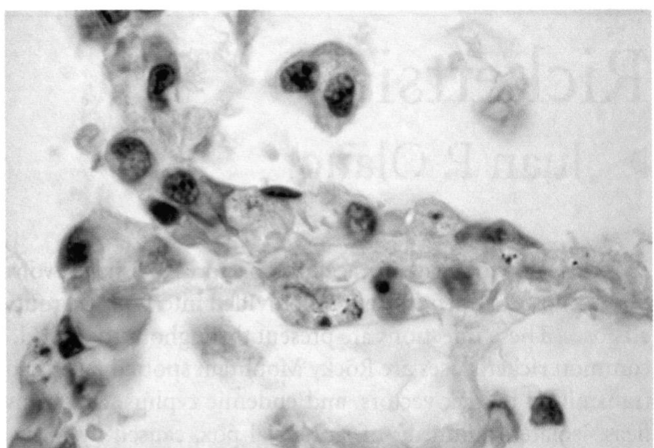

Figure 98.3 Immunostain with rabbit polyclonal antibody against *Rickettsia conorii* showing intracytoplasmic coccobacilli present within endothelial cells lining the capillary vessels of the alveolar septa.

Part 2

Ehrlichia

▶ Juan P. Olano

Ehrlichiae are obligate intracellular organisms that have evolved in association with an arthropod vector. Ehrlichiae have been known mostly as veterinary pathogens. Human ehrlichiosis was described for the first time in 1987. Three forms of human disease have been described to date in this country: human monocytotropic ehrlichiosis (HME) (caused by *Ehrlichia chaffeensis* and transmitted by ticks), human granulocytotropic anaplasmosis (formerly known as human granulocytotropic ehrlichiosis, caused by Anaplasma phagocytophilum), and an unnamed granulocytropic ehrlichiosis (caused by *Ehrlichia ewingii*) that affects mostly immunocompromised patients.

E. chaffeensis targets cells of the mononuclear phagocytic system; *A. phagocytophilum* and *E. ewingii* target polymorphonuclear neutrophils. Clinically, these infections are multisystemic, targeting the lungs, liver, and spleen. Central nervous system involvement is more common in *E. chaffeensis* infections.

Histologic Features:

- Ehrlichiae are small (0.2–1.0 μm), pleomorphic, coccoid, Gram-negative, cell-walled bacteria.
- Lungs show interstitial pneumonitis, perivasculitis, alveolar edema/hemorrhage, and diffuse alveolar damage.
- Intracytoplasmic aggregates of bacteria (seen by immunoperoxidase or immunofluorescence) in intravascular monocytes or tissue macrophages (*E. chaffeensis infections*) or neutrophils (*A. phagocytophilum* and *E. ewingii* infections).

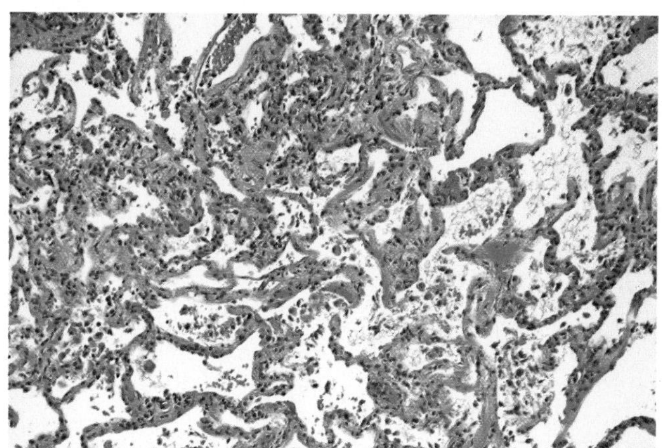

Figure 98.4 Widened and markedly congested alveolar septa with interstitial inflammatory cells, mainly lymphocytes and macrophages, in a fatal case of HME.

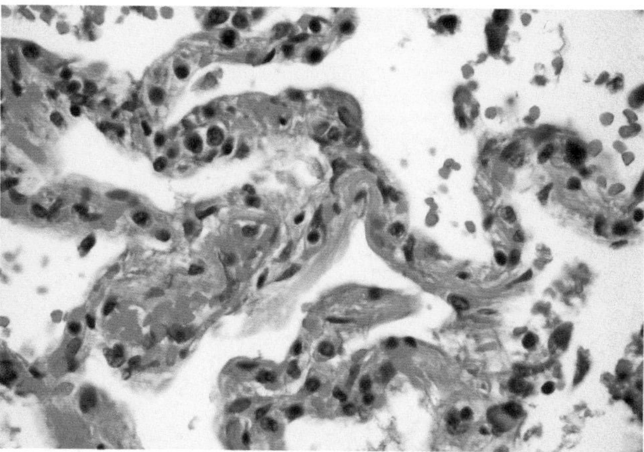

Figure 98.5 Higher power showing macrophages and lymphocytes in the alveolar septa, both intravascularly and extravascularly.

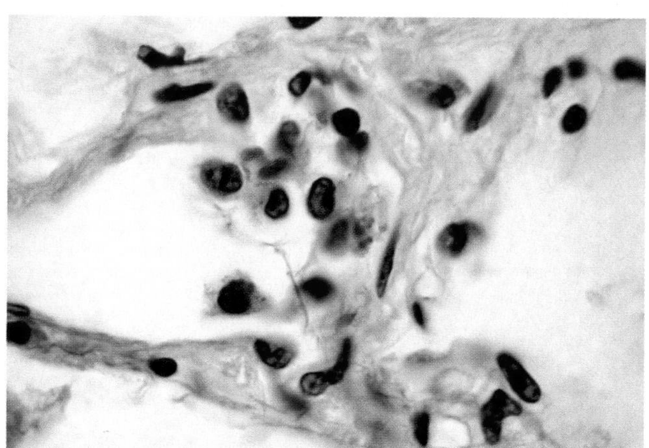

Figure 98.6 Immunostain with rabbit polyclonal antibody against *E. chaffeensis* showing intracytoplasmic *Ehrlichia* within macrophages both in the alveolar space and septa. These structures correspond to the so-called *morules* seen in Giemsa preparations; these morules represent multiple ehrlichial organisms contained in a single cytoplasmic vacuole.

99

Fungus

Pulmonary fungal infections may be endemic or opportunistic. The truly pathogenic (endemic) fungi may infect healthy as well as immunocompromised hosts, whereas the opportunistic fungi usually infect immunocompromised hosts only. Fungal infections are acquired by inhalation of contaminated soil or, less commonly, through a hematogenous route from other infected foci in the body. Once in the lung, the fungi may elicit either an acute exudative reaction or a granulomatous reaction. Depending on the immunocompetence of the host and the pathogenicity of the fungus, the pulmonary lesions may resolve, progress to chronic inflammation, or disseminate systemically.

Diagnosis of fungal infections depends on demonstration of the fungi by histology and culture. Although fungi are often visible on hematoxylin and eosin (H&E)-stained sections, special stains such as Gomori methenamine silver (GMS) or periodic acid–Schiff (PAS) reagent, is often needed for screening and studying the morphologic details. Culture is required for confirmation of diagnosis. Histologically, almost all fungal infections have granulomas with or without a necrotic center, surrounded by lymphocytes, histiocytes, and multinucleated giant cells, with varying degrees of fibrosis in the chronic stage of infection.

Part 1

Aspergillus

▶ Abida Haque

The *Aspergillus* genus has hundreds of species, although three species are most frequently pathogenic: *A. fumigatus, A. flavus,* and *A. niger.* Several forms of pulmonary aspergillosis are seen: surface colonization of bronchial mucosa, formation of aspergilloma (fungus ball) in preexisting cavities, allergic aspergillosis in asthmatics, chronic necrotizing aspergillosis in mildly immunocompromised individuals, and invasive pulmonary aspergillosis in severely immunocompromised individuals.

Invasive aspergillosis is the most aggressive form of *Aspergillus* infection. The early lesions show intense neutrophil response and necrosis, often associated with acute vasculitis, hemorrhage, infarction with formation of targetoid lesions, and cavitation. Occasionally, fungal hyphae are associated with oxalate crystals.

Histologic Features:

- Hyphae are homogenous, uniform, septate, 3 to 6 μm in width, and have parallel contours, with a dichotomous, acute-angle (45-degree) branching.
- The hyphae are basophilic but may appear eosinophilic when degenerated.

- Conidial heads are rare, except when the hyphae are exposed to air as in aspergillomas.
- Aspergilloma is a fungus ball formed by concentric layers of mycelium within a preformed cavity.
- The center of the fungus ball has degenerated hyphae that are swollen and show prominent vesicles.
- Conidial heads may be seen on the surface and oxalate crystals in the fungus ball.
- Necrotizing bronchial aspergillosis is characterized by a pseudomembrane of inflammatory exudates mixed with mucus, inflammatory cells, and abundant hyphae.
- The hyphae often invade and destroy the bronchial wall, but no vascular invasion is present.
- Invasive pulmonary aspergillosis is characterized by vascular invasion and occlusion with a nodular pulmonary infarction.

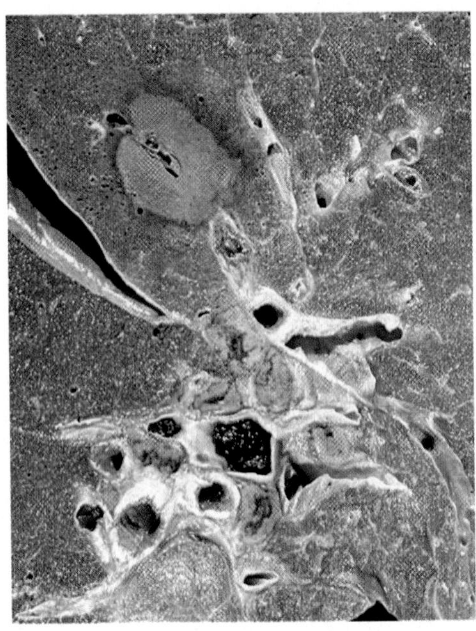

Figure 99.1 Gross figure showing a round area of infarct with a central partially thrombosed vessel characteristic of *Aspergillus* infarct.

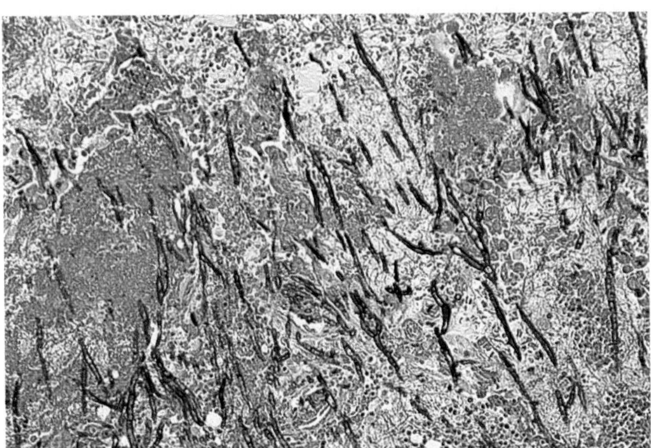

Figure 99.2 Center of the infarct with acutely branching septate hyphae diagnostic of *Aspergillus* sp.

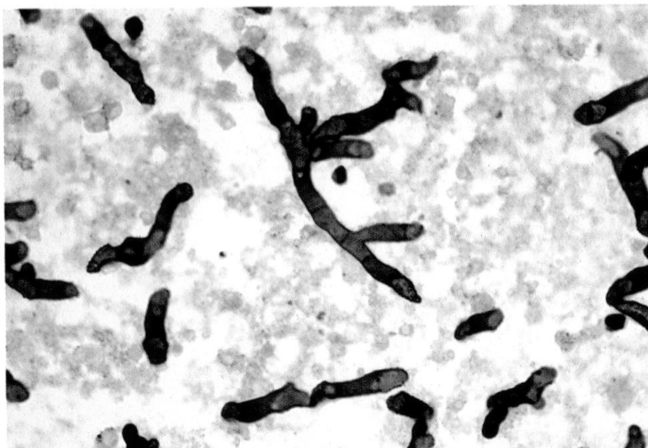

Figure 99.3 GMS stain showing higher power of acutely branching septate hyphae.

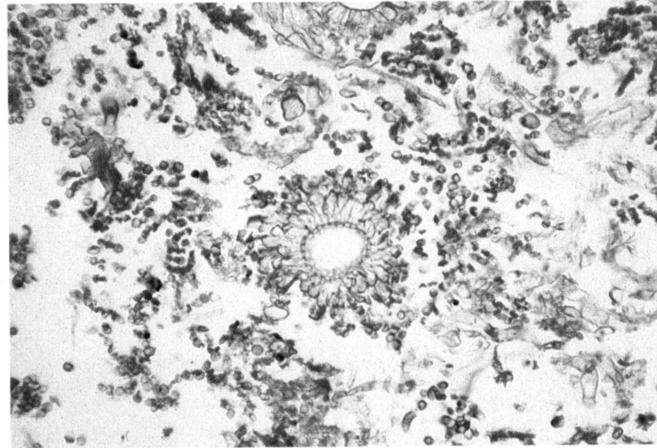

Figure 99.4 Conidial head of *Aspergillus* from a transbronchial biopsy of a cavitary aspergilloma.

Part 2

Mucormycosis

▶ Abida Haque and Mary Ostrowski

Synonyms include phycomycosis, zygomycosis, and hyphomycosis. These are opportunistic infections in immunocompromised or neutropenic individuals caused by a group of bread-mold fungi that include *Mucor, Rhizopus, Absidia,* and *Apophysomyces.* The fungi are angioinvasive, resulting in thrombosis, infarction, and dissemination of the fungi.

Histologic Features:

- The fungi are broad, irregular, pleomorphic, pauciseptate hyphae, 5 to 20 μm wide.
- They show wide-angle and haphazard branching.
- The walls of the hyphae are thin, appear basophilic or amphophilic, and stain weakly with GMS and PAS; they are often seen better with H&E stain.
- Early lesions show neutrophilic infiltrate and necrosis associated with fungal hyphae.
- Foreign body-type giant cells containing fragments of hyphae may be present.

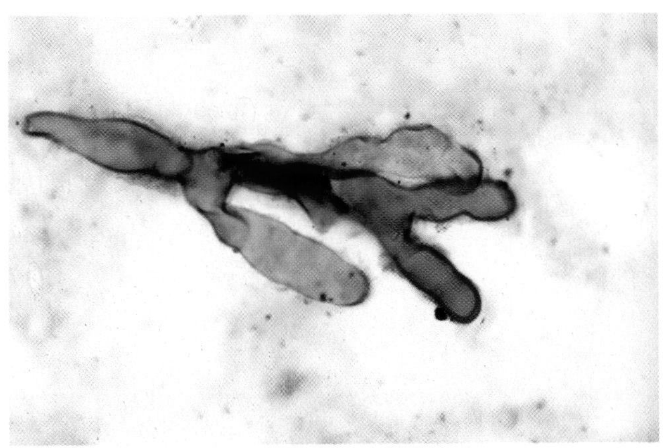

Figure 99.5 Cytology figure showing broad-branching hypha with a pseudoseptation characteristic of *Mucor.*

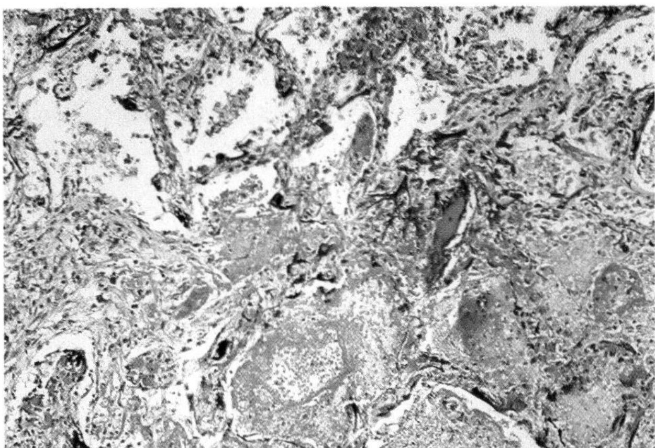

Figure 99.6 Coagulation necrosis associated with mucormycosis in the *lower half* of the figure.

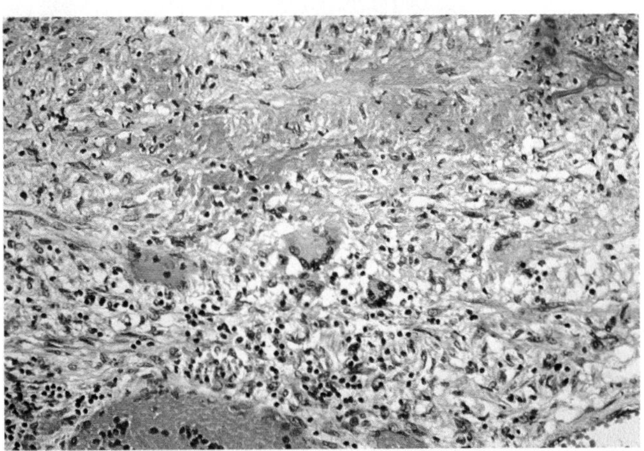

Figure 99.7 The edge of the infarct shows a few centrally located multinucleated giant cells and fungal hyphae in the *upper right corner.*

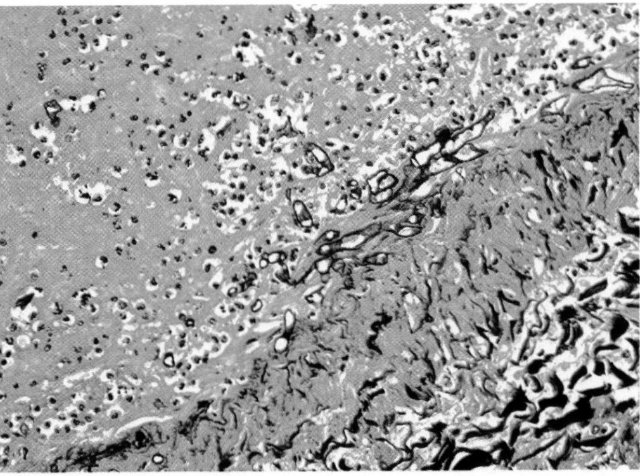

Figure 99.8 GMS stain of a vessel wall invaded by multiple, wide, pauciseptate hyphae.

Part 3

Pneumocystis

▶ Abida Haque and Carlos Bedrossian

Pneumocystosis is an opportunistic pulmonary infection, caused by *Pneumocystis jiroveci* (formerly *carinii*), that occurs almost exclusively in patients with impaired cell-mediated immunity. The most common pulmonary findings are the presence of interstitial infiltrates and alveolar characteristic exudates; rarely nodules, cavities, and pleural effusions are seen. Fatal pulmonary infections may be associated with diffuse alveolar damage (DAD).

Cytologic Features:

- Bronchoalveolar lavage specimens commonly reveal characteristic frothy material, where the outlines of *P. jiroveci* can be seen within the exudate.

Histologic Features:

- The characteristic finding is foamy, eosinophilic alveolar exudates, with mild alveolar wall thickening and alveolar pneumocyte hyperplasia.
- The alveolar exudates has fine, basophilic dots.
- *Pneumocystis* show internal single or paired distinctive foci of enhanced staining with GMS, which help to differentiate *P. jiroveci* from other small fungi.

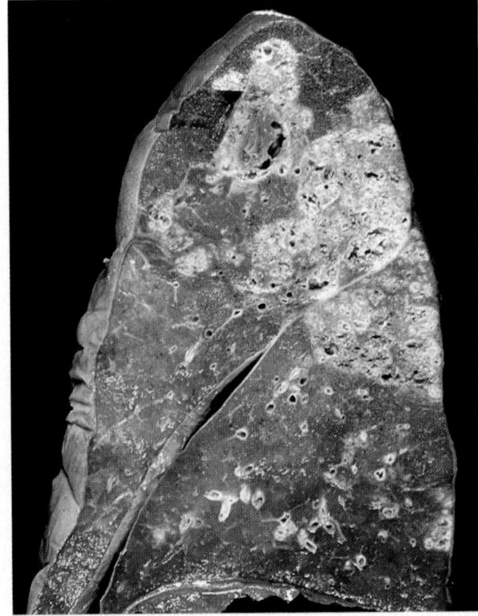

Figure 99.9 Gross figure showing granulomatous and partly cavitary lesions, present predominantly in the upper portions of both lobes, and diffuse consolidation, present predominantly in the lower portions of both lobes.

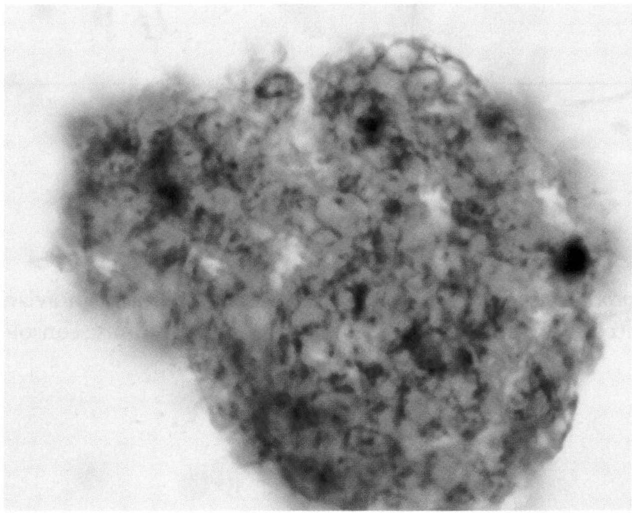

Figure 99.10 Cytology figure of bronchoalveolar lavage specimen showing frothy material characteristic of *Pneumocystis*.

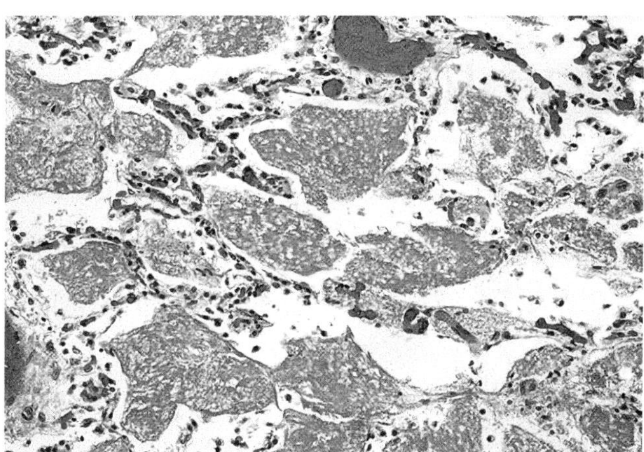

Figure 99.11 Characteristic frothy eosinophilic infiltrate within alveolar spaces.

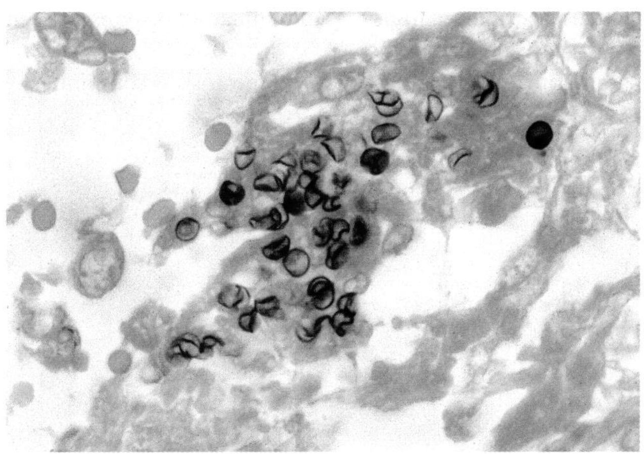

Figure 99.12 GMS stain of the frothy infiltrate containing multiple organisms.

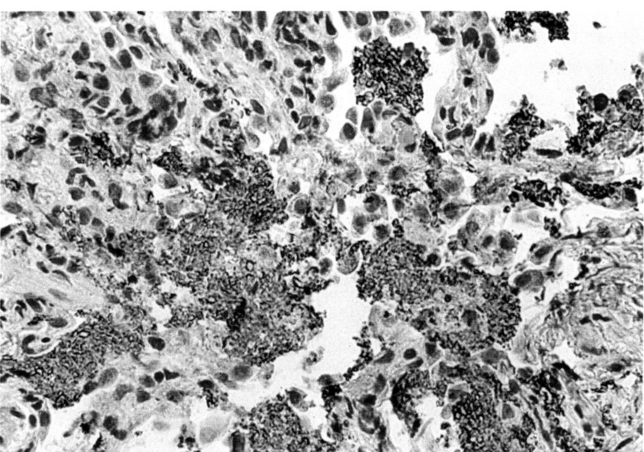

Figure 99.13 Immunostain showing clusters of organisms in alveoli.

Part 5

Histoplasma

▶ Abida Haque and Mary Ostrowski

Histoplasma capsulatum is a dimorphic fungus with yeast and mycelial forms. Infection is seen worldwide. In the United States, it is endemic in the Mississippi and Ohio River valleys. Primary pulmonary infection is acquired with exposure to conidial aerosols from avian habitats. It is often asymptomatic, with formation of small calcified nodules. Heavy exposure in healthy individuals or exposure in immunocompromised patients results in symptomatic infections manifested as either acute pulmonary or disseminated infection. Acute pulmonary infection is characterized by many yeast forms crowding within the cytoplasm of macrophages and is accompanied by mononuclear cell infiltrates and necrosis.

Histologic Features:

- *H. capsulatum* is a narrow-based budding yeast 2 to 5 μm in diameter.
- The rapidly dividing yeast can produce large extracellular collections referred to as *yeast lakes* in immunosuppressed patients.
- In immunocompetent individuals, giant cell granulomas with or without necrosis are formed.
- The residual nodule or histoplasmoma consists of a central zone of caseous necrosis with either a few viable or degenerated ghost forms of the yeast (with GMS stain), surrounded by histiocytes, giant cells, lymphocytes, and a fibrous capsule, with calcification.
- Differential diagnosis includes two yeastlike pathogens of similar size, *Torulopsis glabrata* and *Penicillium marneffei; T. glabrata is* amphophilic and shows budding but is more variable in size than histoplasma; *P. marneffei* is nonbudding.

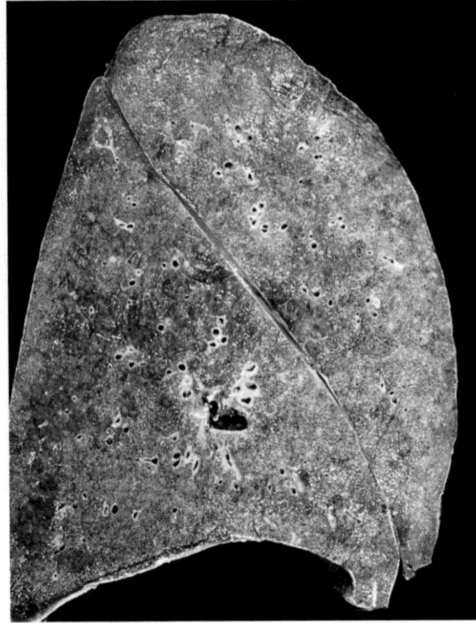

Figure 99.20 Gross figure showing extensive consolidation of both lobes associated with poorly formed small granulomas. A small bronchiectatic cavity is present in the lower lobe.

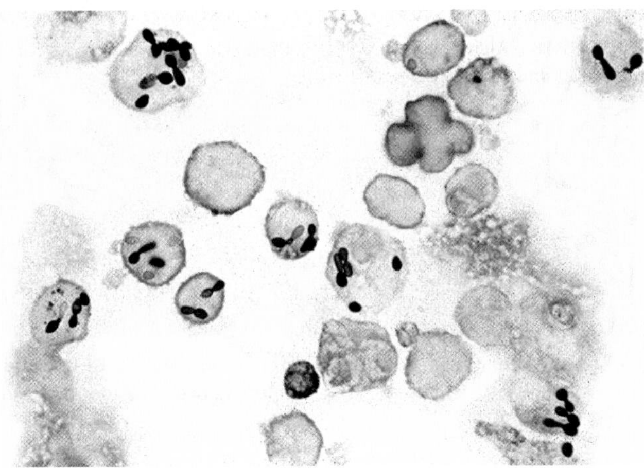

Figure 99.21 Cytology figure showing small budding yeast within macrophages on GMS stain.

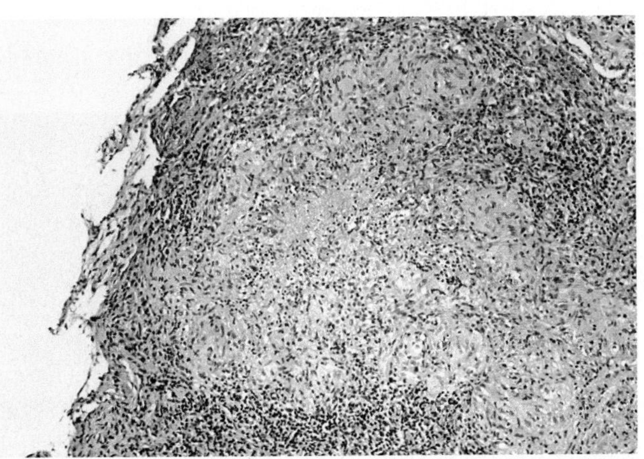

Figure 99.22 Poorly formed cellular granuloma with minimal necrosis in the center.

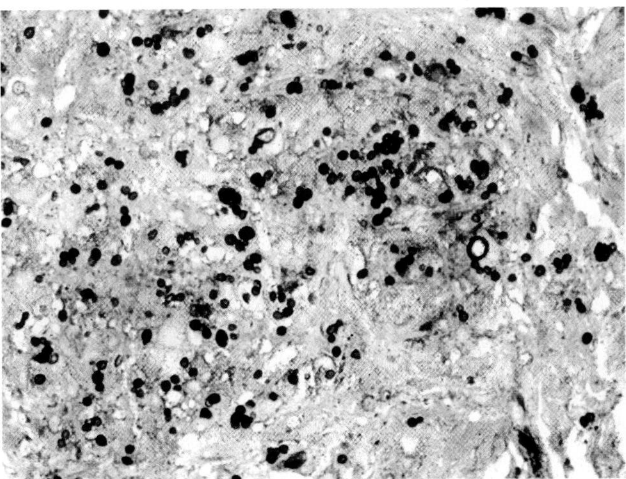

Figure 99.23 GMS stain showing multiple small oval yeast forms. Rare budding yeast forms are seen in the center of the granuloma.

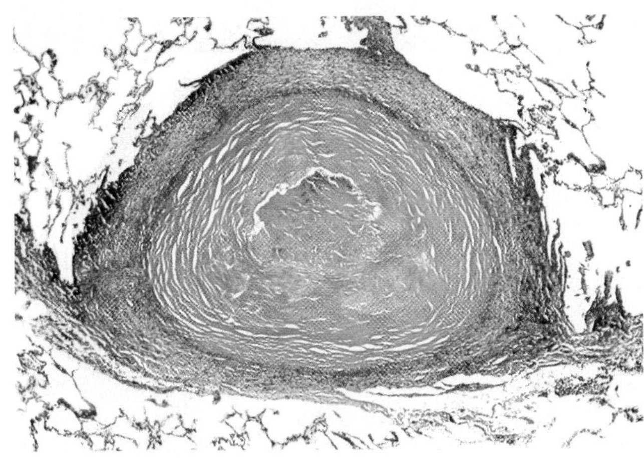

Figure 99.24 Old, healed granuloma with concentric collagen layers characteristic of remote *Histoplasma* infection.

Part 6

Coccidioides

▶ Abida Haque

Coccidioides infection is caused by *Coccidiodes immitis*, a fungus endemic in the southwest United States and South America. Pulmonary infection may present as an acute or a chronic residual form. The fungus consists of large cystlike spherules 20 to 100 μm in diameter and filled with several hundred tiny 1- to 2-μm endospores. Immature spherules are empty. The mature spherules rupture to release the endospherules that enlarge, mature, and repeat the cycle. Rarely, branched septate hyphae and Arthroconidia may be seen in immunosuppressed patients.

Histologic Features:

- Acute pulmonary lesions may be miliary with formation of suppurative reaction to the endospores, with an intense neutrophil response and microabscesses.

- Granulomas are formed in 1 to 2 weeks and show central necrosis surrounded by lymphocytes, epithelioid cells, and multinucleated giant cells.
- Residual pulmonary infection is characterized by fibrocavitary lesions that resemble cavitary tuberculosis.

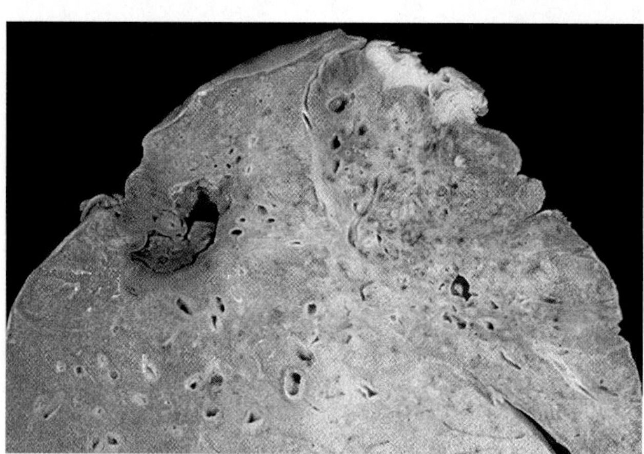

Figure 99.25 Gross figure shows marked fibrosis and contraction in the upper lobe and an acute necrotic cavitary lesion in the lower lobe.

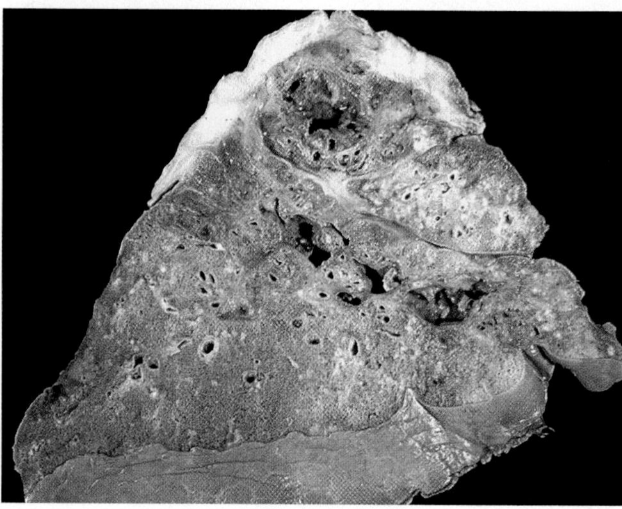

Figure 99.26 Gross figure of chronic cavitary and fibrotic lesions of the upper lobe associated with dense pleural fibrosis, with acute cavities in the lower lobe.

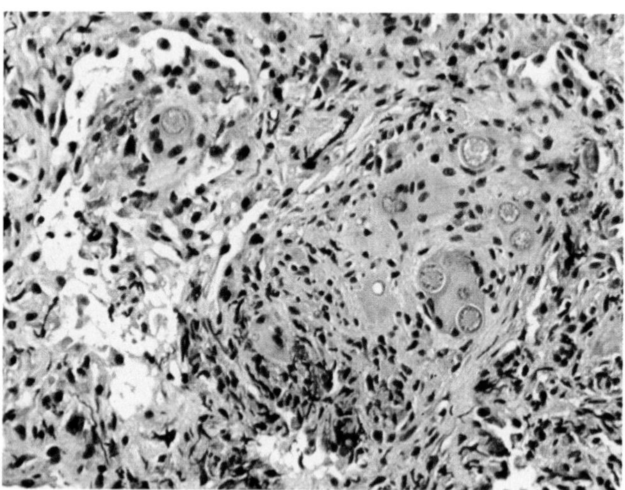

Figure 99.27 Movat stain shows granulomas containing giant cells with fungal spherules, some containing endospores.

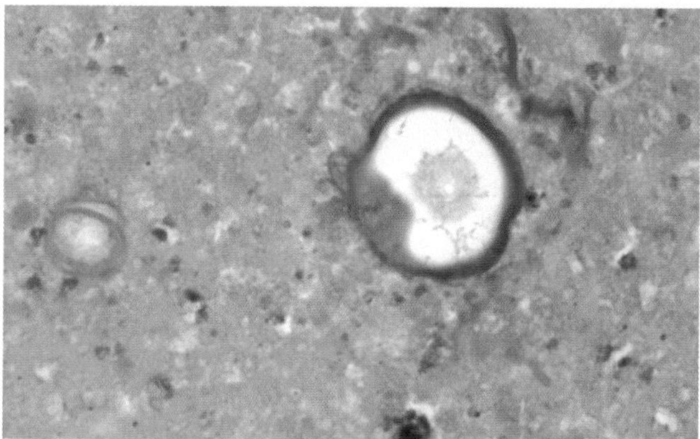

Figure 99.28 High power shows empty thick-walled spherule in necrosis within a granuloma.

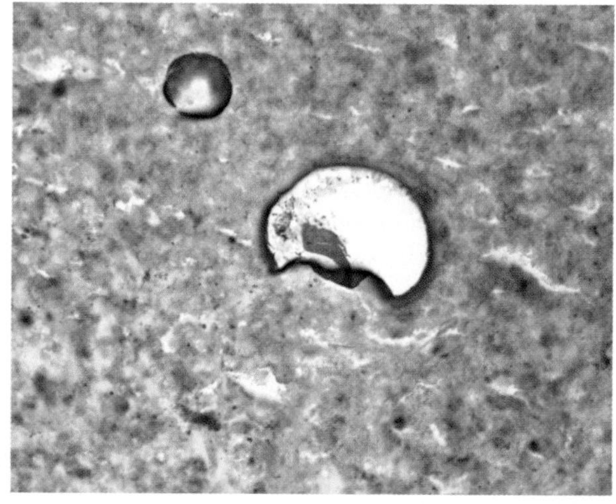

Figure 99.29 High power shows similar empty thick-walled spherule highlighted by GMS stain.

Part 7

Paracoccidioidomycosis

▶ Abida Haque and Carlos Bedrossian

Paracoccidioidomycosis infection is caused by *Paracoccidioides brasiliensis,* which is endemic in South America, Mexico, and Central America. Sporadic cases are seen in southern United States. Pulmonary infections are characterized by infiltrative lesions in the acute form by and granulomatous inflammation with fibrosis in the chronic form.

Histologic Features:

- Granulomas contain the typical fungus, which is spherical, 3 to 30 μm in diameter, with a thick refractile wall and a characteristic multiple budding pattern with a shipwheel appearance, often in the center of the granuloma.
- In tissue sections, large cells are completely covered with small buds, 1 to 3 μm in diameter (steering-wheel forms), may be seen and are considered pathognomonic.
- Older lesions may develop fibrosis.

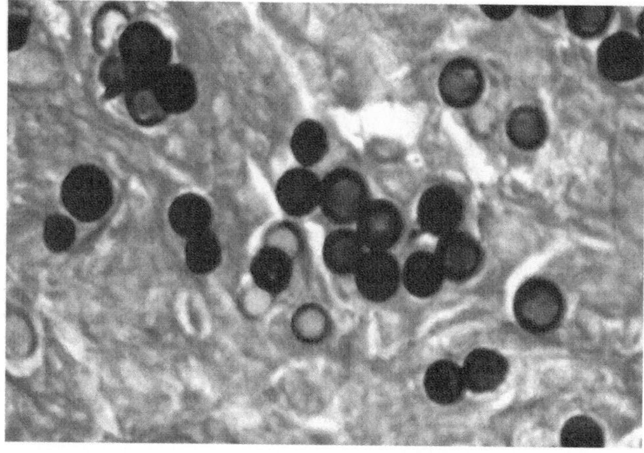

Figure 99.30 GMS stain of Paracoccidioidomycosis showing spherical budding fungi.

Part 8

Blastomycosis

▶ Abida Haque and Carlos Bedrossian

Infection is caused by *Blastomyces dermatitidis,* a dimorphic fungus saprophytic in soil. It is called *North American blastomycosis* and is endemic in the Ohio and Mississippi River valleys. Systemic infection with severe exposure causes diffuse pneumonitis and DAD, even in immunocompetent individuals. It has a high mortality if left untreated. Immunosuppressed patients develop early systemic dissemination of infection.

Histologic Features:

- Pulmonary infection is characterized by suppurative, granulomatous inflammation with numerous single and budding yeast.
- The yeast forms are 8 to 15 μm in diameter, spherical or oval, and have thick double-contoured walls.
- Broad-based budding forms and small "microforms" measuring 2 to 4 μm in diameter are seen in the same lesions, thus presenting a continuous series of fungal sizes.
- Early lesions show an intense neutrophil response around the fungi, with formation of microabscesses surrounded by epithelioid cells and multinucleated giant cells.
- Older lesions show typical granulomas with chronic inflammation and fibrosis.

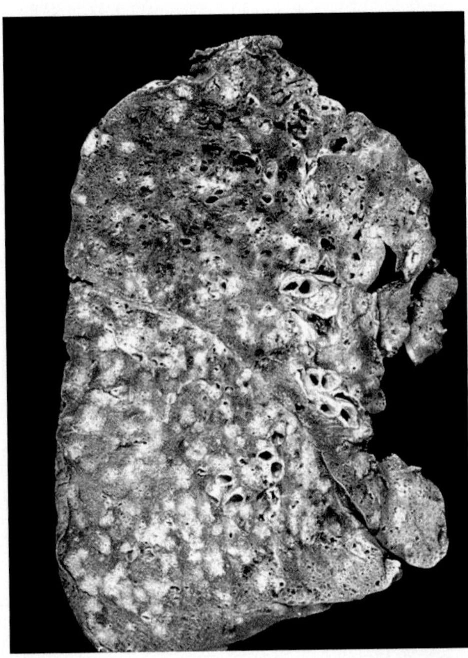

Figure 99.31 Gross figure of blastomycosis showing multiple and extensive granulomas involving the entire lung, with small cavities in the apical area.

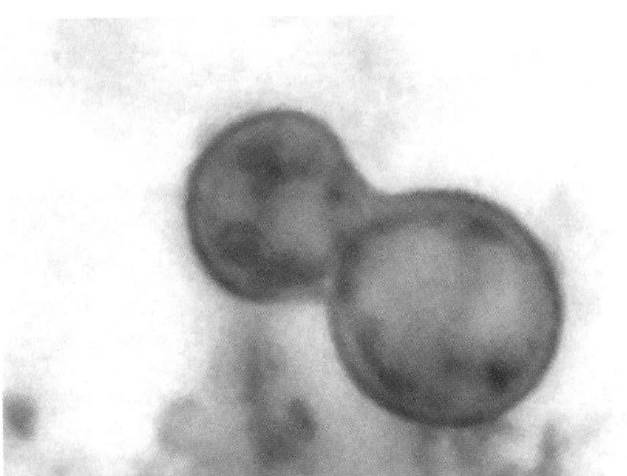

Figure 99.32 *Blastomyces* organism with characteristic broad-based budding forms.

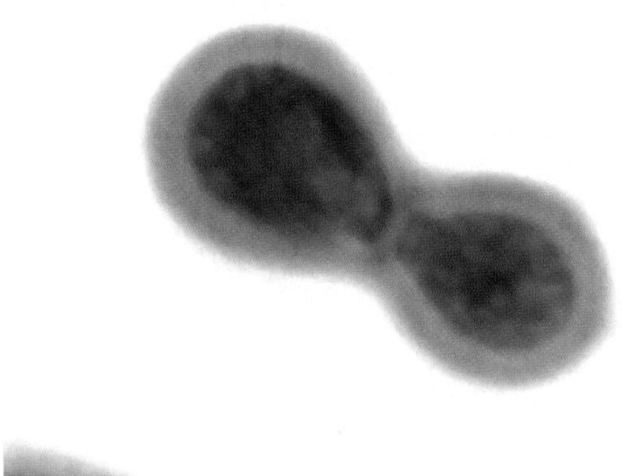

Figure 99.33 *Blastomyces* organism showing thick, double-contoured wall.

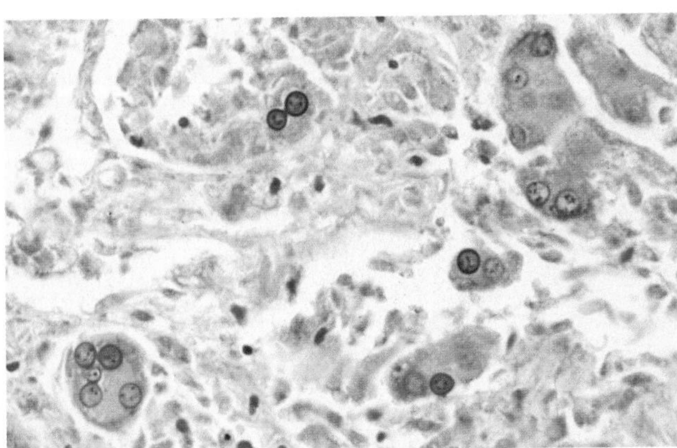

Figure 99.34 *Blastomyces* organisms within giant cells in lung parenchyma.

Part 9

Candida

▶ Abida Haque and Mary Ostrowski

Candida is the most common fungal infection in immunocompromised patients. The lungs are commonly infected in disseminated candidiasis, from seeding through hematogenous spread. Airway infection can result from primary oropharyngeal infection. The most common pathogenic *Candida* species are *C. albicans* and *C. tropicalis.*

Cytologic Features:

- *Candida* may present as both yeast and pseudohyphae or conidiophores.
- The pseudohyphae of *Candida* are not septated but form elongated budding structures that mimic septations.

Histologic Features:

- The lungs typically show bronchopneumonia, often suppurative and associated with acute vasculitis, hemorrhage, and infarction with formation of "targetoid" lesions.
- *Candida* sp. are seen in sections as small oval yeast forms, 2 to 4 μm, pale blue, with budding and pseudohyphae, and rarely true hyphae.
- Early infections are associated with intense neutrophil response and necrosis, and acute vasculitis; rarely, a granulomatous inflammation may be seen.

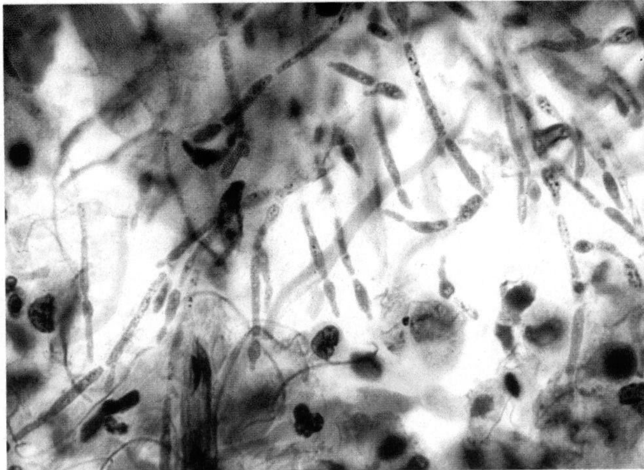

Figure 99.35 Cytology figure shows pseudohyphae and a few budding yeast of *Candida* on Papanicolaou stain.

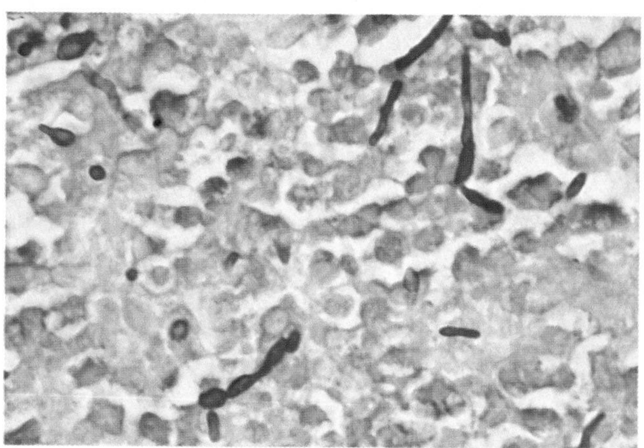

Figure 99.36 PAS stain shows pseudohyphae and budding yeast of *Candida.*

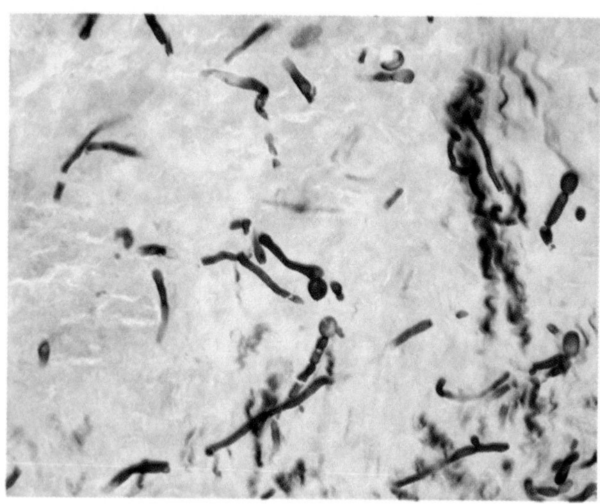

Figure 99.37 GMS stain showing *Candida* pseudohyphae.

Part **10**

Sporotrichosis

▶ Dani S. Zander and Carlos Bedrossian

Sporotrichosis is caused by the dimorphic fungus *Sporothrix schenckii,* a saprophyte found in soil and many types of plants. Most infections are cutaneous and develop from accidental inoculation with an infested thorn or barb in people whose occupations expose them to plants and soil (farmers, gardeners, florists). These infections can spread along draining lymphatics, producing chronic subcutaneous nodules. Inhalation of fungi can rarely cause a primary pulmonary infection. Dissemination from a primary cutaneous infection to the lung can also occur. Primary infections usually produce apical, cavitary, destructive lesions clinically resembling tuberculosis and tend to occur in middle-aged men with chronic obstructive pulmonary disease and alcoholism. Disseminated disease is very rare and occurs primarily in patients with serious underlying diseases, immunocompromise, or alcoholism.

Histologic Features:

- Large necrotizing and nonnecrotizing granulomas that contain scattered or clustered yeastlike cells that usually are not apparent on H&E stain.
- Granulomas may have suppurative centers or become fibrotic.
- Intracavitary fungus balls are unusual.
- Methenamine silver stain highlights the fungi, which appear as spherical, oval, or elongate (cigar-shaped) single or budding yeastlike cells, 2 to 6 μm or more in diameter.
- Yeastlike cells may have elongate "teardrop" or "pipestem" buds, occasionally multiple.
- Hyphae are rarely present in tissue.
- Coating of yeastlike cells with eosinophilic, radially oriented material (Splendore-Hoeppli phenomenon) can occur.
- Isolation by culture or direct immunofluorescence staining in smears or tissue sections is helpful in confirming the diagnosis; serology can also be helpful.

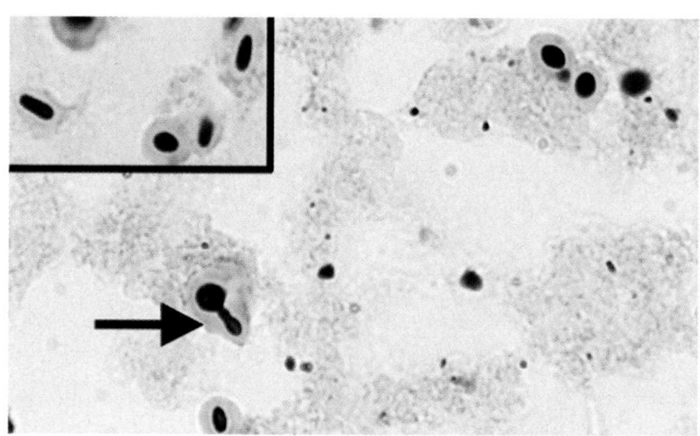

Figure 99.38 Methenamine silver stain showing spherical, oval, and cigar-shaped yeastlike cells in a background of necrotic material. One elongate "teardrop" or "pipestem" bud is present *(arrow)*.

Part 11

Phaeohyphomycosis

▶ Dani S. Zander and Carlos Bedrossian

Phaeohyphomycosis refers to subcutaneous and systemic fungal infections caused by one of numerous species of soil and plant saprophytes that are dematiaceous (naturally pigmented). Infections occur most frequently in immunocompromised or debilitated people and occasionally in healthy patients. The subcutaneous form is more common than the systemic form of infection. Systemic phaeohyphomycosis is usually acquired via inhalation, and the primary pulmonary infection is usually clinically unapparent. The most common species causing systemic phaeohyphomycosis is *Xylohypha bantianum,* a fungus that has a strong propensity to involve the brain. *Alternaria* and *Curvularia* sp. are other agents that cause pulmonary phaeohyphomycosis.

Histologic Features:

- Nonnecrotizing, necrotizing, or suppurative granulomas containing scattered individual or small aggregates of fungi, surrounded by hyalinized fibrous tissue.
- Fungi appear as brown, septate hyphae that are 2 to 6 μm wide, branch, and are constricted at their prominent septations.
- Large thick-walled vesicular swellings and budding yeastlike cells may be present.
- In some cases, the pigmentation may not be obvious, but a stain for melanin can sometimes reveal the presence of melanin or melaninlike pigments in the cell walls.
- Species classification of the organism can be accomplished by culture but not based on morphology, because the individual agents appear morphologically similar in tissue.

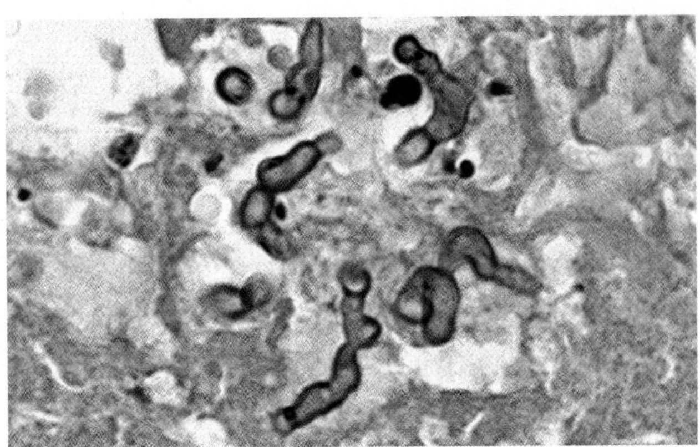

Figure 99.39 In tissue, fungi causing phaeohyphomycosis appear as brown, branching septate hyphae with constrictions at their septations.

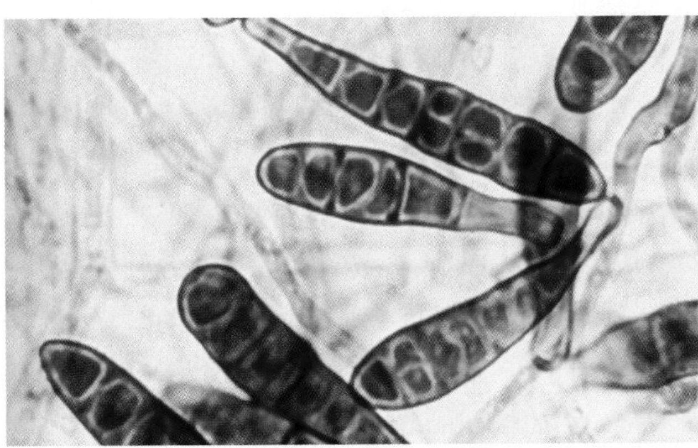

Figure 99.40 Culture showing brown macroconidia, which are drumstick shaped and have transverse and longitudinal septa.

Mycobacteria

100

Mycobacterial infections include tuberculosis, which is a historic and very important infection found worldwide, and atypical mycobacterial infections. The latter are caused by nontuberculous mycobacteria.

Part 1

Tuberculosis

▶ Sajid A. Haque and Abida Haque

Pulmonary tuberculosis is infection caused by *Mycobacterium tuberculosis* and is a classic example of granulomatous inflammation. There is a mild increase in mycobacterial infection, tuberculosis, and atypical mycobacterial infections, the latter almost exclusively in patients with acquired immunodeficiency syndrome (AIDS). Primary pulmonary tuberculosis caused by *M. tuberculosis* is often asymptomatic and results in formation of the Ghon complex in the lower lobes. Reactivation of pulmonary *M. tuberculosis* may manifest as acute necrotizing pneumonia, cavitation, or fibrosis with bronchiectasis.

Histologic Features:

- The hallmark of infection with M. tuberculosis is the formation of granulomas with central caseous necrosis surrounded by lymphocytes, macrophages, and Langerhans-type giant cells (nuclei arranged in horseshoe shape); the caseous areas may have microcalcifications.
- Mycobacteria tend to be at the periphery of the granuloma and not in the caseous area.
- *M. tuberculosis* is a slender, curved, sometimes beaded rod 1.0 to 4.0 μm in length and 0.5 μm in diameter; the bacilli stain intense red with Ziehl-Nielsen or modified Kinyoun stain.
- Fluorescent stain such as auramine or rhodamine may be used (more sensitive than Ziehl-Nielsen) for screening.
- The bacilli are Gram positive, periodic acid–Schiff (PAS) positive, and Gomori methenamine silver (GMS) positive. GMS stain is useful to demonstrate the bacilli after they have lost their acid fastness due to treatment/degeneration.
- Healed tuberculous lesions appear as fibrocalcific nodules.
- Hilar and mediastinal lymph nodes also show caseating granulomas.

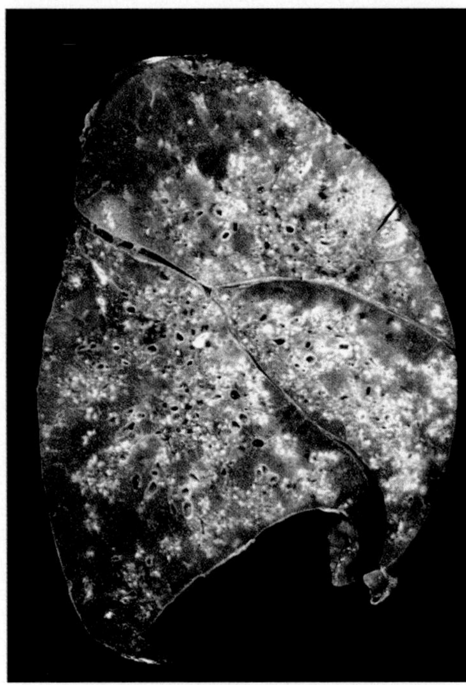

Figure 100.1 Gross figure showing multiple small granulomas fill the lung parenchyma, characteristic of miliary tuberculosis.

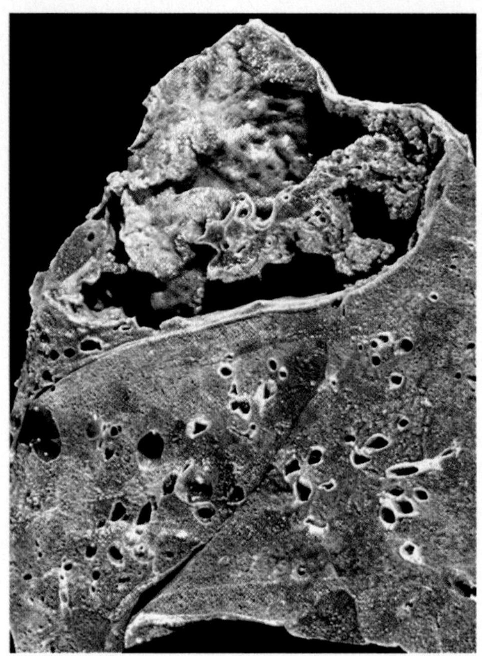

Figure 100.2 Gross figure of reactivated tuberculosis with formation of necrotic cavity involving the entire upper lobe.

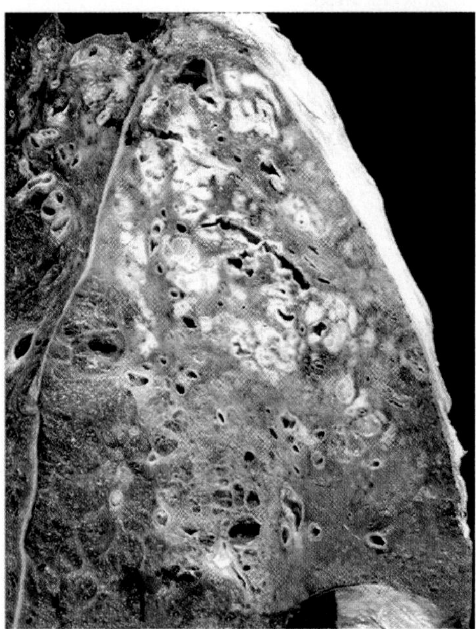

Figure 100.3 Gross figure demonstrating endobronchial spread of tuberculosis, also associated with pleural and pulmonary fibrosis.

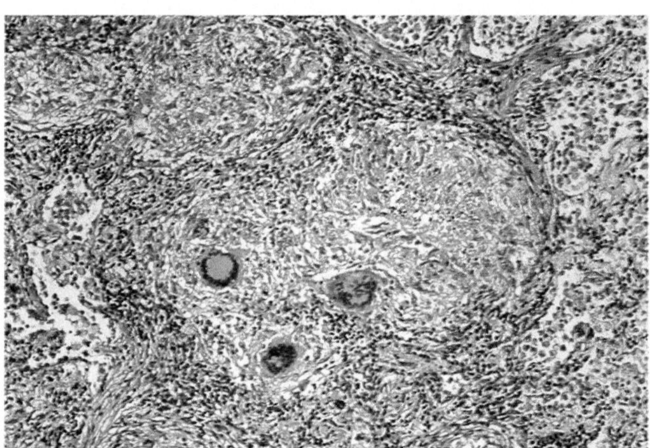

Figure 100.4 Granuloma without conspicuous necrosis and Langerhans-type giant cells.

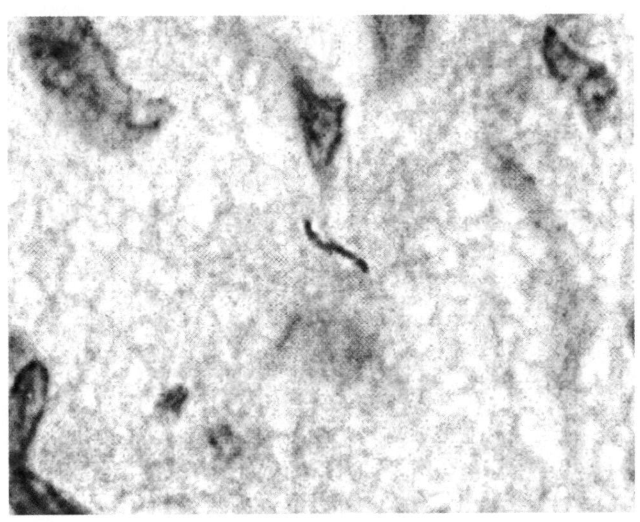

Figure 100.5 Acid fast stain for *M. tuberculosis* showing acid-fast bacillus in the center of the field.

Part 2

Atypical Mycobacteria

▶ Sajid A. Haque and Abida Haque

Atypical mycobacteria are a group of nontuberculous mycobacteria that include *M. avium, M intracellulare* [these two are designated mycobacterium avium complex (MAC)], *M. kansasii, M. scrofulaceum, M. xenopi,* and *M. marinum.* These bacteria are ubiquitous in the environment. Pulmonary infection with atypical mycobacteria is seen in debilitated and immunocompromised subjects. The incidence has increased dramatically with the onset of AIDS. Although there are several species of atypical mycobacteria, infections caused by *M. avium-intracellulare* (MAC) and *M. kansasii* are the most common. Although it is difficult to distinguish these two histologically, *M. kansasii* is longer and shows more distinct cross banding compared to MAC.

Cytologic Features:

- Acid-fast bacilli may be seen within histiocytes and multinucleated giant cells.

Histologic Features:

- Clusters or sheets of foamy histiocytes filled with stacks of acid-fast bacilli.
- Granulomas are present in immunocompetent patients, whereas well-formed granulomas are absent in patients with AIDS; rarely, cavitary lesions may be seen.
- Extrapulmonary lesions are more common than pulmonary lesions.
- MAC are beaded rods, 1.0×4 to 6 μm, and stain intense red with Ziehl-Nielsen and Fite stains; bacilli also stain with PAS and GMS.

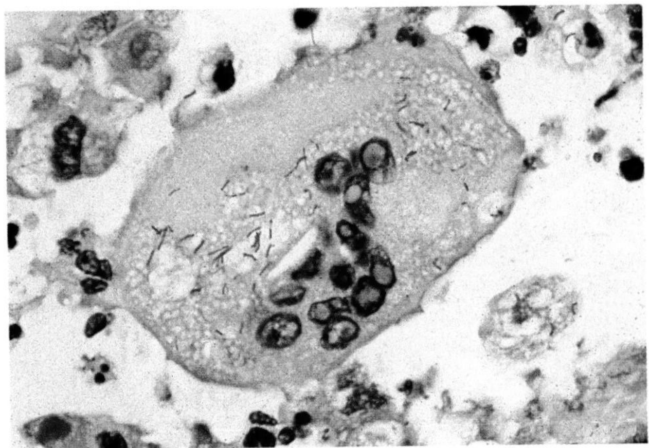

Figure 100.6 Acid fast stain showing multinucleated giant cell with multiple acid-fast bacilli.

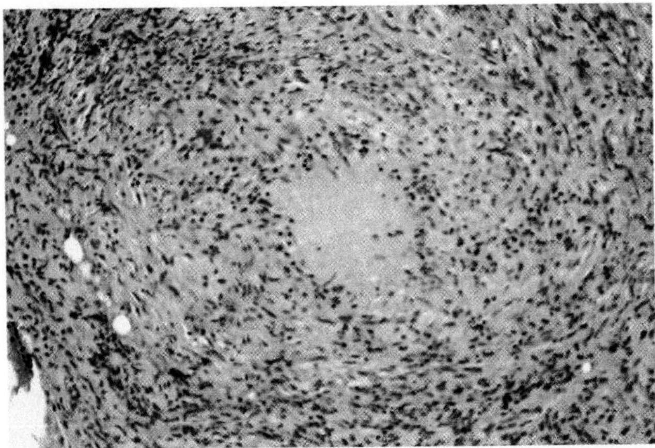

Figure 100.7 Granulomatous inflammation consisting of macrophages is usually seen with MAC infection. However, rarely small necrotic granulomas may be seen, as in this case.

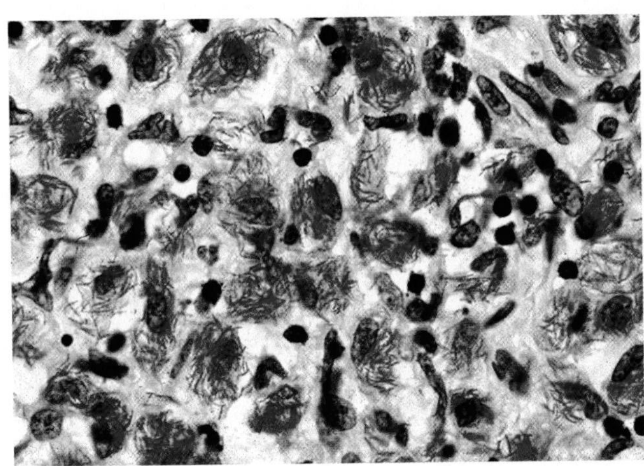

Figure 100.8 Acid fast stain showing sheets of macrophages packed with bundles of acid-fast bacilli, characteristic of atypical mycobacterial infection.

101 Parasites

Several parasites have been found in the lungs and associated tissues of humans. Of these, only two infect human lungs by preference: *Dirofilaria immitis* and *Paragonimus* sp. The remainder are in transit to another organ, in the wrong host or tissue, or disseminated. In this chapter, we illustrate some of the more common parasites that can be encountered in the lung.

Part 1

Dirofilaria

▶ Abida Haque

D. immitis, the dog heartworm, can infect humans when the infective larva is deposited subcutaneously by an infected mosquito's bite. The larvae grow into immature worms and are carried to the pulmonary circulation, where they become trapped and die, producing pulmonary vascular occlusion and infarction.

Histologic Features:

- Characteristic histologic lesion shows a circular or wedge-shaped area of coagulative necrosis with a pulmonary artery branch in the center containing the coiled worm, surrounded by granulomatous reaction.
- The immature worm measures 100 to 360 μm in diameter, with a thick cuticle (5–25 μm), prominent muscular wall, and inconspicuous lateral chords.
- The cuticle projects inward at the lateral chords, forming prominent internal longitudinal ridges.
- The worm may not be easily found in some cases and may require deeper levels and elastic stains.

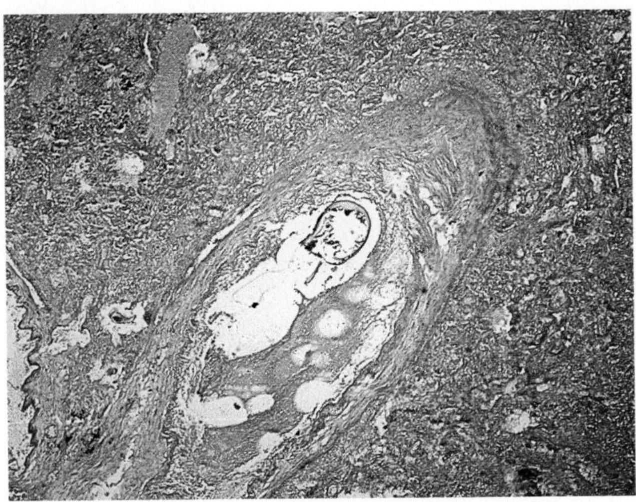

Figure 101.1 The center of an infarct with a pulmonary artery containing a cross section of *Dirofilaria* associated with thrombus.

Part 2

Strongyloides

▶ Abida Haque

Infection with strongyloides is endemic in developing countries, including southern, eastern, and central Europe, and Appalachian United States. Travel to endemic areas can result in acquiring infection. The infection may be latent for years or decades, only becoming active with immunosuppression, particularly with corticosteroid treatment.

Strongyloides stercoralis causes lung infection as the larvae migrate through the pulmonary circulation, enter the alveoli through the capillaries, and molt there as part of their life cycle. In immunocompromised individuals, all stages of maturation can be present in the lung, including the filariform and rhabditiform larvae, eggs, and rarely adult worms. Marked tissue eosinophilia with granulomas should alert one to examine carefully for parasites.

Cytologic Features:

- Filariform larvae may be seen in a background of inflammation, necrosis, and hemorrhage.
- Eggs of *Strongyloides* may be seen in cytologic preparations of sputum specimens.

Histologic Features:

- The lungs show acute inflammation, necrosis, hemorrhage, and abscesses.
- In chronic infection, multiple granulomas with or without larvae in the center are seen in the pulmonary interstitium and alveoli.
- Granulomatous inflammation of the airways and rarely the pulmonary vessels may be seen.
- The filariform larvae are long and slender (500–600 μm long and 10–16 μm in diameter), and most frequently found in extraintestinal sites; the larvae have a cylindrical esophagus occupying almost half of its length, and four lateral alae.
- The rhabditiform larvae (300–380 μm long and 20–25 μm in diameter) are only rarely found in the lungs; the larvae have a short bulbar esophagus and a thin, longer intestine.
- The adult females (1.5–10.0 mm long and 30–95 μm in diameter) are found in the small intestine and very rarely in the lungs; the cuticle of the parasite is finely striated, and cross section may show a muscular esophagus, intestine, ovary, and eggs.

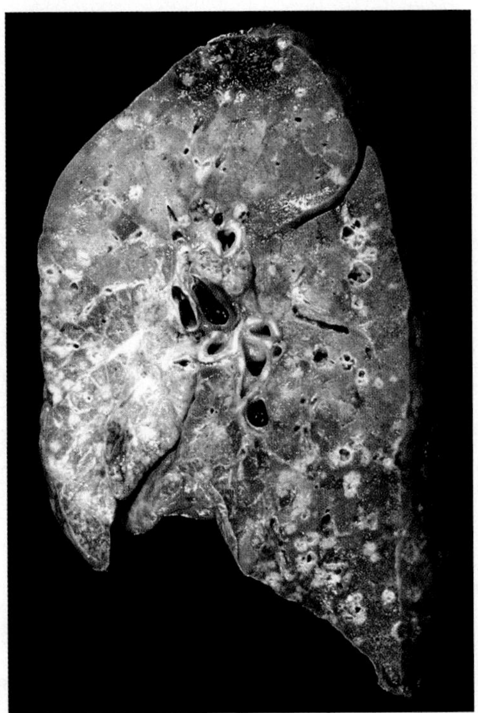

Figure 101.2 Gross figure showing consolidation with multiple areas of necrotizing bronchopneumonia, some with cavities.

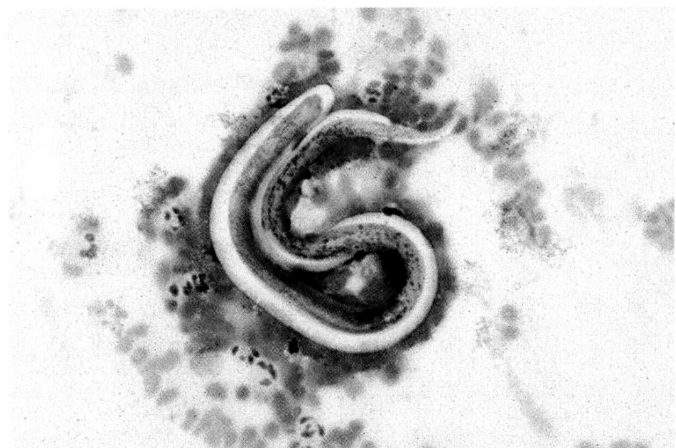

Figure 101.3 Cytology figure of sputum showing filariform larva with basophilic nuclei in the posterior two thirds of the organism.

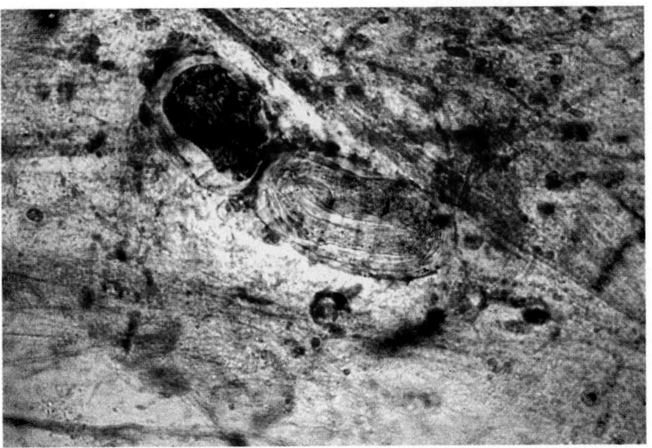

Figure 101.4 Cytology figure of sputum showing eggs of *Strongyloides*.

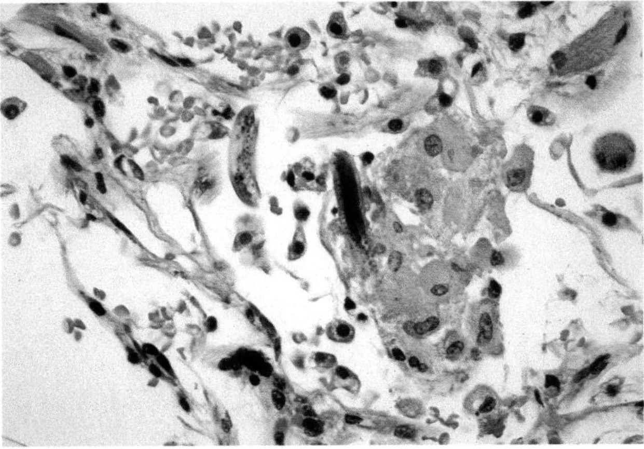

Figure 101.5 High power showing sections of larvae surrounded by macrophages.

Part 3

Malaria

▶ Judith Aronson

Four species of malarial protozoa, *Plasmodium*, cause human infection: *P. vivax*, *P. malariae*, *P. ovale*, and *P. falciparum*. *P. falciparum* causes the most severe form of malaria, including cerebral malaria, which is commonly fatal. During the erythrocytic cycle of parasite replication, human red blood cells become heavily parasitized by trophozoites.

Parasitized red blood cells adhere to microvascular endothelium via knobs on the surface of the infected erythrocytes. This leads to widespread microcirculatory disturbance in virtually all of the visceral organs, including the lung.

Histologic Features:

- Pulmonary congestion is seen, with stasis of parasitized erythrocytes in the capillaries.
- Parasitized erythrocytes are recognized by presence of basophilic "ring forms" of the trophozoite and the presence of malarial pigment, the result of hemoglobin digestion by the parasite.
- Alveolar septa may display mononuclear infiltrates, composed of monocytes, lymphocytes, and plasma cells.

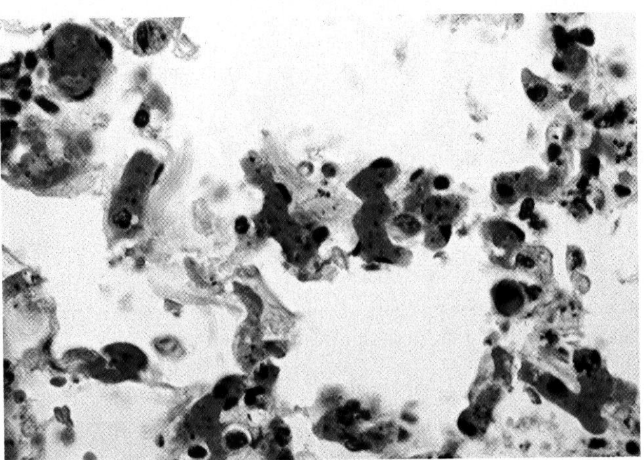

Figure 101.6 Alveolar capillaries containing numerous parasitized red blood cells, from an autopsy of a young, asplenic West African man.

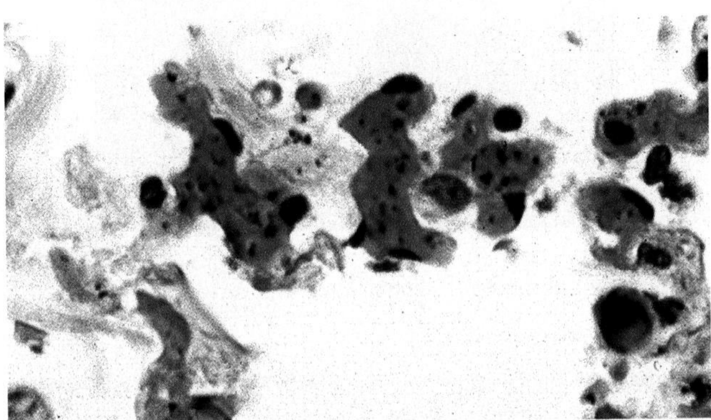

Figure 101.7 Higher power showing alveolar capillaries with parasitized red blood cells.

Part 4

Toxoplasma

▶ Abida Haque

Toxoplasma gondii is an obligatory intracellular protozoon that can parasitize humans, cats, and other mammals. Acute infection is often asymptomatic. Acute infection in immunocompromised subjects or infants results in rapid multiplication of the tachyzoites in host cells. The tachyzoites are contained in a cytoplasmic vacuole, forming tissue cysts measuring 15 to 100 μm. Tachyzoites are crescentic in shape, 4 to 8 μm in length and 2 to 3 μm in width, with one end broader than the other.

Chronic infection is characterized by the presence of infective bradyzoites within tissue cysts. Lung infection is characterized by chronic interstitial pneumonia, but organisms are often difficult to find.

Histologic Features:

- Interstitial pneumonia with mononuclear infiltrate.
- Alveolar pneumocytes and macrophages may show the tachyzoites within cytoplasmic vacuoles.

- Tachyzoites may be seen diffusely in the pulmonary interstitium or within foci of coagulation necrosis.
- The organisms are best seen in smears or touch preparations; they show blue cytoplasm and dark red nucleus with Giemsa stain.
- The lack of kinetoplast differentiates *Toxoplasma* from *Trypanosoma cruzi* and *Leishmania* sp.

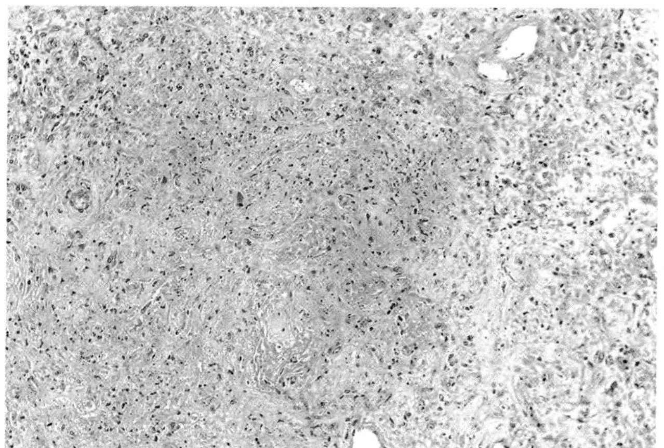

Figure 101.8 Low power showing necrotizing pneumonia with multiple mononuclear cells and abundant nuclear dust.

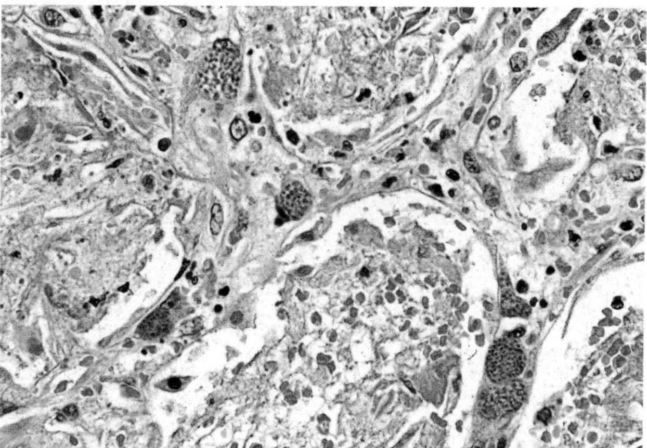

Figure 101.9 Higher power showing multiple cysts filled with bradyzoites within the pulmonary interstitium, and alveolar spaces containing fibrinous exudates, a few macrophages, and red blood cells.

Part 5

Entamoeba Histolytica

▶ Avissai Alcántara-Vázquez

Pulmonary amebiasis is caused by infection of the lung with the protozoan *Entamoeba histolytica.* This disease is found worldwide. Although the most common clinical presentation is as a gastrointestinal infection acquired through ingestion of contaminated food or water, when the patient develops hepatic amebic abscesses, they may open into the thoracic, pleural, or pericardial cavity. The lung abscesses are usually contiguous with those in the liver. The fluid within the abscess appears thick and brown. The center of the abscess consists of necrotic debris with scattered trophozoites.

Histologic Features:

- Abscesses with central necrosis.
- Trophozoites measuring approximately 15 to 25 μm in diameter.
- Trophozoites may contain red blood cells.
- The trophozoites are strongly periodic acid-Schiff (PAS) positive and contain a small nucleus (2–3 μm).
- An iron stain may help demonstrate the cellular organelles of the trophozoites and facilitate the distinction of cells in the surrounding tissue.
- Trophozoites may be confused with histiocytes.

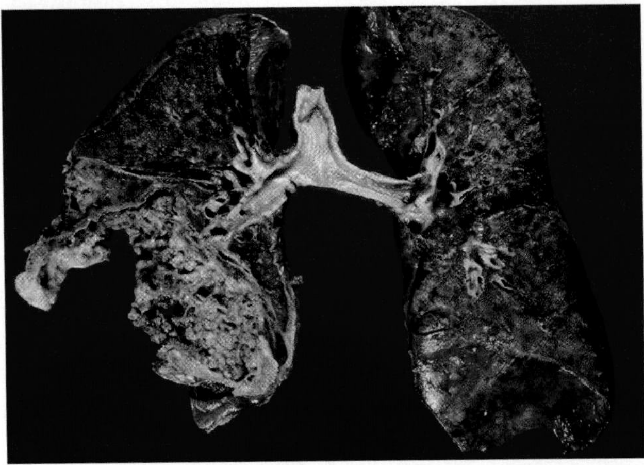

Figure 101.10 Gross figure of an amebic abscess opened to the pulmonary parenchyma, with a central area of cavitation surrounded by extensive necrosis.

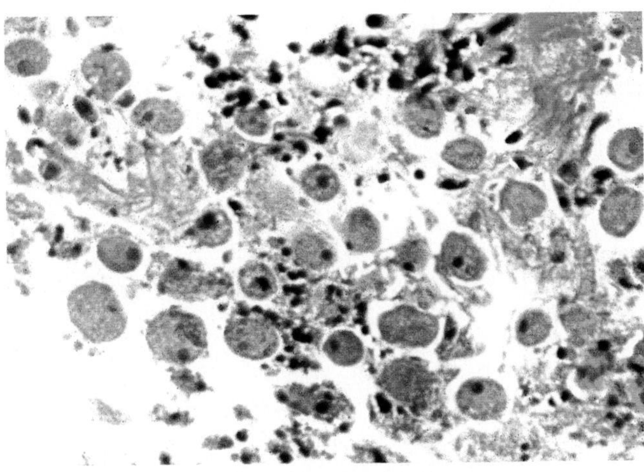

Figure 101.11 Amebic abscess containing trophozoites that are round to oval, with small nuclei and occasional red blood cells within their cytoplasm.

Part 6

Acanthamoeba

▶ Abida Haque

At least three genera of free-living amebae besides *Entameba histolytica* are known to cause disease in humans and animals. These include *Naegleria, Acanthamoeba,* and *Balamuthia mandrillaris;* all three are ubiquitous in the environment, particularly in fresh water and soil. *N. fowleri* can infect healthy individuals via the nasal passages, causing fulminant meningoencephalitis. *Acanthamoeba* and *Balamuthia* often infect immunocompromised hosts and cause a chronic granulomatous inflammation. Histologically, *Acanthamoeba* and *Balamuthia* have trophozoite and cyst forms in tissues, but *Naegleria* have only trophozoite forms. Disseminated infections have been seen only with *Acanthamoeba* and *Balamuthia.*

Histologic Features:

Acanthamoeba and Balamuthia

- Trophozoites are 15 to 35 μm in diameter, with granular or vacuolated cytoplasm and a single nucleus with a prominent "targetoid" karyosome.
- Cyst forms are 12 to 30 μm in diameter, have a thick wall, are intensely basophilic, and show an undulating or wrinkled external wall and a spherical internal wall.

Naegleria

- Trophozoites are 10 to 20 μm in diameter and have a granular or vacuolated cytoplasm, an indistinct nucleus, and a prominent "targetoid" karyosome.
- The nuclear membrane lacks peripheral chromatin in all amebic trophozoites.

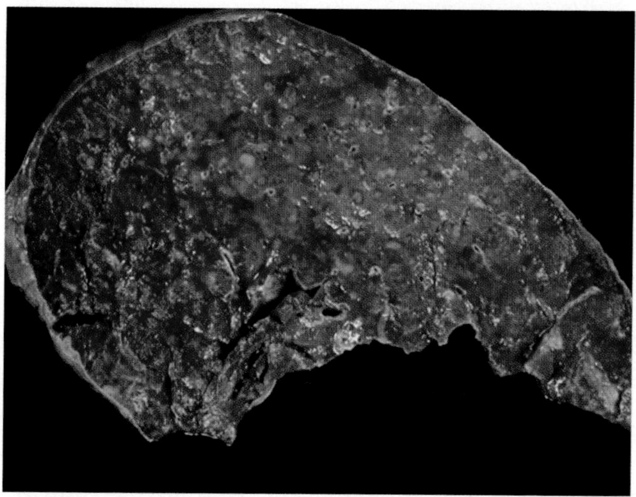

Figure 101.12 Gross figure from a patient with heart transplant who developed disseminated infection showing extensive bronchopneumonia, with focal hemorrhages.

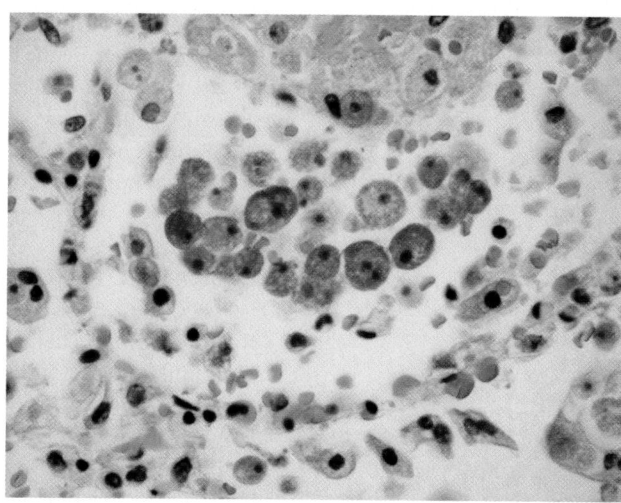

Figure 101.13 Clusters of trophozoites within the alveolar space, without any inflammatory infiltrate.

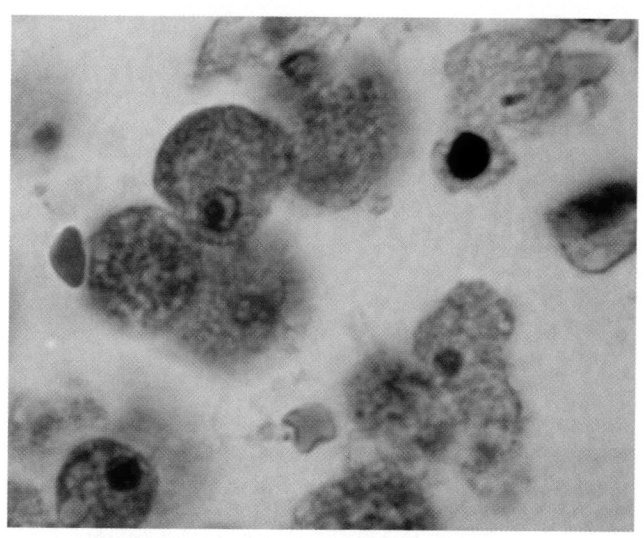

Figure 101.14 Higher power of the trophozoites with granular and vacuolated cytoplasm, and a single nucleus with prominent "targetoid" karyosome.

Part 7

Paragonimus

▶ Rodolfo Laucirica and Alvaro C. Laga

Paragonimiasis is an infection caused by a lung fluke (trematode) of the genus *Paragonimus.* These are the only helminthic parasites of man that, as adult worms, infect the lungs as part of their natural cycle. Paragonimiasis causes chronic lung disease and is more common in Asia, Africa, and South America. Approximately 48 species and subspecies have been described and only 9 are thought to cause disease in humans. The most common species infecting humans is *Paragonimus westermani.*

Humans contract the disease by eating infected raw crabs or crayfish. Once ingested, the larvae penetrate the intestinal wall, subsequently the diaphragm, and finally settle in the lung parenchyma or pleura. The worms provoke inflammation and fibrosis, and egg lying starts in about 70 days.

Patients frequently present with cough, hemoptysis, severe chest pain, and night sweats. Diffuse pulmonary infiltrates and ring shadows are generally seen on chest x-ray films.

Histologic Features:

- Adult worms usually settle near bronchi or large bronchioles.
- An inflammatory infiltrate with eosinophils surrounds groups of worms or rarely single worms.
- A fibrous-walled cyst usually develops around the worm and may become several millimeters thick.
- Eggs of *Paragonimus* show characteristic operculum.

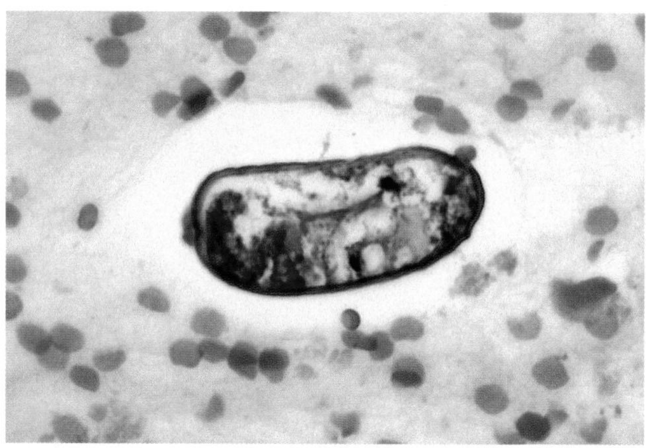

Figure 101.15 Cytology figure containing a structure consistent with *P. westermani.*

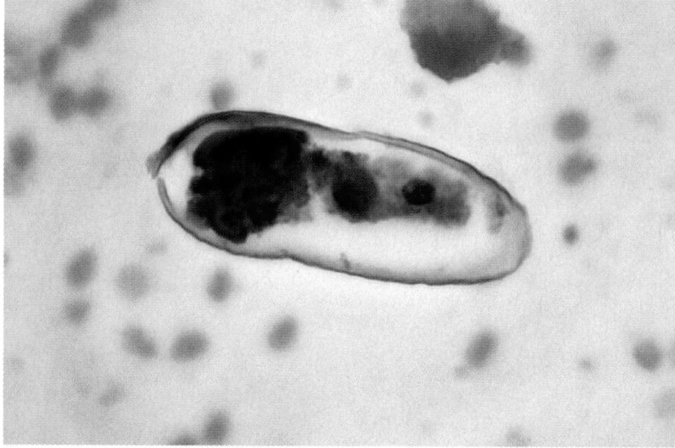

Figure 101.16 Cytology figure showing *P. westermani* with outer tegument and a portion of intestine inside.

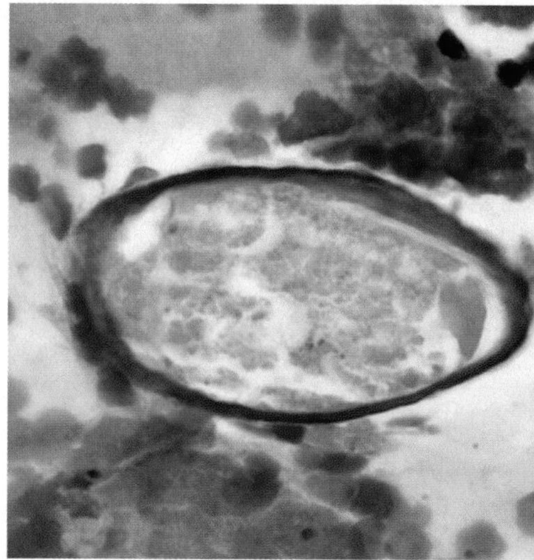

Figure 101.17 Cytology figure showing egg of *P. westermani* with characteristic operculum.

Part 8

Ascaris

▶ Rodolfo Laucirica and Alvaro C. Laga

Ascaris lumbricoides is a nematode that infects humans and causes ascariasis. This entity is particularly common in tropical and subtropical areas with abundant moisture and fecal contamination of the soil. It is ordinarily an innocuous disease; most people are unaware of it. The most common complication of ascariasis is pneumonitis due to migrating larvae, which provoke an allergic reaction that causes an asthmalike transient syndrome. Clinically, it presents with dyspnea, cough, wheezing, low-grade fever, and transient eosinophilia. These signs and symptoms are collectively known as *Loeffler syndrome.* Humans contract the disease by ingesting eggs of *A. lumbricoides* that contain larvae. Grossly, the lungs infected with larvae of *A. lumbricoides* have small areas of consolidation in the lower lobes.

Histologic Features:

- Interstitial pneumonitis and areas of bronchopneumonia may be seen around larvae.
- Larvae may be encountered in alveoli, alveolar septa, bronchioles, and bronchi.
- Larvae are frequently surrounded by eosinophils and histiocytes.

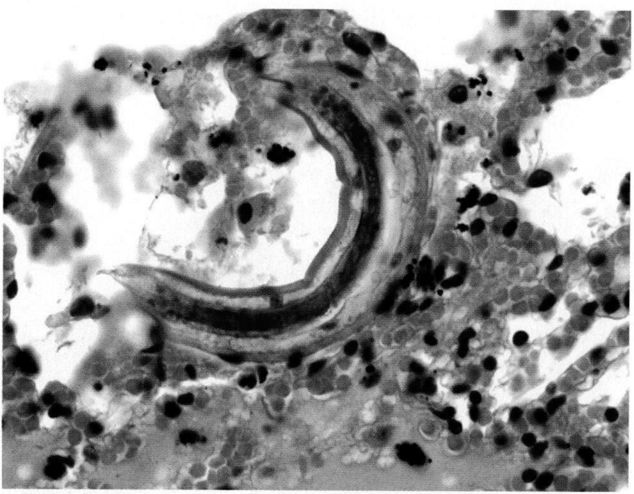

Figure 101.18 Longitudinal section of *A. lumbricoides* larva within a background of inflammation and hemorrhage.

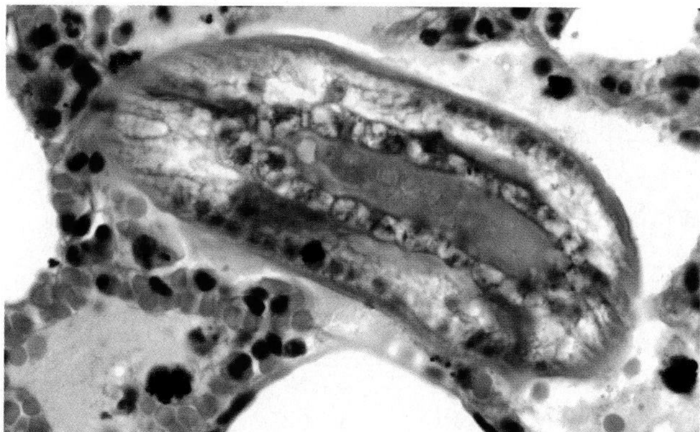

Figure 101.19 Portion of *A. lumbricoides* larva.

Part 9

Schistosoma

▶ Rodolfo Laucirica and Alvaro C. Laga

Schistosoma infection is a tropical disease caused by a blood fluke (trematode). In the past, it was limited to endemic countries. However, with the increase in migration and travel, it is now seen more frequently in nonendemic, developed countries. Five species can infect humans: *S. mansoni, S. japonicum, S. haematobium, S. intercalatum,* and *S. mekongi.* Lung involvement occurs with migration of schistosomula (metamorphosed cercariae) via the hemolymphatic system through the heart to the lungs. Humans acquire the disease by swimming, drinking, or washing with contaminated water containing cercariae. Cercariae penetrate the skin, enter capillaries in the dermis, and travel through the venous circulation through the heart to the lungs. They squeeze through the pulmonary capillaries and travel back to the heart and then to the liver, where they mature to egg-lying adults. Pulmonary manifestations such as dyspnea and pulmonary hypertension develop in only a small number of infected individuals, usually after years of persistent infestation.

Histologic Features:

- Eggs are usually surrounded by epithelioid cells and a rim of collagen.
- Eggs may cause granulomatous endarteritis.
- Aneurysmal dilation of the pulmonary artery may be seen.
- Adult schistosomes are occasionally found within the lumen of pulmonary vessels.

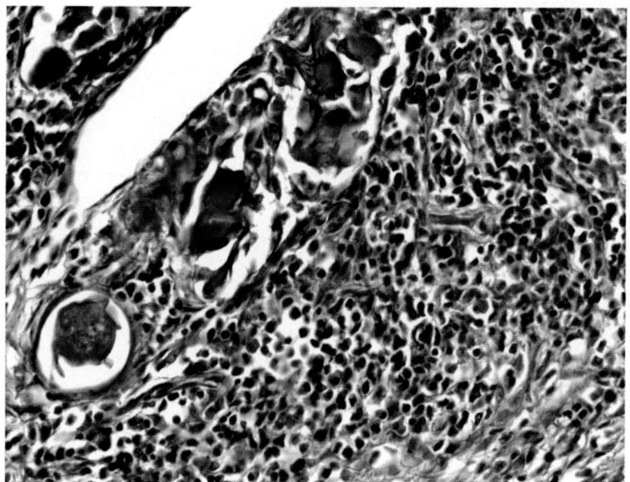

Figure 101.20 *S. mansoni* eggs within a focus of intense lymphoplasmacytic inflammatory infiltrate.

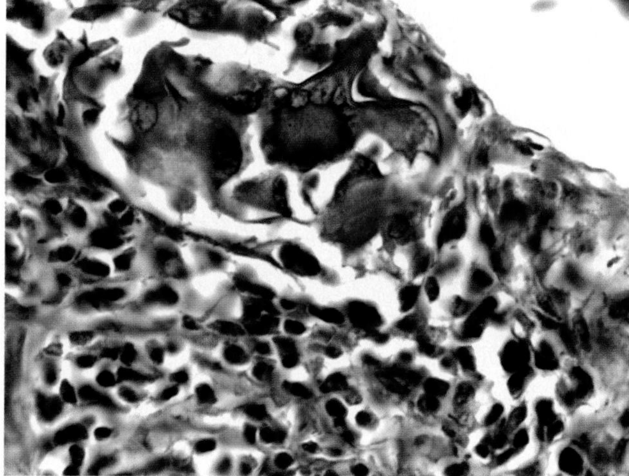

Figure 101.21 Higher power of *S. mansoni* egg showing characteristic strong lateral spine.

Part 10

Leishmania

▶ Alvaro C. Laga and Charles Stager

Leishmania donovani causes visceral leishmaniasis (kala azar) in Africa, Asia, and South America. Leishmaniasis may cause skin lesions or systemic disease. Pulmonary disease is rare in immunocompetent individuals. The parasites multiply in the phagocytic cells of the spleen, bone marrow, Kupffer cells, and lymph nodes. *L. donovani* amastigotes are frequently present in histiocytes within the pulmonary interstitium. Serology may assist in excluding other parasitoses.

Histologic Features:

- Noncaseating granulomas may occur.
- Endobronchial biopsies may show acute and chronic inflammation.
- *L. donovani* amastigotes may be found in macrophages in the pulmonary interstitium.

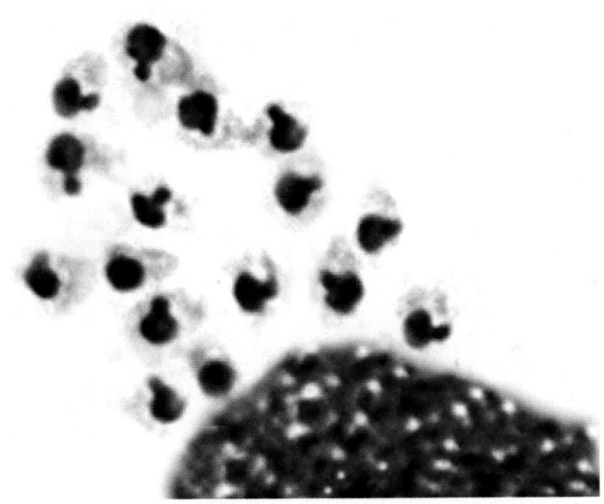

Figure 101.22 *Leishmania* sp. amastigotes bursting out of a macrophage, with characteristic nucleus and kinetoplast.

Part 11

Echinococcus

▶ Alvaro C. Laga and Charles Stager

Echinococcosis involving the lung is caused by *Echinococcus granulosus* in the vast majority of cases. This disease is acquired in humans by consuming eggs from the feces of a definitive host, including dogs. When ingested, these eggs develop into larvae that penetrate the duodenum and go to the liver via the portal circulation. The majority of the larvae remain in the liver. Of those that escape the liver, most are ensnared in alveolar capillaries, where they develop into cysts containing immature worms.

Histologic Features:

- Cysts of *E. granulosus* are usually surrounded by a fibrous wall of host tissue.
- Scolices and protoscolices may be found in lung parenchyma and/or sputum after rupture of hydatid cyst.
- Cysts may rupture into bronchi, causing suppurative inflammation and/or abscess.
- Fragments of cysts may cause necrotizing granulomas in the lung.

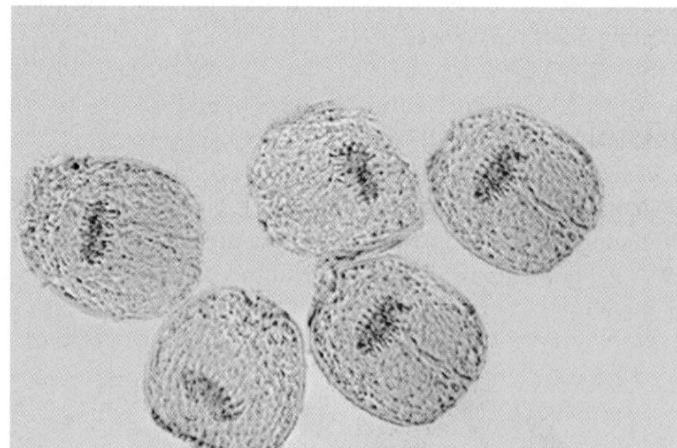

Figure 101.23 *E. granulosus* free scolices with hooklets liberated from cyst.

Agents of Biologic and Chemical Warfare

102

Biologic and chemical agents have been weaponized to produce diseases. Many of these agents are not commonly encountered by clinicians or pathologists in their daily practices but have received greater attention as potential threats in recent years. Chemical warfare agents include nerve agents such as sarin, tabun, soman, and VX gas; vesicants such as sulfur mustard and nitrogen mustard; pulmonary agents such as phosgene and chlorine; and cyanides, among others. Potential biologic warfare agents include small pox, anthrax, plague, botulism, tularemia, Ebola hemorrhagic fever, Marburg hemorrhagic fever, Lassa fever, and Argentine hemorrhagic fever.

Part 1

Anthrax

▶ Abida Haque

Anthrax, primarily a disease of herbivores, is a zoonotic disease due to infection with *Bacillus anthracis.* Exposure to the bacteria may result in cutaneous, gastrointestinal, or pulmonary disease. Pulmonary disease results from inhalation of infective spores and was particularly common in wool sorters. Clinically, a severe respiratory distress develops with shock and death within 24 to 48 hours of onset. Chest radiographs show a characteristic expansion of mediastinum.

Histologic Features:

- The hallmark lesions of anthrax are edema and hemorrhage.
- The lungs show extensive suppurative and hemorrhagic bronchopneumonia with abundant Gram-positive rods measuring 1 to 1.25 × 3 to 5 μm.
- The bacilli are described as "boxcar" or "bamboo rod."
- The mediastinum shows massive edema and enlarged hemorrhagic lymph nodes.

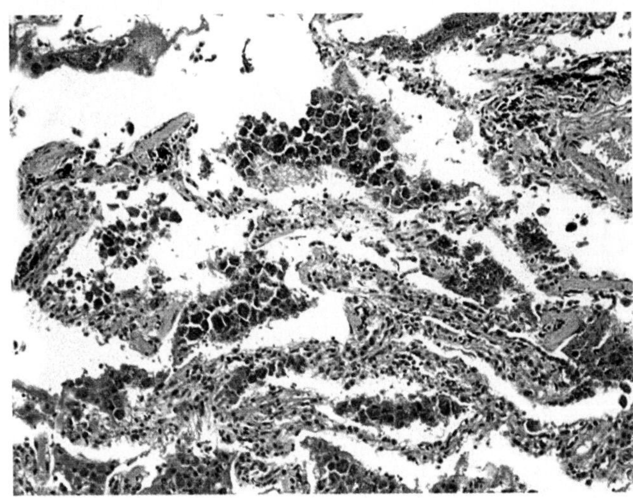

Figure 102.1 Hyaline membranes and pigment-filled macrophages associated with interstitial inflammation.

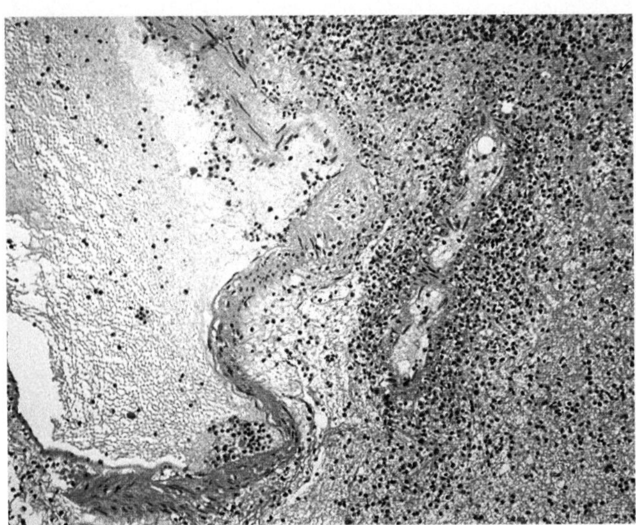

Figure 102.2 Mediastinal tissues with severe edema, inflammation, and hemorrhage. An extremely dilated blood vessel is also present.

Part 2

Tularemia

▶ Dani S. Zander

Tularemia is caused by *Francisella tularensis,* a small pleomorphic Gram-negative coccobacillus that is acquired by contact with an infected animal (usually a rabbit or squirrel) or from a bite by an infected tick or deer fly. Inhalation of organisms on aerosolized droplets leads to primary pulmonary tularemia. Pneumonia may develop secondary to septicemia. Hilar lymphadenopathy and pleural effusion may accompany the pneumonia.

Histologic Features:

- Edema, fibrin, and mononuclear cells in alveoli.
- Parenchymal necrosis resembling an infarct or geographic focus of caseation.
- Granulomatous response may be present, but giant cells are usually absent.
- Organization and calcification can occur.
- Thrombosis and necrosis of medium and small arteries and veins.
- Bacteria stain poorly with tissue Gram stain but stain well with silver impregnation techniques (Steiner, Warthin-Starry, Dieterle); bacteria are usually found within macrophages.
- Diagnosis can be established by culture, serology, or direct fluorescent antibody identification of the organism in lesional exudate smears or tissue sections.

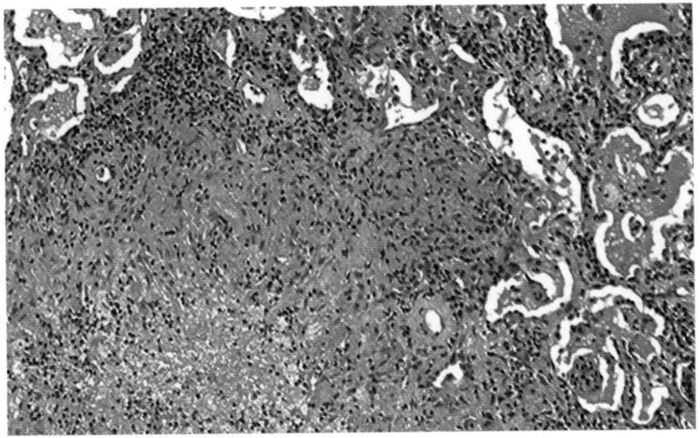

Figure 102.3 Necrotizing granulomatous reaction to the infection, with nearby alveoli containing fibrinous material and small numbers of mononuclear inflammatory cells within alveolar spaces and infiltrating the interstitium.

Part 3

Chemicals

▶ Alvaro C. Laga, Timothy Allen, and Philip T. Cagle

Chemical agents that affect the lung parenchyma are known as *pulmonary damaging agents* or *choking agents*. These include phosgene, diphosgene, chlorine, and chloropicrin. Phosgene is the prototypical and most dangerous agent of this group. It is a colorless gas under ordinary conditions of temperature and pressure with a boiling point of 8.2°C, making it a highly volatile and nonpersistent agent. It has a density 3.4 times that of air; therefore, it may remain for long periods in low-lying areas such as trenches. In low concentrations it has a smell of new-mown hay. It readily reaches the respiratory bronchioles and alveoli, causing direct toxicity by disrupting the alveolar-capillary membrane when hydrochloric acid is released as phosgene interacts with intraalveolar water. Clinical presentation depends on the level of exposure. Symptoms include cough, dyspnea, chest tightness, and substernal discomfort. With exposures to very high concentrations, pulmonary edema ensues within 12 hours, followed by death in 24 to 48 hours.

Histologic Features:

- Massive pulmonary edema.
- Tracheobronchitis and hyaline membranes may be seen, especially in cases of chlorine exposure.

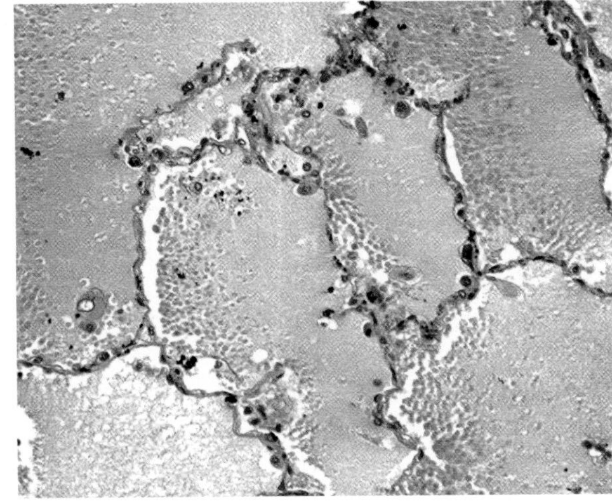

Figure 102.4 Pulmonary edema with eosinophilic proteinaceous material occupying alveolar spaces.

Section 18

Transplant-Related Pathology

Table 103.2. Grading of Airway Inflammation (B Grade)

Grade	Features
B0 (no airway inflammation)	No mononuclear cells
B1 (minimal airway inflammation)	Rare mononuclear cells in bronchial or bronchiolar submucosa
B2 (mild airway inflammation)	Circumferential mononuclear cell infiltrate ± occasional eosinophils in bronchial or bronchiolar submucosa; small numbers of intraepithelial lymphocytes may be present
B3 (moderate airway inflammation)	Dense grade B2 mononuclear cell infiltrate with numerous intraepithelial lymphocytes, lymphocyte satellitosis, epithelial cell apoptosis
B4 (severe airway inflammation)	Grade B3 features with epithelial detachment, ulceration, fibrinopurulent exudate
BX (ungradeable)	Grade cannot be assigned because of sampling or technical problem or other existing pathology (e.g., infection)

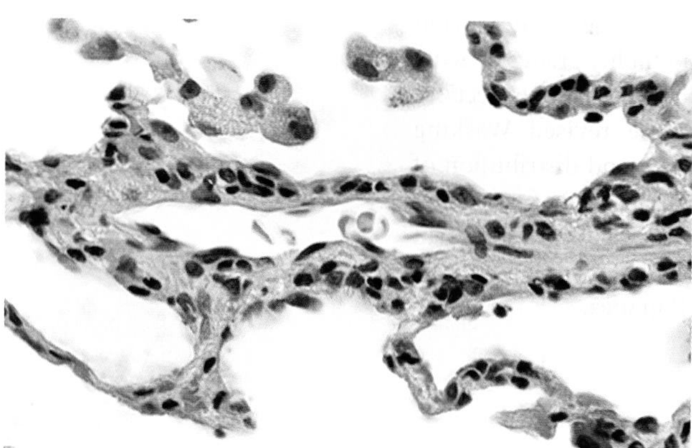

Figure 103.1 Acute cellular rejection, grade A1. A scant perivascular lymphocytic infiltrate is present.

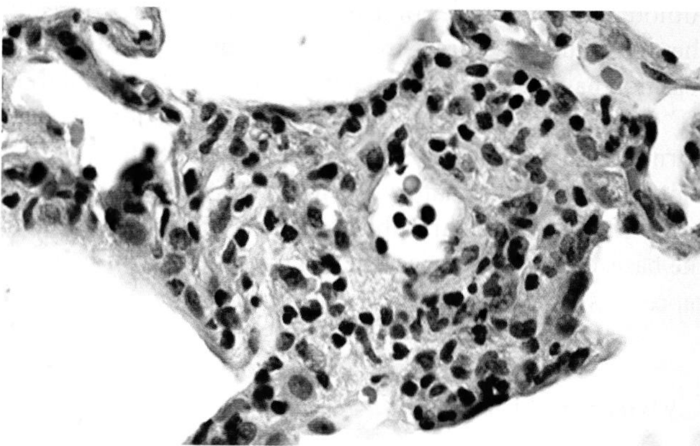

Figure 103.2 Acute cellular rejection, grade A2. A thick cuff of lymphocytes surrounds this venule.

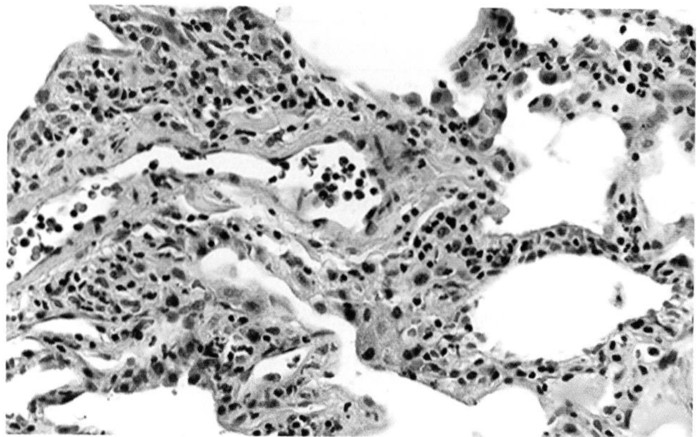

Figure 103.3 Acute cellular rejection, grade A3. The perivascular mononuclear cell infiltrate extends into adjacent alveolar septa.

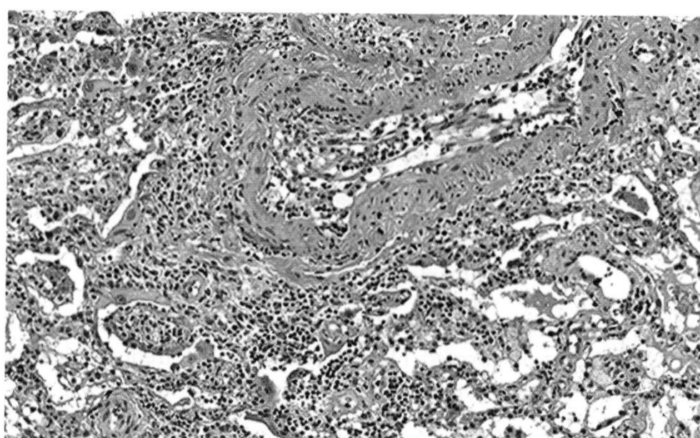

Figure 103.4 Airway inflammation, grade A4. Extensive perivascular, interstitial, and alveolar mononuclear cell infiltrates are present with alveolar fibrinous exudate. There is prominent endothelialitis (shown at higher power in Fig. 103.5). Alveolar pneumocyte injury, loss, and proliferation are present in different areas.

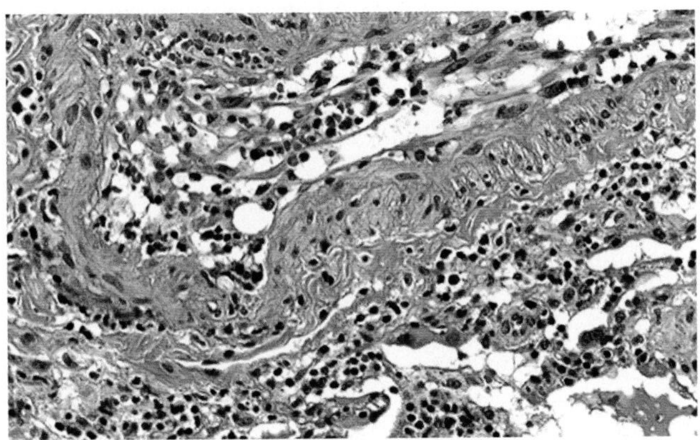

Figure 103.5 Airway inflammation, grade A4. Lymphocytic infiltration of the endothelium is associated with endothelial cell vacuolization and proliferation.

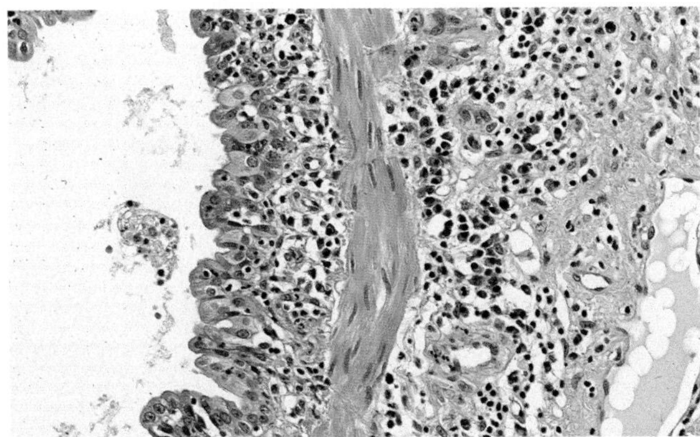

Figure 103.6 Airway inflammation, grade B3. Numerous lymphocytes and plasma cells infiltrate the mucosa and submucosa, with associated apoptosis of epithelial cells.

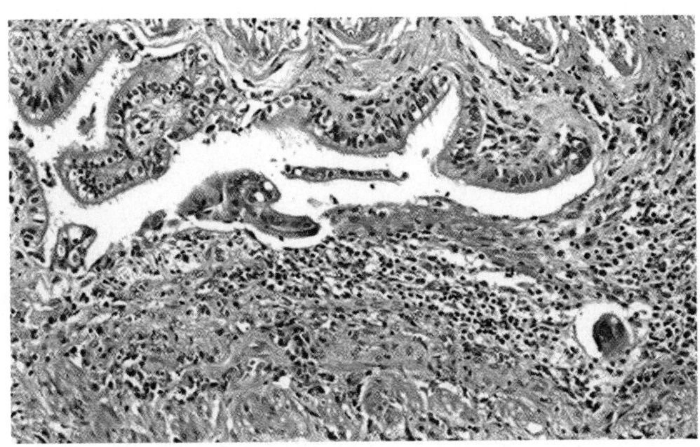

Figure 103.7 Airway inflammation, grade B4. Bronchiolar ulceration has occurred in association with prominent mononuclear inflammatory cell infiltrates. The lumen contains fibrinous exudate with early organization.

104 Chronic Lung Transplant Rejection

▶ Dani S. Zander

Chronic rejection of transplanted lungs is manifested primarily as obliterative bronchiolitis (chronic airway rejection) and accelerated graft vascular sclerosis (chronic vascular rejection), and it probably accounts, at least in part, for some cases of large airway fibrosis. The reported prevalence of this complication ranges from 30% to 60% and is influenced by the definition of the at-risk patient group and whether the diagnosis is made clinically (bronchiolitis obliterans syndrome) or histologically (obliterative bronchiolitis). Obliterative bronchiolitis is the most frequent cause of death in long-term survivors of lung transplantation. Multiple risk factors have been implicated in its genesis, including the number and severity of acute rejection episodes, lymphocytic bronchitis/bronchiolitis, cytomegalovirus (CMV) infection, human leukocyte antigen (HLA) mismatching, decreased immunosuppression, longer ischemia times, young and older recipient age, and excessive recipient body mass index. Chronic airway rejection is most often diagnosed near the end of the first posttransplantation year or later. Symptoms include dyspnea and cough, and physiologic evidence of airway obstruction is present.

Cytologic Features:

- Lymphocytosis and neutrophilia in bronchoalveolar lavage fluid.

Histologic Features:

Obliterative Bronchiolitis

- Dense collagen in the submucosa of small airways, either concentric or eccentric, leading to luminal narrowing or obliteration.
- Mononuclear cell infiltrates may be present in airway submucosa, luminal connective tissue, and/or peribronchiolar connective tissue; if these inflammatory cell infiltrates are present, the obliterative bronchiolitis is termed *active;* the modifier *inactive* is used if the infiltrates are absent.
- Epithelial cell injury is often present in active obliterative bronchiolitis.
- Airway smooth muscle may be fragmented or replaced by collagen.
- May be accompanied by foamy macrophages in bronchiole and/or alveoli (endogenous lipoid pneumonia).

Accelerated Graft Vascular Sclerosis

- Fibrointimal thickening of arteries and veins with variable accompanying subendothelial, intimal, and/or medial mononuclear cell infiltrates.
- Coexisting obliterative bronchiolitis is usually present.

Large Airway Fibrosis

- Dense collagen in the bronchial submucosa, with variable accompanying submucosal and epithelial mononuclear cell infiltrates.
- Bronchiectasis is usually present.
- Fungal colonization, especially with *Aspergillus* sp., may be present.

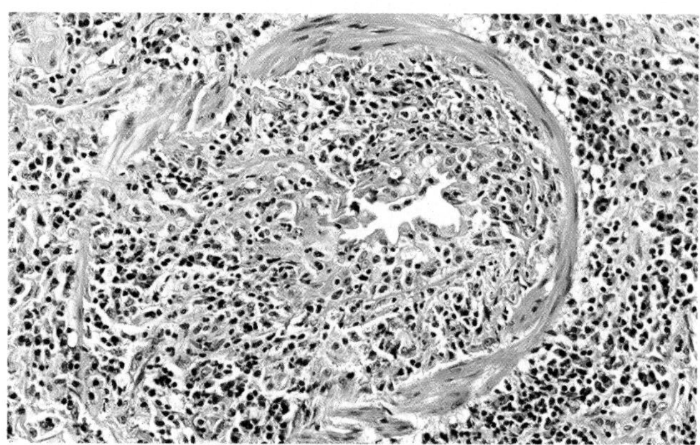

Figure 104.1 Histology figure of active obliterative bronchiolitis. There is concentric narrowing of the bronchiolar lumen due to fibrous thickening of the submucosa, with accompanying submucosal and peribronchiolar lymphoplasmacytic infiltrates. Respiratory epithelial cell injury is also present.

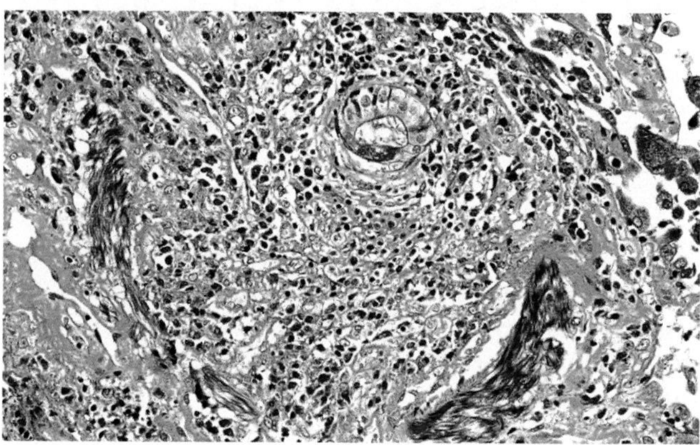

Figure 104.2 Masson trichrome stain of active obliterative bronchiolitis. This stain is helpful for highlighting the presence of the mature collagen, which is necessary to apply the diagnosis of obliterative bronchiolitis.

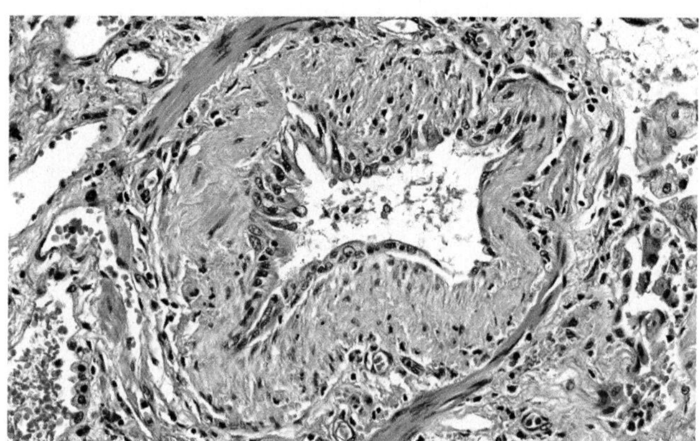

Figure 104.3 Histology figure of inactive obliterative bronchiolitis. This bronchiole demonstrates concentric deposition of subepithelial collagen without associated inflammation. There is focal epithelial cell loss and repair (flattened epithelial cells). Partial loss of airway smooth muscle is also evident.

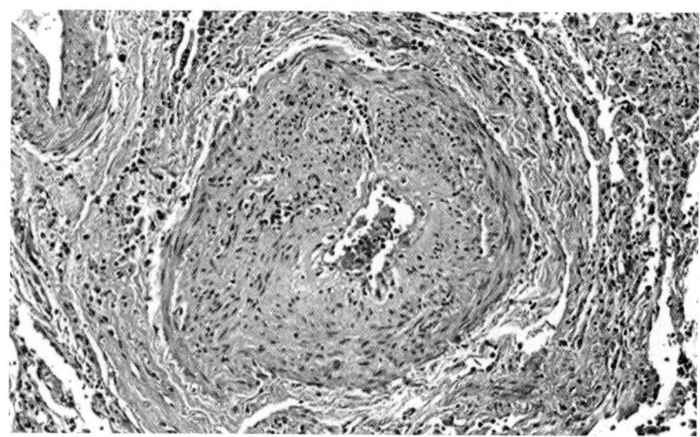

Figure 104.4 Histology figure of chronic vascular rejection. This artery manifests fibrointimal thickening and luminal narrowing.

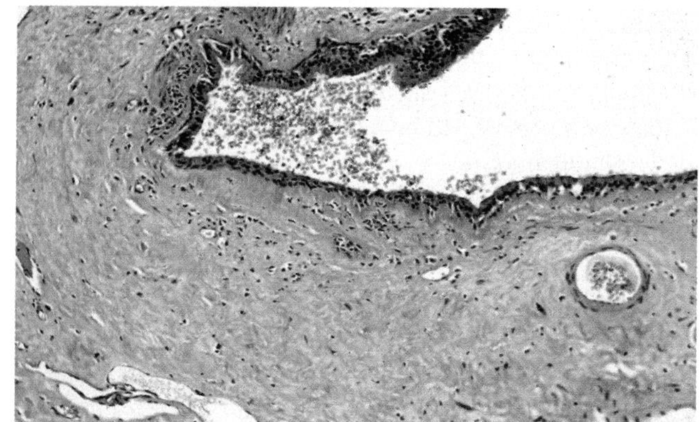

Figure 104.5 Histology figure of large airway fibrosis. Normal bronchial structures (cartilage, smooth muscle, submucosal glands) have been replaced by hyalinized collagen. There is a sparse mononuclear inflammatory cell infiltrate and focal squamous metaplasia.

Hyperacute Rejection of the Transplanted Lung

105

▶ Dani S. Zander

Hyperacute rejection is very rare and has not yet been precisely defined. Most reported cases have been fatal and share the following features: onset of pulmonary edema and hemorrhage during or immediately after transplantation, presence of antibodies to class I or II human leukocyte antigen (HLA), and the histologic findings described in the following.

Histologic Features:

- Increased interstitial neutrophils and mononuclear cells, with some neutrophils in alveolar spaces.
- Extensive alveolar hemorrhage.
- Edema and hyaline membranes.
- Alveolar septal necrosis, platelet/fibrin thrombi, fibrinoid necrosis of arterioles, bronchiolar epithelial cell necrosis, and neutrophil infiltration are variably present.
- Immunofluorescence staining for immunoglobulin G (IgG) may be present along alveolar septa.

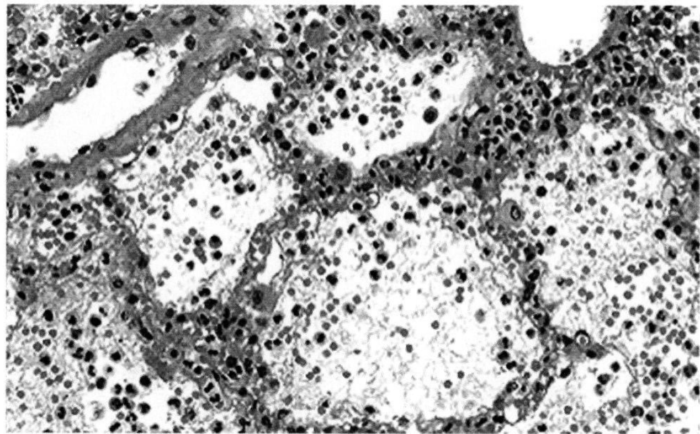

Figure 105.1 Alveolar septa containing neutrophils and mononuclear cell infiltrates; congestion and alveolar hemorrhage and fibrin are present, with alveolar neutrophils and apoptotic cells.

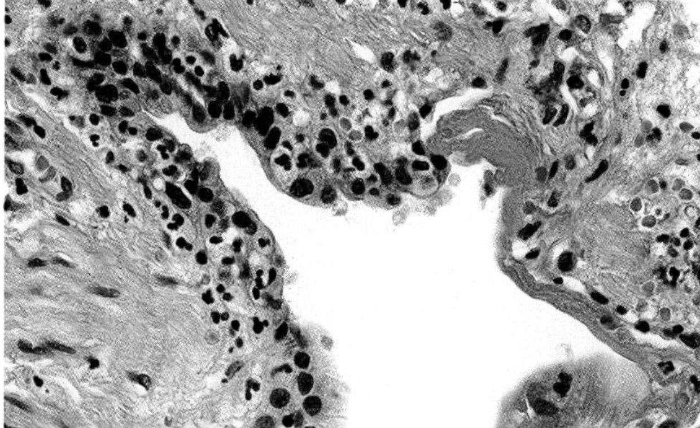

Figure 105.2 Partial replacement of bronchiole lining by a hyaline membrane, with neutrophils and mononuclear inflammatory cells infiltrating the remaining bronchiole epithelium.

Lung Transplant Anastomotic Complications

106

▶ Dani S. Zander

Loss of the bronchial artery blood supply renders the bronchial anastomosis vulnerable to ischemic and infectious complications. Not infrequently, ischemic necrosis of the airway develops early after transplantation, predisposing to infections and rarely leading to dehiscence. Common agents responsible for anastomotic infections include *Pseudomonas* spp., other Gram-negative bacilli, coagulase-positive staphylococci, *Candida* spp., and *Aspergillus* spp. With therapy, infections can usually be controlled, allowing the necrotic tissues to heal with formation of granulation tissue and fibrosis. Uncommon later complications include bronchomalacia and stenosis.

Vascular anastomotic complications are currently very rare and include pulmonary venous and arterial obstructions due to thrombosis, excessive or inadequate length and distortion of vessels, and restrictive suture.

Histologic Features:

Airway Anastomotic Complications

- Coagulative necrosis of the bronchial mucosa, submucosa, and sometimes cartilage.
- Bacteria and/or fungi may be visible on routine hematoxylin and eosin stain, but a methenamine stain is also recommended to more thoroughly assess for the presence of fungi.
- Neutrophil infiltrates are usually present when a bacterial or fungal infection exists.

Vascular Anastomotic Complications

- Thrombosis is common.

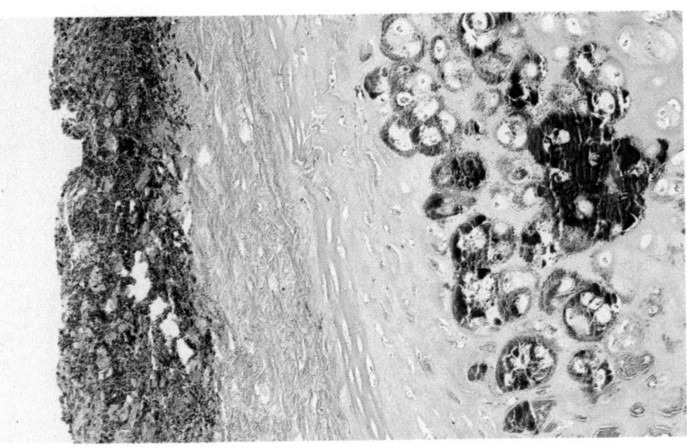

Figure 106.1 Ischemic necrosis of the bronchial anastomosis showing all layers of the bronchial wall have undergone coagulative necrosis. The bronchial cartilage shows loss of nuclei and calcification, and an inflammatory exudate covers the necrotic mucosal surface.

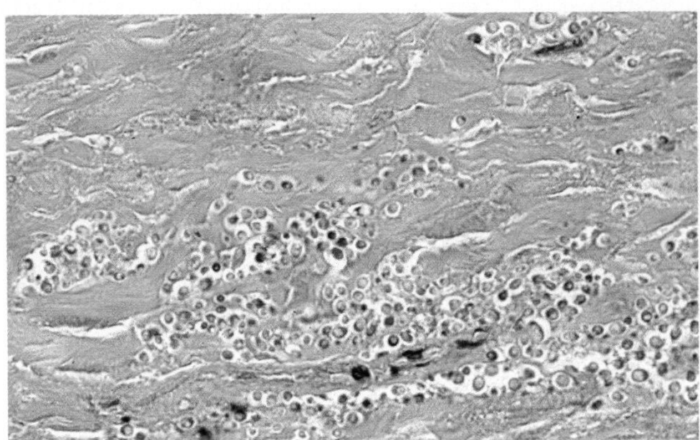

Figure 106.2 *Candida albicans* infection of the bronchial anastomosis, with numerous yeasts permeating the necrotic bronchial submucosa.

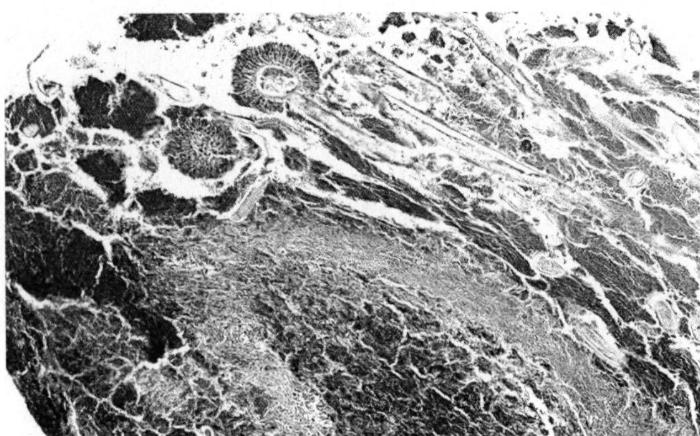

Figure 106.3 *Aspergillus niger* infection of the bronchial anastomosis showing the conidial heads ("fruiting heads") consisting of a globose vesicle that is completely covered by phialides, which in turn produce conidia. The fungi lie amidst necrotic debris covering the anastomotic site. Fruiting heads can sometimes be found in infected sites that are exposed to ambient air.

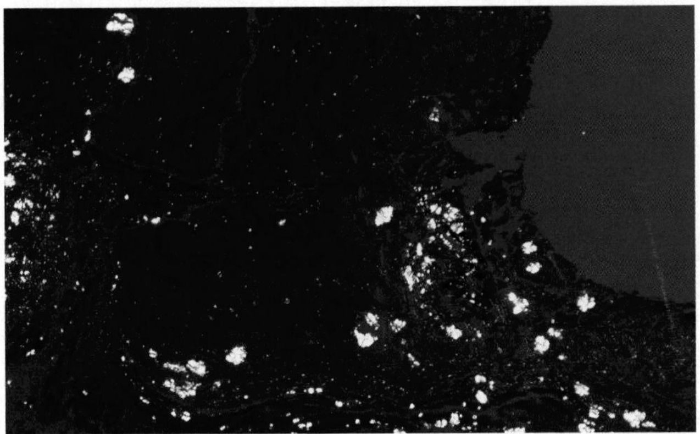

Figure 106.4 *A. niger* infection of the bronchial anastomosis, under polarized light, with numerous oxalate crystals apparent under polarized light. Oxalic acid produced by *A. niger* combines with host-derived calcium ions to form the crystals.

Transplant-Related Infections

107

▶ Dani S. Zander

Solid organ and bone marrow transplant recipients are vulnerable to infections caused by a wide spectrum of opportunistic pathogens, as well as agents capable of producing disease in healthy hosts. Predisposing factors include the use of immunosuppressive agents, the presence of other types of lung injury induced by chemotherapeutic agents or radiation, and in lung transplant recipients, loss of the cough reflex in the allograft and airway anastomotic ischemia. In recipients of transplanted lungs, most infections involve the allograft, but occasionally a remaining native lung is the site of the infection. Pulmonary infections usually are acquired via inhalation or hematogenous spread, but in lung transplant recipients, the donor lung may also be the source of the infection (bacteria, tuberculosis, fungi).

Pathogens, usual patterns of injury, and some of the unique presentations in transplant patients are listed in Table 107.1. It should be noted, however, that the severity and nature of the manifestations for many of these agents can vary substantially because of host factors, variables related to the exposure, and therapeutic regimens. Most of these agents are discussed more extensively in other sections of this book. Representative illustrations of some of these agents are also shown here.

Table 107.1

Agents	Usual Patterns of Injury
Bacterial infections, especially *Pseudomonas* sp, other Gram-negative bacilli, coagulase-positive staphylococci	Airway anastomotic infection (localized) in lung transplant recipient Acute/necrotizing bronchitis/bronchopneumonia Abscess Diffuse alveolar damage
Cytomegalovirus	Interstitial pneumonia Diffuse alveolar damage
Herpes simplex virus	Ulcerative tracheobronchitis Necrotizing pneumonia (bronchocentric or hematogenous) Diffuse alveolar damage
Human herpes virus 6	Interstitial pneumonia
Varicella zoster virus	Necrotizing pneumonia (hematogenous)
Adenovirus	Necrotizing bronchocentric pneumonia Diffuse alveolar damage
Respiratory syncytial virus parainfluenza	Acute bronchiolitis Interstitial pneumonia Diffuse alveolar damage
Influenza	Acute/necrotizing bronchitis/bronchopneumonia Diffuse alveolar damage
Candida spp.	Airway anastomotic infection (localized) in lung transplant recipient Airway colonization Acute/necrotizing bronchitis/bronchopneumonia, abscesses Diffuse alveolar damage

Continued

Table 107.1, cont'd

Agents	Usual Patterns of Injury
Aspergillus sp.	Airway anastomotic infection (localized) in lung transplant recipient
	Airway colonization and invasive airway infection
	Colonization of a parenchymal cavity
	Bronchocentric granulomatous infection
	Chronic necrotizing aspergillosis
	Angioinvasive pneumonia
	Diffuse alveolar damage
Mucormycosis	Necrotizing bronchitis
	Abscess
	Angioinvasive pneumonia
Pneumocystis jiroveci	Interstitial pneumonia, occasionally with granuloma formation
	Diffuse alveolar damage
M. tuberculosis and nontuberculous mycobacteria	Granulomatous infection
Toxoplasma gondii	Necrotizing pneumonia

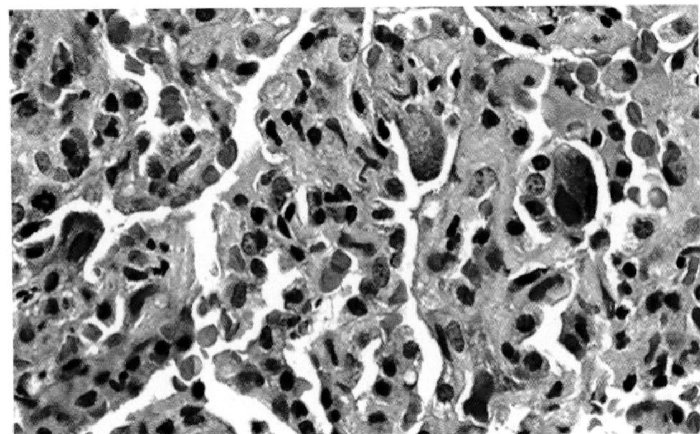

Figure 107.1 Cytomegalovirus infection showing characteristic cellular alterations caused by cytomegalovirus (cytomegaly, nucleomegaly, intranuclear inclusions, intracytoplasmic inclusions) evident in several infected cells. A mild interstitial lymphocytic infiltrate represents the host response to the infection.

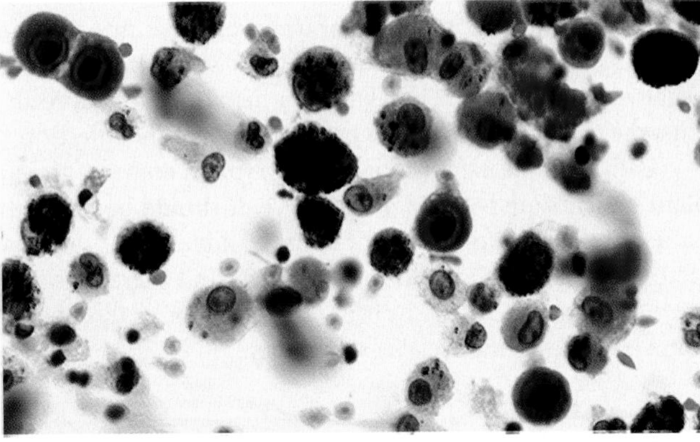

Figure 107.2 Cytology figure of cytomegalovirus infection from a bronchoalveolar lavage fluid showing several cells containing large intranuclear inclusions characteristic of cytomegalovirus. Abundant pigment-laden macrophages are also present.

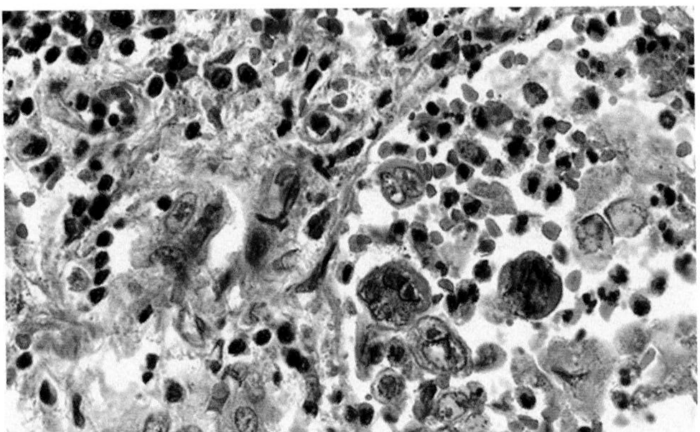

Figure 107.3 Herpes simplex virus pneumonia with multinucleated giant cells containing eosinophilic intranuclear inclusions or ground glass chromatin within an alveolus, accompanied by a mixed inflammatory infiltrate and apoptotic cells.

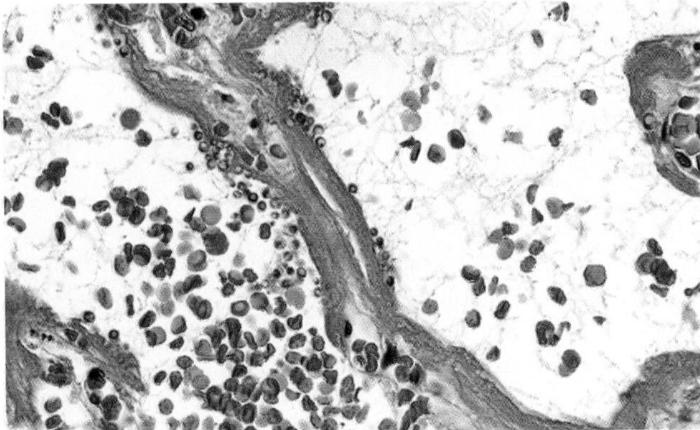

Figure 107.4 Diffuse alveolar damage due to *Candida albicans* (granulocytopenic bone marrow transplant recipient), with hyaline membranes covered by numerous small yeasts.

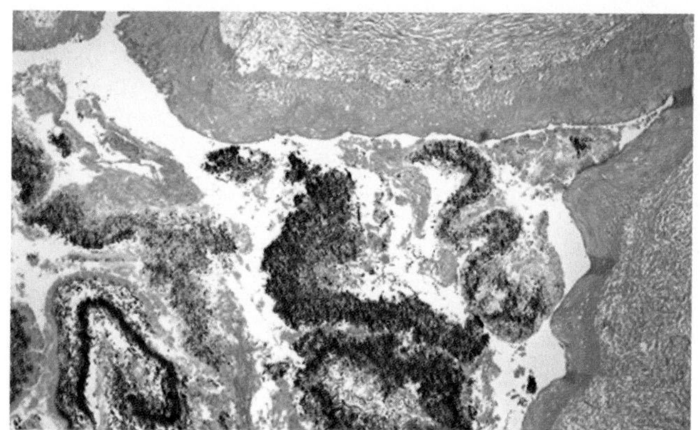

Figure 107.5 Methenamine silver stain of an intrabronchial aspergilloma (transplanted lung) showing masses of aspergillus filling the lumen of an ectatic bronchus and replacement of the respiratory epithelium by metaplastic squamous epithelium.

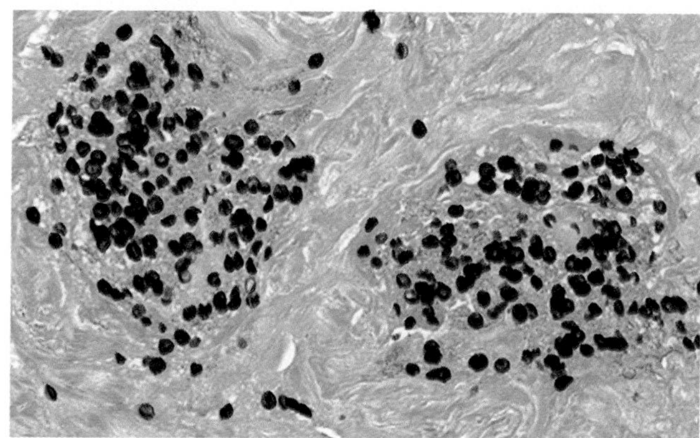

Figure 107.6 Methenamine silver stain of *Pneumocystis jiroveci.* Numerous small cysts lie enmeshed in alveolar exudate.

Ischemia-Reperfusion Injury in the Transplanted Lung

108

▸ Dani S. Zander

Ischemia-reperfusion injury is a significant cause of early posttransplant morbidity and mortality and is one of the etiologies of primary graft failure. Onset of symptoms occurs within 72 hours after lung transplantation. The clinical presentation ranges from mild hypoxemia with few radiographic infiltrates to an acute respiratory distress syndromelike picture. Pathologic findings likewise range from focal acute alveolar injury to diffuse alveolar damage. The process can undergo resolution or can organize, leading to an organizing pneumonia or organizing diffuse alveolar damage pattern.

Histologic Features:

- Histologic features of diffuse alveolar damage are present but may be focal, patchy, or diffuse.
- Differential diagnosis includes acute alveolar injury/diffuse alveolar damage secondary to acute rejection, which is much more lymphocyte rich, or infections.

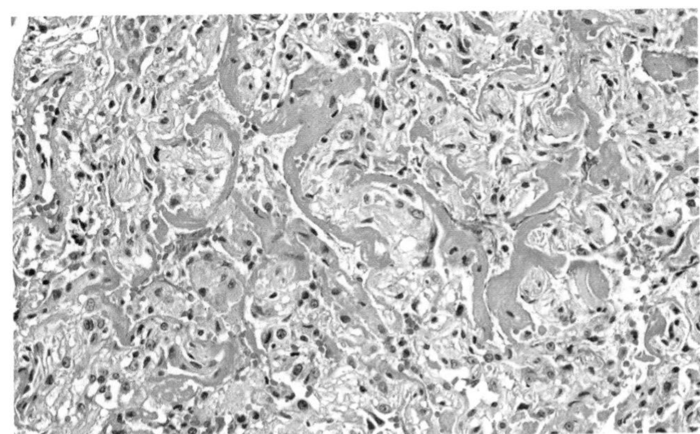

Figure 108.1 Prominent hyaline membranes line alveolar septa, which appear slightly thickened but have no significant inflammatory infiltrates.

109 Organizing Pneumonia in the Transplanted Lung

Dani S. Zander

In lung transplant biopsies, organizing pneumonia occurs in several clinicopathologic settings. Most frequently, it accompanies ongoing acute rejection or reflects an earlier, resolved, episode of acute rejection. It may coexist with obliterative bronchiolitis (chronic airway rejection). Pneumonias caused by cytomegalovirus, herpes simplex virus, respiratory viruses, *Pneumocystis jiroveci, Aspergillus,* and bacteria can be associated with this reaction pattern. The reaction also can be seen as a sequel to initially diffuse acute ischemia-reperfusion injury.

Histologic Features:

- Granulation tissue in alveolar spaces and respiratory bronchioles and, to a lesser extent, the alveolar interstitium; granulation tissue consists of fibroblasts with spindle-shaped nuclei in an acid mucopolysaccharide-rich matrix.
- Variable collagen deposition.
- Small numbers of lymphocytes and macrophages, including some containing hemosiderin, in the alveolar connective tissue.
- Increased mononuclear cells, particularly if they have a perivascular distribution, may indicate the presence of acute cellular rejection.
- Reactive alveolar pneumocytes.

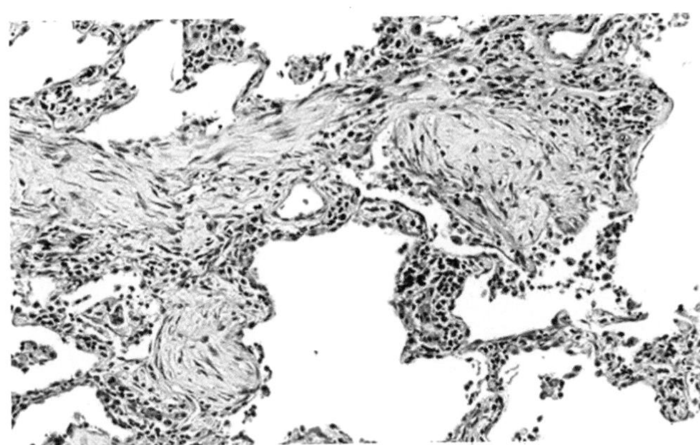

Figure 109.1 Young connective tissue with some collagen deposition fills alveolar spaces. Perivascular and interstitial lymphocytic infiltrates indicate the presence of high-grade acute cellular rejection.

Other Lung Transplant-Related Pathology

110

▸ Dani S. Zander

Recurrence of native disease in the transplanted lung is very uncommon. Diseases reported to recur include the following:

- Sarcoidosis.
- Lymphangioleiomyomatosis.
- Desquamative interstitial pneumonia.
- Giant cell interstitial pneumonia.
- Langerhans cell histiocytosis.
- Alveolar proteinosis.
- Diffuse panbronchiolitis.
- Idiopathic pulmonary hemosiderosis.
- Bronchioloalveolar carcinoma.

Alveolar proteinosis also represents an unusual complication of lung transplantation that may stem from an impairment in macrophage processing of lipoprotein and fibrinous material, predisposed to by immunosuppressive therapy and repeated alveolar injury.

Alveolar hemosiderosis occurs to varying degrees in transplanted lungs. Patients with multiple bouts and higher grades of rejection or bleeding abnormalities tend to accumulate more hemosiderin-laden macrophages in alveoli. Sites of earlier infection and prior biopsy sites also commonly show increased numbers of hemosiderin-laden macrophages.

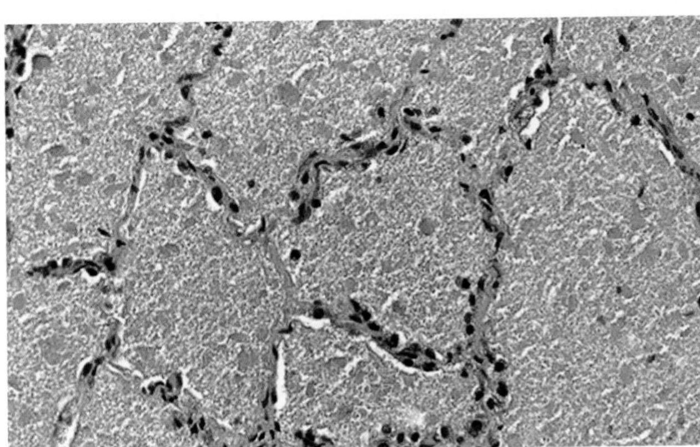

Figure 110.1 Alveolar proteinosis, with eosinophilic proteinaceous material filling alveolar spaces.

Posttransplant Lymphoproliferative Disorders

111

▶ Dani S. Zander

Posttransplant lymphoproliferative disorders (PTLDs) are a morphologically heterogeneous group of lymphoid proliferations that includes both hyperplasias and neoplasms. Most cases arise within the first 2 years after transplantation, in the allograft itself, lymph nodes, or other lymphoid tissues. In transplanted lungs, most appear as nodules that may be visualized during bronchoscopy as ulcerated and necrotic masses in airways. PTLDs can be multicentric, representing either advanced-stage disease or multiple independent primary tumors. Although most PTLDs are of B-lymphocyte origin, cases with a T- or natural killer (NK)-cell origin have also been reported. In solid organ transplant recipients, most PTLDs arise from recipient cells, whereas the reverse is true for patients with bone marrow transplants. Approximately 90% of PTLDs contain Epstein-Barr virus (EBV).

Major categories of PTLDs include (i) hyperplastic PTLDs ("early lesions")—reactive plasmacytic hyperplasia, infectious mononucleosis, atypical lymphoid hyperplasia with architectural retention; (ii) polymorphic lymphoproliferative disorders; and (iii) lymphomatous or monomorphic PTLDs—B-cell lymphomas (diffuse large cell and Burkittlike lymphomas, MALToma) and T-cell lymphomas (peripheral T-cell, anaplastic large cell, hepatosplenic γ-δ T-cell lymphomas). Other less common categories include plasmacytoma, myeloma, and T-cell–rich/Hodgkin diseaselike large B-cell lymphoma. Most hyperplastic PTLDs are polyclonal, but they may contain one or more minor clonal subpopulations. These lesions usually regress after reduction or withdrawal of immunosuppression. The malignant lymphomas are monoclonal, manifest alterations involving the N-*ras* or c-*myc* protooncogenes or the p53 tumor suppressor gene, and often progress despite aggressive therapy. The polymorphic lymphoproliferative disorders are also monoclonal but demonstrate variable clinical behavior.

Pathologic approach to diagnosis should incorporate morphologic, phenotypic, and clonality assessment, as well as information about EBV status. Phenotypic and clonality evaluation can be performed using immunohistochemistry, flow cytometry, and/or molecular methodologies. EBV status can be assessed by immunohistochemistry (EBV latent membrane protein) or *in situ* hybridization (EBV EBER1 RNA). In difficult cases in which the differential diagnosis includes acute rejection or non-EBV infection, the presence of EBV in lymphoid cells favors PTLD. Nonetheless, EBV positivity should not be considered equivalent to a diagnosis of PTLD if morphologic, phenotypic, and clonal criteria for PTLD are not fulfilled.

Histologic Features:

Features of the most common types of PTLDs are presented here. The referenced articles provide more information about the less common categories.

Plasmacytic Hyperplasia

- Retention of underlying tissue architecture.
- Infiltration of tissue or expansion of nodal interfollicular area by a population of plasmacytoid lymphocytes, plasma cells, and sparse immunoblasts.
- Germinal centers may be hyperplastic, involuted, or absent.

Polymorphic PTLD

- Infiltration of tissues and replacement of normal structures by a mixture of cells, including plasmacytoid lymphoid cells, immunoblasts with or without cytologic atypia and plasmacytoid features, and plasma cells.
- Confluent areas of coagulative necrosis, single-cell necrosis, or necrosis of small areas may be present.

Monomorphic PTLD (Diffuse Large Cell Lymphoma)

- Infiltration of tissues and replacement of normal structures by a monomorphic population of large transformed lymphoid cells with vesicular chromatin, round to oval nuclei, and one or two nucleoli.
- Some cases include numerous immunoblasts (large transformed cells with large central nucleoli and amphophilic/basophilic cytoplasm).
- In some cases, cells may have plasmacytoid features.
- Confluent areas of coagulative necrosis, single-cell necrosis, or necrosis of small areas may be present.

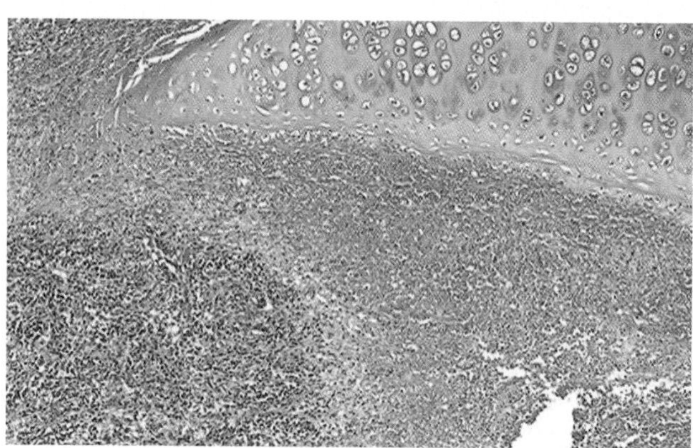

Figure 111.1 Monomorphic PTLD (diffuse large cell lymphoma) forming an extensively necrotic endobronchial mass.

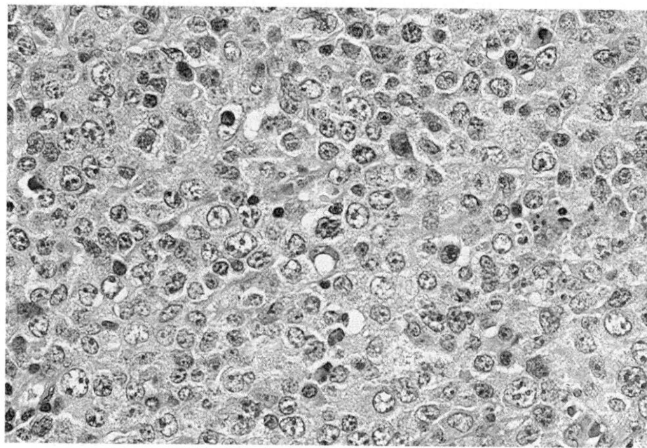

Figure 111.2 Monomorphic PTLD (diffuse large cell lymphoma) showing large transformed lymphoid cells replacing normal structures. Nuclei are ovoid or irregular, with vesicular chromatin and one or more small nucleoli.

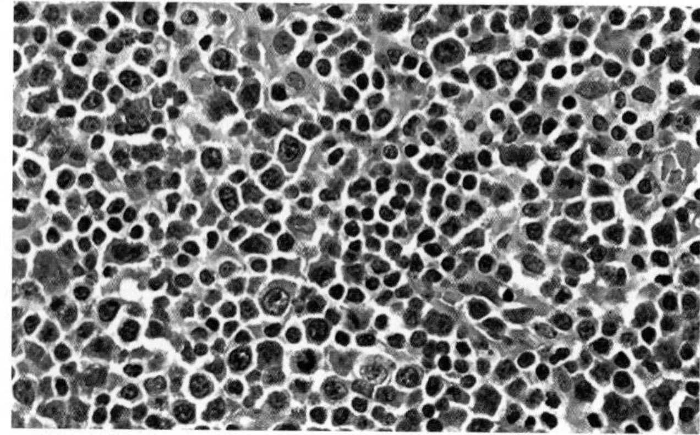

Figure 111.3 Polymorphic PTLD showing a mixture of cell types, including small lymphocytes, large plasmacytoid lymphocytes, and plasma cells.

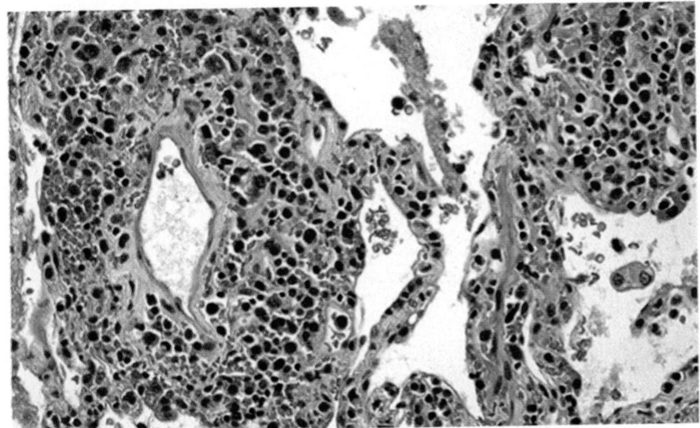

Figure 111.4 Polymorphic PTLD showing a perivascular infiltration by lymphoid cells, a common feature. In cases with little cytologic atypia, acute lung transplant rejection may be considered in the differential diagnosis if the patient is a lung transplant recipient.

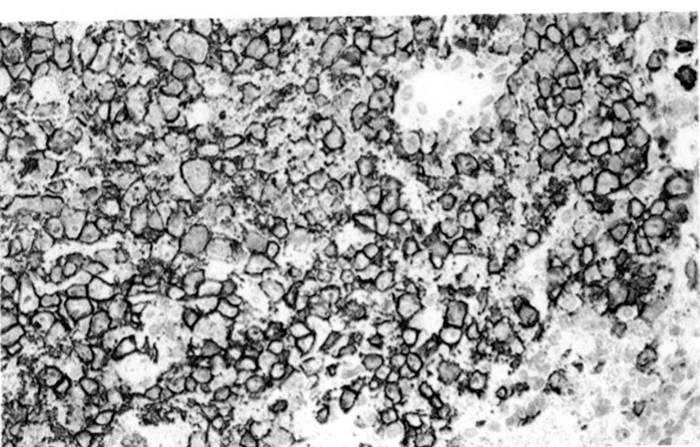

Figure 111.5 Immunohistochemistry of CD20; the overwhelming predominance of CD20-staining cells, in combination with the lack of CD3 expression (see Fig. 111.6), supports a diagnosis of B-cell lymphoma.

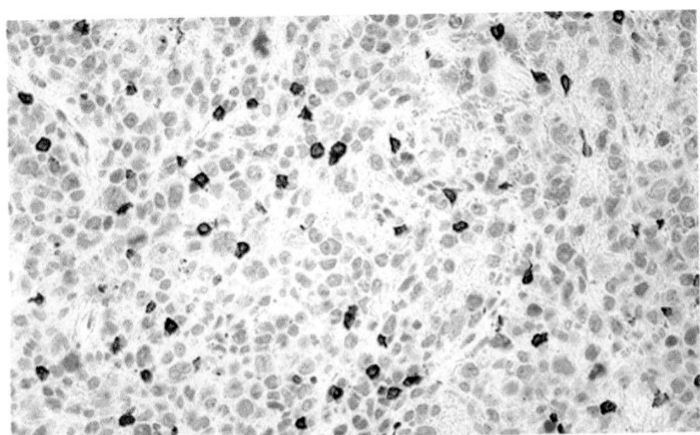

Figure 111.6 Immunohistochemistry of CD3. CD3-staining cells are much scantier than cells expressing CD20 (see Fig. 111.5), supporting a diagnosis of B-cell lymphoma.

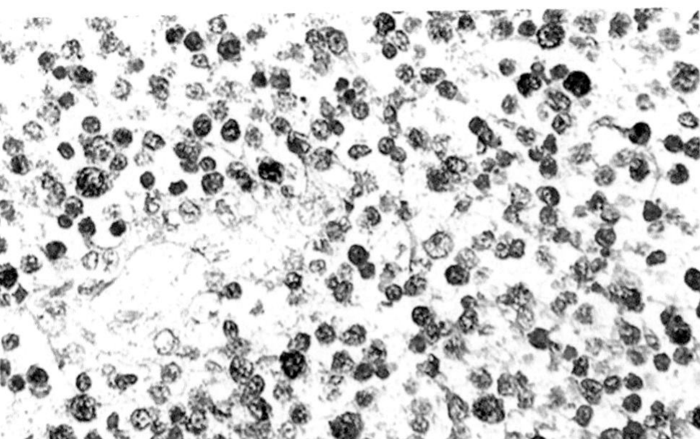

Figure 111.7 *In situ* hybridization for EBV EBER1 RNA; nuclear signal (brown) indicates the presence of EBV infection.

112 Graft Versus Host Disease

Dani S. Zander

Pulmonary manifestations of graft versus host disease (GVHD) usually occur in patients who have extrapulmonary GVHD (most commonly skin or gastrointestinal involvement), but occasionally it can represent the sole manifestation of GVHD. The spectrum of histologic abnormalities resembles that associated with acute and chronic lung transplant rejection and includes infiltration of perivascular regions and alveolar septa by mononuclear cells, lymphocyte-mediated airway injury, and chronic sequelae. The pathogenesis of this process is complex but involves donor-derived T-cell–mediated injury and destruction of cells expressing host human leukocyte antigen (HLA) and other antigens, including endothelial cells and epithelial cells. Serum components leak into airspaces and become organized into granulation tissue. The granulation tissue may resorb or progress to fibrosis.

Categories of morphologic changes representing cellular and fibrotic manifestations of GVHD are listed here. Infections, drug reactions, and radiation-associated pneumonia can produce similar pathologic findings and should be considered in the differential diagnosis when appropriate.

Histologic Features:

- Interstitial and perivascular mononuclear cell infiltrates.
- Lymphocytic bronchitis/bronchiolitis.
- Diffuse alveolar damage.
- Organizing pneumonia.
- Obliterative bronchiolitis.

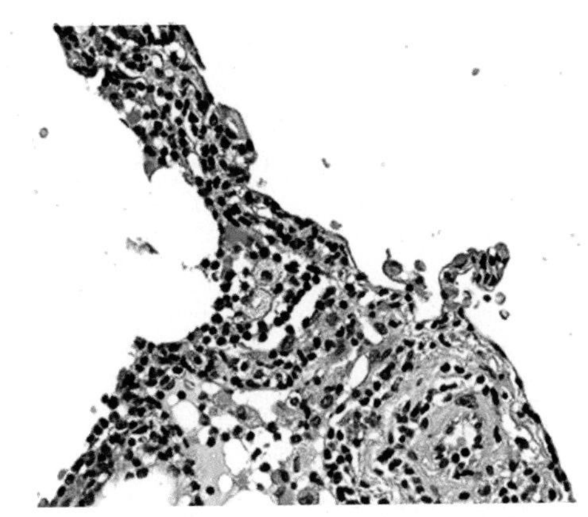

Figure 112.1 Manifestations of GVHD include interstitial and perivascular lymphocytic infiltrates.

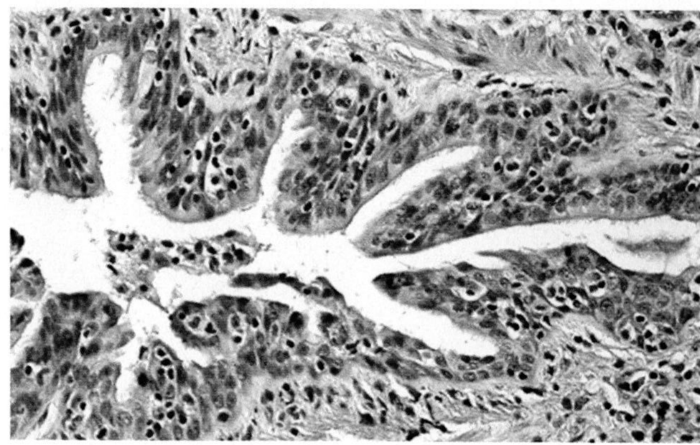

Figure 112.2 Lymphocytic bronchiolitis showing characteristic intraepithelial lymphocytes and respiratory epithelial cell apoptosis.

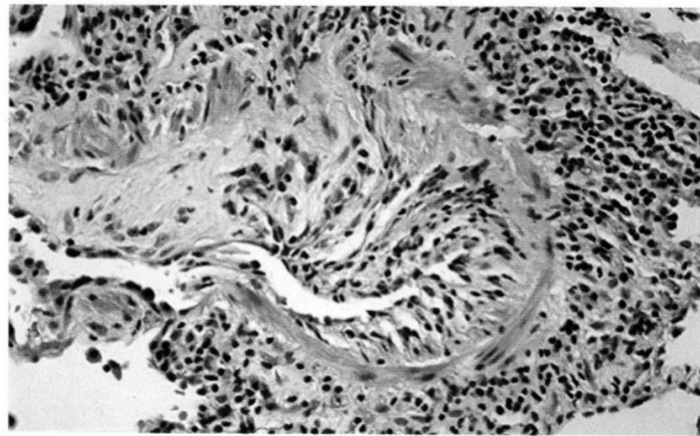

Figure 112.3 Obliterative bronchiolitis lesion showing marked luminal narrowing by connective tissue that includes substantial mature collagen and scattered lymphocytes. Peribronchiolar lymphocytic infiltrates are also present.

Section 19

Lung Pathology in Collagen Vascular Diseases

113 Lung Pathology in Collagen Vascular Diseases

Dani S. Zander

Pulmonary involvement by collagen vascular diseases can take a variety of forms. The individual diseases tend to be associated with a particular set of pathologic manifestations that may occur individually, in combination, or not at all, in individual patients. Conversely, most of the pathologic manifestations are associated with more than one disease. The spectrum of pathologic manifestations associated with the collagen vascular diseases is listed here. More information about specific diseases can be obtained from the referenced books.

Lung disease in these patients can develop as a consequence of therapy. Because collagen vascular diseases are often treated with immunosuppressive therapy, evaluation for opportunistic infections is an important responsibility of the pathologist. Reactions to therapeutic drugs may also be considered in the differential diagnosis, particularly if there is a temporal relationship between symptomatology and drug administration.

Histologic Features:

Pleural Abnormalities

- Chronic or fibrinous pleuritis.
- Pleural fibrosis.
- Pleural effusions.
- Rheumatoid nodules (rheumatoid arthritis).

Diffuse Interstitial and Alveolar Abnormalities

- Usual interstitial pneumonia.
- Nonspecific interstitial pneumonia.
- Diffuse alveolar damage.

Focal or Patchy Parenchymal Lesions

- Organizing pneumonia.
- Aspiration pneumonia.
- Rheumatoid nodule.

Vascular Lesions

- Vasculitis with or without diffuse alveolar hemorrhage (see Chapter 50, Part 1).
- Pulmonary hypertension.

Airway Lesions

- Follicular bronchitis/bronchiolitis.
- Lymphocytic infiltration of submucosal glands, atrophy (Sjögren syndrome).
- Obliterative (constrictive) bronchiolitis.

Amyloidosis

Malignancies

- Lung cancer (scleroderma).
- Lymphoma (Sjögren syndrome).

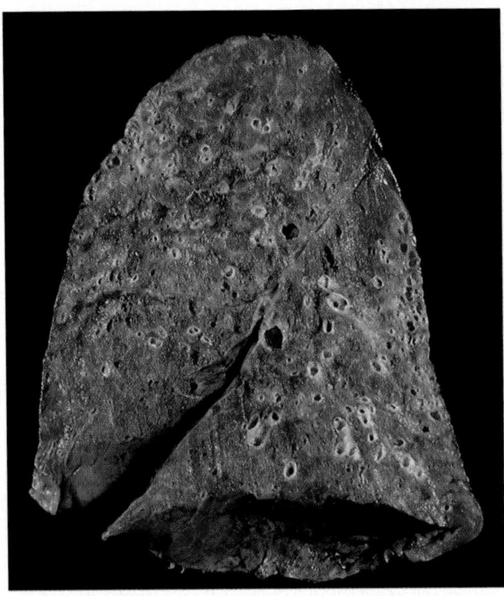

Figure 113.1 Gross figure of rheumatoid arthritis with usual interstitial pneumonia showing subpleural honeycomb change and extensive interstitial fibrosis.

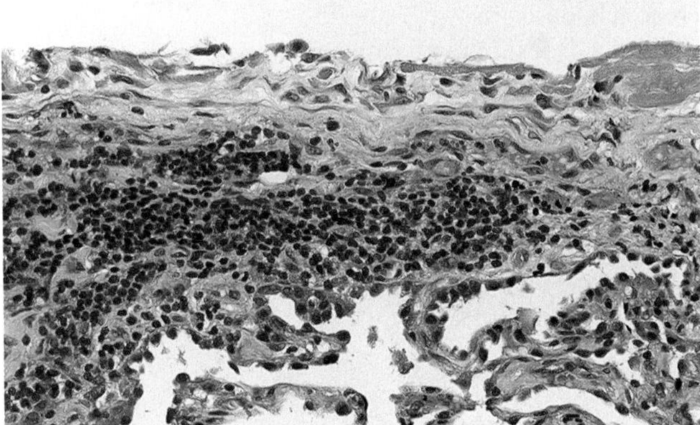

Figure 113.2 Rheumatoid pleuritis with pleural infiltration by lymphocytes and a partially covering pleural fibrinous exudate.

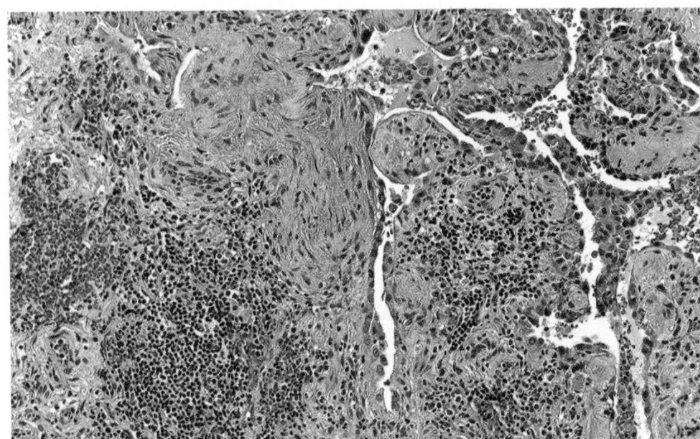

Figure 113.3 Usual interstitial pneumonia in rheumatoid arthritis, with marked interstitial fibrosis containing several lymphoid aggregates, a fibroblast focus, type 2 pneumocyte proliferation, and alveolar macrophage aggregation.

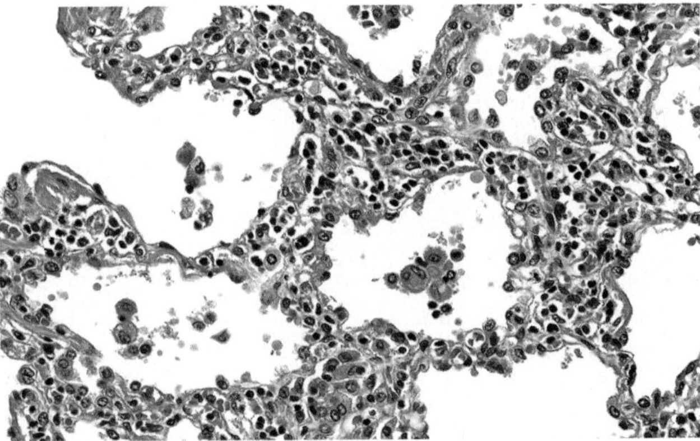

Figure 113.4 Nonspecific interstitial pneumonia, cellular type, in systemic lupus erythematosus showing an interstitium widened by an infiltrate consisting of lymphocytes and plasma cells, with little fibrosis.

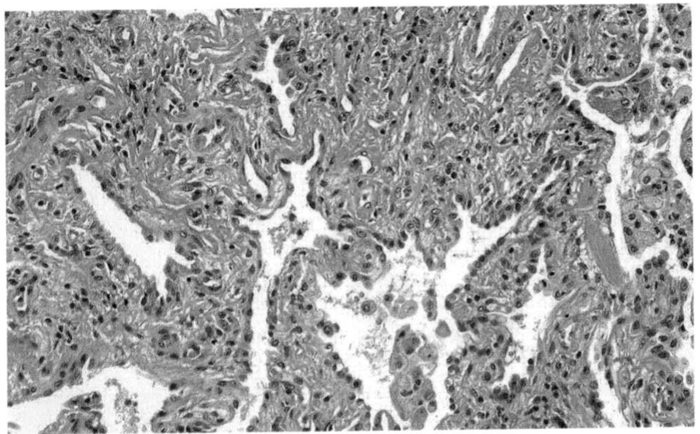

Figure 113.5 Nonspecific interstitial pneumonia, fibrosing type, in scleroderma showing uniform fibrotic thickening of the interstitium, with some type 2 pneumocyte proliferation.

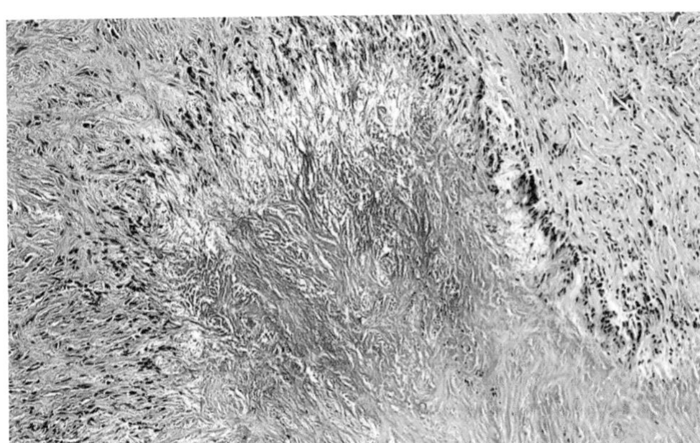

Figure 113.6 Rheumatoid nodule with a rim of palisaded histiocytes and a center of collagen with fibrinoid degeneration; the nodule is surrounded by dense fibrous tissue.

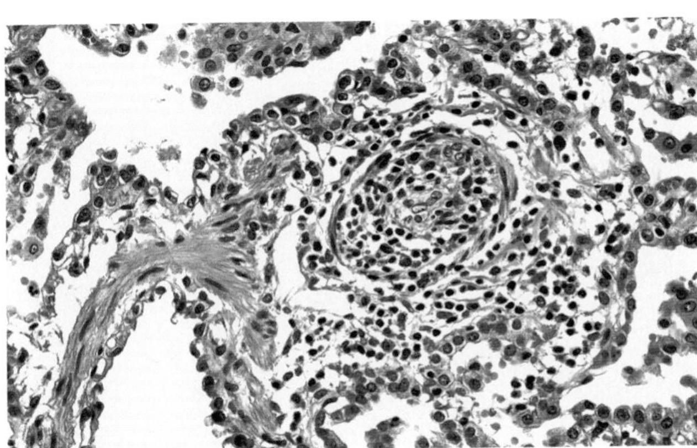

Figure 113.7 Vasculitis in rheumatoid arthritis, with a small artery infiltrated by mononuclear inflammatory cells.

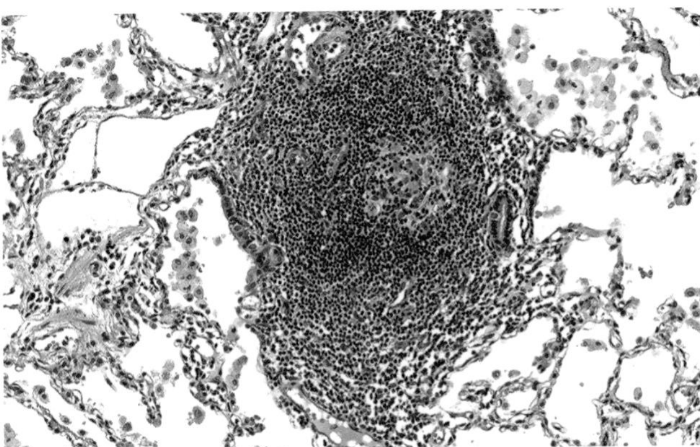

Figure 113.8 Follicular bronchiolitis in rheumatoid arthritis, with a lymphoid aggregate containing a germinal center distorting the wall of a respiratory bronchiole. The bronchiole contains smoker's macrophages (respiratory bronchiolitis).

114

Amiodarone

▶ Roberto Barrios
▶ Hakan Cermik

Amiodarone is a frequently used antiarrhythmic drug. It causes lung changes that are largely reversible but which may become permanent over time.

Cytologic Features:

- Finely vacuolated foamy macrophages, with or without neutrophils.

Histologic Features:

- Lymphocytic alveolitis.
- Alveolar macrophages with lamellar inclusions.
- Varying degrees of interstitial fibrosis.
- Diffuse alveolar damage.

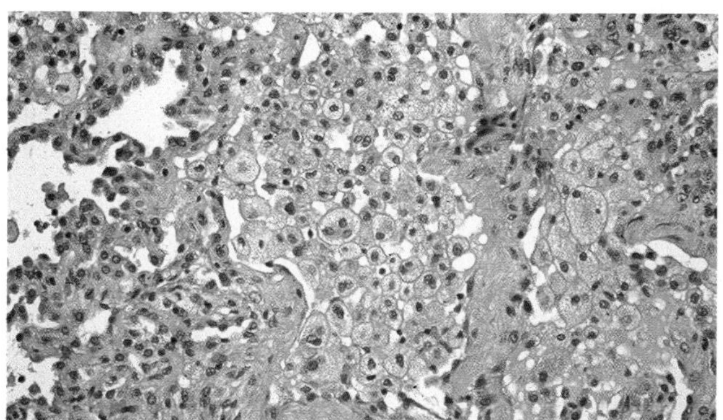

Figure 114.1 Low power shows intraalveolar accumulation of foamy macrophages and mild lymphoplasmacytic inflammation.

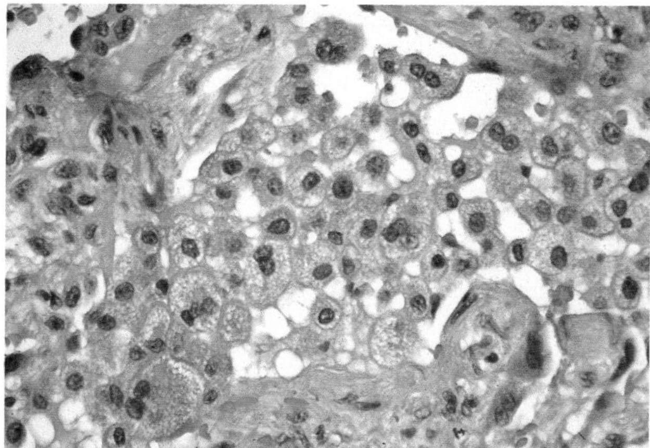

Figure 114.2 High power shows typical alveolar macrophages with finely vacuolated cytoplasm.

115 Methotrexate

Roberto Barrios
Hakan Cermik

Methotrexate is a folic acid antagonist that has been used as an antineoplastic and antiinflammatory drug. Methotrexate pneumonitis is an unpredictable and sometimes life-threatening side effect of methotrexate therapy. Lung lesions associated with this compound include interstitial infiltrates, granulomas, and changes consistent with diffuse alveolar damage associated with perivascular inflammation.

Histologic Features:

- Lymphocytic alveolitis (predominance of suppressor/cytotoxic T cells with a reduced $CD4^+/CD8^+$ ratio is common in methotrexate-induced pneumonitis).
- Neutrophilic alveolitis consisting of less than 5% neutrophils; this may reflect fibrosis.
- Eosinophilic alveolitis consisting of less than 5% eosinophils.
- Changes consistent with diffuse alveolar damage with perivascular infiltrates.
- Occasional focal isolated granulomas.

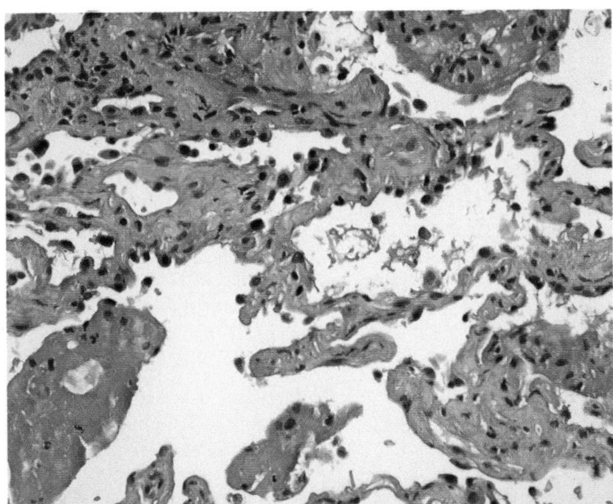

Figure 115.1 In addition to the interstitial changes, intraalveolar deposits of fibrin, occasional polymorphonuclear leukocytes, and eosinophils are present.

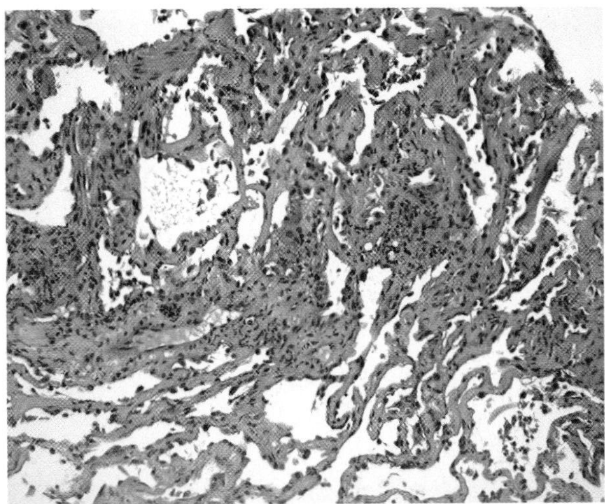

Figure 115.2 Changes secondary to methotrexate administration, including interstitial pneumonitis and fibrosis.

116

Phen-fen

- Roberto Barrios
- Timothy Allen

Phen-fen, a combination of the amphetamine analogs phentermine and fenfluramine, has been used to treat obesity and substance abuse disorders. Primary pulmonary hypertension has been reported to occur in patients treated with phen-fen.

Histologic Features:

- Plexiform arteriopathy is present in about 60% of pulmonary hypertension cases associated with phen-fen.
- Fibroproliferative intimal lesions in all arteries, including the main pulmonary arteries, and elastic, muscular, and small arteries.
- Diffuse and segmental thickening of intima and elastic media.

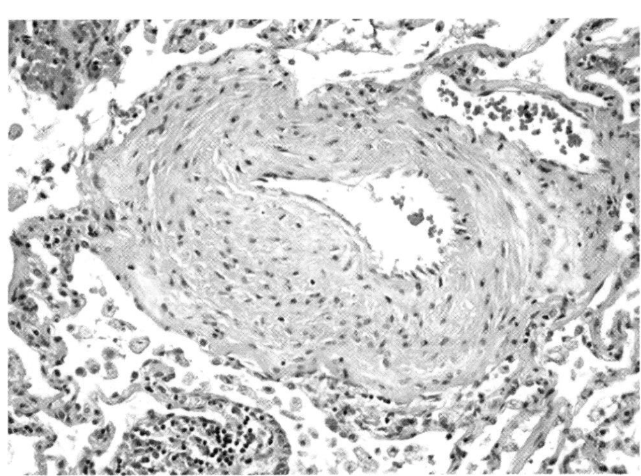

Figure 116.1 Lung parenchyma from a patient exposed to phen-fen shows a blood vessel with fibroproliferative intimal and medial thickening.

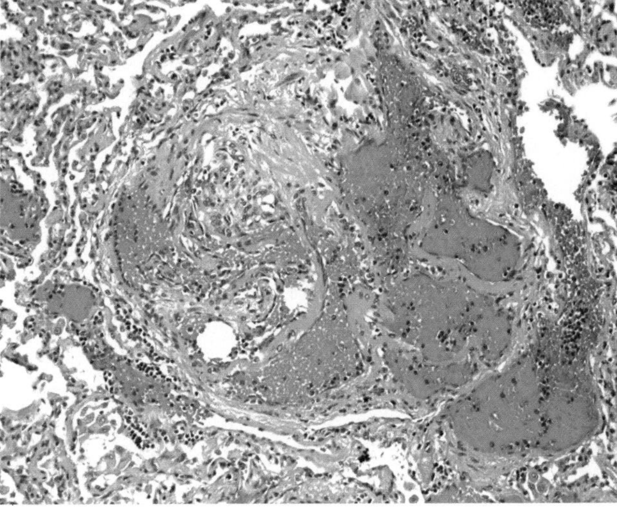

Figure 116.2 Plexiform arteriopathy in a patient exposed to phen-fen.

117

Mesalamine

▶ Dani S. Zander

In patients with inflammatory bowel diseases (IBDs) who are treated with mesalamine (5-aminosalicylic acid), lung disease can develop as a reaction to the mesalamine. Insidious and progressive dyspnea, nonproductive cough, fatigue, and low-grade fevers are the most common symptoms, and patients can have hypoxemia ranging from mild to severe. The onset of the reaction ranges widely from days to several years after the introduction of mesalamine therapy, and the likelihood of lung disease does not appear to be related to the dose of the medication. Lymphocyte stimulation tests suggest that mesalamine causes immune-mediated alveolitis.

Pulmonary function tests usually reveal a restrictive ventilatory defect with reduced diffusing capacity. Chest radiographs manifest a variety of abnormalities, including interstitial infiltrates, consolidation, and pleural effusions. Although pathologic features overlap with other lung diseases, particularly Crohn disease, the combination of interstitial mononuclear cell infiltrates and poorly formed nonnecrotizing granulomas should prompt consideration of mesalamine-related lung disease in a patient receiving this medication. Improvement of the lung disease upon withdrawal of mesalamine provides further support for a diagnosis of mesalamine-related lung disease.

Histologic Features:

- Interstitial mononuclear cell infiltrates.
- Nonnecrotizing granulomas and/or multinucleated giant cells.
- Alveolar fibrinous exudates, granulation tissue, or fibrosis may be present.
- Alveolar foamy macrophages may be present.
- Alveolar eosinophil infiltrates may be present.
- Lymphocytic airway inflammation or granulation tissue may be present.
- Differential diagnosis: IBD-associated lung disease, hypersensitivity pneumonia, other drug reactions, sarcoidosis, granulomatous infections.

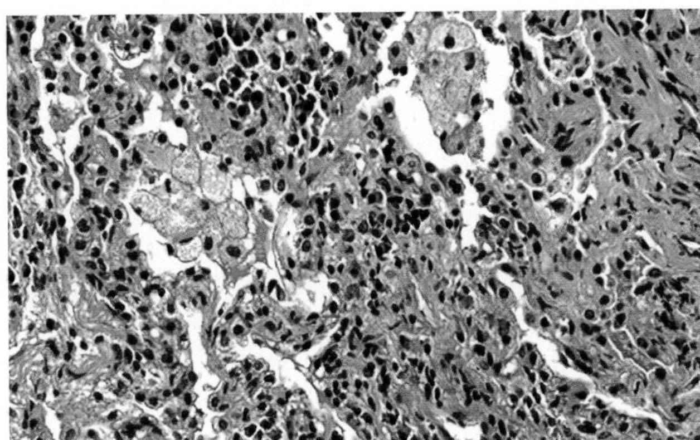

Figure 117.1 Lymphocytic and plasma cell infiltrates within alveolar septa and airspaces containing foamy macrophages.

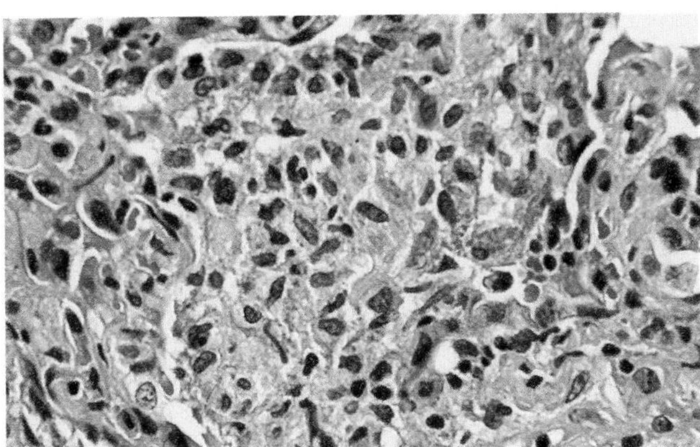

Figure 117.2 Poorly formed nonnecrotizing granuloma within an alveolar space.

Other Drugs

118

▶ Roberto Barrios
▶ Alvaro C. Laga
▶ Mary Ostrowski
▶ Carlos Bedrossian
▶ Hakan Cermik

Other drugs that may induce pulmonary toxicity include cyclophosphamide, bleomycin, busulphan, sulfasalazine, and nitrofurantoin, among others. Cyclophosphamide pulmonary toxicity is more common in combination chemotherapy regiments. According to various reports, the incidence of busulphan pulmonary toxicity in patients treated with this chemotherapeutic agent ranges widely. Nitrofurantoin is a drug with multiple pulmonary manifestations; toxicity is generally acute in onset, with presentation occurring within a few weeks of initiating the therapy.

Cytologic Features:

- Cellular atypia including large and hyperchromatic nuclei with coarse granular or smudged chromatin.
- Intranuclear vacuoles, binucleation, or multinucleation are frequently seen.

Histologic Features:

Cyclophosphamide

- Interstitial pneumonia.
- May present as diffuse alveolar damage or organizing pneumonia.

Bleomycin

- Intracellular edema and blebbing of endothelial cells.
- Necrosis of type 1 pneumocytes, loss of lamellar inclusions in type 2 pneumocytes, and pneumocyte atypia.
- Fibroblast proliferation and fibrosis.

Busulphan

- Interstitial pneumonia.
- Diffuse alveolar damage.

Sulfasalazine

- Eosinophilic pneumonia.
- Interstitial pneumonialike pattern.
- May present as diffuse alveolar damage or organizing pneumonia.

Nitrofurantoin

- Acute or chronic interstitial pneumonitis.
- Pulmonary hemorrhage, bronchoconstriction, or anaphylaxis.
- Usual interstitial pneumonia or desquamative interstitial pneumonialike reactions.
- Pleural effusion.

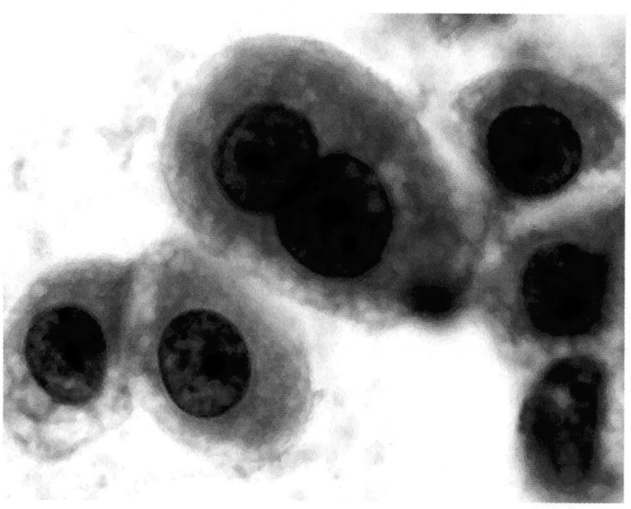

Figure 118.1 Cytology figure of chemotherapy effects shows atypical cells, one of which is binucleated, with enlarged nuclei containing coarse chromatin and prominent nucleoli.

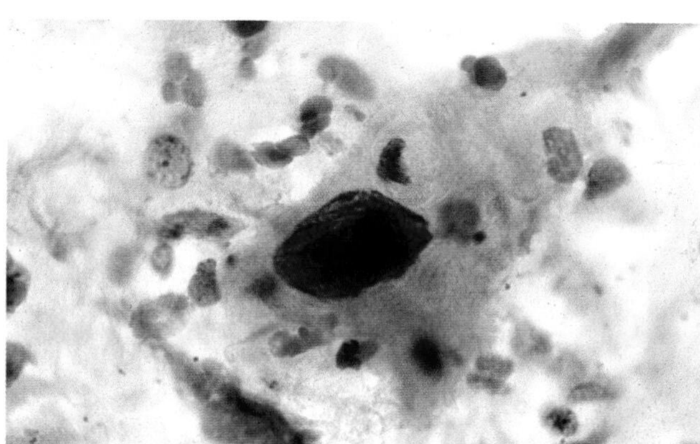

Figure 118.2 Cytology figure of squamous cell with chemotherapy effect shows enlarged hyperchromatic nuclei with irregular contours.

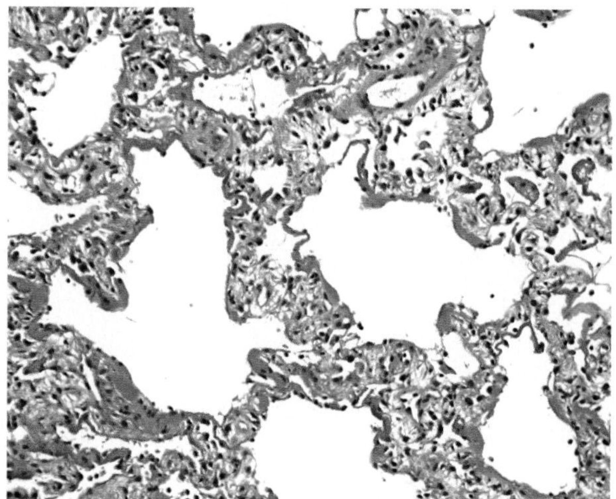

Figure 118.3 Bleomycin toxicity appears as acute diffuse alveolar damage in this case.

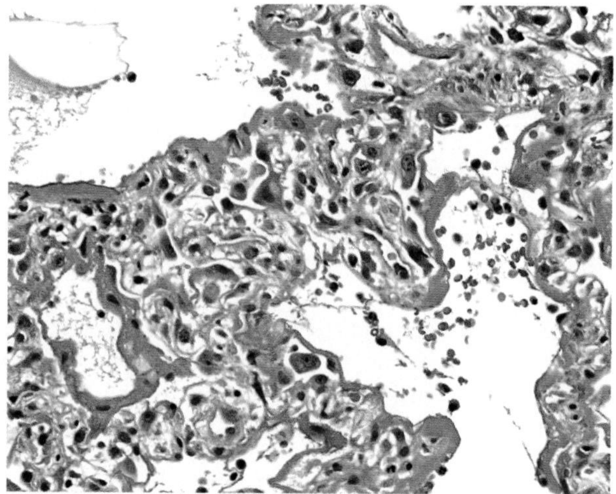

Figure 118.4 Higher power shows interstitial widening, edema, and fibrin layering the airspaces in bleomycin toxicity.

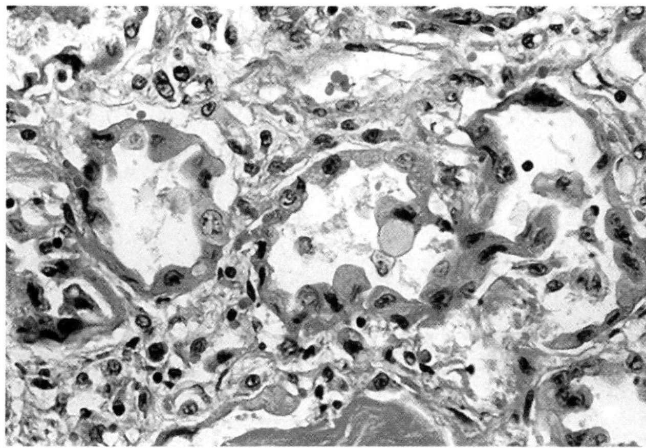

Figure 118.5 Lung parenchyma in bleomycin toxicity shows intracellular edema and blebbing of endothelial cells, fibroblast proliferation, and pneumocyte atypia.

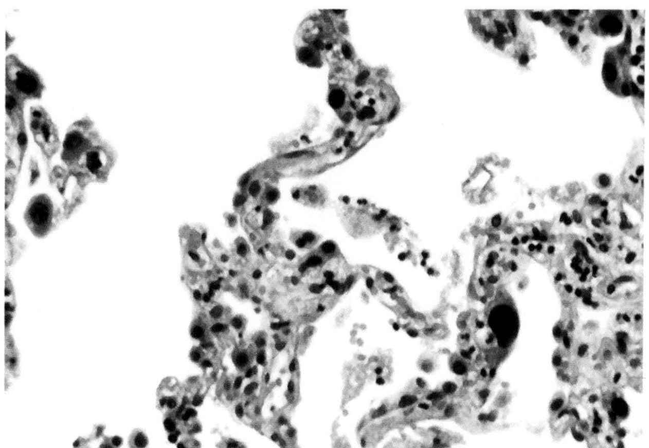

Figure 118.6 Cytotoxic effects of busulphan therapy show enlarged pulmonary epithelial cells with atypical nuclei and abundant eosinophilic cytoplasm.

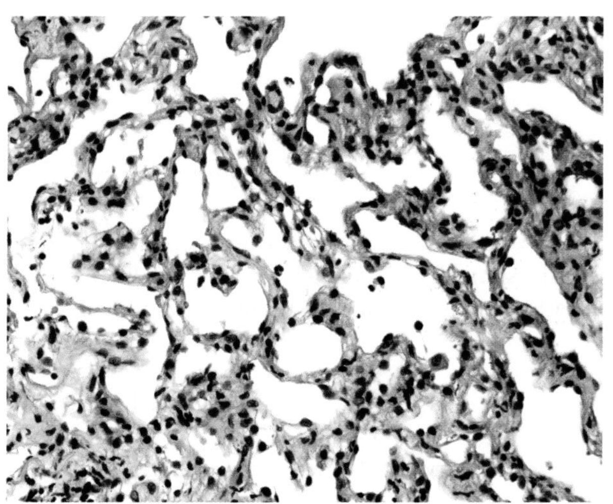

Figure 118.7 Nitrofurantoin toxicity shows interstitial lymphocytic infiltrate.

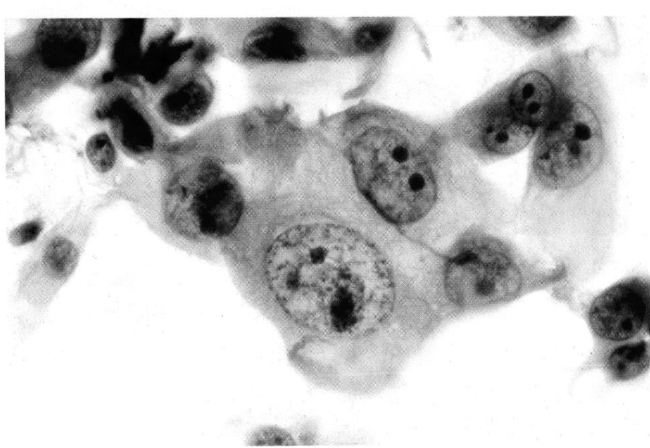

Figure 119.1 Cytology figure showing a small cluster of markedly enlarged cells with abundant cytoplasm, slightly increased nuclear-to-cytoplasmic ratio and nucleoli.

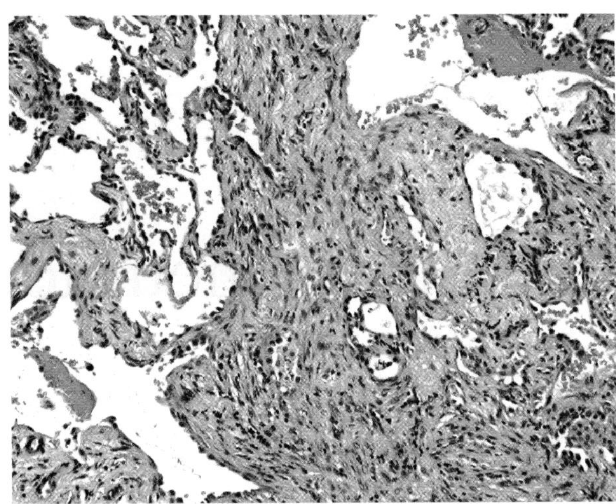

Figure 119.2 Lung parenchyma in radiation pneumonitis with areas of radiation-induced fibrosis.

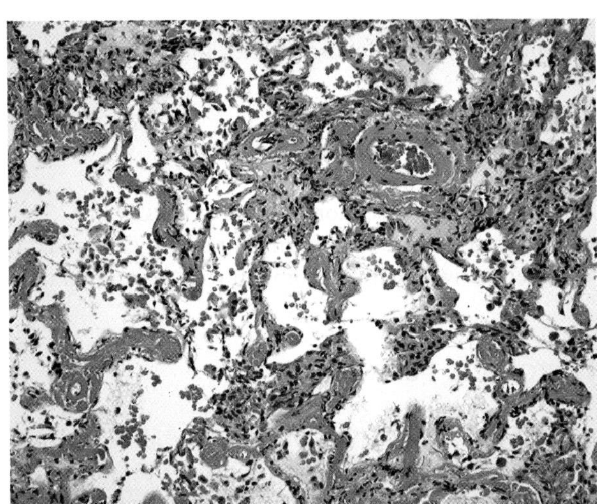

Figure 119.3 Dense paucicellular fibrosis involving alveolar septa and blood vessel walls.

Section 21

Forensic Pathology

120

Drowning

▶ Abida Haque

Drowning is a common cause of accidental deaths, particularly in children. The lungs are edematous in both fresh and salt water drowning; however, "dry lungs," or absence of edema, is well known in some cases of drowning. The hemodynamic changes and hypoxemia are the cause of death and are determined by the type of aspirated water. Because of the hyperosmolality, salt water drowning results in exudation of fluid from the circulation into the alveolar spaces. Fresh water drowning, on the other hand, results in influx of the hypotonic fluid from the lungs into the circulation.

Histologic Features:

- Lungs are edematous, with alveolar spaces expanded and filled with eosinophilic fluid.
- Presence of diatoms and other foreign particles is highly indicative of death by drowning.
- In cases of delayed death after resuscitation, superimposed changes of infection, barotraumas, and acute respiratory distress syndrome may be present.

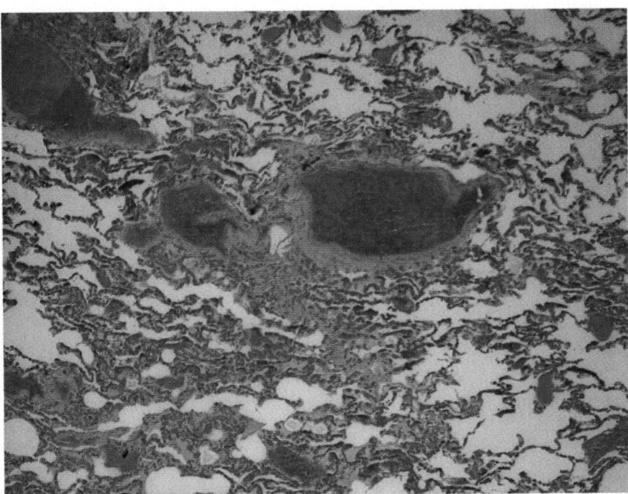

Figure 120.1 Severe pulmonary edema, congestion, and hemorrhage characteristically present in drowning victims.

Fires and Smoke Inhalation

121

▶ Abida Haque

Respiratory complications are a major cause of death in victims of fire and inhalation injury. The presence of inhalation injury dramatically increases mortality, even in the presence of relatively small burns. Thermal injury to the respiratory tract is usually associated with facial burns, steam inhalation, and inhalation of explosive gases. Inhaled smoke results in necrosis and desquamation of the respiratory epithelium, and alveolar pneumocytes, the latter resulting in alveolar edema and acute respiratory distress syndrome (ARDS). Patients who survive the initial injury may develop pneumonia and sepsis, with ARDS occurring later. Those who survive may develop bronchiolitis obliterans and hyperreactive airways.

Histologic Features:

- Pulmonary edema, mucosal necrosis, and mucosal shedding resulting in bronchial and bronchiolar casts.
- Soot deposits on the airway mucosal surface and alveoli.
- Neutrophil infiltrates, often within 12 to 24 hours, followed by macrophages.
- Diffuse alveolar damage, either early with inhalation injury or later with sepsis or barotrauma.
- Bronchiolitis obliterans and alveolar fibrous plugs occur later in those who survive.

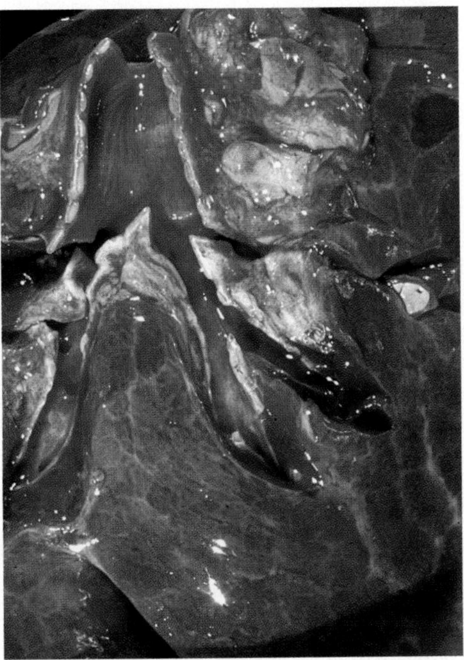

Figure 121.1 Gross specimen of lung showing marked pulmonary edema associated with airway congestion and hemorrhage, characteristic of inhalation injury.

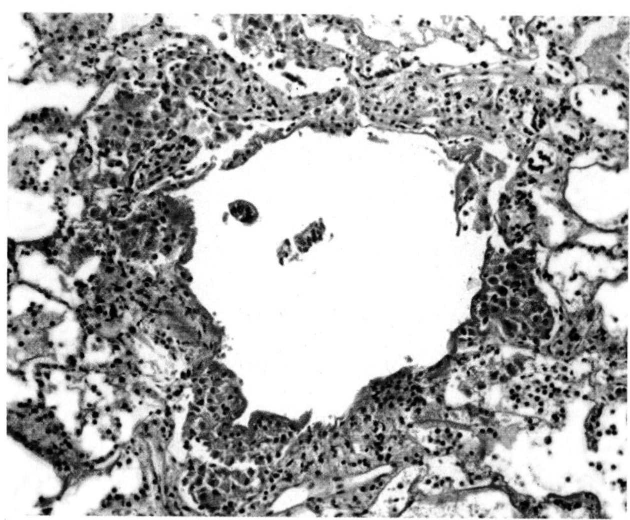

Figure 121.2 Acute inflammation with necrosis of respiratory bronchiolar epithelium is associated with a small particle of inhaled soot.

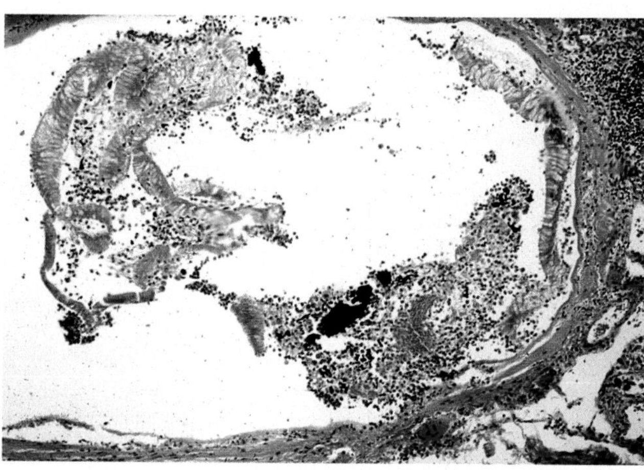

Figure 121.3 Small airway demonstrates necrosis and denudation of the epithelium forming necrotic casts. Particles of soot are mixed with the denuded mucosa.

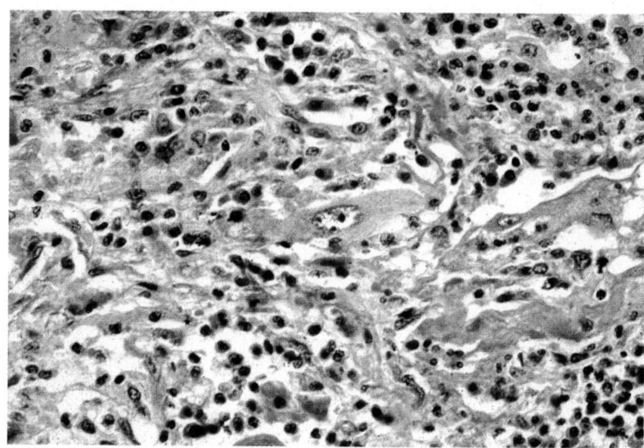

Figure 121.4 High magnification of exudative stage of ARDS showing hyaline membranes, large atypical type 2 pneumocytes, and inflammatory cells. The alveolar structures are obscured by the intense inflammatory infiltrate.

122 Contusions

▶ Abida Haque

Pulmonary contusions can occur as a result of rapid deceleration injury, explosions, or high-velocity projectile injury to the chest or abdomen. Often, there is no obvious injury, such as rib fractures seen in the chest wall. Pulmonary contusions and lacerations may be diagnosed by computed tomography of the chest.

Histologic Features:

- Lesions may appear as intraparenchymal hematoma, lacerations, and/or blood-filled cavities.

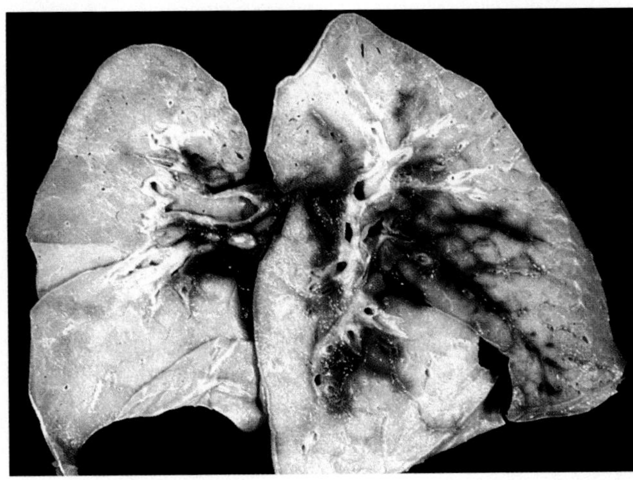

Figure 122.1. Lungs of a child killed in a motor vehicle accident shows pulmonary hemorrhage along the bronchovascular bundles.

123 Intravenous Drug Abuse

▶ Alvaro C. Laga
▶ Timothy Allen
▶ Philip T. Cagle

Drug abusers may inject drugs intended for oral use. The drugs often contain filler substances such as talc, microcrystalline cellulose, cornstarch, and crospovidone that play different functions in tablets, such as binding, providing volume, or acting as a tablet disintegrant (crospovidone). Talc or other powdery substances may also have been used by the drug dealer to dilute ("cut") the pure drug and thus increase profits. When these substances are injected, they lodge in the lung capillaries because of their size and may cause angiothrombosis or elicit a foreign body reaction. The physiologic consequence of widespread occlusion of small pulmonary arteries is pulmonary hypertension.

Histologic Features:

- Foreign body granulomas ("talc granulomas") may be observed both intravascularly and extravascularly.
- Birefringent talc particles are generally 0.5 to 50 μm in size.
- Most tablet filler and binder substances are brightly birefringent and can be identified using crossed polarizers.
- Some patients may develop fibrosis in the middle and upper zones of the lung resembling progressive massive fibrosis; birefringent material can be identified within the fibrous tissue.
- Emphysema with or without bullae may be encountered in some cases.
- Embolized crospovidone appears as basophilic coral-like material within a foreign body giant cell reaction.

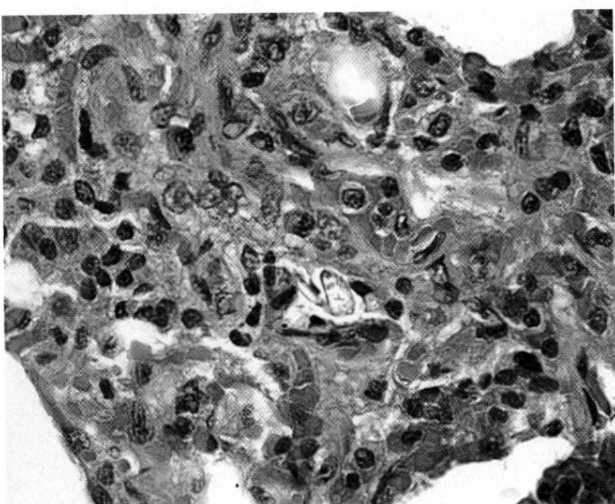

Figure 123.1 Thickened alveolar septum with talc particles in a case of intravenous drug abuse.

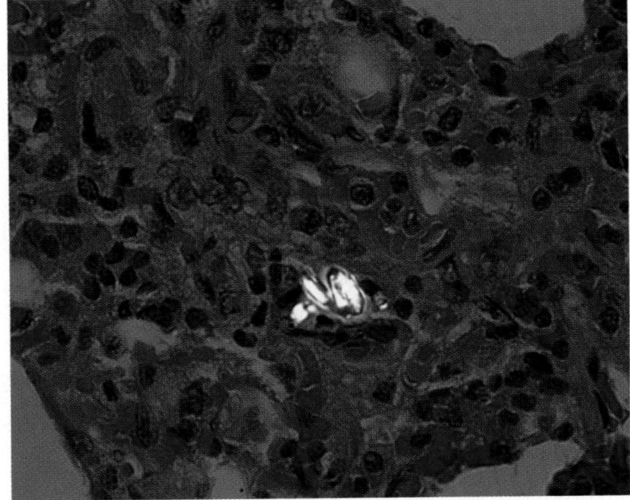

Figure 123.2 Brightly birefringent talc particles are identified under polarization.

124 Cocaine Abuse

- Alvaro C. Laga
- Timothy Allen
- Carlos Bedrossian
- Philip T. Cagle

Patients who abuse cocaine, either intravenously or by smoking it (crack cocaine), may have pulmonary disease. Pulmonary hemorrhage occurs more frequently than is suggested by hemoptysis. Interstitial fibrosis may develop in long-term abusers.

Histologic Features:

- Acute hemorrhage.
- Chronic hemorrhage.
- Interstitial lymphocytic infiltrates and/or interstitial fibrosis.
- Congestion.
- Intraalveolar edema.

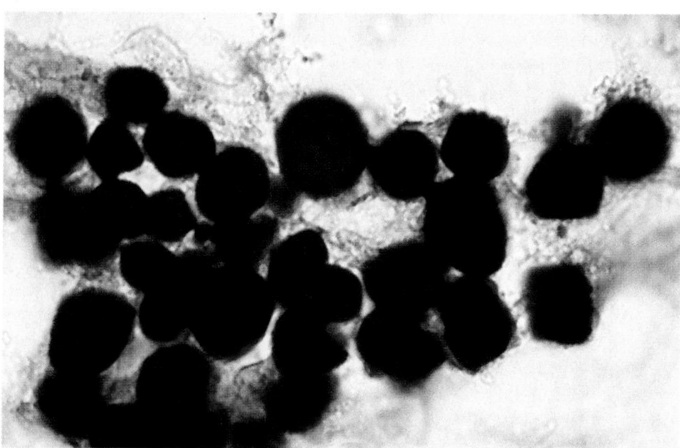

Figure 124.1 Cytology figure shows heavily pigmented macrophages in sputum of a crack cocaine smoker.

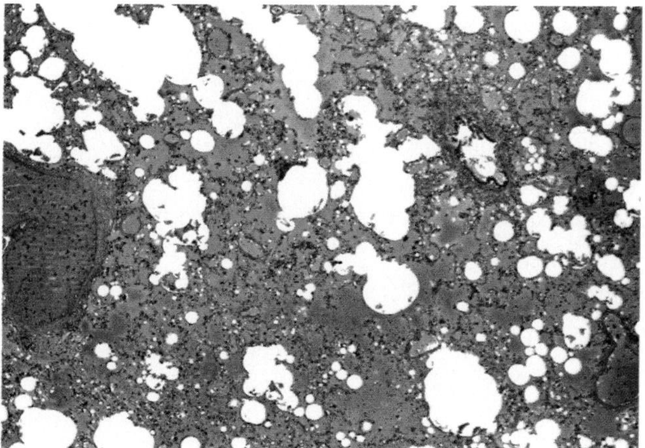

Figure 124.2 Low power shows acute hemorrhage and edema.

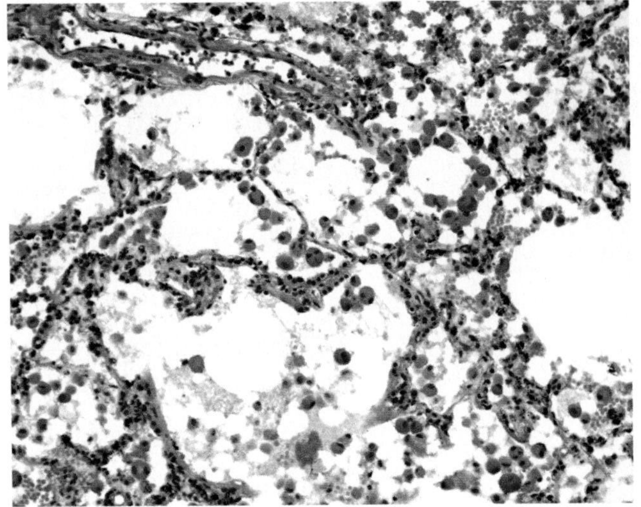

Figure 124.3 Acute hemorrhage, edema, and hemosiderin-laden macrophages in cocaine lung.

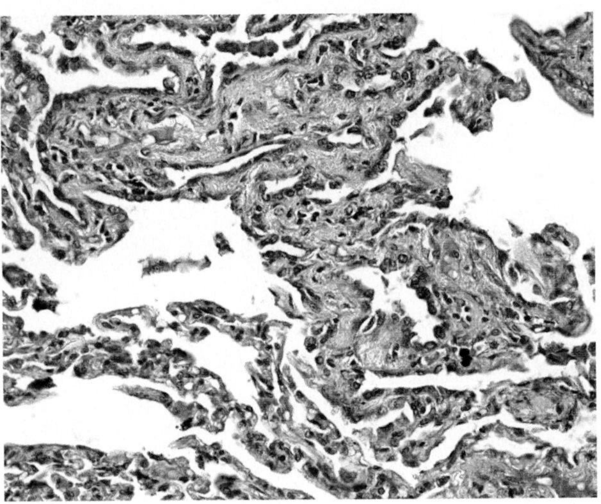

Figure 124.4 Interstitial fibrosis in a long-term cocaine user.

Section 22

Metabolic Disorders/ Storage Diseases

125 Pulmonary Alveolar Microlithiasis

▶ Roberto Barrios

Alveolar microlithiasis is a rare idiopathic alveolar filling disorder. It is characterized by intraalveolar accumulation of calcium phosphate, which forms laminated concretions. Microscopically there are heavily calcified laminar microspheres within the alveolar spaces. These lesions progress slowly and may reach diameters of 0.01 to 3.0 mm. Fibrosis develops over time and eventually the lungs become rock hard. It has been speculated that the disease may be due to a genetically determined metabolic disorder or acquired defects in calcium and phosphorous metabolism. A familial association has been described, but some cases are sporadic. Some authors have proposed an autosomal recessive pattern of inheritance. Alveolar microlithiasis is seen in the third to fifth decades, although it can occur in children. There is no sex predilection. Occasionally microliths can be found by bronchoalveolar lavage. Grossly, the lungs appear gritty and hard. Primary differential diagnosis includes corpora amylacea and intraalveolar lamellar bodies commonly seen in the lungs of older individuals or patients with left heart failure. Corpora amylacea are not calcified or ossified, although they are birefringent with polarized light, and they consist of carbohydrates.

Histologic Features:

- Alveoli occupied by calcospherites within alveolar spaces.
- Microliths measuring 250 to 750 μm in diameter with a lamellar appearance and a concentric onion-skin pattern.
- Alveolar walls may be normal; in longstanding cases there may be interstitial fibrosis.
- Diagnosis may be established by transbronchial biopsy.

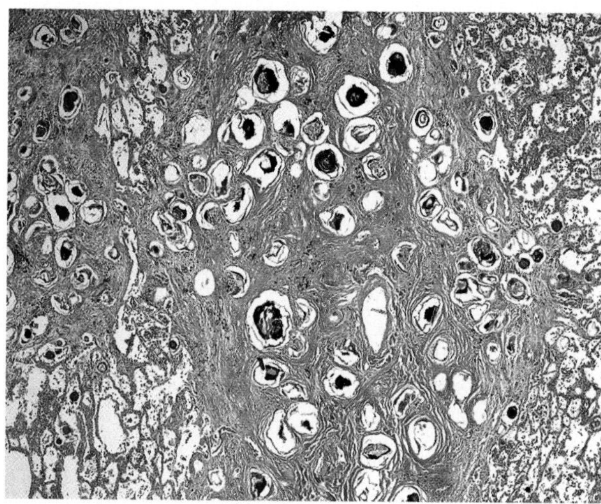

Figure 125.1 Parenchyma showing alveoli occupied by microliths, which elicit septal fibrosis and foreign body reaction. The central portion shows advanced lesions with dense fibrosis.

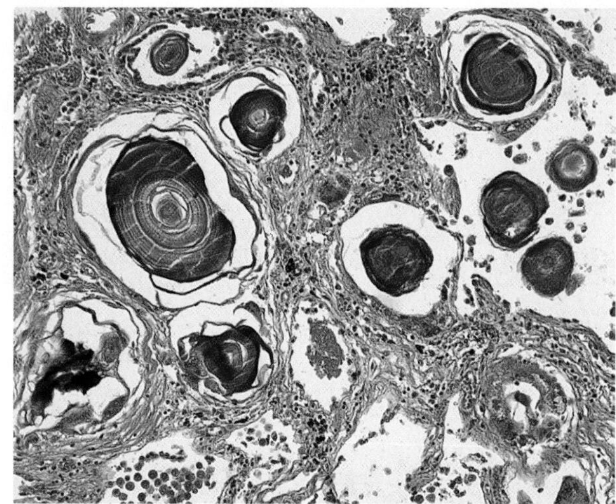

Figure 125.2 Higher power illustrates the presence of laminated concentric calcifications (microliths) surrounded by fibrosis and mild focal chronic inflammation.

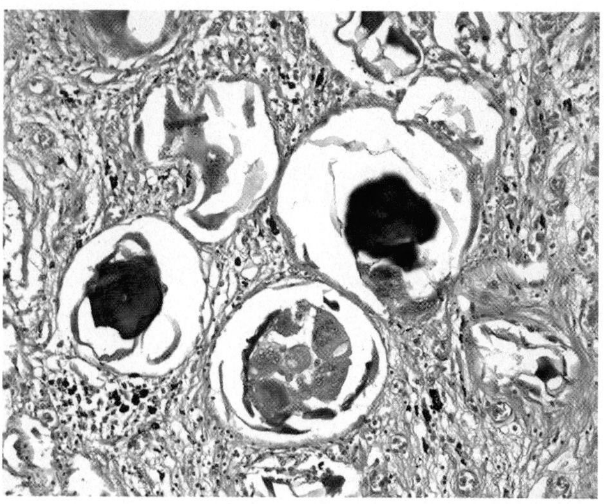

Figure 125.3 High power of a microlith with prominent foreign body reaction. Multinucleated foreign body giant cells are seen adjacent to the microlith.

Pulmonary Calcification

126

▶ Alvaro C. Laga
▶ Roberto Barrios
▶ Dani S. Zander

Pulmonary calcification refers to deposition of calcium salts in the lung. It can be broadly divided into dystrophic calcification, in which calcification occurs in previously injured lung tissue, and metastatic calcification, in which calcium deposits in normal tissue as a result of abnormal serum levels of calcium and phosphate.

Dystrophic calcification in the lungs is frequently seen in old healed granulomas, and it may follow pneumonias, parasitic infections, silicosis, berylliosis, and many other inflammatory conditions. Ossification may also occur in foci of dystrophic calcification. Other than being a marker of tissue injury, dystrophic calcification is of little clinical consequence.

Metastatic calcification is the presence of calcium salt deposits in the pulmonary parenchyma. It is most common in patients with chronic renal insufficiency, especially those chronically treated with hemodialysis, but it can also develop in association with hyperparathyroidism, hypervitaminosis D, sarcoidosis, systemic sclerosis, neoplasms with extensive osseous involvement, or a paraneoplastic syndrome caused by elaboration of a substance with parathormonelike activity. The heart, stomach, and kidneys are other sites that are frequently involved by this process. Patients are usually asymptomatic, but respiratory failure develops in a small number of patients.

Histologic Features:

Metastatic Calcification

- Deposits of basophilic material (calcium salts) in alveolar walls, blood vessel walls, and small airways.
- Fine granular deposits occur early in the process, particularly along elastic fibers.
- As the process advances, the deposits usually become more platelike, with associated fibrosis.
- Deposits stain with von Kossa and Alizarin red S stains.
- Accompanying alveolar organization can be present.
- Metaplastic ossification can occur.

Dystrophic Calcification

- Dystrophic calcification appears as basophilic deposits of calcium salts in previous sites of injury, such as necrosis, organizing exudates, old scars, and granulomas.

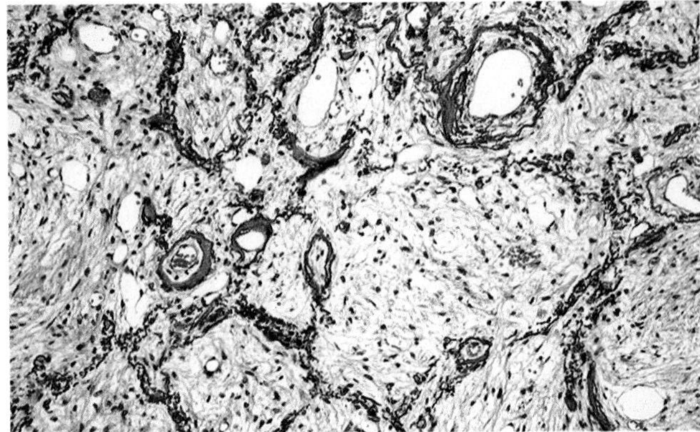

Figure 126.1 Basophilic calcium salt deposits outline alveolar septa in metastatic calcification. There is extensive fibroblast proliferation in the alveolar spaces.

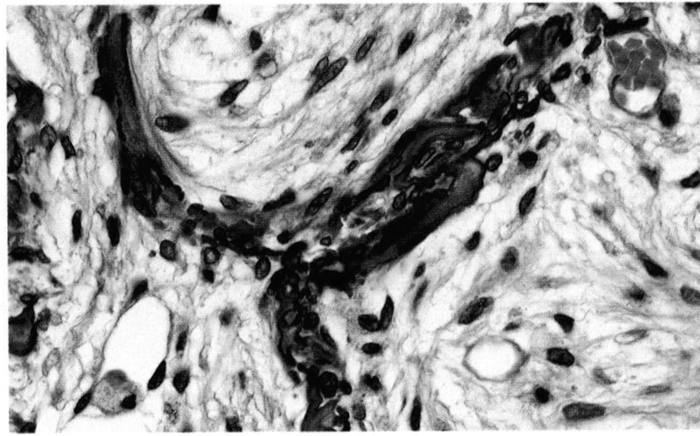

Figure 126.2 Higher power of metastatic calcification of alveolar septa with fibroblast proliferation in the alveolar spaces.

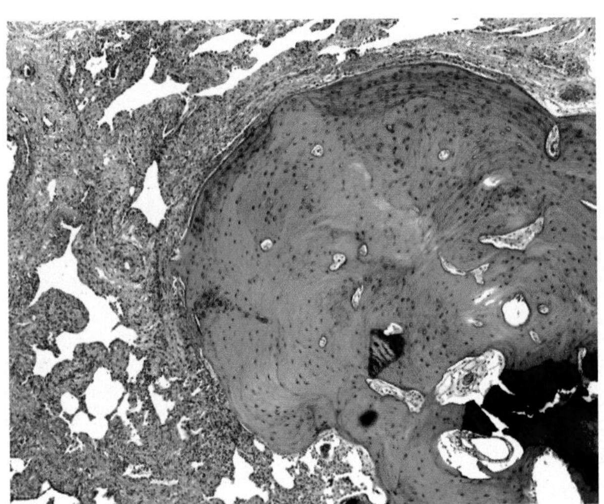

Figure 126.3 Low power shows ossification within lung parenchyma.

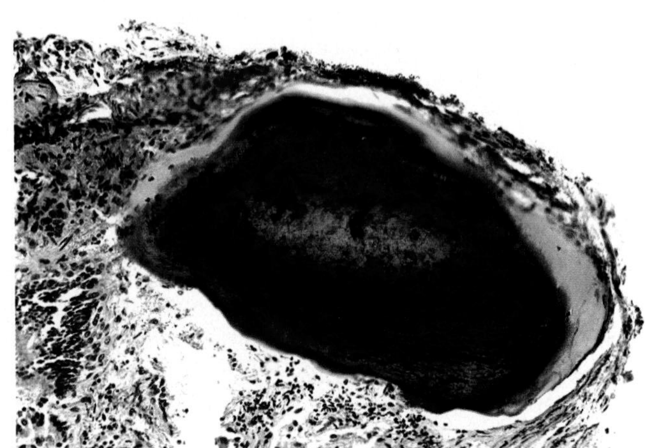

Figure 126.4 Dystrophic calcification with ossification.

127 Storage Diseases

Alvaro C. Laga
Timothy Allen
Megan Dishop
Philip T. Cagle

Several storage diseases may involve the lungs, and some of these diseases cause significant pulmonary disease. Extrapulmonary manifestations generally account for most of the signs and symptoms of storage diseases, and involvement of the lung is common although clinically inapparent. When signs and symptoms of lung involvement by storage diseases occur, they most commonly present as diffuse interstitial lung disease. In this chapter, we discuss two examples of such diseases.

Niemann-Pick disease is a lipid storage disease associated with the deficiency or absence of acid sphingomyelinase. Although patients with type A disease generally die within a few years of birth, patients with type B disease often live into adulthood. Progressive pulmonary infiltration may occur with disease progression typical of type B patients and is a major cause of mortality and morbidity in these patients. Chest x-ray film often shows diffuse or finely nodular reticular infiltrates.

Cholesteryl ester storage disease (CESD) is a rare form of inherited lysosomal lipid storage disease due to deficiency of acid lipase. It results in an accumulation of neutral lipids, predominantly cholesterol esters, within different cells, including pulmonary interstitial cells, alveolar macrophages, fibroblasts, and hepatocytes. CESD is associated with extensive systemic atherosclerosis with prominent involvement of the pulmonary vasculature and consequent pulmonary hypertension.

Histologic Features:

Niemann-Pick Disease

- Alveolar filling by foamy macrophages.
- Foamy macrophages contain generally uniform lipid droplets arranged in a "honeycomb" or "mulberrylike" pattern.
- Ultrastructurally, the foamy macrophages contain giant lamellar structures within the cytoplasm.

CESD

- Cytoplasmic lipid deposits in pulmonary interstitial cells and alveolar macrophages.
- Focal concentric intimal deposits of foam cells, extracellular lipid, and reactive fibrosis in arteries.

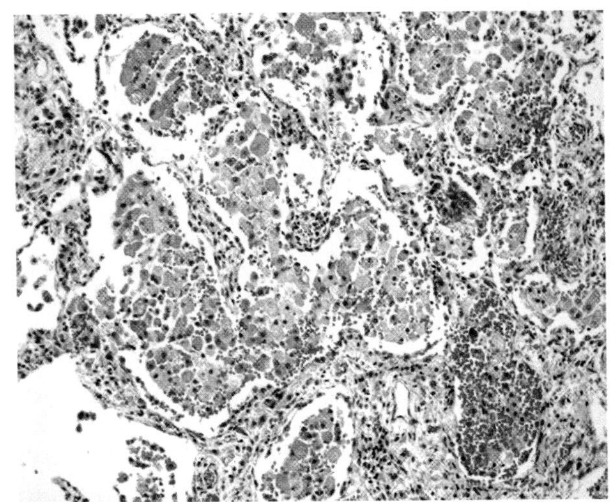

Figure 127.1 Low power shows alveolar spaces filled with foamy macrophages in Niemann-Pick disease.

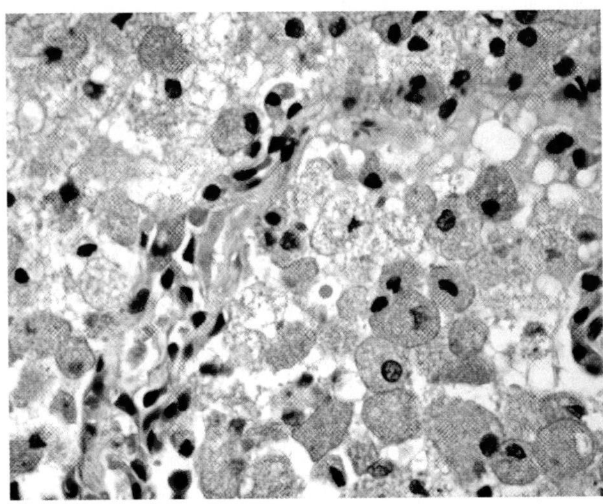

Figure 127.2 Higher power shows foamy macrophages with uniform-appearing lipid droplets in Niemann-Pick disease.

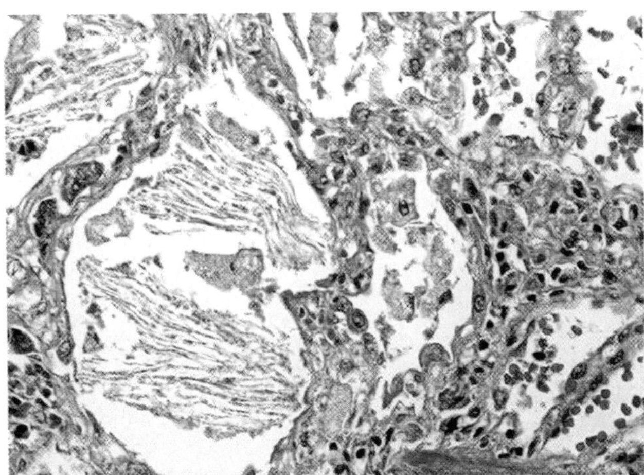

Figure 127.3 Numerous cholesterol clefts are seen within alveoli in CESD.

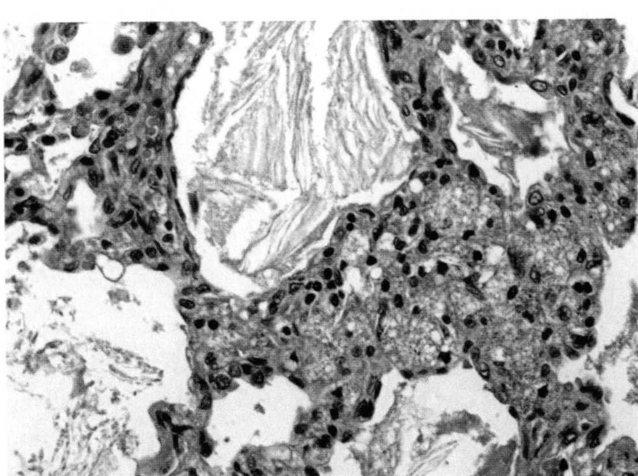

Figure 127.4 Numerous macrophages with vacuolated cytoplasm that thickens the alveolar septa and numerous cholesterol clefts within alveoli in CESD.

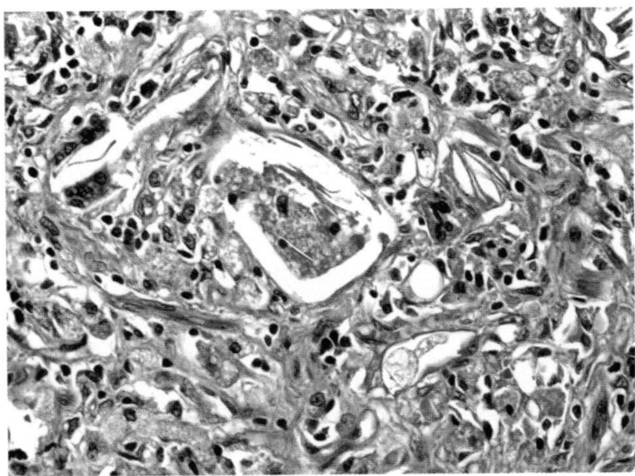

Figure 127.5 Foamy cells with finely vacuolated cytoplasm occupying the interstitium and alveolar spaces and cholesterol clefts within multinucleated giant cells in CESD.

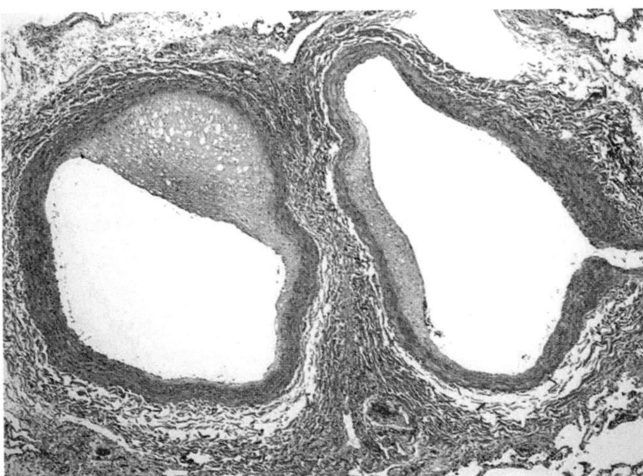

Figure 127.6 Pulmonary artery with focal intimal lipid deposits consisting of foamy macrophages and extracellular lipid in CESD.

Section 23

Non-Neoplastic Lesions of the Pleura

Fibrinous and Fibrous Pleuritis

128

▶ Alvaro C. Laga
▶ Timothy Allen
▶ Philip T. Cagle

Pleuritis may exhibit fibrinous exudates on the visceral and/or parietal pleural surfaces. Over time, the fibrinous exudates are often organized by granulation tissue. Fibrinous and fibrous pleuritis may be accompanied by inflammation, particularly lymphoid aggregates in the pleura and subpleural tissues. The granulation tissue of the organizing fibrous pleuritis may mature into fibrous tissue, resulting in a thickened, fibrotic pleura. A variety of conditions may cause fibrinous pleuritis, including pneumonia, pericarditis, hepatitis, peritonitis, pancreatitis, collagen-vascular disease, drug reactions, and cancer.

In some cases, the fibrous tissue may organize into pleural plaque. Grossly, pleural plaque is a thick, firm, yellow-tan to off-white tissue on the surface of the parietal or visceral pleura. Microscopically, pleural plaque consists of virtually acellular collagen bundles in a characteristic basketweave pattern. Pleural plaques, especially when bilateral, lower zone, and symmetrical, may be markers of asbestos exposure. Pleural plaques may also be seen as a result of infections, surgery, trauma and apical caps (see Chapter 33). Pleural plaques may undergo calcification or ossification.

Sarcomatous or desmoplastic mesothelioma may sometimes enter into the differential diagnosis of fibrous pleuritis. Fibrous pleuritis is generally limited to or oriented along the pleural surface, whereas sarcomatoid mesothelioma tends to involve the full thickness of the pleura. Keratin immunostains may assist in this differential diagnosis by indicating the location of the mesothelial cells within a thickened pleura (keratin-positive reactive mesothelial cells are generally found toward the pleural surface, whereas keratin-positive mesothelioma cells may be found in the full thickness of the pleura and invade underlying tissues). Another feature of benign reactive pleuritis is that the blood vessels in the granulation tissue tend to be parallel to one another and perpendicular to the pleural surface.

Histologic Features:

- Pleuritis may consist of fibrinous exudates on the pleural surface, organizing granulation tissue, or fibrous tissue.
- Blood vessels in organizing pleuritis tend to be parallel to one another and perpendicular to the pleural surface.
- Inflammatory cells, particularly lymphoid aggregates, may be present.
- Pleural plaque consists of dense virtually acellular collagen bundles arranged in a basketweave pattern.
- Pleural plaques may be calcified or ossified.

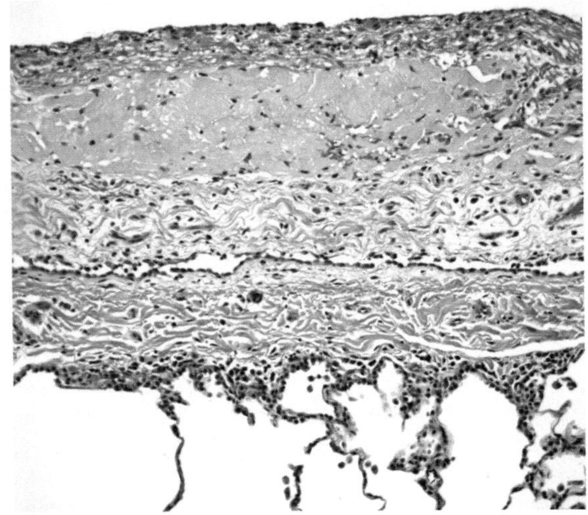

Figure 128.1 Pleuritis with fibrinous exudate and fibrous tissue overlying the pleural surface with entrapped reactive mesothelial cells.

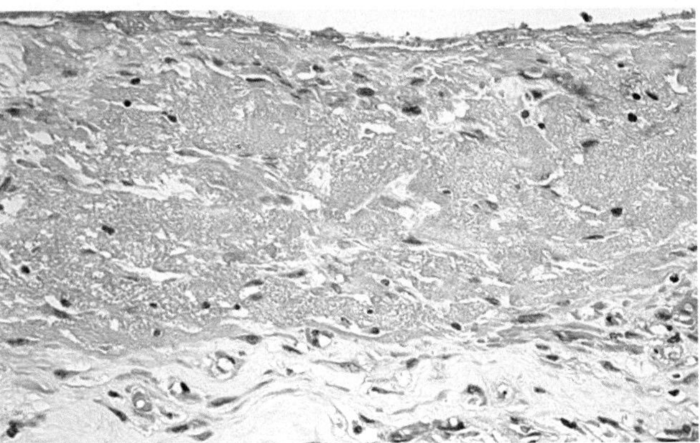

Figure 128.2 Fibrinous and fibrous tissue on the pleural surface.

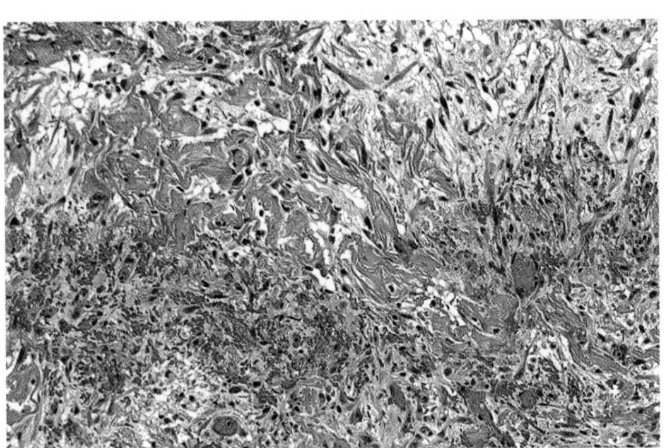

Figure 128.3 Organization of fibrinous exudates by granulation tissue consisting of proliferating capillaries and fibroblasts.

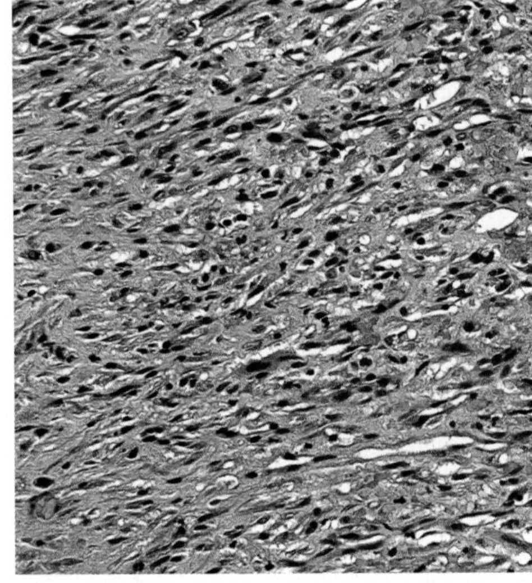

Figure 128.4 Proliferating blood vessels and fibroblasts of organizing pleuritis show reactive atypia but are parallel to each other.

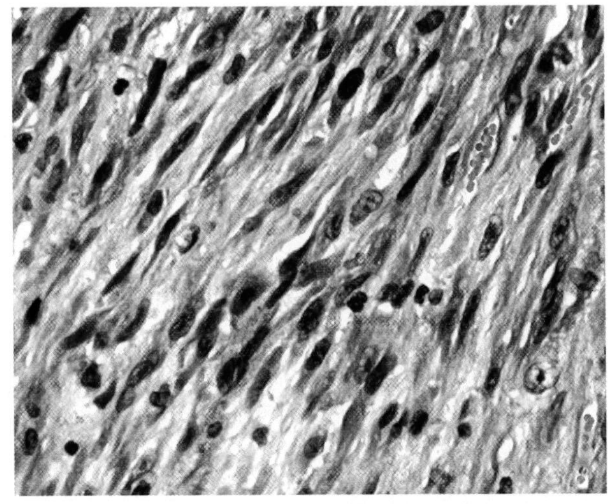

Figure 128.5 Higher power of parallel blood vessels and fibroblasts in organizing pleuritis.

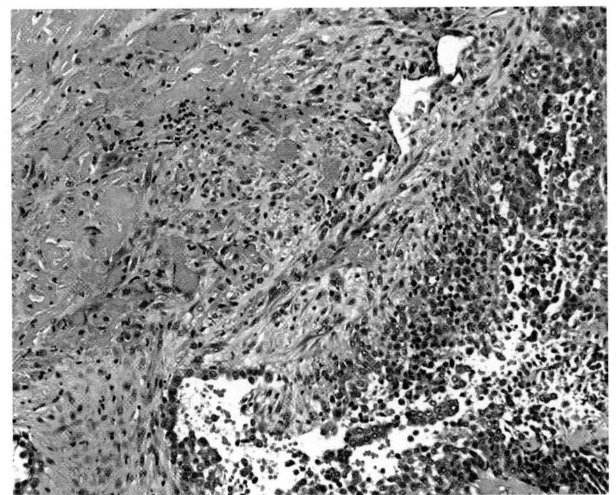

Figure 128.6 Organizing pleuritis with florid reactive mesothelial cell proliferation.

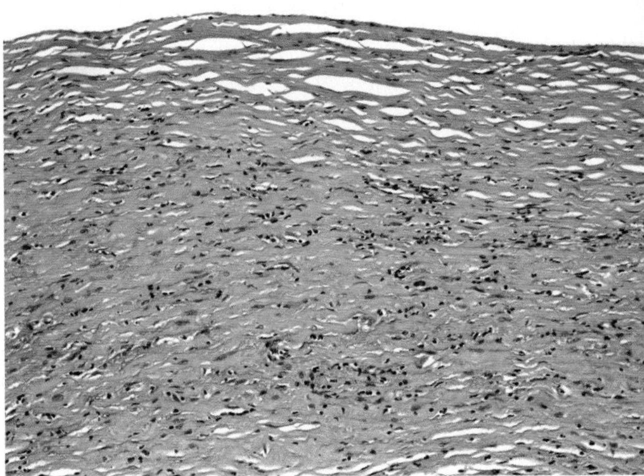

Figure 128.7 Fibrous pleuritis shows early plaque formation on the surface where the fibrous tissue is virtually acellular and arranged in a basketweave pattern.

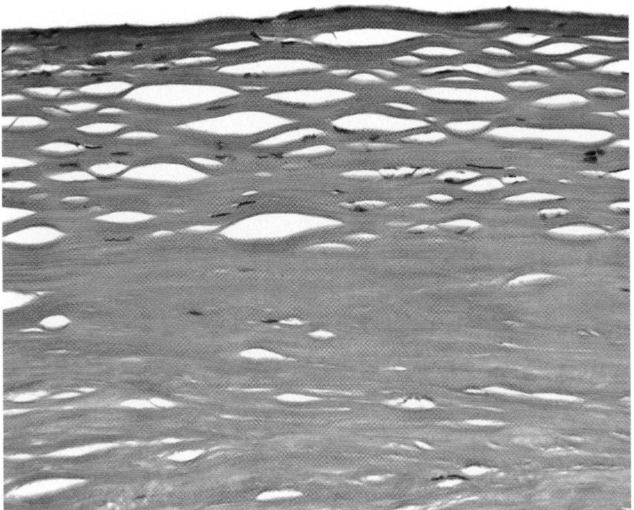

Figure 128.8 Pleural plaque shows dense, virtually acellular collagen bundles in a basketweave pattern.

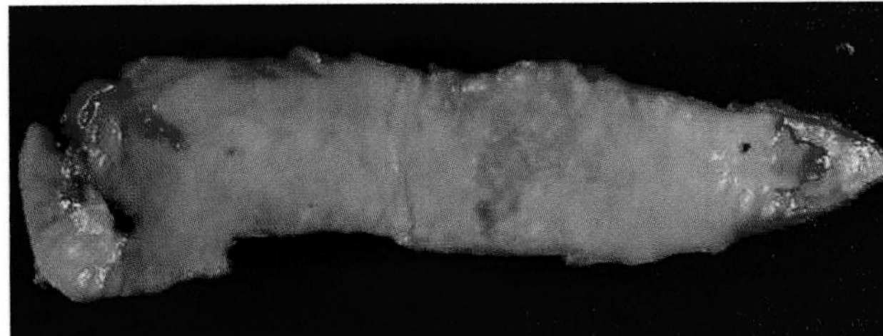

Figure 128.9 Grossly pleural plaque stripped from the pleural surface consists of dense, firm, yellow-tan tissue.

129 Specific Forms of Pleuritis

▶ Alvaro C. Laga
▶ Timothy Allen
▶ Philip T. Cagle

Eosinophilic pleuritis is characterized by abundant eosinophils in the pleural tissue and fluid. Eosinophilic pleuritis occurs as a reaction to pneumothorax or hemothorax from a wide variety of causes. Other etiologies of eosinophilic pleuritis include drug reactions and infections (tuberculosis, parasites, fungus, certain bacteria). It is commonly identified in patients undergoing pleurectomy and/or excision of blebs and bullae. In these cases, the eosinophilic pleuritis may be associated with bullae or focal honeycombing of the underlying lung parenchyma. In women of childbearing age, the underlying lung may be affected by lymphangioleiomyomatosis.

Granulomatous pleuritis may be seen in association with infection (tuberculosis or fungus), sarcoidosis, and Wegener's granulomatosis. Foreign body granulomatous reactions may occur in the pleura as the result of iatrogenic instillation of foreign material into the pleural cavity to cause its obliteration for the purpose of treating recurrent pleural effusions.

Histologic Features:

Eosinophilic Pleuritis

- Infiltrate of eosinophils in the pleural tissue and fluid may include reactive mesothelial cells, histiocytes, lymphocytes, and giant cells.
- Adjacent lung may show focal eosinophilic infiltrates within small vessels.
- Underlying lung may show bullae, focal honeycombing, or lymphangioleiomyomatosis.

Granulomatous Pleuritis

- Areas of granulomatous inflammation or well-formed granulomas with or without central necrosis.
- Special stains for organisms, such as Gomori methenamine silver are helpful when positive but a negative special stain does not rule out infection.
- Foreign material such as talc may be identified on polarized light when deliberately instilled into the pleura to cause fibrosis as a treatment for recurrent pleural effusion.

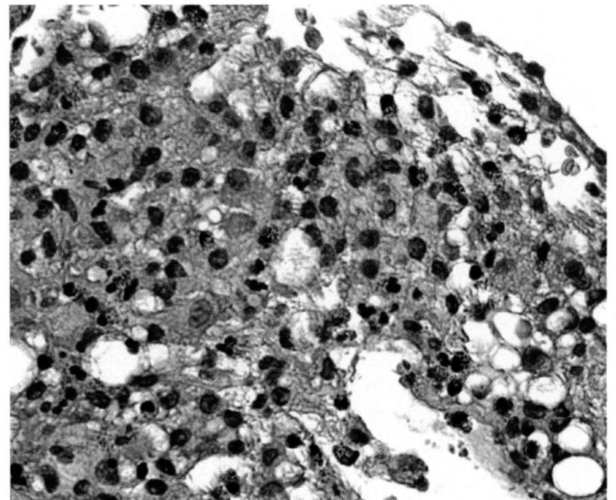

Figure 129.1 Pleural fluid in eosinophilic pleuritis with eosinophils and reactive mesothelial cells.

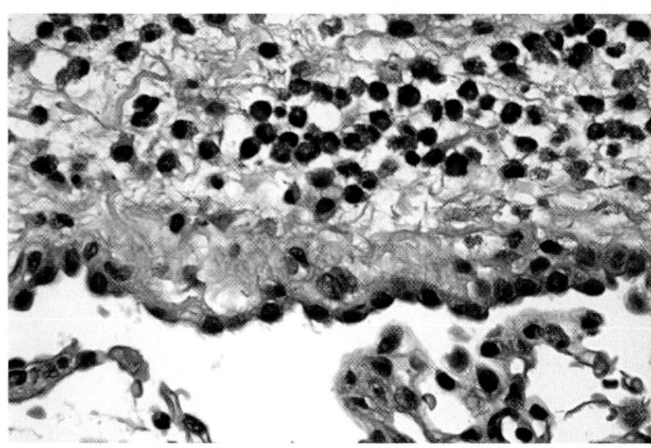

Figure 129.2 Eosinophils in the visceral pleura in eosinophilic pleuritis.

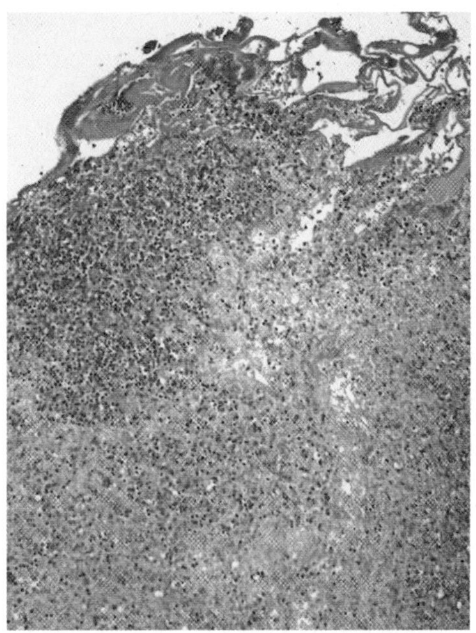

Figure 129.3 Low power of pleuritis with "dirty" necrosis composed of basophilic nuclear and cellular debris commonly seen with infections.

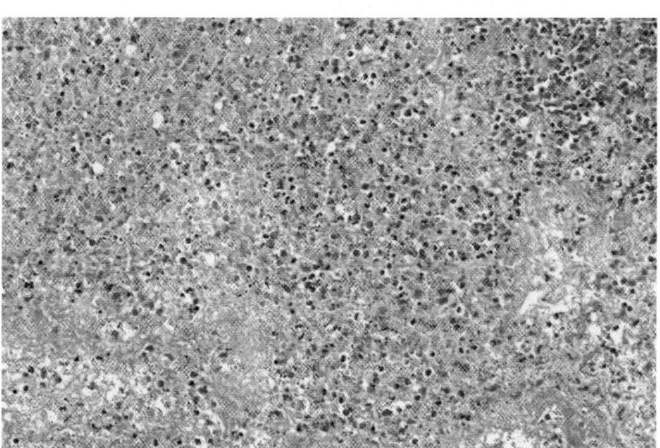

Figure 129.4 Higher power shows that "dirty" necrosis is composed of basophilic nuclear debris and cellular debris admixed with neutrophils and other inflammatory cells.

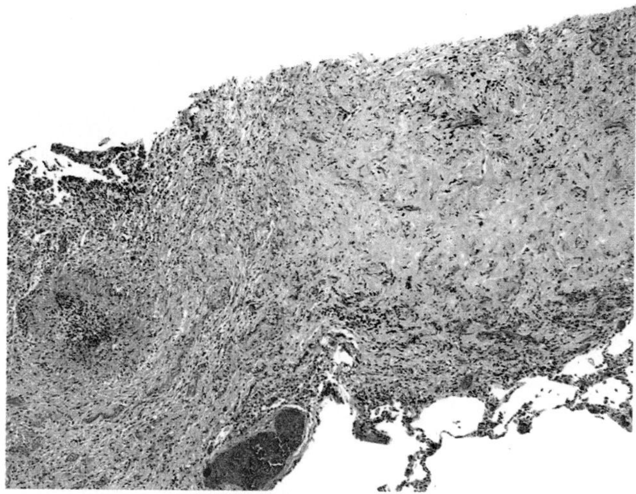

Figure 129.5 Thickened fibrotic pleura has a granuloma composed of histiocytes and central necrosis in the **left** of the figure.

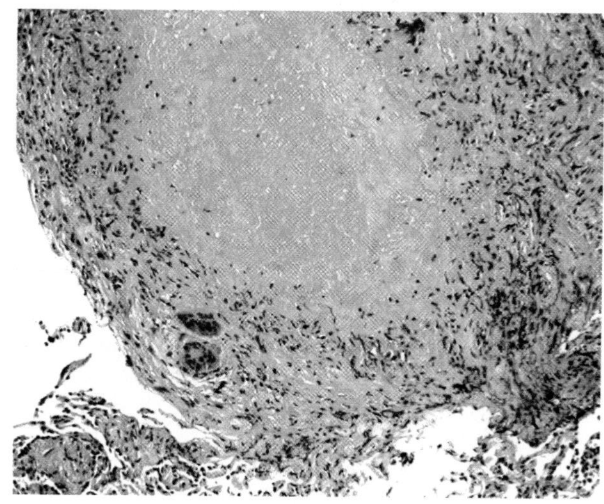

Figure 129.6 Pleural granuloma with central necrosis and multinucleated giant cells due to pleural tuberculosis.

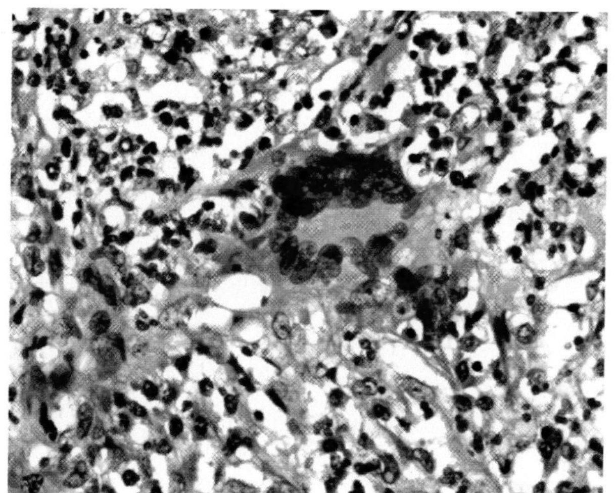

Figure 129.7 Multinucleated giant cells mixed with acute inflammatory cells in granulomatous pleuritis.

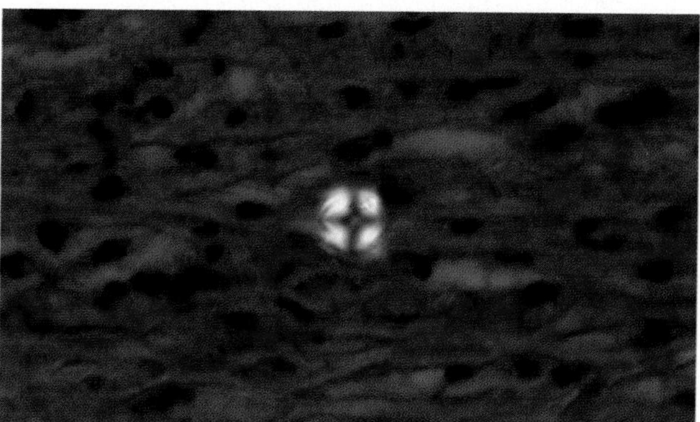

Figure 129.8 Polarized light shows iatrogenically instilled birefringent talc with a central cross in a pleura deliberately fibrosed to treat recurrent pleural effusion (pleurodesis).

Reactive Mesothelial Hyperplasia

130

- Alvaro C. Laga
- Timothy Allen
- Carlos Bedrossian
- Rodolfo Laucirica
- Philip T. Cagle

Reactive mesothelial cell hyperplasia is often seen in association with pleural effusion, including infections, collagen-vascular diseases, drug reactions, pneumothorax, chest surgery, and trauma. Reactive mesothelial cells proliferate along the pleural surface and may shed into pleural fluid. Benign reactive mesothelial cells may have cytologic atypia and mitoses, may proliferate in papillary tufts or other structures, and may be entrapped by overlying organizing pleuritis or pleural fibrosis mimicking invasion. Distinguishing reactive mesothelial cell hyperplasia from diffuse malignant mesothelioma may be a diagnostic dilemma, especially with small biopsies.

Histologic Features

- The mesothelial cells are generally cuboidal, with round nuclei, prominent nucleoli, and abundant eosinophilic cytoplasm.
- Depending on the severity of the reaction, the mesothelial cells may exhibit cytologic atypia and mitoses.
- Entrapment of proliferating reactive mesothelial cells by fibrin, granulation tissue, and/or fibrous tissue overlying the pleural surface in pleuritis may mimic invasion; the entrapped mesothelial cells are typically arranged linearly parallel to the pleural surface and lack invasion into the deeper pleural and underlying tissues.

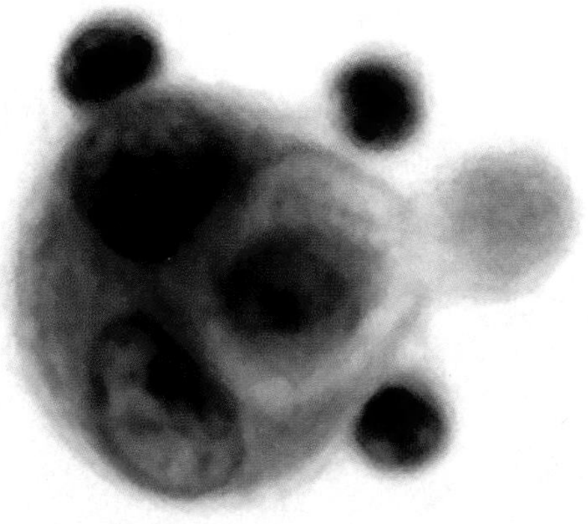

Figure 130.1 Cluster of enlarged, cytologically atypical reactive mesothelial cells in a pleural fluid may mimic neoplastic mesothelial cells.

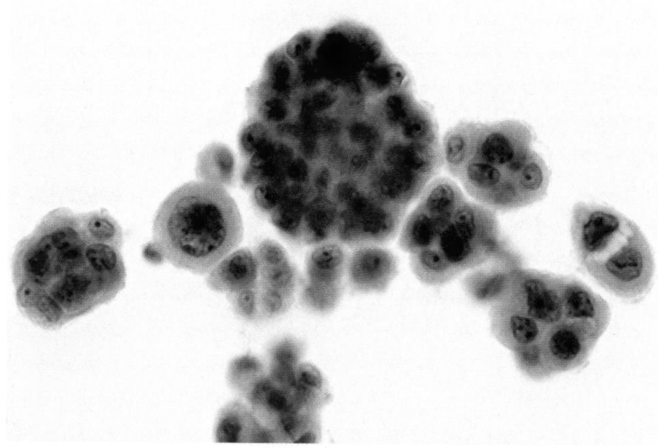

Figure 130.2 Collections of proliferating reactive mesothelial cells in a pleural fluid are suggestive of malignant morulae. Note the "window" or space between the two mesothelial cells on the right.

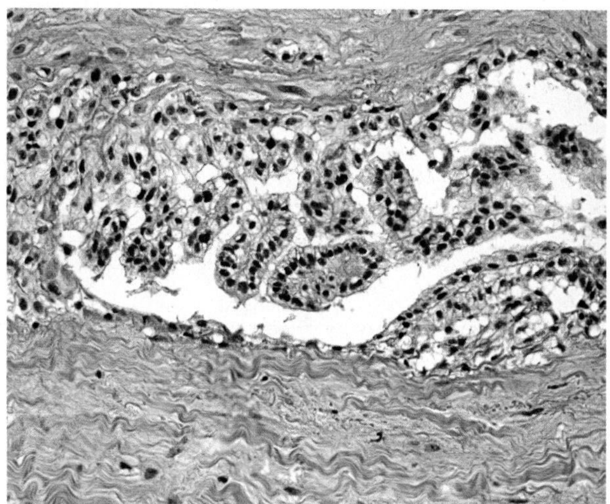

Figure 130.3 Proliferating mesothelial cells entrapped by overlying fibrous tissue must be differentiated from invasive malignant mesothelial cells.

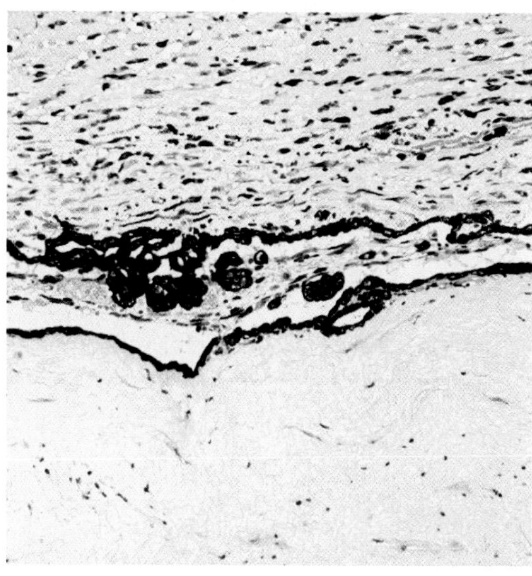

Figure 130.4 Keratin immunostain demonstrates linear array of benign hyperplastic mesothelial cells entrapped beneath pleuritis containing proliferating spindled mesothelial cells. The keratin-positive mesothelial cells do not invade the underlying pleural tissue.

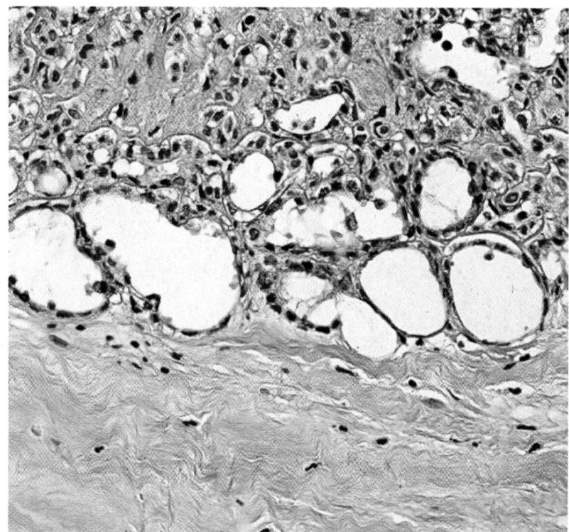

Figure 130.5 Entrapped reactive mesothelial cells at the interface of the pleural surface and overlying pleuritis gives a false impression of invasion.

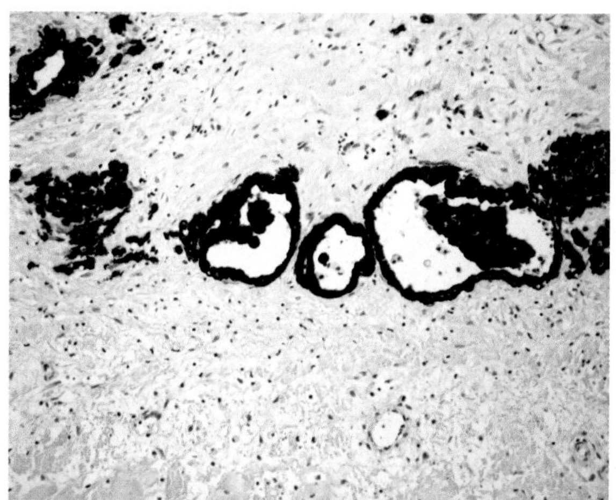

Figure 130.6 Keratin immunostain of same case as shown in Figure 130.5 highlights the proliferating mesothelial cells arranged in a line at the interface of the pleural surface and overlying pleuritis. The cells line the residual pleural space beneath the pleuritis, creating an impression of lumens of glands. There is no invasion of the underlying pleura by keratin-positive mesothelial cells.

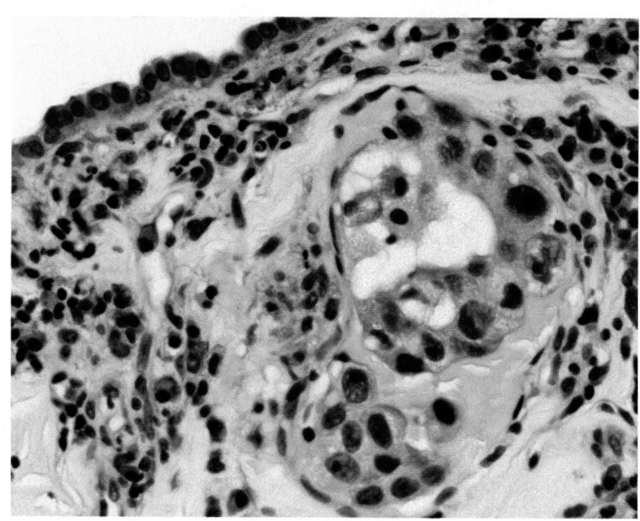

Figure 130.7 High power of vascular invasion of the pleura by a carcinoma with reactive hyperplastic cuboidal mesothelial cells lining the overlying pleural surface.

131

Endometriosis

▶ Rodolfo Laucirica

Endometriosis is defined as extrauterine growth of endometrial tissue. It usually is confined to the pelvic cavity but can occur elsewhere, including the pleura. It usually causes chest pain and dyspnea and sometimes is associated with catamenial (simultaneous with menses) pneumothorax and pleural effusion.

Cytologic Features:

- Benign columnar cells and glands in a bloody background may be seen.
- Stromal cells may resemble reactive mesothelial cells.
- Decidual change may be observed occasionally.

Histologic Features:

- Focal endometrial glands with surrounding stroma.
- Fibrosis, inflammation, hemorrhage, and hemosiderin-laden macrophages.
- Decidual reaction may be seen.

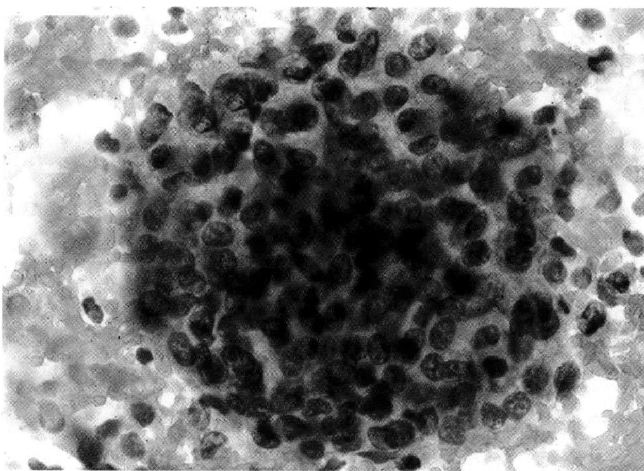

Figure 131.1 Cytology figure of pleural fluid shows endometrial glands and blood in a patient with endometriosis of the pleura.

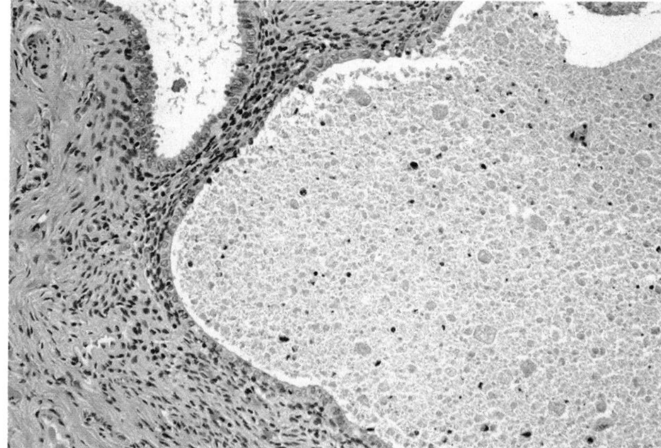

Figure 131.2 Biopsy of pleura shows endometrial glands filled with hemosiderin, blood, and debris in endometriosis of the pleura.

132

Splenosis

▶ Andras Khoor

Pulmonary parenchymal (thoracic) splenosis is a rare condition resulting from seeding of splenic tissue in the pleura and/or pulmonary parenchyma after lacerating trauma to the spleen. The majority of cases present as pleural-based nodules and may masquerade as a metastatic neoplasm.

Cytologic Features:

- Lymphoid tissue with abundant vascularity is seen in fine-needle aspiration specimens.

Histologic Features:

- Nodules of splenic tissue with red and white pulp are present.
- Adjacent lung tissue may show type 2 cell hyperplasia.

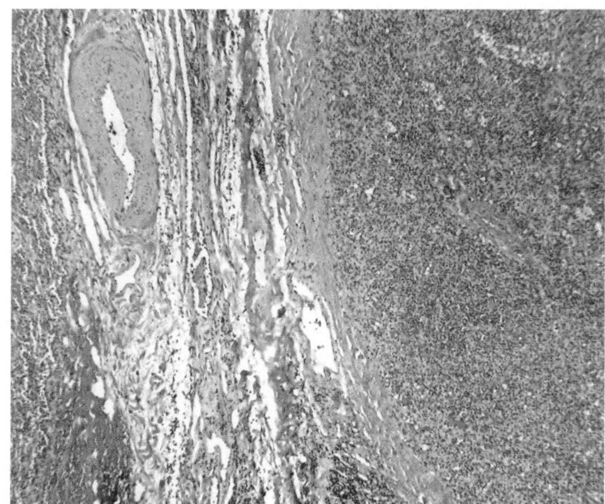

Figure 132.1 Low power shows a nodule of splenic tissue embedded in the pleura and compressing underlying pulmonary parenchyma.

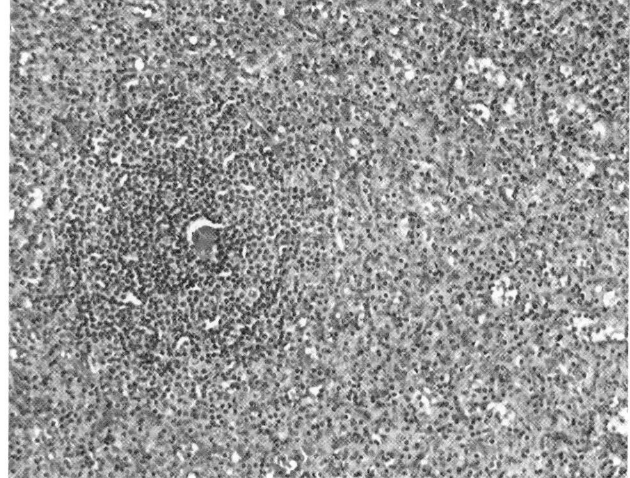

Figure 132.2 Medium power reveals splenic red and white pulp.

Section 24

Pediatric Pulmonary Pathology

133

Childhood Asthma

▶ Megan Dishop
▶ Claire Langston

Asthma is a common disease usually with onset in childhood. It is characterized by airway hyperreactivity with acute episodic narrowing, particularly following environmental triggers. This disease affects approximately 3% to 8% of the population and, despite medical management, results in 2,000 to 3,000 deaths annually in the United States. Based on autopsy findings, an acute attack results in alternating areas of atelectasis and hyperexpansion of the lungs. Microscopic features of asthma include marked thickening of airway smooth muscle, submucosal edema and vascular dilation, thickening of the basal lamina of the mucosa, increased numbers of mucosal goblet cells, and mucus plugs within small to medium bronchi. The airway walls typically show a mixed inflammatory infiltrate that includes numerous eosinophils, as well as plasma cells, lymphocytes, and neutrophils. Adjacent alveolar infiltrates may be present. The mucous plugs and sputum from asthmatic patients may contain admixed inflammatory cells, particularly eosinophils, and may also show Curschmann spirals, Charcot-Leyden crystals (formed from degranulated eosinophils), or Creola bodies (sloughed respiratory epithelium).

Histologic Features:

- Bronchial smooth muscle thickening.
- Thickening of basal lamina.
- Increased number of mucosal goblet cells.
- Submucosal edema.
- Mixed inflammatory infiltrate with numerous eosinophils.
- Mucus plugs, Curschmann spirals, Charcot-Leyden crystals, and Creola bodies.

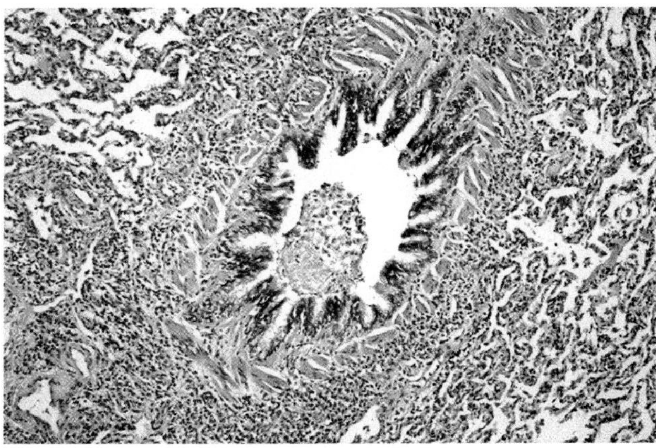

Figure 133.1 Asthma. The airways typically show mucus plugging.

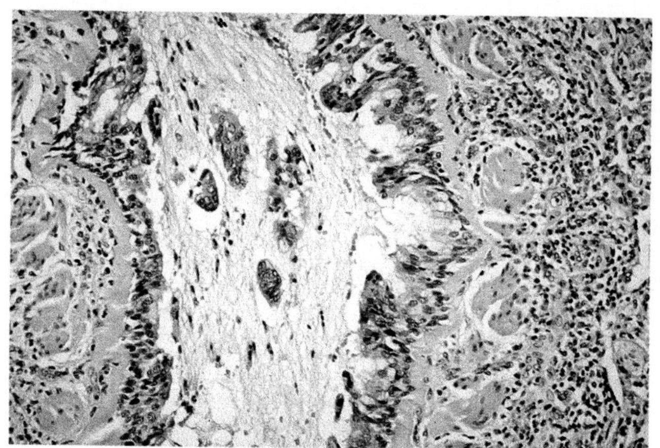

Figure 133.2 Asthma. Mucous plug with intraluminal inflammatory cells and hyperplasia of airway smooth muscle.

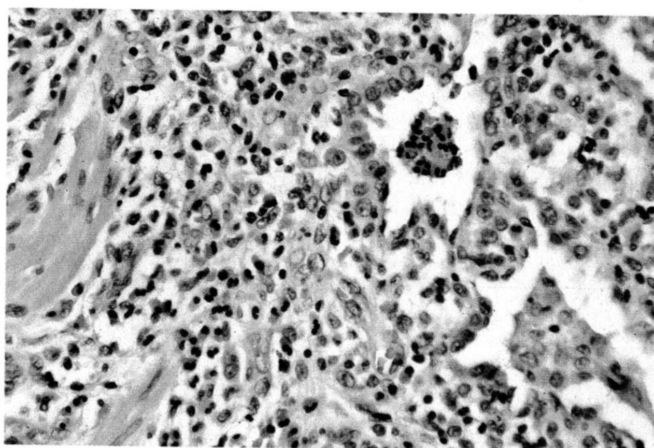

Figure 133.3 Asthma. The inflammatory cell infiltrate, predominantly eosinophils, extends focally into airspaces.

Bronchial Atresia and Intralobar Sequestration

134

▸ Megan Dishop
▸ Claire Langston

Bronchial atresia may be lobar, segmental, or subsegmental, and it may be isolated or associated with systemic arterial connection (intralobar sequestration) and, more rarely, abnormal venous connection. Those cases with systemic arterial connection may occasionally have connection to the gastrointestinal tract (intralobar sequestration and communicating bronchopulmonary foregut malformation).

Isolated bronchial atresia usually involves a segmental bronchus, most commonly in the left upper lobe and rarely in the right upper or lower lobe. Bronchial atresia is said to typically present in late childhood or adolescence with dyspnea, recurrent pneumonia, or as an incidental finding on chest x-ray film. With increasing application of prenatal ultrasonography, diagnosis *in utero* is becoming more common. Grossly, the atretic bronchus results in a mucocele, which may appear as a bulge at the hilum of the lung. The parenchyma beyond the atresia and mucocele contains abundant mucus and shows other obstructive changes, including airspace enlargement and decreased density of airways and vessels. The distal parenchyma often shows maldevelopment in the form of pulmonary hyperplasia or microcystic maldevelopment. Microcystic maldevelopment occurs in approximately 50% of cases and resembles the small cyst type of congenital cystic adenomatoid malformation (Stocker type II). There may also be superimposed chronic inflammatory infiltrates when diagnosis and definitive surgery are delayed.

Bronchial atresia involving the lower lobes, especially the left lower lobe, is often associated with aberrant systemic arterial connection, forming an "intralobar sequestration" in which a region of parenchyma is functionally isolated from the remainder of the lung. Despite investment by the same pleura, one region of the lobe is "sequestered" from the surrounding parenchyma by both the absence of connection with the tracheobronchial tree and an aberrant vascular supply. The arterial supply may be from single or multiple vessels arising from the distal thoracic or proximal abdominal aorta, celiac, splenic, intercostal, or subclavian arteries. Although venous drainage is usually by the pulmonary vein, the aberrant vessels may include systemic venous connection. Intralobar sequestration is infrequently associated with other anomalies and is rarely identified at birth, although, like other developmental abnormalities of the lung, it is increasingly being recognized by prenatal ultrasonography. The morphologic features of bronchial atresia with systemic arterial connection (intralobar sequestration) are similar to isolated bronchial atresia, including the presence of a mucocele and histologic evidence of obstructive changes with parenchymal maldevelopment.

It should be noted that the term *sequestration* has been expanded in common usage to denote the larger group of lung malformations with aberrant vascular supply, including those with normal bronchial communication. In the strict sense, however, *pulmonary sequestration* refers to lack of normal airway connection and aberrant vascular supply, and it may be either intralobar or extralobar.

Histologic Features:

- Mucocele.
- Obstructive parenchymal changes.
- Airspace enlargement, abundant mucus, with or without chronic inflammatory infiltrates.
- Pulmonary hyperplasia.
- Microcystic maldevelopment.

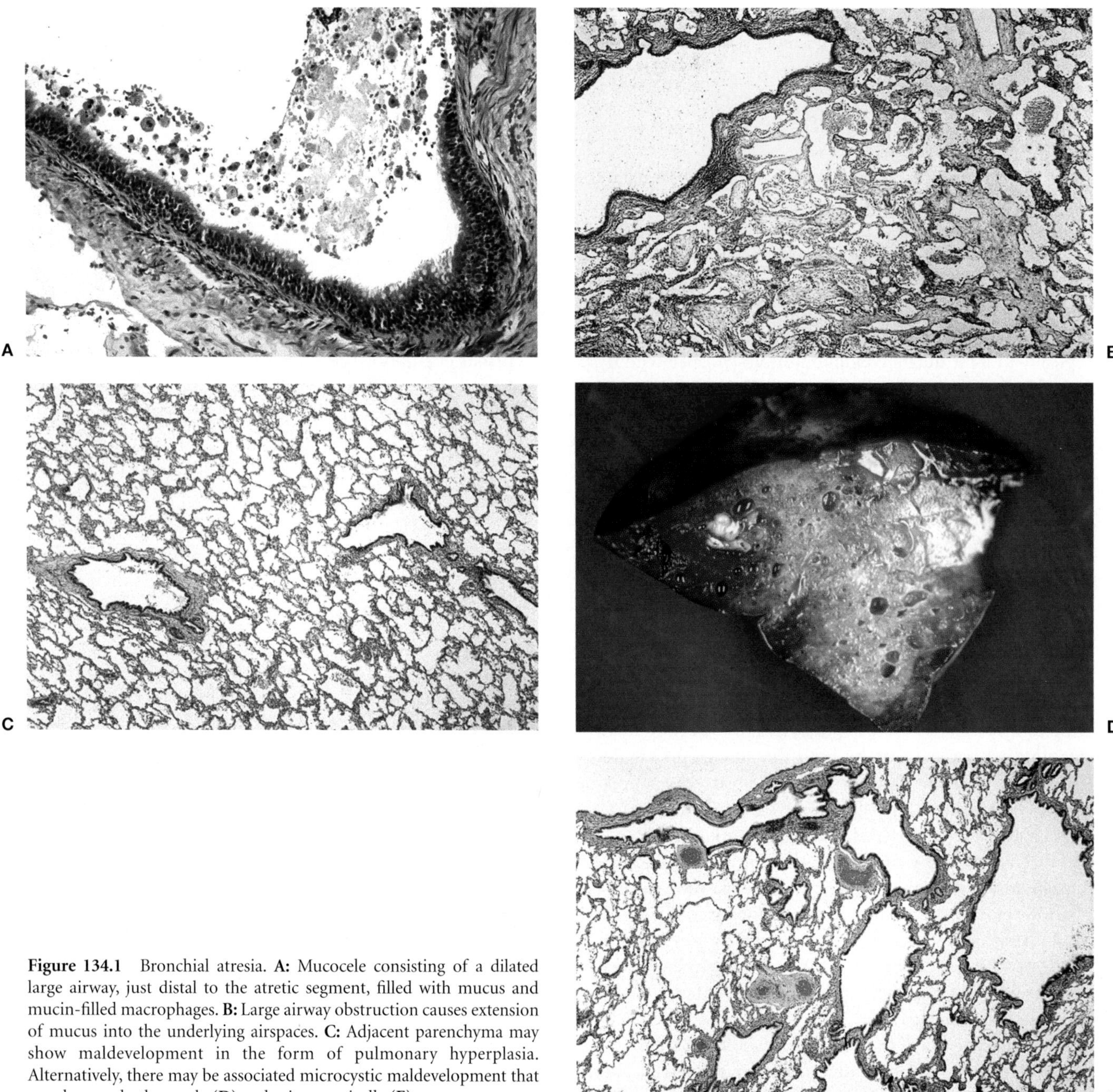

Figure 134.1 Bronchial atresia. **A:** Mucocele consisting of a dilated large airway, just distal to the atretic segment, filled with mucus and mucin-filled macrophages. **B:** Large airway obstruction causes extension of mucus into the underlying airspaces. **C:** Adjacent parenchyma may show maldevelopment in the form of pulmonary hyperplasia. Alternatively, there may be associated microcystic maldevelopment that may be seen both grossly (**D**) and microscopically (**E**).

A 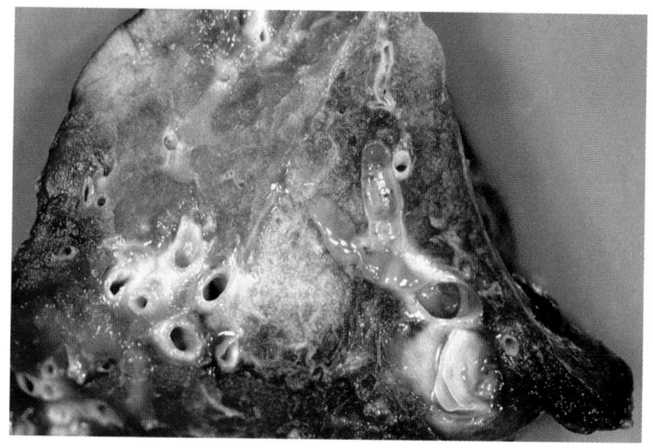

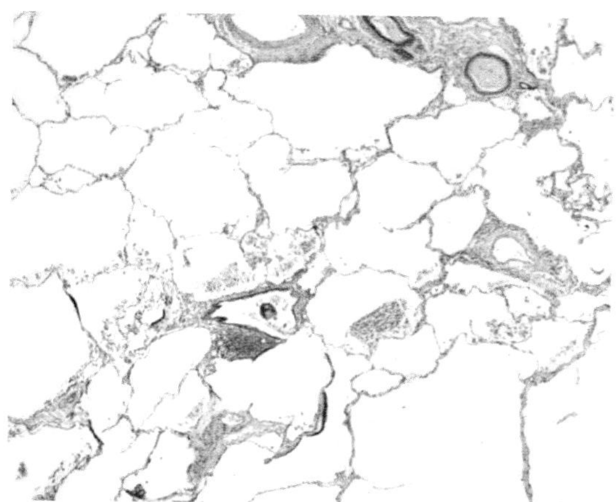 B

Figure 134.2 Intralobar pulmonary sequestration. **A:** Gross appearance shows a dilated airway and distal pale parenchyma. **B:** Microscopically, overinflation and simplification of airspaces are typical.

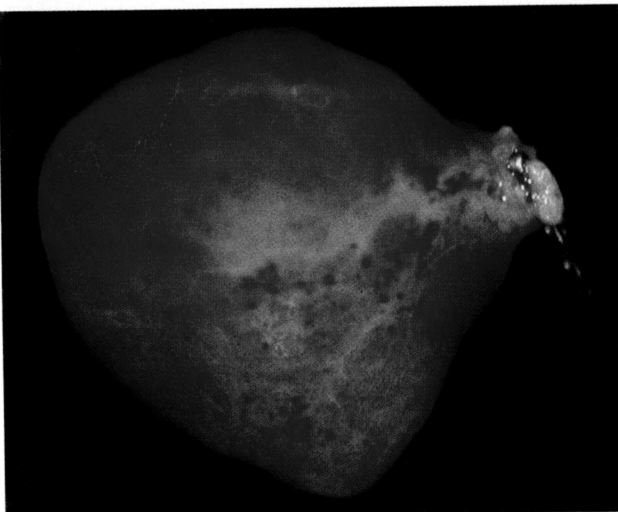

Figure 135.1 Extralobar sequestration. Typical gross appearance of a wedge-shaped piece of lung tissue invested in its own visceral pleura. The surgical clip identifies the vascular pedicle. This small extralobar sequestration was identified incidentally adjacent to the left diaphragmatic surface in an infant undergoing excision of a bronchogenic cyst.

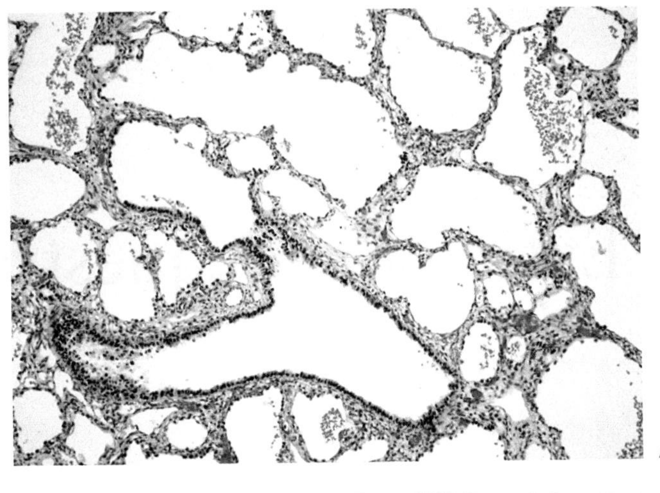

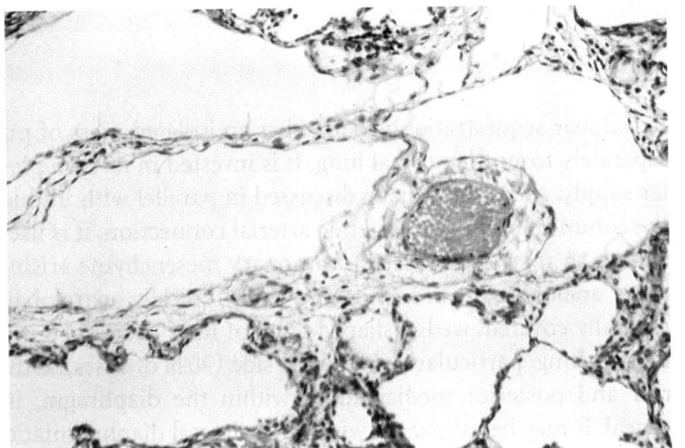

Figure 135.2 Extralobar sequestration. Microscopically, the lung parenchyma is simplified with distention of airspaces (**A**). Some cases may also show associated lymphangiectasis (**B**).

Bronchogenic Cyst

136

▸ Megan Dishop
▸ Claire Langston

Bronchogenic cysts are usually solitary unilocular cystic structures filled with either fluid or mucus and are usually attached to the trachea or major bronchi. Although they do not communicate with the foregut, they are thought to originate from an aberrant supernumerary bud of the developing foregut. The most common location is in the mediastinum above the tracheal bifurcation, but bronchogenic cysts may occur at the hilum of the lung or any paramidline site from suprasternal to infradiaphragmatic and rarely have been reported in extrathoracic locations. Although usually associated with the extrapulmonary tracheobronchial tree, bronchogenic cysts may also be located within the lung parenchyma. In these cases, no connection to adjacent airways can be demonstrated, unless there is disruption of the wall due to secondary infection and necrosis. Because of localized compressive effects, the surrounding parenchyma may show obstructive changes including airspace enlargement but otherwise normal architecture. Bronchogenic cysts have been reported in association with congenital lobar overinflation, bronchial atresia, and extralobar sequestration.

Bronchogenic cysts may present in infancy with respiratory distress from mass effect or later with symptoms of infection. Many are asymptomatic and fortuitously discovered. They gradually increase in size with age and somatic growth, and they may reach a diameter of 10 cm in older patients. Late complications include infection, cyst rupture, and, rarely, hemoptysis or pneumothorax.

Histologic Features:

- The wall of a bronchogenic cyst replicates the bronchial wall, including the presence of hyaline cartilage plates and, less commonly, bronchial glands.
- Presence of cartilage is a helpful feature in distinguishing these lesions from enteric duplication cysts and neurenteric cysts.
- Although usually lined by gastric or esophageal epithelium, enteric cysts may contain ciliated epithelium, especially in young children.
- Bronchial-type pseudostratified ciliated columnar epithelium with goblet cells.
- Smooth muscle and fibrovascular tissue; presence of bronchial glands is variable.
- Cartilage plates must be present.
- Differential diagnosis includes enteric duplication cyst, neurenteric cyst, pericardial cyst, and cystic teratoma.

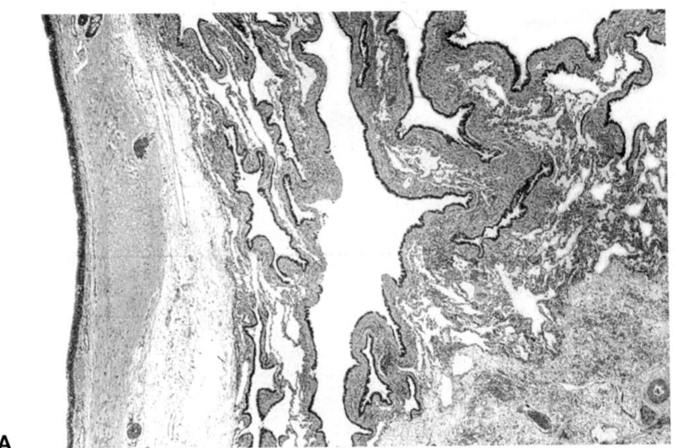

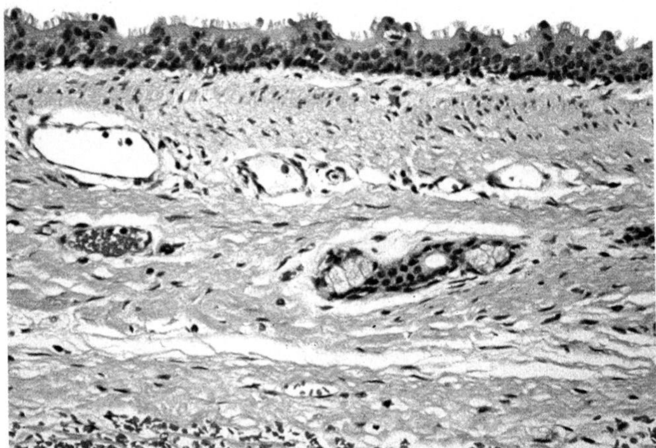

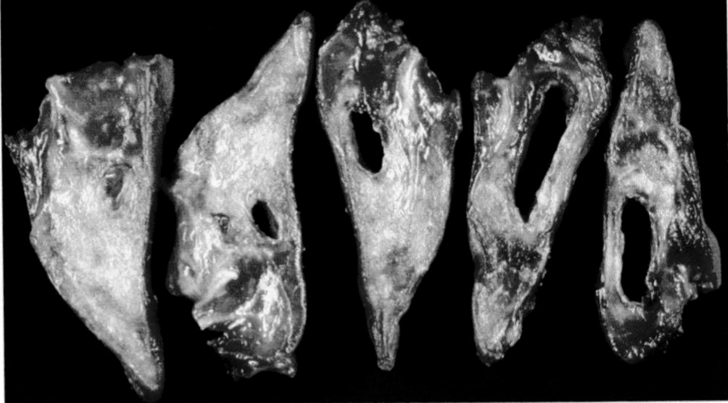

Figure 136.1 Bronchogenic cyst. **A:** The wall contains a cartilaginous plate. This bronchogenic cyst within the lung parenchyma is associated with parenchymal maldevelopment. **B:** The cyst is lined by bronchial-type ciliated columnar epithelium. **C:** Bronchogenic cysts may become infected, as in this case with consolidation and purulent material at the periphery of the cyst. In such situations, their true nature may be difficult to identify.

Congenital Cystic Adenomatoid Malformation, Large Cyst Type

137

▸ Megan Dishop
▸ Claire Langston

The classification of cystic lesions of the lung remains problematic as attempts at classification based on size of cysts do not satisfactorily address pathogenesis and do not easily accommodate lesions with overlapping features. In 1977, Stocker described three types of congenital cystic adenomatoid malformations (CCAM, types I-III) based on their gross appearance: type I (large, often multiloculated cysts >2 cm in diameter), type II (more uniform small cysts <2 cm), and type III (solid "adenomatoid" type, not grossly cystic). This classification has been helpful in pointing out the varied nature of developmental lesions of the lung and is useful as long as one recognizes that not all developmental cystic lesions of the lung can be fit into this classification. In fact, the type III lesion is now known to represent pulmonary hyperplasia. Of the two major types—large cyst (i.e., Stocker type I) and small cyst (i.e., Stocker type II)—the large cyst is more common and more easily recognized. It should be noted that the small cyst type is likely part of a malformation sequence resulting from airway obstruction during development. An obstructive lesion, most commonly bronchial atresia, is identified in virtually all cases with the microcystic pattern of maldevelopment, although the obstructing lesion may easily be overlooked (see Bronchial Atresia, Chapter 134). In cases in which an obstructive lesion is identified, the microcystic area should not be considered as a separate entity but rather as part of a malformation sequence. In contrast, the pathogenesis of the large cyst type remains uncertain, and it is considered a distinct malformation.

The large cyst type of CCAM usually presents in infancy with progressive respiratory distress due to air trapping within the malformation. In some cases, there may be associated pulmonary hypoplasia due to compression by mass effect. Increasingly, these lesions are identified *in utero* by ultrasonography; however, occasionally they are not recognized clinically until late childhood or adulthood. Typically, large cyst CCAM affects only one lobe and consists of a large (>2 cm), often multiloculated cystic structure, occasionally with smaller cysts or microcystic maldevelopment at the periphery merging with the adjacent lung. Microscopically, these lesions are not true cysts, and there is always communication with the surrounding parenchyma and the proximal airways. The lining is composed of respiratory epithelium with a small amount of underlying smooth muscle but no cartilage. Some also contain mucigenic epithelium resembling gastric mucinous epithelium. The distal lung parenchyma shows a pattern of secondary changes similar to that described for other obstructing lesions. A significant proportion (up to 25%) has a systemic arterial supply.

Differential diagnosis includes low-grade cystic pleuropulmonary blastoma, cystic intraparenchymal lymphangioma, and pneumatocele. In addition, there are reports of bronchioloalveolar carcinoma originating in previously unrecognized or incompletely resected large cyst type CCAM in older children or adults.

Histologic Features:

- Respiratory epithelial lining.
- Sometimes including mucigenic epithelium.
- Small amount of smooth muscle but no cartilage.
- Connections to adjacent parenchyma, distal and proximal, are always present.

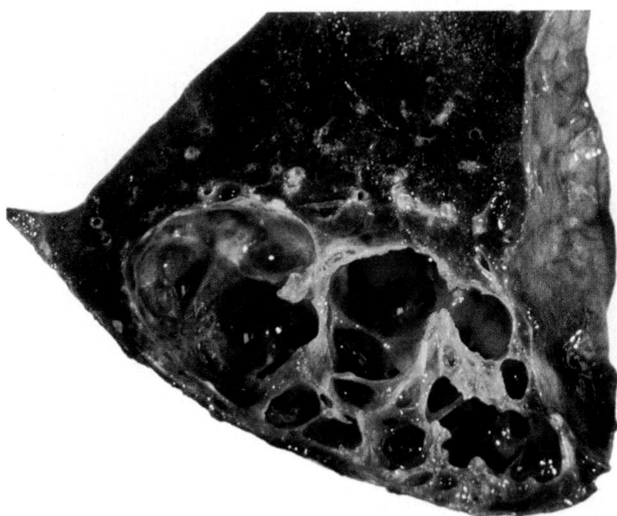

Figure 137.1 Cystic adenomatoid malformation, large cyst type. The typical gross morphology consists of a large cystic space with variable septation, forming a mass lesion within the lung parenchyma.

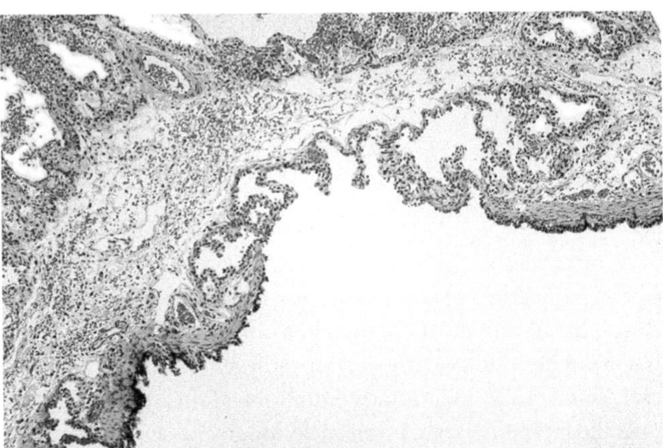

A

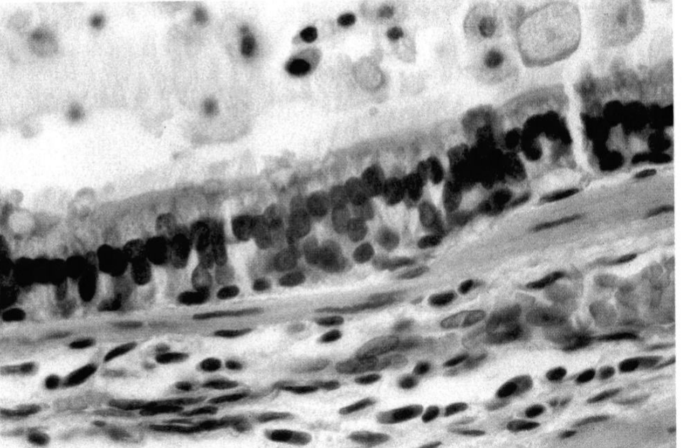

B

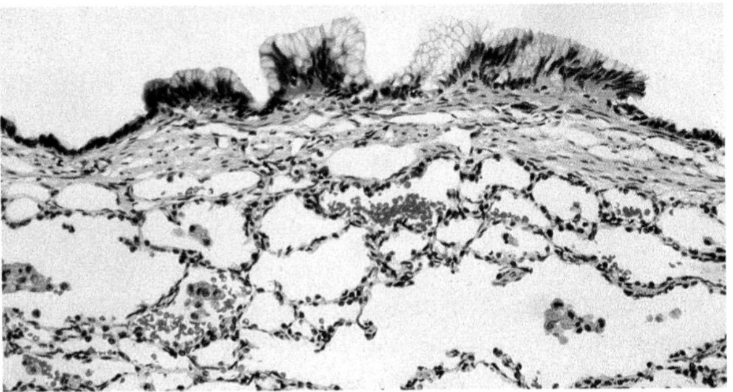

C

Figure 137.2 Cystic adenomatoid malformation, large cyst type. **A:** Microscopically, the cyst wall shows at least focal connection to the distal alveolar spaces. **B:** The lining is comprised of ciliated respiratory-type epithelium. **C:** The lining may contain foci of mucigenic epithelium.

138 Pulmonary Hyperplasia and Related Disorders

▶ Megan Dishop
▶ Claire Langston

Pulmonary hyperplasia refers to abnormal overgrowth of lung parenchyma, reflected by increased number and enlargement of airspaces. It is always a secondary phenomenon and is thought to be a response to airway obstruction during development. Pulmonary hyperplasia may affect both lungs equally, as in fetal laryngeal atresia, but more commonly affects a single lung or portion of one lung. Laryngeal atresia may be an isolated anomaly or syndromic, as in Fraser syndrome (cryptophthalmos, ear anomalies, syndactyly, renal anomalies, and cryptorchidism). The bilateral pulmonary hyperplasia in this setting is related to obstructed outflow of fluid from both lungs *in utero.* The lungs may weigh 150% to 300% normal and are characterized histologically by airspaces that are increased in number, enlarged, and poorly subdivided.

In its most dramatic form, pulmonary hyperplasia has been described as the solid (or "adenomatoid") form of cystic adenomatoid malformation (Stocker type III), a rare lesion recognized as massive enlargement of one or more lobes in fetuses and stillborn infants. By ultrasound, these are large brightly echogenic masses, which may enlarge or regress *in utero.* Grossly, the lung parenchyma appears uniform and solid, except for scattered tiny cystic spaces. The histologic features are similar to those described in the setting of fetal laryngeal atresia, with markedly increased numbers of alveolar structures that are mildly enlarged and poorly subdivided. The airways are widely separated by the increased lobular parenchyma but are otherwise normal. Interlobular septa are infrequent to absent. The parenchyma is often also described as having an immature appearance, although this is explained by the immaturity of the fetuses and premature stillborns in whom these lesions are identified. Although not clearly documented to date, airway obstruction during development likely accounts for the pathogenesis of these rare lesions.

Polyalveolar lobe is another form of pulmonary hyperplasia in which there is enlargement of a lobe due to increased numbers of alveoli. Most often involving the left upper lobe, the polyalveolar lobe is typically markedly enlarged, in some cases causing compression of adjacent lobes and mediastinal shift. There is a marked increase in alveolar number with large areas devoid of bronchioles. As in parenchyma associated with obstructing lesions, the alveolar spaces tend to be simplified without prominent subdivision.

In addition to these more striking manifestations, pulmonary hyperplasia may affect smaller regions of the lung due to local obstruction, as in bronchial atresia or bronchogenic cysts.

Histologic Features:

- Increased alveolar number.
- Enlargement of airspaces with simplification and lack of subdivision.
- Widely spaced bronchioles.
- Parenchyma may appear immature, as in the solid form of congenital cystic adenomatoid malformation (Stocker type III).
- Differential diagnosis includes congenital lobar overinflation.

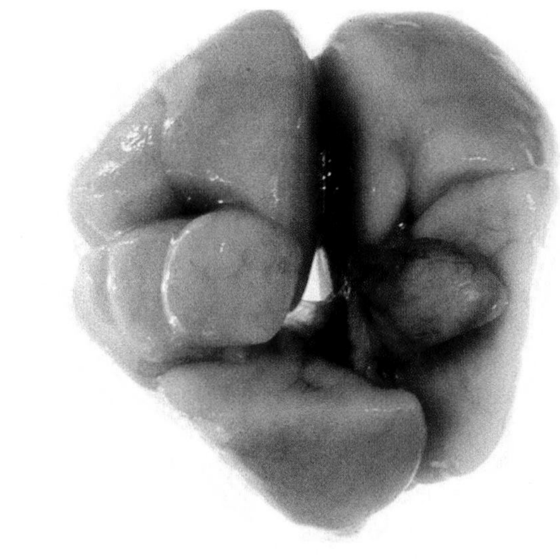

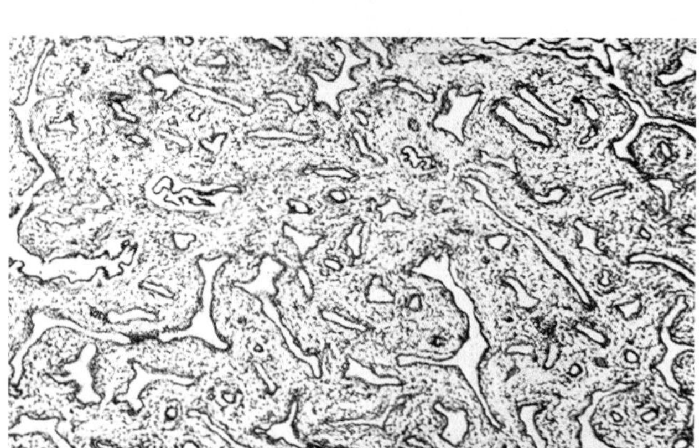

Figure 138.1 Pulmonary hyperplasia. **A:** This 17-week-gestation fetus with tracheal atresia had markedly enlarged lungs bilaterally, which is underscored by the relatively small size of the heart. **B:** The immature lung shows a marked increase in small irregular airspaces, many of which may be bronchiolar in nature, as the lung is largely formed of airways rather than airspaces at this gestational age.

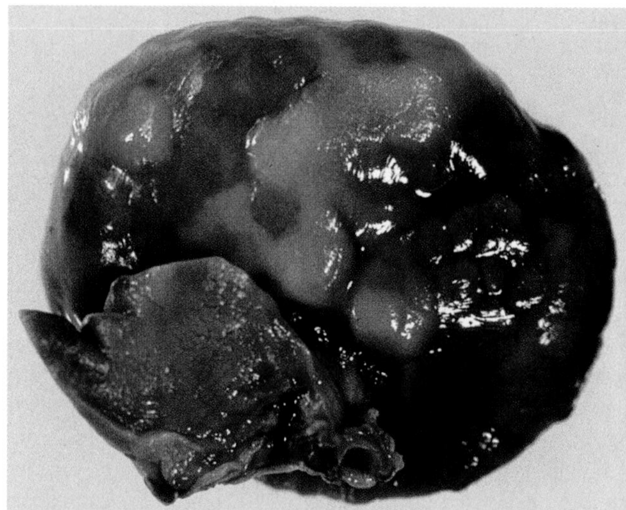

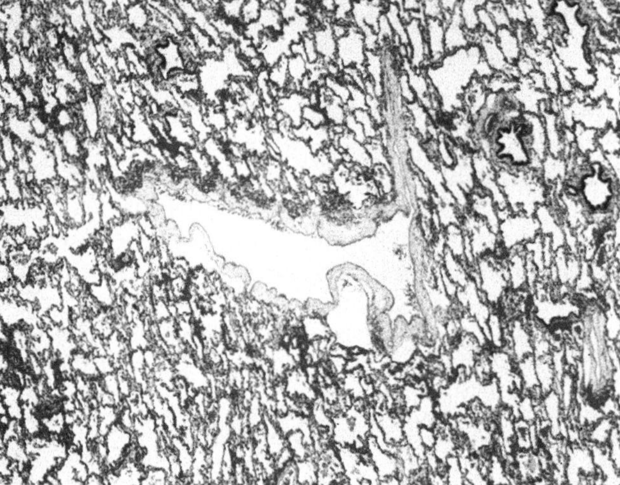

Figure 138.2 Pulmonary hyperplasia presenting as congenital cystic adenomatoid malformation, Stocker type III. **A:** The external surface of the lung is enlarged because of the underlying parenchymal maldevelopment and overgrowth. **B:** Microscopically, the airspaces are increased in number and poorly subdivided.

Congenital Lobar Overinflation

139

▶ Megan Dishop
▶ Claire Langston

Congenital lobar overinflation, often called *congenital (or infantile) lobar emphysema,* refers to marked enlargement of a lobe due to airspace enlargement. It most often affects the upper lobes, particularly the left upper lobe. It is an uncommon cause of respiratory distress in infancy and in only a very few cases has been detected by prenatal ultrasound. Affected infants usually become symptomatic within the first month of life, and presentation after 6 months of age is unusual. Although there may be partial regression in size *in utero,* lobectomy may be necessary because of excessive air trapping postnatally.

Congenital lobar overinflation is thought to be caused by partial obstruction, either intrinsic or extrinsic, to a lobar bronchus. Complete obstruction is rare but has been identified; obstruction is most often partial and may be due to bronchomalacia, mucus plugs, webs or stenoses, bronchial torsion, or extrinsic compression by vascular structures, bronchogenic cysts, or postinflammatory strictures. Defective or absent bronchial cartilage may also cause expiratory collapse and hyperinflation. The lobe is typically markedly enlarged but, in contrast to polyalveolar lobe, shows only airspace enlargement rather than increased numbers of alveoli. Polyalveolar lobe may be a variant of congenital lobar overinflation or may be a separate condition. It is much less common than congenital lobar overinflation.

Histologic Features:

- Airspace enlargement.
- Normal numbers of alveoli.
- No evidence of parenchymal maldevelopment.
- Differential diagnosis includes polyalveolar lobe and pulmonary hyperplasia (solid or "adenomatoid" type of cystic adenomatoid malformation).

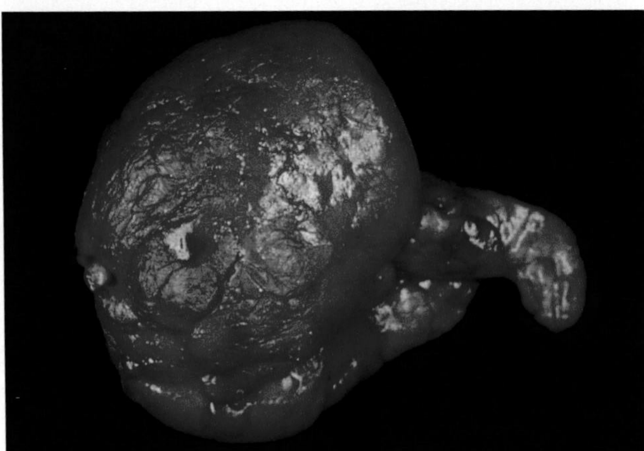

Figure 139.1 Congenital lobar overinflation. From the external surface, the majority of this left upper lobe is markedly hyperinflated relative to the more normal appearing lingula (**bottom right**).

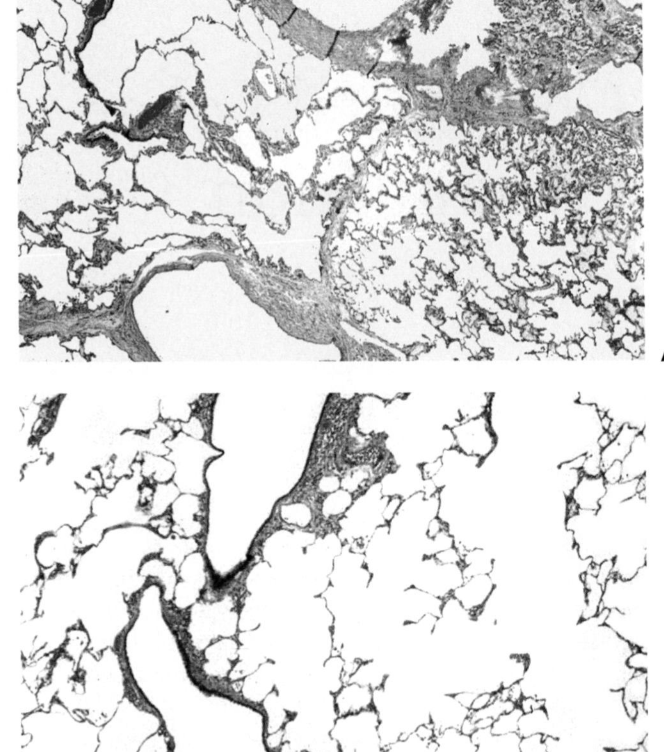

Figure 139.2 Congenital lobar overinflation. **A:** The overinflation of the airspaces is best appreciated at the junction with normal parenchyma. **B:** The airspaces are distended but not increased in number.

Complications of Prematurity

140

▶ Megan Dishop
▶ Claire Langston

Hyaline Membrane Disease

Hyaline membrane disease, the histologic counterpart of severe respiratory distress syndrome, is the major cause of neonatal respiratory distress in premature infants and more rarely occurs in term infants, usually with a variety of underlying conditions. It is caused by lung immaturity with its developmental deficiency of surfactant, which is necessary to lower alveolar surface tension and maintain open alveoli after expiration. It is usually complicated by poor resorption of lung fluid leading to edema. Lack of surfactant causes collapse of alveoli, and high ventilatory pressures may become necessary to adequately expand the lungs. Grossly, the lungs are typically red and firm, with a solid appearance due to extensive atelectasis. Although lung immaturity with inadequate surfactant is the primary problem in clinically severe cases, therapeutic support with mechanical ventilation and supplemental oxygen may also play a role. Hyaline membranes form along terminal bronchioles as well as alveolar ducts and respiratory bronchioles. They are composed of cellular debris, fibrin and other exudate, and amniotic fluid material and appear microscopically as homogeneous granular to linear eosinophilic material. The hyaline membranes are not usually visible histologically until 6 hours after birth, but they can form as early as 2 to 3 hours after birth if there is prenatal injury. They are well formed by 8 to 12 hours. In the absence of conditions that may foster continual lung injury, they may resorb by 48 hours.

Pulmonary Interstitial Emphysema

One of the complications of hyaline membrane disease is pulmonary interstitial emphysema(PIE). Because of the high ventilatory pressures sometimes required to maintain oxygenation, barotrauma may cause disruption of the terminal bronchiolar wall or at the lobular periphery, with consequent dissection of air into interlobular septa and peribronchial spaces. The air may dissect either centrally, causing pneumomediastinum, pneumopericardium, and/or pneumoperitoneum, or peripherally, causing pneumothorax. Grossly, air bubbles may be seen on the pleural surface within interlobular septa. Microscopically, the dissection of air results in dilated empty spaces within bronchovascular bundles, interlobular septa, and the pleura. The spaces have no epithelial or endothelial lining. When present for a prolonged period, interstitial air may lead to a foreign body-type reaction, and these spaces may be partially lined by histiocytes and histiocytic giant cells.

Chronic Neonatal Lung Injury (Bronchopulmonary Dysplasia)

With continual lung injury and repair in severe respiratory distress syndrome, chronic changes become superimposed on acute hyaline membrane disease. As a consequence, the lung begins to remodel, and this may begin as early as 36 hours after birth. This remodeling occurs in three major ways. The first to appear is early fibroplasia in the lobular interstitium. The second is variable plugging of small airways by necrotic debris, with some lobules becoming overexpanded and others collapsed and compressed. This results in uneven ventilation and, when prolonged, fixed collapse and even virtual disappearance of lobules, marked only by linear retractions on the pleural surfaces (accessory fissures). This results in a "cobblestone" appearance of the visceral pleura. The third is fibrous obliteration of the lumens of some small airways, with resultant protection of the distal parenchyma in these regions but lack of access to it via the airways for ventilation. Microscopically, there are variable areas of hyperinflation and collapse. The airway epithelium may show hyperplasia, regenerative changes, or squamous metaplasia, and there may be residual debris within the bronchi and bronchioles. These changes are analogous to diffuse alveolar damage, particularly in its later stages.

The progression from hyaline membrane disease to chronic neonatal lung injury (bronchopulmonary dysplasia) has been divided into four stages: acute exudative (I), early subacute reparative (II), late subacute fibroproliferative (III), and chronic fibroproliferative (IV). In individual examples, these stages may be present together in a varied fashion as the result of ongoing injury, or some features of stages may not be present.

Histologic Features:

Stages of Evolution from Hyaline Membrane Disease to Chronic Neonatal Lung Injury

- Stage I (0–4 Days): Acute Exudative.
  - Hyaline membrane formation.
  - Hyperemia, atelectasis.
  - Necrosis of bronchiolar mucosa; patchy loss of ciliated cells.
  - Edema.
  - Lymphatic dilation.

- Stage II (4–10 Days): Early Subacute Reparative.
  - Hyaline membranes persist.
  - Necrosis of bronchiolar mucosa with eosinophilic exudate in lumen.
  - Evidence of early repair of airway epithelium with metaplastic and regenerative changes.
  - Interstitial edema.
  - Early alveolar septal fibroplasia.

- Stage III (10–20 Days): Late Subacute Fibroproliferative.
  - Few hyaline membranes.
  - Irregular aeration with alternating hyperinflation and atelectasis.
  - Alveolar epithelial injury with type 2 cell hyperplasia/regeneration.
  - Squamous metaplasia of airway mucosa.
  - Bronchiolectasis and bronchiolitis obliterans.
  - Increased interstitial and perialveolar duct fibrosis (centrilobular fibrosis).
  - Airway smooth muscle proliferation and intralobular extension.
  - Extension of pulmonary arterial smooth muscle into intralobular vessels.

- Stage IV (>1 Month): Chronic Fibroproliferative.
  - Groups of hyperinflated alveoli.
  - Increased interstitial collagen fibrosis.
  - Septal fibrosis is characteristic.
  - Thickened airspace walls.
  - Capillaries at a distance from alveolar epithelium or festooned along the alveolar wall.
  - Tortuous dilated lymphatics.
  - Hyperplasia of pulmonary arterial smooth muscle.

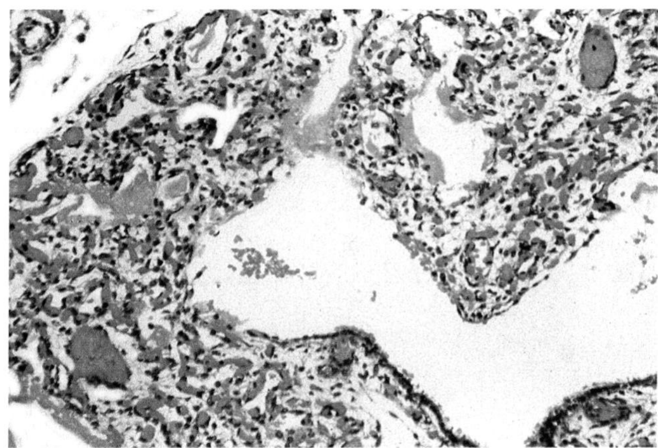

Figure 140.1 Hyaline membrane disease. Hyaline membranes lining the terminal bronchioles and alveolar ducts are well developed in this premature infant.

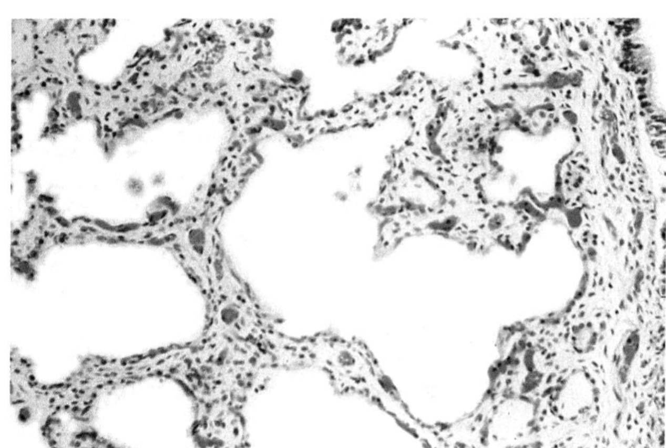

Figure 140.2 Hyaline membrane disease with early fibroplasia. As the hyaline membranes resorb, the interstitium is mildly expanded by edema, and the stellate mesenchymal cells become bipolar or spindled elongated fibroblasts.

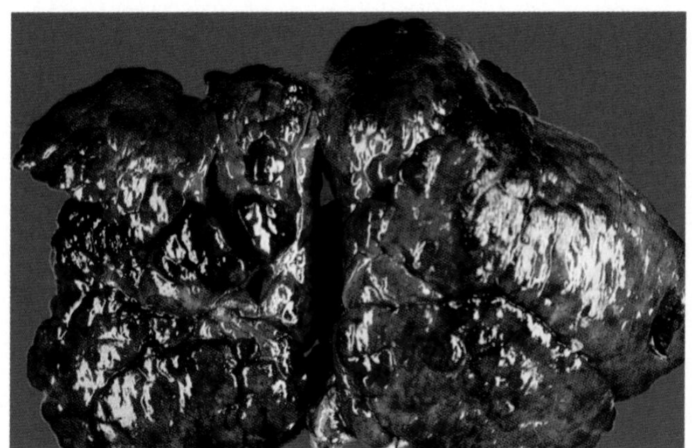

Figure 140.3 Chronic neonatal lung injury (bronchopulmonary dysplasia). The external surfaces of the lungs in bronchopulmonary dysplasia are characterized by alternating areas of hyperinflation and collapse with linear areas of contraction of the visceral pleural (accessory fissures). The child, a former 25-week-gestation premature infant, died at age 10 months.

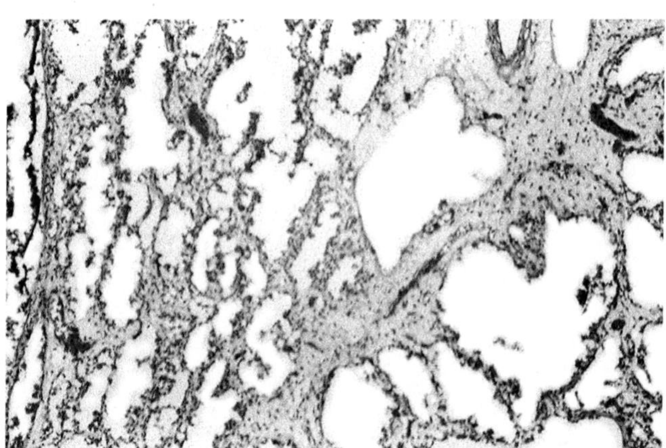

Figure 140.4 Chronic neonatal lung injury (bronchopulmonary dysplasia). Microscopically, the lungs also typically show hyperexpanded alveoli adjacent to areas of collapse. The interstitium shows variable degrees of fibrosis.

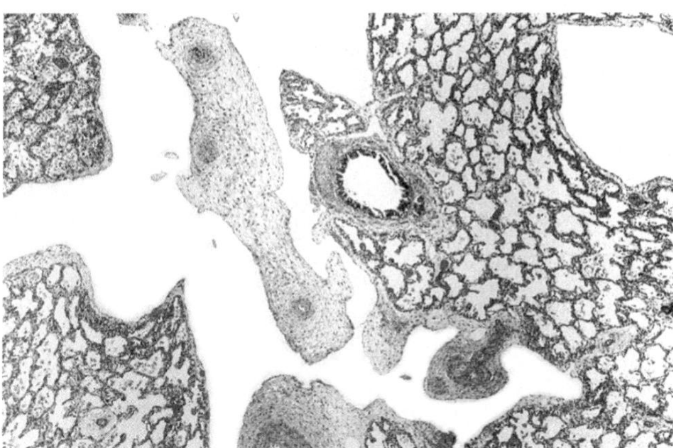

Figure 140.5 Pulmonary interstitial emphysema. Dissecting air-filled spaces are present in interlobular septa and the pleura.

141

Lymphatic Disorders

▶ Megan Dishop
▶ Claire Langston

Congenital pulmonary lymphangiectasis is a rare primary disorder that causes respiratory distress in the newborn. In severe cases it may be fatal within the first few days of life; however, there are less severe cases with prolonged survival with optimal management. Although usually sporadic, congenital pulmonary lymphangiectasis may be associated with malformation syndromes such as Turner, Noonan, and Down syndrome. It is often accompanied by a chylous pleural effusion, suggesting an intrinsic abnormality of lymphatic development in such cases. Grossly, the lungs are firm and bosselated, with visible distention of lymphatics across the pleural surface. Microscopically, the lymphatics in the interlobular septa and subpleural region are cystically dilated, forming empty spaces lined by a thin endothelium. If necessary, the endothelial lining may be demonstrated with the aid of immunohistochemistry using antibodies to CD31 or factor VIII-related antigen.

Pulmonary lymphangiectasis may be a secondary condition or may be part of a systemic lymphatic maldevelopment. It is categorized into three main groups: primary, secondary, and generalized. Primary lymphangiectasis is thought to result from failure of pulmonary lymphatics to connect with systemic lymphatics, for example, via the thoracic duct. Secondary pulmonary lymphangiectasis is associated with cardiac maldevelopment with obstruction of pulmonary venous drainage (e.g., total anomalous pulmonary venous return). Generalized lymphangiectasis is a systemic abnormality that involves not only the lung but also the soft tissue, viscera, or bone of the thorax, and sometimes extrathoracic sites.

Lymphangiomas rarely occur in the lung, but when they do, they produce local mass lesions. They resemble lymphangiomas in other locations, being composed of thin-walled vascular spaces of variable size, which may contain proteinaceous lymph fluid. In contrast, diffuse pulmonary lymphangiomatosis is a generalized process in the lung with widespread lymphatic proliferation consisting of complex anastomosing spaces along the usual lymphatic pathways without an associated mass lesion. Smooth muscle associated with these lymphatic channels may be prominent in some cases. Although lymphangiectasis refers to dilation of preexisting vascular spaces, diffuse pulmonary lymphangiomatosis denotes lymphatic proliferation with more numerous and smaller lymphatics. In addition, some cases have a kaposiform morphology with proliferation of spindle cells, endothelial hyperplasia, and hemosiderin deposition. Lymphangiomatosis may also involve other thoracic tissues, including soft tissues of the mediastinum, pericardium, chest wall, and bones.

Histologic Features:

- Congenital pulmonary lymphangiectasis consists of cystically dilated lymphatic channels in interlobular septa and the pleura.
- Lymphangioma is a localized proliferation of lymphatics forming a mass lesion.
- Diffuse lymphangiomatosis is a proliferation of complex anastomosing lymphatics within interlobular septa and the pleura.
- May have kaposiform morphology.

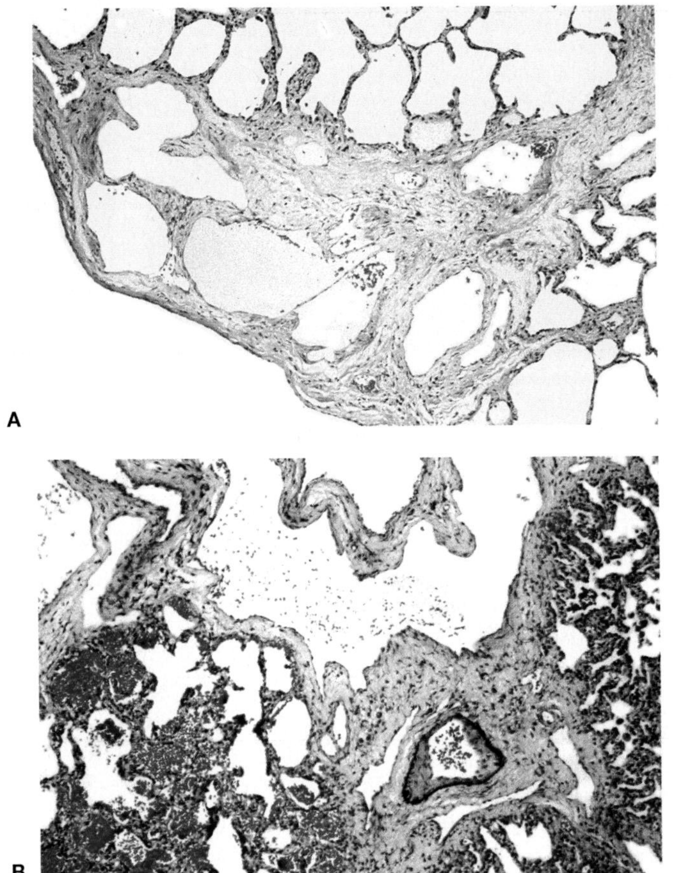

A

B

Figure 141.1 Pulmonary lymphangiectasis. **A:** Dilated lymphatics within the pleura. **B:** Dilated peribronchial lymphatics (Movat pentachrome).

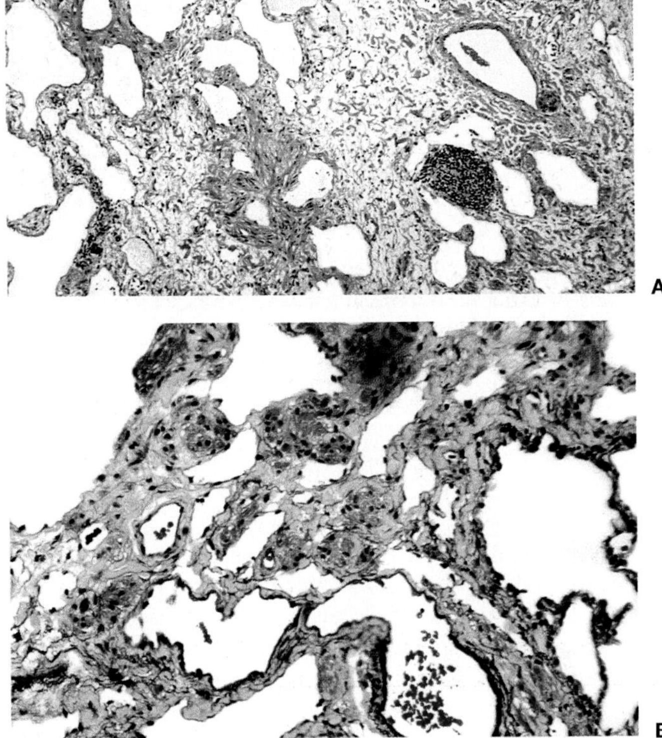

A

B

Figure 141.2 Diffuse pulmonary lymphangiomatosis. **A:** Lymphatic proliferation is present within the interlobular septa, and focal lymphoid aggregates may be present. **B:** Smooth muscle may be focally prominent (Movat pentachrome).

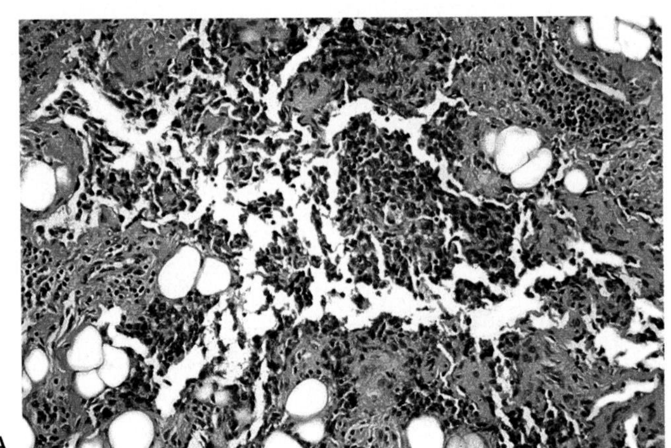

A

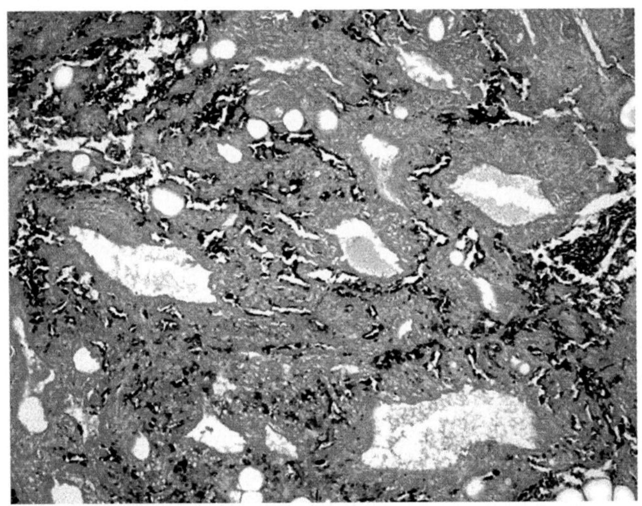

B

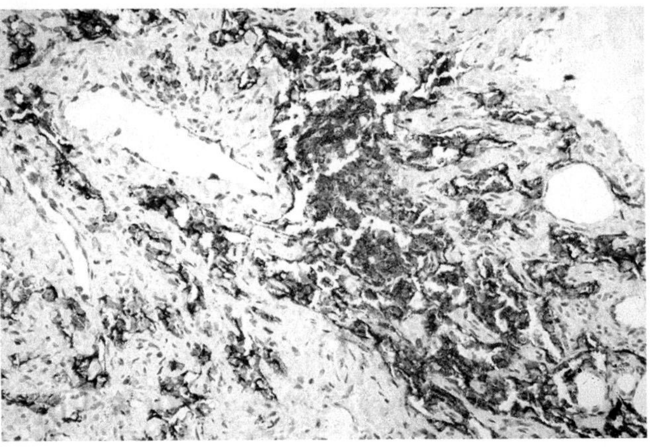

C

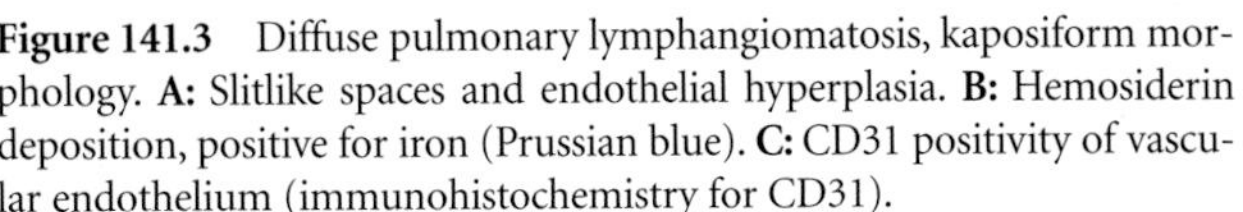

Figure 141.3 Diffuse pulmonary lymphangiomatosis, kaposiform morphology. **A:** Slitlike spaces and endothelial hyperplasia. **B:** Hemosiderin deposition, positive for iron (Prussian blue). **C:** CD31 positivity of vascular endothelium (immunohistochemistry for CD31).

Tissue Heterotopia and Related Abnormalities

142

▶ Megan Dishop
▶ Claire Langston

Although rare, a variety of heterotopic tissues in the lung have been described, including striated muscle, adrenal tissue, thyroid, pancreas, and liver. Glial tissue has also been observed uncommonly. Most cases are associated with anencephaly or other open neural tube defects, presumably from fetal aspiration of brain tissue *in utero*.

Rhabdomyomatous dysplasia is a rare phenomenon that consists of diffuse infiltration of striated muscle fibers within the interstitium of the lung. It is always seen in association with some other pulmonary developmental abnormality, particularly extralobar sequestration and less commonly cystic adenomatoid malformation and other abnormalities. It has also been reported in association with complex cardiopulmonary malformations. Alternate names in the literature include adenorhabdomyoma, hemangiorhabdomyoma, rhabdomyomatoid dysplasia, and diffuse heteroplasia of striated muscle.

Histologic Features:

- Rhabdomyomatous dysplasia consists of a diffuse interstitial infiltrate of striated muscle, usually in the setting of maldeveloped lung.
- Glial tissue in the lung may be seen in airways or alveoli of fetus with anencephaly.
- Adrenal tissue may present with adrenal cytomegaly.

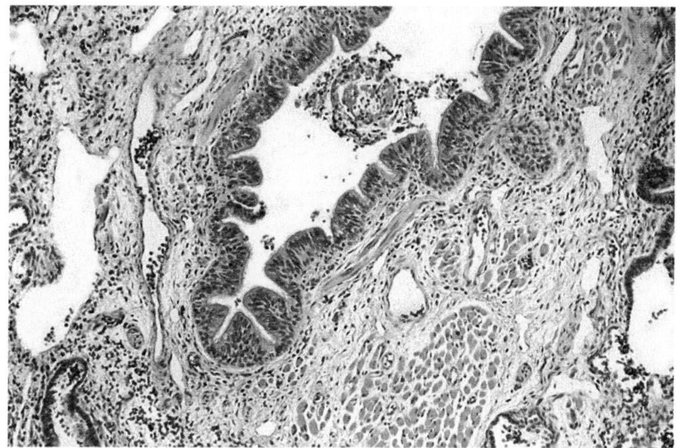

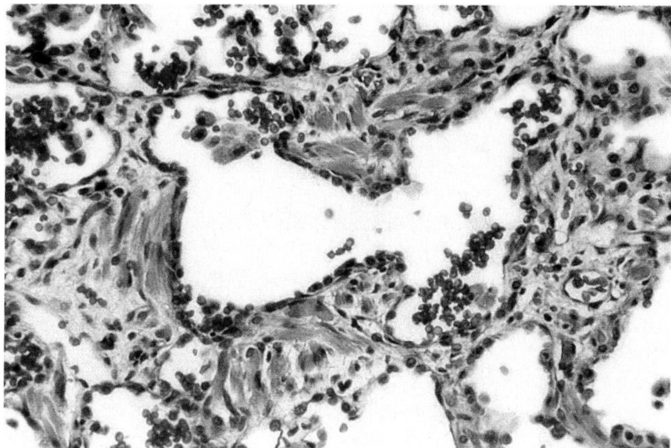

Figure 142.1 Rhabdomyomatous dysplasia. Foci of skeletal muscle are seen in this abnormally developed lung from an infant with scimitar syndrome.

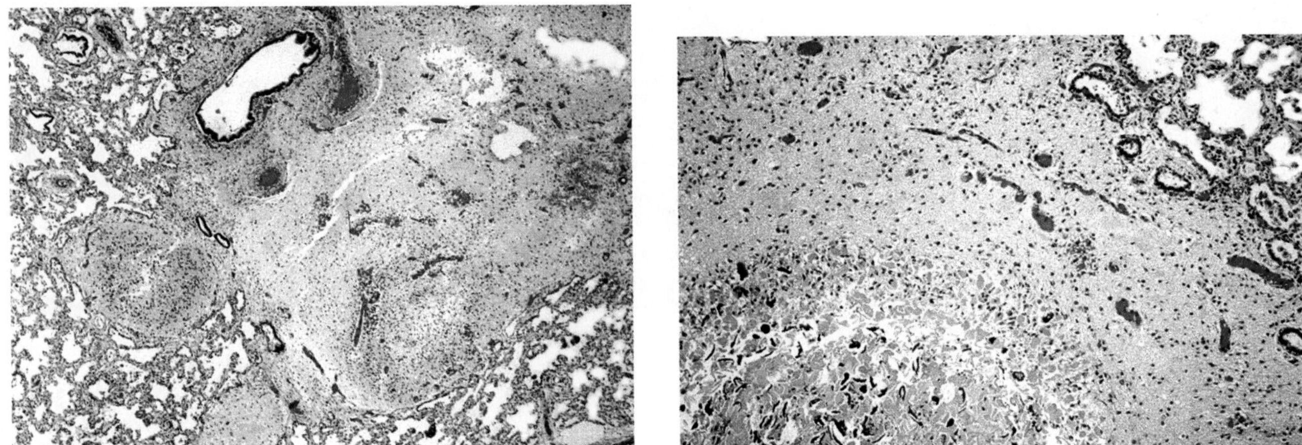

Figure 142.2 Ectopic glial tissue. This infant showed deposits of glial tissue with vascularization and overgrowth within otherwise normally developed lung parenchyma. The infant's twin died *in utero* and was the presumed source of aspirated brain tissue from within the shared amniotic fluid sac.

Neuroendocrine Hyperplasia of Childhood (Persistent Tachypnea of Infancy)

143

▸ Megan Dishop
▸ Claire Langston

Neuroendocrine hyperplasia of childhood is the pathologic correlate of the clinical syndrome persistent tachypnea of infancy. Persistent tachypnea of infancy occurs in term or near-term infants who, after an initial period of well-being, present with tachypnea, wheezing, chest retractions, exercise intolerance, or decreased oxygen saturation and supplemental oxygen requirement. Chest x-ray film typically shows hyperinflation and interstitial infiltrates. The infants usually remain stable or show gradual improvement in symptoms over a period of months to years.

Microscopically, it has been observed that babies with persistent tachypnea have minimal changes on lung biopsy, except for increased numbers of neuroendocrine cells (or "clear cells") in the mucosa of their airways. Although visible on sections stained with hematoxylin and eosin, the neuroendocrine cells are best demonstrated using immunohistochemistry for bombesin, where they may be seen in the airways in markedly increased numbers and in the parenchyma as prominent clusters ("giant" neuroendocrine bodies). It should be noted that other conditions known to be associated with neuroendocrine cell hyperplasia were absent from the children studied, including bronchopulmonary dysplasia, acute lung injury, extreme altitude, smoke exposure, cystic fibrosis, and sudden infant death syndrome. Although the pathogenesis of persistent tachypnea of infancy remains unproved at this point, neuroendocrine cell hyperplasia may mediate bronchoconstriction in these children.

Histologic Features:

- Mild increase in airway smooth muscle.
- Mild increase in alveolar macrophages.
- Increased numbers of clear cells in bronchiolar epithelium, highlighted using immunohistochemistry for bombesin.

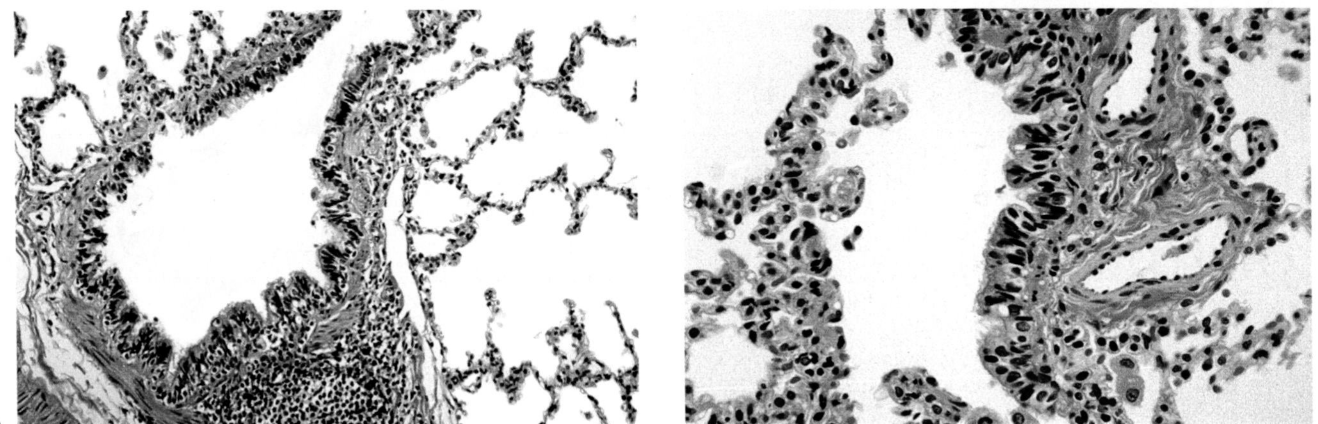

Figure 143.1 Neuroendocrine hyperplasia of childhood. Clear cell hyperplasia of airway epithelium.

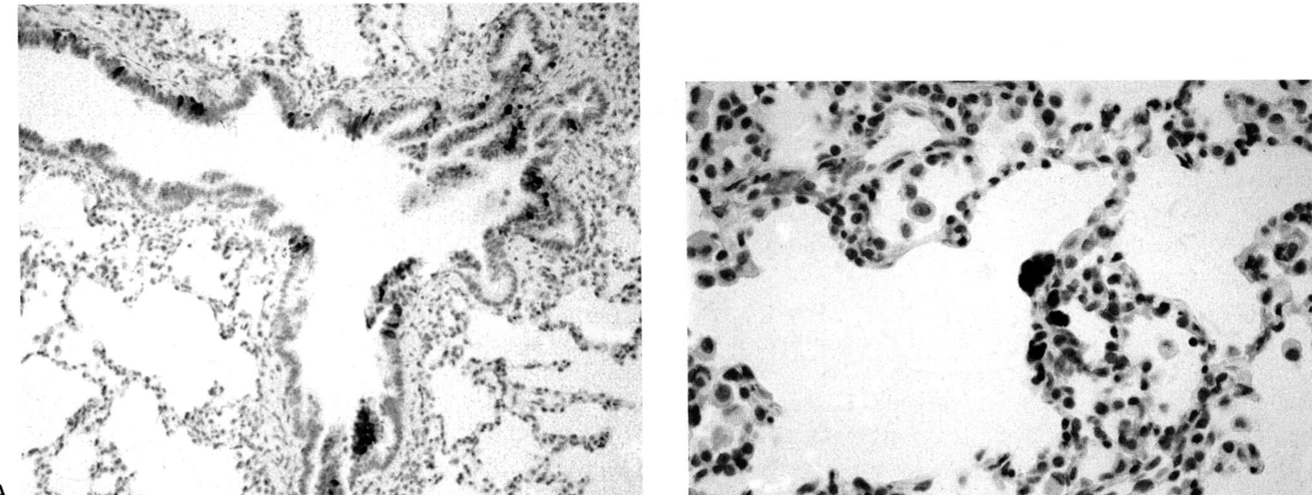

Figure 143.2 Neuroendocrine hyperplasia of childhood. Immunohistochemistry for bombesin highlights increased numbers of neuroendocrine cells in the airways (**A**) and neuroendocrine bodies within the alveolated parenchyma (**B**).

Surfactant Protein B Deficiency and Pulmonary Alveolar Proteinosis

144

▸ Megan Dishop
▸ Claire Langston

Pulmonary alveolar proteinosis, sometimes called *lipoproteinosis,* in infants and young children may be associated with a genetic disorder of surfactant protein B. When pulmonary alveolar proteinosis is seen histologically in an infant, an evaluation for surfactant protein B deficiency should always be done. This can be done on blood, bronchoalveolar lavage (BAL) fluid, or on tissue samples. Surfactant protein B deficiency is an autosomal recessive disorder, so the diagnosis has implications for the family. Currently, the only available treatment is lung transplantation. The histology of pulmonary alveolar proteinosis may also be seen in immunocompromised and immunosuppressed infants and young children both spontaneously and in the setting of infection. In these circumstances, the proteinosis is likely related to macrophage dysfunction, either congenital or acquired.

Most infants with a genetic abnormality leading to surfactant protein B deficiency do not have the classic histologic picture of pulmonary alveolar proteinosis. Rather, they have a variant histology in which there is widening of alveolar walls by mild to moderate uniform alveolar epithelial hyperplasia and mildly increased structural components, without significant inflammatory infiltrate. The airspaces contain mildly increased numbers of macrophages and a variable amount of periodic acid–Schiff (PAS) positive material. The PAS-positive material may be quite scanty, but some should be present and should be extracellular. There is no lobular remodeling, and the vasculature appears normal.

Histologic Features:

Classic Histology

- Pulmonary alveolar proteinosis.

Typical Histology

- Alveolar epithelial hyperplasia.
- Widened alveolar walls without significant inflammation.
- Mild to minimal PAS-positive intraalveolar material.
- No significant remodeling.

Table 144.1. Surfactant Protein B

- Hydrophobic protein with expression confined to the lung.
- Functions in surfactant metabolism include the following:
  - Intracellular packaging.
  - Formation of tubular myelin.
  - Presentation of surfactant/phospholipid monolayer to air-fluid interface.
- Deficiency results in hypoxemic respiratory failure.

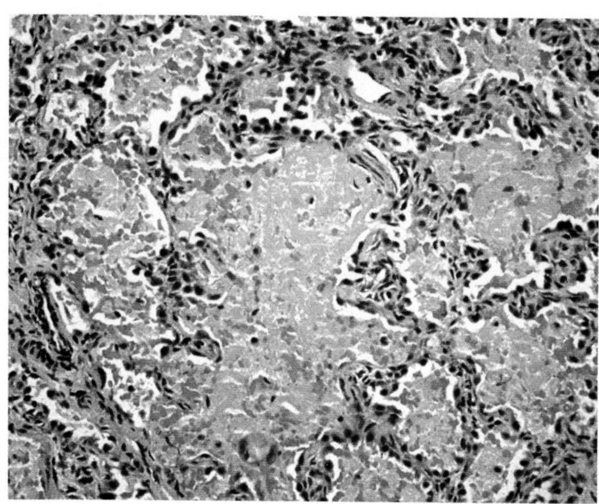

Figure 144.1 Congenital pulmonary alveolar proteinosis. Airspaces are filled with eosinophilic slightly granular acellular material. There is mild alveolar epithelial hyperplasia without interstitial inflammation.

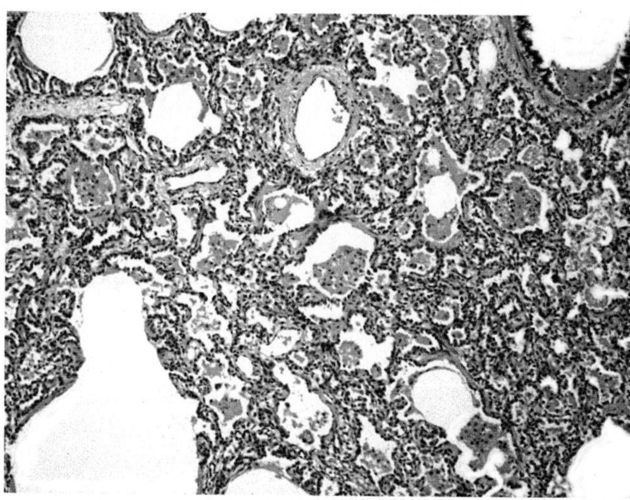

Figure 144.2 Surfactant protein B deficiency, variant histology. There is prominent alveolar epithelial hyperplasia and mild alveolar wall widening without remodeling. Airspaces contain variable amounts of eosinophilic material intermixed with macrophages.

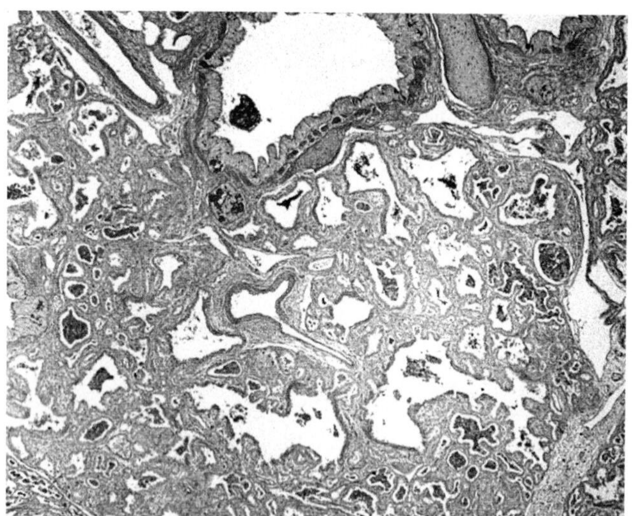

Figure 144.3 PAS stain of surfactant protein B deficiency, variant histology. Relatively small amounts of intraalveolar PAS-positive material is present.

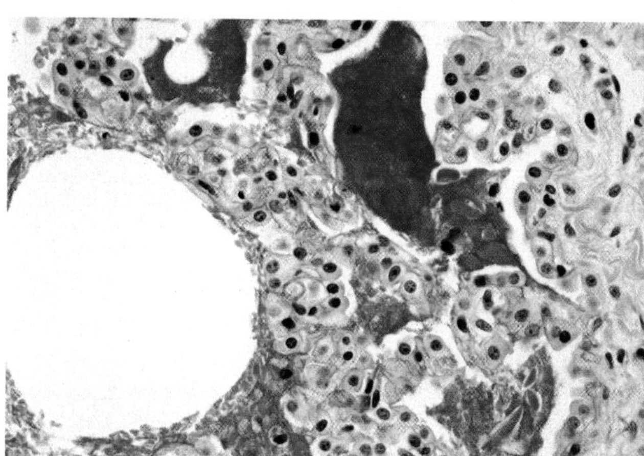

Figure 144.4 Acquired pulmonary alveolar proteinosis. This lung biopsy from a boy with treated acute lymphocytic leukemia in second relapse with active infection shows focal regions of pulmonary alveolar proteinosis with concomitant alveolar epithelial hyperplasia and virtual absence of macrophages. This process is thought to be due to macrophage depletion and dysfunction related to chemotherapy and is seldom of clinical significance.

Surfactant Protein C Deficiency and Chronic Pneumonitis of Infancy

145

▶ Megan Dishop
▶ Claire Langston

Chronic pneumonitis of infancy was described in 1995 by Katzenstein et al. A similar picture in somewhat older children had previously been described by Fischer et al. as a constellation of findings rather than a specific entity. In both reports, the clinical picture was variable and the histologic changes somewhat nonspecific. The affected infants are usually term or near term. They initially are well for weeks to months before they develop cough, respiratory distress, and failure to thrive. The course and outcome of these infants has been highly variable, with some remaining stable but with continued symptomology, and others deteriorating, with several of the infants dying of respiratory disease. Many of the infants had been evaluated and treated for aspiration without improvement in their symptomology.

None of the infants were evaluated for abnormalities of surfactant proteins, but the histologic picture is not that of the typical or variant histology of surfactant protein B (Sp-B) deficiency. However, some infants with identical histologic findings have since been shown to have abnormalities of surfactant protein C with a variety of genetic abnormalities. Additionally, surfactant protein C deficiency has been shown to be associated with chronic lung disease in both children and older individuals and may be associated with many different forms of interstitial lung disease. In infants it has been seen with the histologic picture of chronic pneumonitis of infancy, as well as with a more lipoid pneumonia and cholesterol pneumonialike picture. In older children and adults it has been associated with chronic lung disease with interstitial fibrosis and with chronic lipoid/cholesterol pneumonias without known etiology. These diverse presentations may be related to different genetic abnormalities of the surfactant protein C gene.

Histologic Features:

- Lungs show a very similar picture, with alveolar wall widening by prominent alveolar epithelial hyperplasia and increased structural cells; some have generally mild infiltrates of lymphocytes and plasma cells.
- Macrophages, eosinophilic periodic acid-Schiff (PAS) positive globules, and occasional cholesterol clefts are present within alveolar spaces.

Table 145.1. Surfactant Protein C

- Hydrophobic protein with expression confined to the lung.
- Functionally similar to Sp-B.
- Deficiency results in milder forms of respiratory failure than Sp-B deficiency in infants and familial interstitial lung disease in older children and adults.

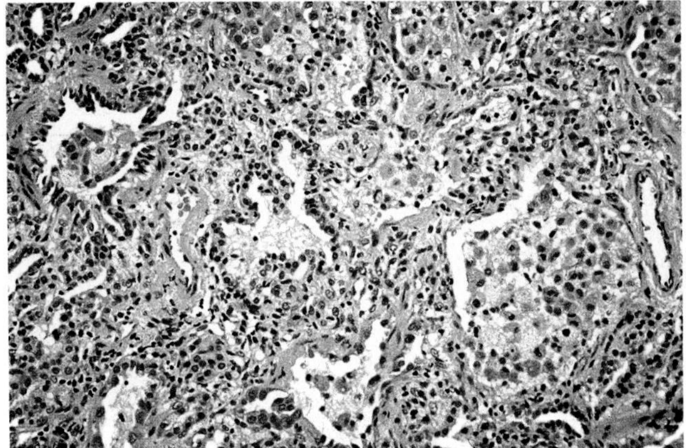

Figure 145.1 Chronic pneumonitis of infancy. Lung parenchyma shows more evidence of remodeling than seen in Sp-B deficiency, including prominent alveolar epithelial hyperplasia with moderate alveolar wall widening by predominantly structural cells and a variably prominent airspace exudate of macrophages, acellular material, hyalin globules, and cholesterol clefts.

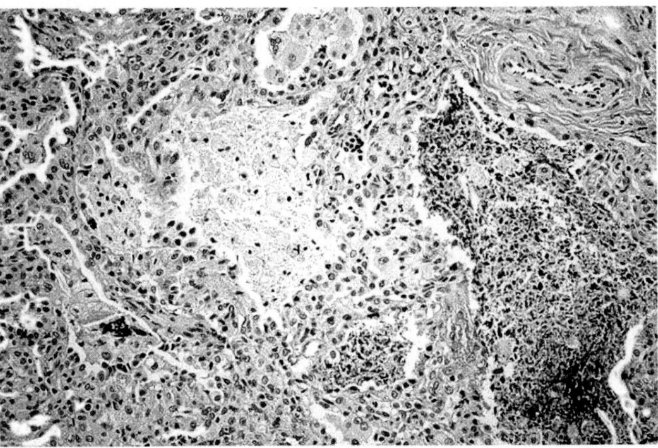

Figure 145.2 Surfactant protein C deficiency presenting in infancy. The histology is identical to that seen in chronic pneumonitis of infancy in this particular case.

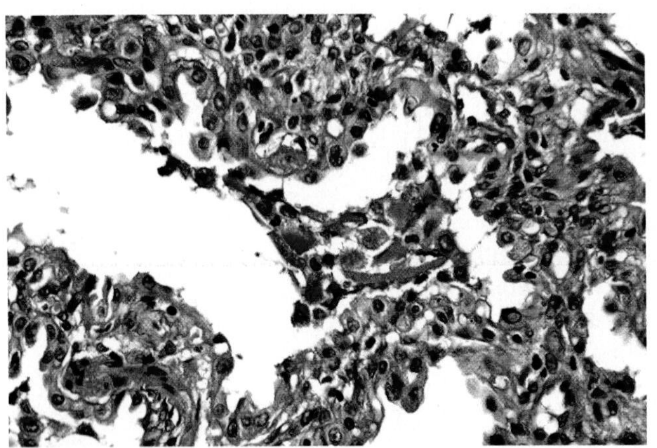

Figure 145.3 PAS stain of surfactant protein C deficiency presenting in infancy. Small amounts of PAS-positive material can be found within airspaces but must be searched for carefully.

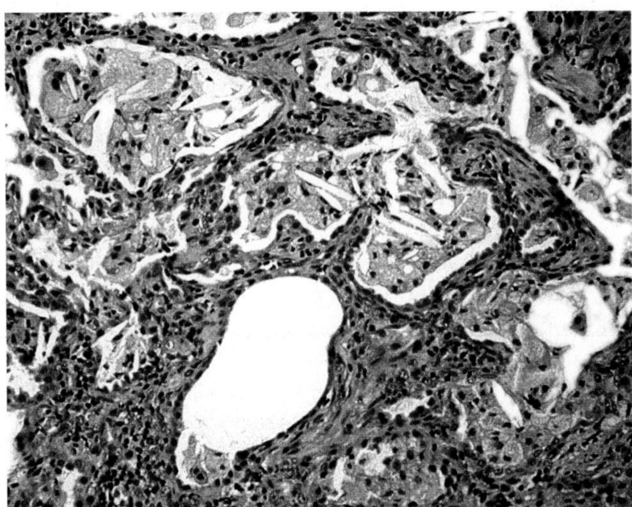

Figure 145.4 Surfactant protein C deficiency presenting in infancy. In some cases cholesterol clefts are quite prominent, both free and within macrophages in airspace.

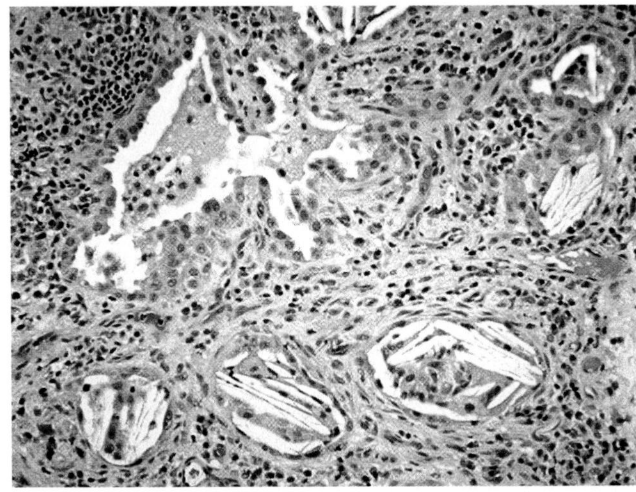

Figure 145.5 Surfactant protein C deficiency presenting in infancy. If biopsied somewhat later, fibrosis and foci of cholesterol pneumonia may be seen.

146

Cystic Fibrosis

▶ Megan Dishop
▶ Claire Langston

Cystic fibrosis is the major cause of severe chronic lung disease in children. It also is the principal reason for lung transplantation in this age group. Cystic fibrosis is an autosomal recessive disorder of exocrine glands caused by homozygous or compound heterozygous mutations in the cystic fibrosis transmembrane conductance regulator *(CFTR)* gene. It results in high viscosity of mucoid secretions with plugging of ducts and organ damage. Although outcome has improved remarkably over the last few decades, pulmonary infection remains the most common cause of morbidity and mortality in these children (median survival is 32 years in the United States).

Chronic lung disease in these patients results from inspissation of mucus in airways, leading to bacterial colonization and chronic bronchocentric infection with bronchiectasis. Common organisms include *Staphylococcus aureus, Haemophilus influenzae, Pseudomonas aeruginosa* (particularly mucigenic strains), and *Burkholderia cepacia.* Fungal organisms, especially *Candida* and *Aspergillus* species, also infect approximately 20% of cystic fibrosis patients, and allergic bronchopulmonary aspergillosis is a feature in approximately 10%. Other life-threatening pulmonary complications include pneumothorax, massive hemoptysis, and cor pulmonale.

Pathologically, the lungs are characterized by mucus plugs beginning in infancy, followed by progressive infection, inflammation, and mucosal necrosis of the airways, resulting in severe bronchiectasis, which is the hallmark of cystic fibrosis. The areas of bronchiectasis are often most accentuated in the upper lobes and may extend nearly to the pleural surface, where they terminate in fibrous-walled cavities (bronchiectatic cysts). Grossly, the central airways contain thick tenacious yellow mucus, and there are often areas of surrounding parenchymal consolidation. Microscopically, the central airways contain adherent mucus material admixed with inflammatory cells and debris and may show squamous metaplasia or increased numbers of goblet cells. Characteristically, the submucosal glands show areas of hyperplasia associated with mucus-filled ducts alternating with areas of glandular atrophy. The mucosa of ectatic airways is frequently ulcerated and replaced by granulation tissue with a surrounding dense lymphoplasmacytic inflammatory infiltrate. Small airways are also affected, showing bronchiolar stenosis or obliteration. Hyperinflation and patchy bronchopneumonia are common parenchymal features.

Histologic Features:

- Bronchiectasis and mucus plugging.
- Dense eosinophilic secretions admixed with acute inflammation and debris.
- Bacterial colonization.
- Fungal organisms or allergic bronchopulmonary aspergillosis may be present.
- Mucosal ulceration and granulation tissue.
- Chronic bronchitis and bronchiolitis.

- Lymphoplasmacytic infiltrate.
- Submucosal gland hyperplasia alternating with atrophy.
- Small airway stenosis/obliteration.
- Patchy bronchopneumonia (variable).

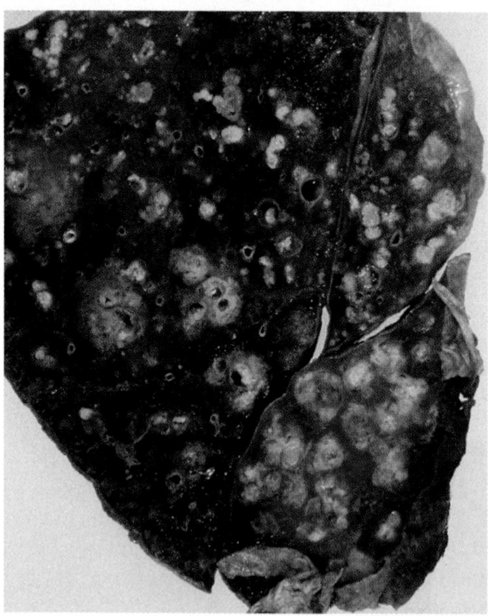

Figure 146.1 Gross figure of end-stage cystic fibrosis lung.

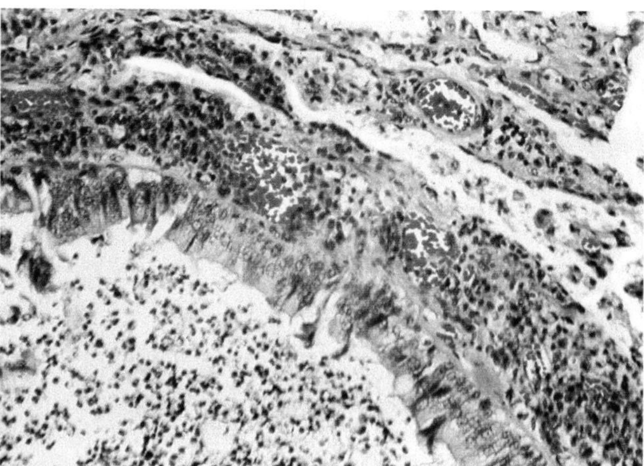

Figure 146.2 Cystic fibrosis showing a large bronchus containing mucus and acute inflammatory debris.

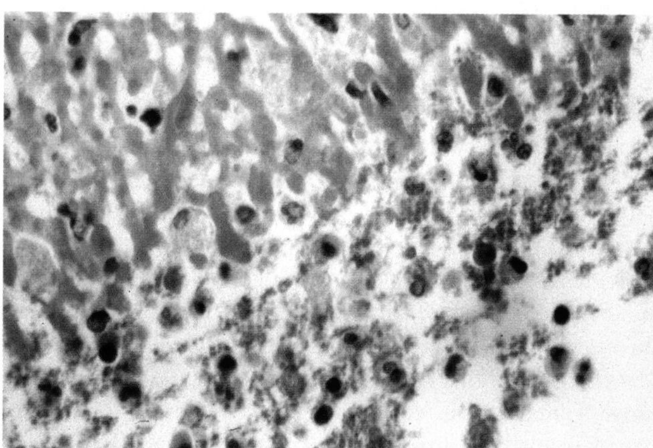

Figure 146.3 Cystic fibrosis with dense eosinophilic mucus and bacterial colonies within a large airway.

Alveolar Capillary Dysplasia with Misalignment of Pulmonary Veins

147

▶ Megan Dishop
▶ Claire Langston

Alveolar capillary dysplasia with misalignment of pulmonary veins is an increasingly recognized cause of persistent pulmonary hypertension in the newborn. Although initially seen only at autopsy, there are now many examples of lung biopsy in young infants in whom this developmental abnormality has been recognized. Affected infants are usually term or near term, and they present with persistent pulmonary hypertension in the first few postnatal days. Although they may initially respond to therapeutic measures, a sustained response is never achieved and most die before they are 1 month old. There are many exceptions, however, with later presentations and longer survival, but all eventually succumb to pulmonary hypertension or its complications. There have been a number of familial cases with affected sibling pairs, indicating that, at least in some families, this condition is likely to be autosomal recessive in nature. Many affected infants have abnormalities of other organ systems, predominantly the heart and gastrointestinal and genitourinary tracts. Several limb abnormalities have also been described. No consistent pattern of associated malformation has been identified. The genetic abnormality of this unusual condition has yet to be identified. This uniformly lethal condition may be amenable to treatment by lung transplantation, but none has been reported.

Although it has been suggested that alveolar capillary dysplasia can occur without misalignment of pulmonary veins, such cases more likely represent other conditions modified by prolonged supportive measures and not this developmental abnormality.

Histologic Features:

- Grossly, the lung usually appears deeply congested; lung weight is normal to increased.
- The lung shows striking abnormalities of the vascular and lobular architecture.
- There is striking muscularization of small pulmonary arteries both adjacent to airways and in the lobular parenchyma.
- The abnormally muscularized arteries in both of these locations are accompanied by dilated veins and venules.
- The veins are often markedly congested as well as dilated.
- There is a striking reduction in the alveolar capillary bed and a reduction in smaller veins in interlobular septa.
- Larger veins are usually normally positioned.
- Lobular architecture is abnormal, but the changes in the lobule are somewhat more variable from case to case and occasionally within the same lung.
- Changes include a simplified appearance with a reduced radial alveolar count, moderate alveolar epithelial hyperplasia, widened alveolar walls with absent capillaries, and centrally placed, often dilated, sinusoidal channels.
- About one third of cases have associated pulmonary lymphangiectasia.

Table 147.1. Clinical and Histologic Features of Alveolar Capillary Dysplasia with Misalignment of Pulmonary Veins

Clinical Features	Histologic Features
■ Term or near-term neonate. ■ Respiratory failure at early, but variable, postnatal age. ■ Elevated pulmonary artery pressure. ■ No sustained response to therapy. ■ Half of affected infants have other, usually minor, anomalies.	■ Malpositioned pulmonary vein branches. ■ Markedly increased medial smooth muscle in small pulmonary arteries. ■ Extreme muscularization of lobular arterioles. ■ Deficient alveolar development, variable. ■ Deficient capillary development. ■ Pulmonary lymphangiectasis is one third of cases.

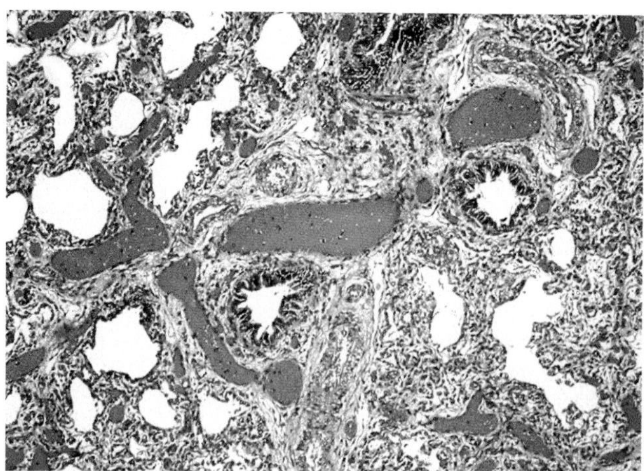

Figure 147.1 Alveolar capillary dysplasia. Excessively muscularized small pulmonary arteries and markedly dilated and congested veins are present adjacent to membranous bronchioles and extend together into the lobular parenchyma.

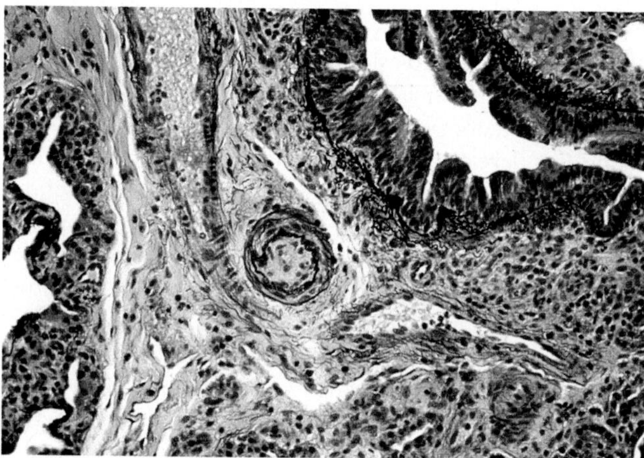

Figure 147.2 Movat stain showing a small pulmonary artery with a markedly thickened wall and a pinpoint lumen sharing the same connective tissue sheath with a dilated and congested vein. Both are adjacent to a membranous bronchiole.

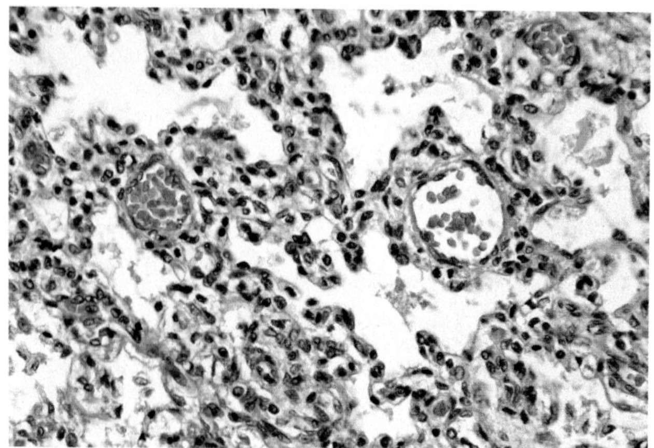

Figure 147.3 Lobular maldevelopment with widened alveolar walls, alveolar epithelial hyperplasia, deficient capillaries, and centrally located sinusoidal channels.

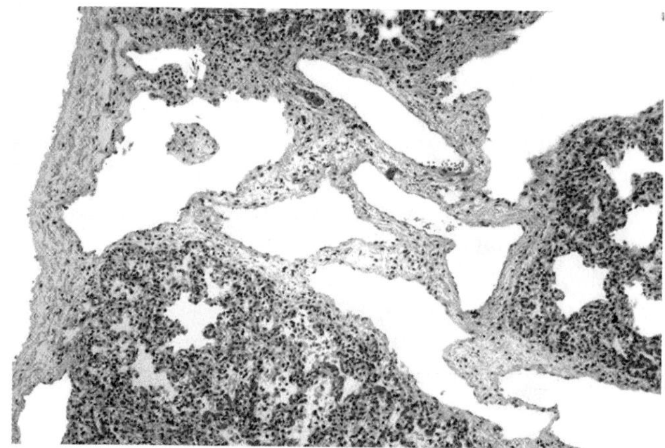

Figure 147.4 Pulmonary lymphangiectasia associated with alveolar capillary dysplasia with misalignment of pulmonary veins.

Acinar Dysgenesis/Aplasia

148

▶ Megan Dishop
▶ Claire Langston

This condition is an exceedingly rare but quite striking form of pulmonary maldevelopment with arrest of lung development at an immature stage that varies from case to case. Almost all affected infants have been female. They are born at or near term and usually appear to be normally developed. They develop respiratory distress rapidly after birth and die within a few hours because they cannot be adequately oxygenated or ventilated. At autopsy, the lungs are usually somewhat small, about 50% of predicted volume and weight. Sometimes other minor abnormalities are found at autopsy. Two familial cases have been described.

The pathogenesis of this developmental abnormality is unknown, but an abnormality in epithelial/mesenchymal interaction has been postulated. Whether the cases with somewhat later developmental arrest have a similar pathogenesis is unclear. Some of these infants have a somewhat longer course, but they usually die of respiratory failure within 1 month. It can be difficult to separate these cases from those with acquired abnormalities related to prolonged and extensive therapeutic support.

Histologic Features:

- Lung development is strikingly abnormal, with abundant loose mesenchyme in which sometimes only airways are present; this suggests developmental arrest at the pseudoglandular stage, the period in which all airways are formed.
- The airway structures (bronchi and bronchioles) have continued to mature across the rest of gestation and usually show normal cytodifferentiation without evidence of airspace development.
- Some infants show arrest of lung development at somewhat later stages (late canalicular or early saccular), again with cytodifferentiation of the structures formed.
- Airway smooth muscle can be identified by immunohistochemistry in abundance in quite peripheral locations.
- Many have ectopic cartilage formation with nodules of cartilage in the pleura and not associated with airways.

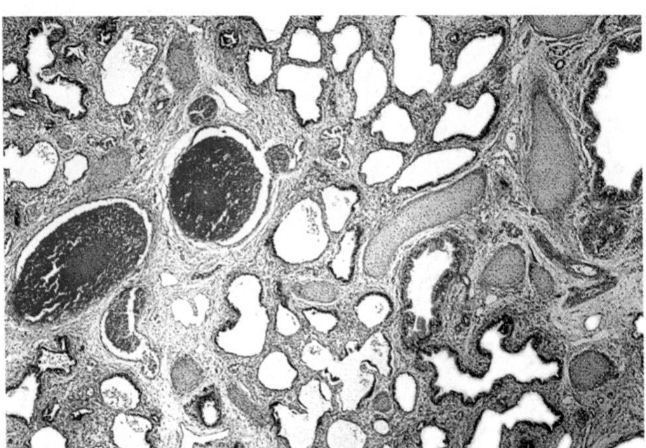

Figure 148.1 Overview of the lung parenchyma in acinar dysplasia showing multiple, apparently well-developed bronchi with abundant cartilage. Cartilage not associated with these bronchi is also evident. There is no evidence of alveolar development. Large dilated spaces with a variable lining are present between well-formed bronchi.

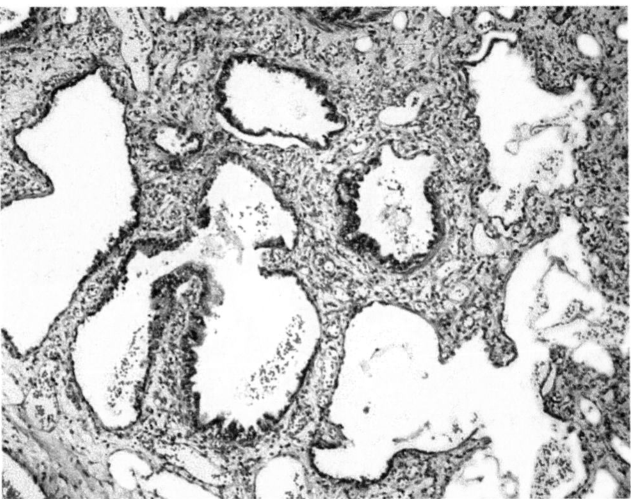

Figure 148.2 The dilated intervening spaces are variably lined by ciliated respiratory epithelium, bronchiolar-type epithelium, or low cuboidal epithelium. The intervening tissue is abundant loose mesenchyme.

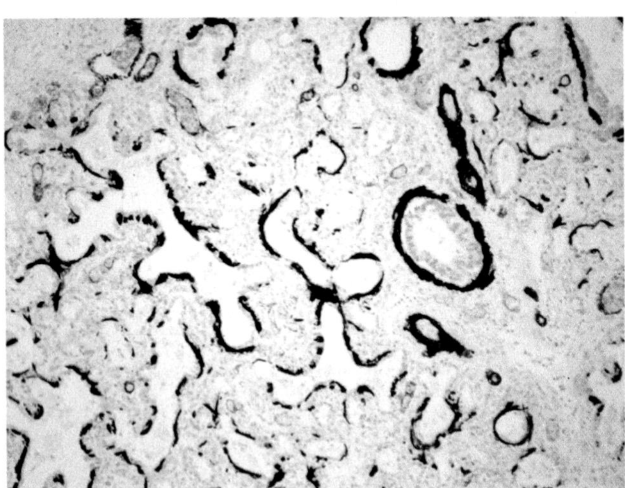

Figure 148.3 Immunostain for smooth muscle actin showing abundant smooth muscle present around bronchioles and in the walls of normally placed arteries and extending around the other dilated structures, which show predominantly airway differentiation even at the periphery of the lung and adjacent to interlobular septa.

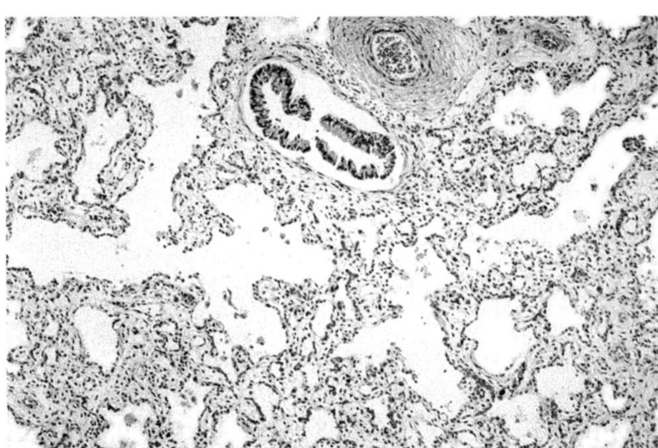

Figure 148.4 Arrested development at the early saccular stage. The airways appear normal, but lobular parenchyma shows no evidence of alveolar development; only simple saccular spaces with thick walls of loose mesenchyme are seen.

149

Pleuropulmonary Blastoma

▶ Megan Dishop
▶ Claire Langston

Pleuropulmonary blastoma, a relatively recently recognized childhood malignancy, is an embryonal tumor of the lung, pleura, or mediastinum derived from the thoracic splanchnopleural or somatopleural mesoderm. Although uncommon (both benign and malignant primary lung tumors are rare in childhood), pleuropulmonary blastoma is actually one of the more common primary lung tumors of childhood. It usually presents in infancy or early childhood, generally before age 3 and almost always before age 12 (as with other embryonal tumors, rare cases have been reported in adults), as a cystic or solid peripheral pulmonary mass. In some children there are multiple or bilateral cystic lesions.

Pleuropulmonary blastoma has a spectrum of differentiation, ranging from low-grade cystic (type I), to partially cystic (type II), to solid tumors (type III). It is separated from adult pulmonary blastoma (which may also rarely occur in childhood) by the exclusively stromal nature of the malignant component in pleuropulmonary blastoma. This malignant component may be present as blastemal tissue or mesenchymal sarcomatous changes.

Grossly, the low-grade cystic lesions often protrude from the pleura surface and are largely covered by pleura. They have often been simply amputated at surgery with only a small pedicle of the underlying lobe attached under the mistaken impression that they are benign developmental cystic lesions. They are exclusively cystic, without any solid regions or nodules. The intermediate or partially cystic lesions are a mixture of cystic and solid components. The high-grade lesions are solid tumors with occasional foci of cystic degeneration related to hemorrhage and necrosis.

The low-grade cystic lesions may be cured by surgery alone but should be followed closely because there have been local recurrences in this setting. Higher-grade lesions require chemotherapy following surgery. Local recurrence or metastases are seen in about half of cases, with local recurrence being more common. Metastases occur late in the disease course and are more common in the brain and bone, although other sites have rarely been described. In recurrence the lesion may be of a higher grade than the initial lesion. Low-grade cystic lesions that are incompletely excised or are followed over an extended period of time without surgical excision may become higher-grade lesions.

It is important to differentiate the low-grade lesions both grossly and histologically from the large cyst type of cystic adenomatoid malformation. Grossly, the low-grade lesions usually present as cystic lesions extending beyond the pleural surface, a quite unusual presentation for cystic adenomatoid malformation, which generally remains within the lobar confines. The low-grade cystic lesions largely account for the multiple reports of sarcomas arising in cystic adenomatoid malformations. Low-grade cystic pleuropulmonary blastoma has been confused with large cyst type cystic adenomatoid malformation, particularly when the stromal malignant component is relatively minor. Review of these reports when relevant histology is available shows the typical histologic appearance of low-grade cystic pleuropulmonary blastoma. The trabeculae in low-grade cystic pleuropulmonary blastoma have a quite different appearance from those seen in large cyst type cystic adenomatoid malformation, being thicker and often having distinctive larger vessels present centrally. The higher-grade lesions have been diagnosed previously as rhabdomyosarcoma. It is likely that most, if not all, rhabdomyosarcoma primary to the lung is the solid variant of pleuropulmonary blastoma. The lesion known as *mesenchymal hamartoma of the lung* likely also belongs in the spectrum of pleuropulmonary blastoma.

Cytogenetic analysis of some pleuropulmonary blastomas has shown a variety of abnormalities, including trisomy 8, trisomy 2, and 17p deletions, as well as frequent occurrence of p53 mutations. Pleuropulmonary blastoma is associated with other embryonal tumors; cystic renal disease, both concurrently and preceding or following the development of pleuropulmonary blastoma in the patient and in other family members; and certain adult tumors.

Histologic Features:

- Low-grade pleuropulmonary blastoma is a cystic lesion with multiple trabeculae composed of poorly cellular mesenchymal tissue and blood vessels, covered by essentially normal alveolar or bronchiolar epithelium.
- Variable amounts of the malignant stromal component can be seen within the trabeculae and may form a "cambium" layer, similar to that seen in botryoid type rhabdomyosarcomas.
- Other mesenchymal elements, usually immature cartilage or rhabdomyoblasts, may be present.
- In low-grade lesions, this malignant mesenchymal tissue may be a quite minor component and should be sought for in multiple sections of cystic lesions with otherwise typical histology.
- High-grade solid pleuropulmonary blastomas contain sheets of malignant mesenchymal cells, sometimes blastemal and sometimes spindled, often with evidence of rhabdomyoblastic differentiation both ultrastructurally and immunohistochemically.
- Between these two ends of the spectrum are partially cystic lesions with features of both low- and high-grade types.

Table 149.1. Pleuropulmonary Blastoma Versus Pulmonary Blastoma

Features	Pleuropulmonary Blastoma	Pulmonary Blastoma
Age at diagnosis (years)	3	43
Gender (male:female)	1:1	2.5:1
Tobacco use	None	Frequent
Origin	Peripheral lung, parietal pleura, mediastinum	Lung, intrabronchial
Neoplastic component	Blastema/ mesenchyme	Epithelium, blastema/ mesenchyme
Tumor pattern	Rhabdomyosarcoma, undifferentiated sarcoma, other sarcomas	Carcinosarcoma, fetal adenocarcinoma
Familial dysplasia/ neoplasia	25%	0%

Table 149.2. Immunohistochemistry of Pleuropulmonary Blastoma

Rhabdomyoblasts	Vimentin, desmin, muscle-specific actin, smooth muscle actin, myogenin, myoglobin
Blastemal cells	Vimentin
Mesenchymal/ spindle cells	Vimentin, muscle-specific actin
Cartilage	S-100 protein
Histiocytoid and bizarre giant cells	α_1-antitrypsin, α_1-antichymotrypsin, lysozyme, CD68
Epithelium (cyst lining or entrapped)	Cytokeratin, epithelial membrane antigen

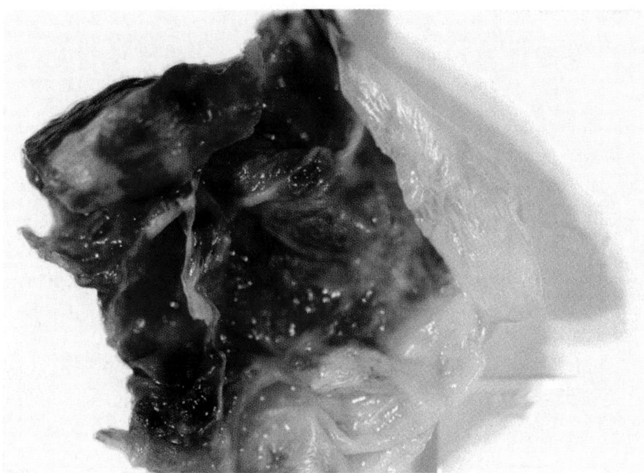

Figure 149.1 Gross figure of low-grade cystic pleuropulmonary blastoma showing multilocular cystic appearance, delicate trabeculae, and thickened overlying pleura.

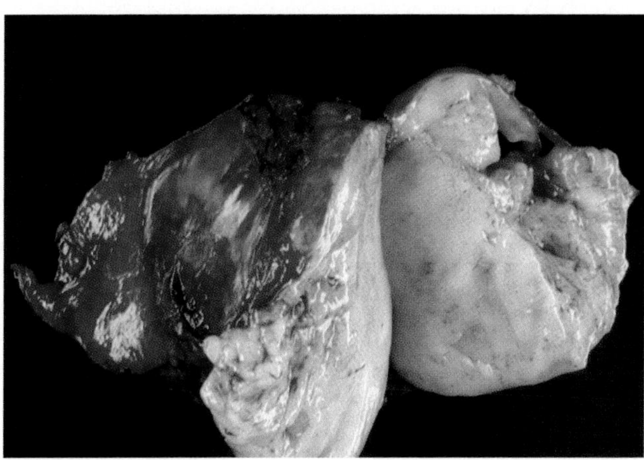

Figure 149.2 Gross figure of a partially cystic pleuropulmonary blastoma showing prominent solid regions with a sarcomatous appearance, as well as multiple nodular regions in the cystic component.

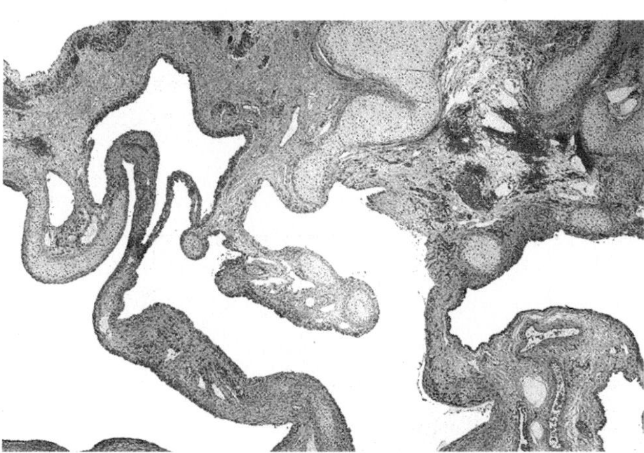

Figure 149.3 Low-grade cystic pleuropulmonary blastoma with multiple wide septa, abundant cartilaginous nodules, and peculiar large vessels.

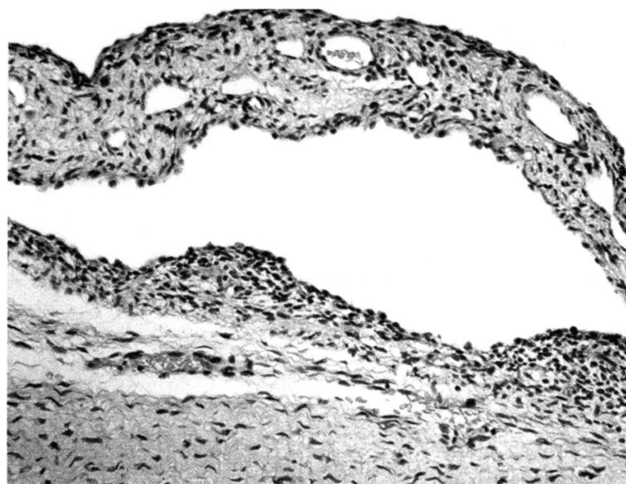

Figure 149.4 Low-grade cystic pleuropulmonary blastoma with cambiumlike layer of undifferentiated blastemal cells beneath the prominent cuboidal alveolar epithelium.

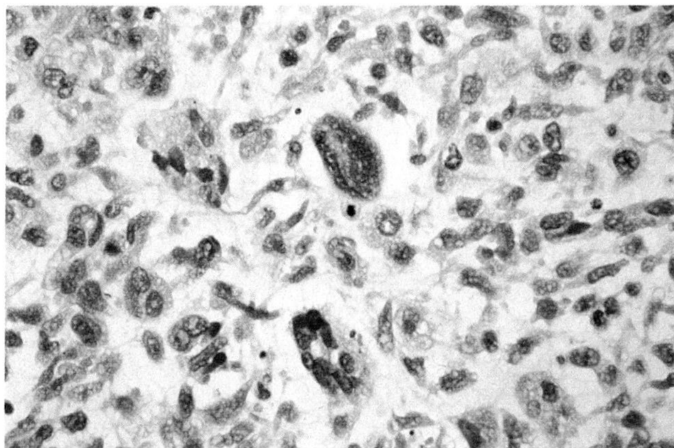

Figure 149.5 Partially cystic pleuropulmonary blastoma with loose undifferentiated mesenchyma tissue containing bizarre giant cells.

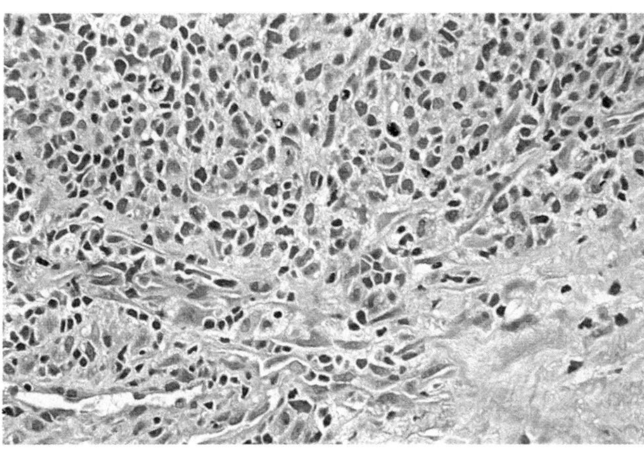

Figure 149.6 Solid pleuropulmonary blastoma with rhabdomyosarcoma-like features.

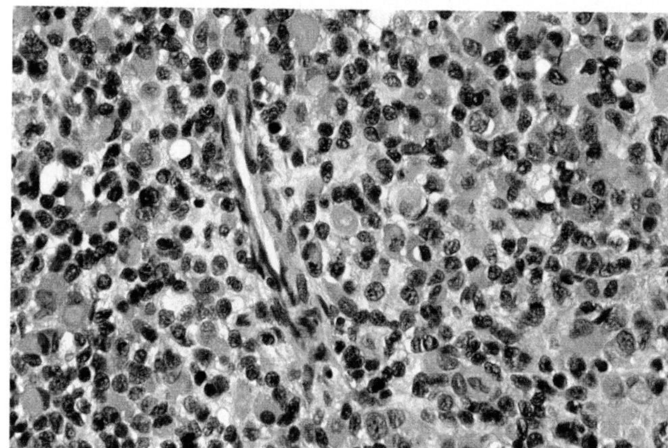

Figure 149.7 Solid pleuropulmonary blastoma post chemotherapy with prominent rhabdomyoblastic differentiation.

Pulmonary Leiomyoma and Leiomyosarcoma in Childhood

150

▶ Megan Dishop
▶ Claire Langston

Smooth muscle tumors—leiomyoma and leiomyosarcoma—are exceedingly rare in children at all sites. They have become somewhat more common recently because of the increasing number of children with human immunodeficiency virus (HIV), solid organ transplantation, and prolonged survival of children with certain forms of congenital immune compromise. Such children are at risk for development of Epstein-Barr virus (EBV)-associated smooth muscle tumors, predominantly of the gastrointestinal and respiratory tracts.

Histologic Features:

- These tumors have typical features of smooth muscle tumors, being circumscribed with pushing borders and rounded outlines.
- They are composed of spindled cells and may vary somewhat in cellularity; both clearly benign and malignant lesions may occur.
- Probes to EBV DNA within the tumor show striking positivity within virtually every smooth muscle cell.
- The EBV present in these tumors has been shown to be clonal, suggesting that the virus plays a role in the development of these lesions.

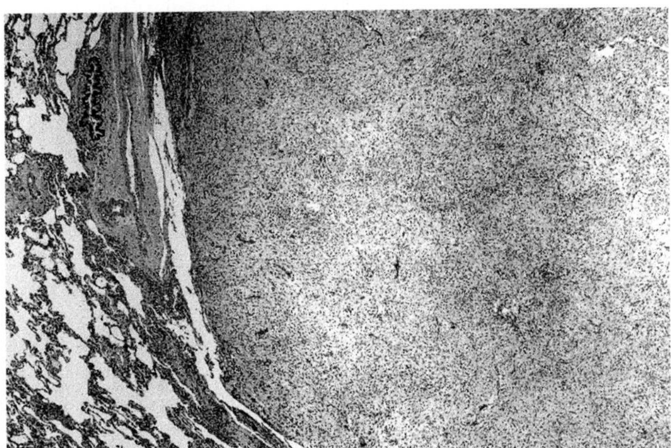

Figure 150.1 Circumscribed pulmonary leiomyoma with pushing borders from a girl 3 years post orthotopic liver transplant.

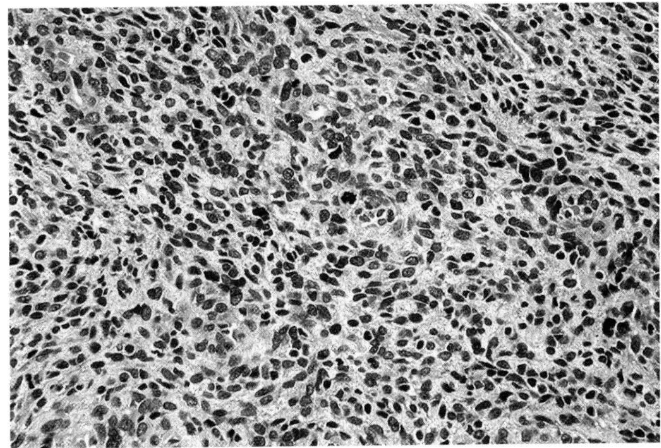

Figure 150.2 Cellular region of a pulmonary leiomyoma with increased mitoses.

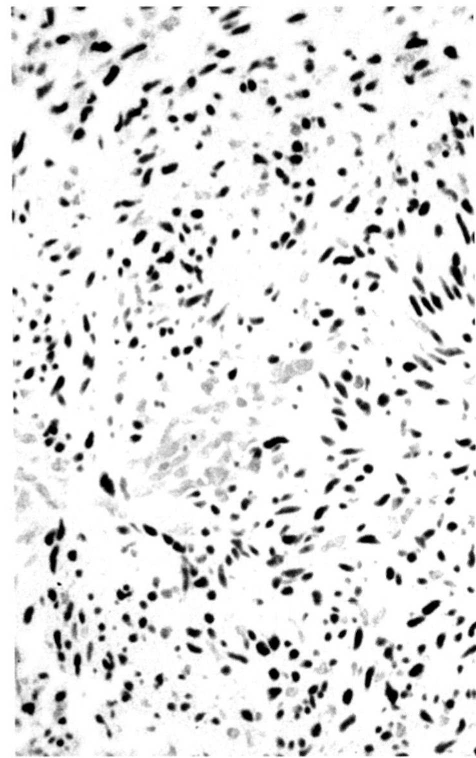

Figure 150.3 Epstein-Barr virus encoded RNA (EBER) *in situ* hybridization showing pulmonary leiomyoma with spindle cells that are all EBV positive by *in situ* hybridization. The vasculature is EBV negative.

Bibliography

Section 1: Normal Cytology and Histology

Colby TV, Yousem SA. Lungs. In: Sternberg SS, ed. *Histology for Pathologists,* 2nd ed. Philadelphia: Lippincott Williams & Wilkins, 1997:433–435.

Gartner LP, Hiatt JL, eds. *Color Atlas of Histology,* 3rd ed. Philadelphia: Lippincott Williams & Wilkins, 2000.

Junqueira LC, Carneiro J, Kelley RO, eds. *Basic Histology,* 9th ed. New York: McGraw-Hill, 1998.

Kuhn C III. Normal anatomy and histology. In: Thurlbeck WM, Churg A, eds. *Pathology of the Lung,* 2nd ed. New York: Thieme, 1995:4–10.

Silverman JF, Atkinson BF. Respiratory cytology. In: Atkinson B, ed. *Atlas of Diagnostic Cytopathology.* Philadelphia: WB Saunders, 1992:137–193.

Wang NS. Anatomy. In: Dail DH, Hammar SP, eds. *Pulmonary Pathology,* 2nd ed. New York: Springer-Verlag, 1994:21–44.

Section 2: Artifacts and Age-Related Changes

Anton R, Cagle PT. Intracellular and extracellular structures. In: Cagle PT, ed. *Diagnostic Pulmonary Pathology.* New York: Marcel Dekker, 2000:501–523.

Cagle PT. Endobronchial and transbronchial biopsies. In: Cagle PT, ed. *Diagnostic Pulmonary Pathology.* New York: Marcel Dekker, 2000:11–18.

Section 3: Malignant Neoplasms

Aguayo SM, Miller YE, Waldron JA Jr, et al. Brief report: idiopathic diffuse hyperplasia of pulmonary neuroendocrine cells and airways disease. *N Engl J Med* 1992;327:1285–1288.

Allen TC, US–Canadian Mesothelioma Reference Panel. Localized malignant mesothelioma. 2004 *(in press).*

Anton R, Schwartz MR, Kessler M, Cagle PT. Metastatic carcinoma of the prostate mimicking primary carcinoid tumor of the lung and mediastinum. *Pathol Res Pract* 1998;194(11):753–758.

Attanoos RL, Appleton MAC, Gibbs AR. Primary sarcomas of the lung: a clinicopathologic and immunohistochemical study of cases. *Histopathology* 1996;29:29–36.

Attanoos RL, Galateau-Salle F, Gibbs AR, et al. Primary thymic epithelial tumours of the pleura mimicking malignant mesothelioma. *Histopathology* 2002;41:42–49.

Bagwell SP, Flynn SD, Cox PM, et al. Primary malignant melanoma of the lung. *Am Rev Respir Dis* 1989;139:1543–1547.

Banks PM, Warnke RA. Primary effusion lymphoma. In: Jaffe ES, Harris NL, Stein H, Vardiman JW eds. *Pathology and Genetics of Tumours of Haematopoietic and Lymphoid Tissues.* Lyon: IARC Press, 2001:179–180.

Beasley MB, Thunissen FB, Brambilla E, et al. Pulmonary atypical carcinoid: predictors of survival in 106 cases. *Hum Pathol* 2000;31(10):1255–1265.

Bertoni F, Bacchini P, Hogendoorn PCW. Chondrosarcoma. In: Fletcher DM, Unni KK, Mertens F, eds. *World Health Organization Classification of Tumours. Pathology and Genetics of Tumours of Soft Tissue and Bone.* Lyon: IARC Press, 2002:247–251.

Bini A, Ansaloni L, Grani G, et al. Pulmonary blastoma: report of two cases. *Surg Today* 2001;31:438–442.

Bodner SM, Koss MN. Mutations in the p53 gene in pulmonary blastomas: immunohistochemical and molecular studies. *Hum Pathol* 1996;27:1117–1123.

Boroumand N, Raja V, Jones D, et al. SYT-SSX2 variant of primary pulmonary synovial sarcoma with focal expression of CD117 (c-Kit) protein and a poor clinical outcome. *Arch Pathol Lab Med* 2003;127(4):e210–e204.

Brambilla E, Moro D, Veale D, et al. Basal cell (basaloid) carcinoma of the lung: a new morphologic and phenotype entity with separate prognostic significance. *Hum Pathol* 1992;9:993–1003.

Brown RW, Campagna LB, Dunn JK, Cagle PT. Immunohistochemical identification of tumor markers in metastatic adenocarcinoma: a diagnostic adjunct in the determination of primary site. *Am J Clin Pathol* 1997;107:12–19.

Butnor K, Sporn T, Hammar S, Roggli V. Well-differentiated papillary mesothelioma. *Am J Surg Pathol* 2001;25:1304–1309.

Cagle PT. Bronchogenic carcinoma. In: Churg AM, ed. *Pathology of the Lung,* 3rd ed. New York: Thieme Medical Publishers, 2004 *(in preparation).*

Cagle PT. Tumors of the lung (excluding lymphoid tumors): uncommon tumors of the lung. In: Thurlbeck WM, Churg A, eds. *Pathology of the Lung,* 2nd ed. New York: Thieme Medical Publishers, 1995:523–526.

Cagle PT. Differential diagnosis between primary and metastatic carcinomas. In: Brambilla C, Brambilla E, eds. *Lung Tumors: Fundamental Biology and Clinical Management.* New York: Marcel Dekker, 1999:127–137.

Cagle PT. Pleural histology. In: Light RW, Lee YCG, eds. *Pleural Disease: An International Textbook.* London: Arnold, 2003:249–255.

Cagle PT, Fraire AE, Greenberg SD, et al. Potential utility of p53 immunopositivity in differentiation of adenocarcinomas from reactive epithelial atypias of the lung. *Hum Pathol* 1996; 27:1198–1203.

Cagle PT, Mace ML, Judge DM, et al. Pulmonary melanoma primary vs. metastatic. *Chest* 1984; 85:125–126.

Catalan RL, Murphy T. Primary primitive neuroectodermal tumor of the lung. *AJR Am J Roentgenol* 1997;169:1201–1202.

Churg AM. Diseases of the pleura. In: Thurlbeck WM, Churg AM, eds. *Pathology of the Lung,* 2nd ed. New York: Thieme, 1995:1067–1110.

Churg A. Localized pleural tumors. In: Cagle PT, ed. *Diagnostic Pulmonary Pathology.* New York: Marcel Dekker, 2000:719–734.

Churg AM, Cagle PT, Roggli V. Tumors of the serosal membranes. In: *Atlas of Tumor Pathology, 4th series, Fascicle X.* Washington, DC: Armed Forces Institute of Pathology, 2004 *(in press).*

Churg A, Colby TV, Cagle PT, et al. US–Canadian Mesothelioma Reference Panel. The separation of benign and malignant mesothelial proliferations. *Am J Surg Pathol* 2000;24:1183–1200.

Colby TV, Koss MN, Travis WD. Miscellaneous mesenchymal tumors. In: *Tumors of the Lower Respiratory Tract.* Washington, DC: Armed Forces Institute of Pathology, 1994:348–353.

Colby TV, Koss MN, Travis WD. Lymphoreticular disorders. In: *Tumors of the lower respiratory tract. Atlas of Tumor Pathology, series III.* Washington, DC: Armed Forces Institute of Pathology, 1995:422–431.

Corrin B. Pleura and chest wall. In: Corrin B, ed. *Pathology of the Lungs.* London: Churchill Livingstone, 2000:607–642.

Crotty TB, Myers JL, Katzenstein A, et al. Localized malignant mesothelioma. *Am J Surg Pathol* 1994;18:357–363.

Dail DH. Uncommon tumors. In: Dail DH, Hammar SP, eds. *Pulmonary Pathology,* 2nd ed. New York: Springer-Verlag, 1994:1279–1462.

Dail DH. Metastases to and from the lung. In: Dail DH, Hammar SP, eds. *Pulmonary Pathology, 2nd* ed. New York: Springer-Verlag, 1994:1581–1616.

Evans HL, Shipley J. Leiomyosarcoma. In: Fletcher DM, Unni KK, Mertens F, eds. *World Health Organization Classification of Tumours. Pathology and Genetics of Tumours of Soft Tissue and Bone.* Lyon: IARC Press, 2002:131–134.

Fisher C, de Bruijin DRH, van Kessel AG. Synovial sarcoma. In: Fletcher DM, Unni KK, Mertens F, eds. *World Health Organization Classification of Tumours. Pathology and Genetics of Tumours of Soft Tissue and Bone.* Lyon: IARC Press, 2002:200–204.

Fisher C, van den Berg E, Molenaar WM. Adult fibrosarcoma. In: Fletcher DM, Unni KK, Mertens F, eds. *World Health Organization Classification of Tumours. Pathology and Genetics of Tumours of Soft Tissue and Bone.* Lyon: IARC Press, 2002:100–101.

Fletcher CDM, van den Berg E, Molenaar WM. Pleomorphic malignant fibrous histiocytoma/undifferentiated high grade pleomorphic sarcoma. In: Fletcher DM, Unni KK, Mertens F, eds. *World Health Organization Classification of Tumours. Pathology and Genetics of Tumours of Soft Tissue and Bone.* Lyon: IARC Press, 2002:120–122.

Flieder DB, Koss MN, Nicholson A, et al. Solitary pulmonary papillomas in adults: a clinicopathologic and in situ hybridization study of 14 cases combined with 27 cases in the literature. *Am J Surg Pathol* 1998;22(11):1328–1342.

Flieder DB, Yousem SA. Pulmonary lymphomas and lymphoid hyperplasias. In: Knowles DM, ed. *Neoplastic Hematopathology.* Philadelphia: Lippincott Williams & Wilkins, 2001:985.

Folpe AL. Glomus tumours. In: Fletcher DM, Unni KK, Mertens F, eds. *World Health Organization Classification of Tumours. Pathology and Genetics of Tumours of Soft Tissue and Bone.* Lyon: IARC Press, 2002:136–137.

Fraire A. Nonmalignant versus malignant proliferations on lung biopsy. In: Cagle PT, ed. *Diagnostic Pulmonary Pathology.* New York: Marcel Dekker, 2000:525–543.

Gaertner EM, Steinberg DM, Travis WD, et al. Pulmonary and mediastinal glomus tumors: report of five cases including a pulmonary glomangiosarcoma: a clinicopathologic study with literature review. *Am J Surg Pathol* 2000;24:1105–1114.

Galateau-Salle F, Cagle PT. Non-malignant versus malignant proliferations on pleural biopsy. In: Cagle PT, ed. *Diagnostic Pulmonary Pathology.* New York: Marcel Dekker, 2000:555–567.

Gallateau-Salle F. Well-differentiated papillary mesothelioma. *Histopathology* 2002;4[Suppl 2]:154–156.

Gatter KC, Warnke RA. Intravascular large B-cell lymphoma. In: Jaffe ES, Harris NL, Stein H, et al, eds. *Pathology and Genetics of Tumours of Haematopoietic and Lymphoid Tissues.* Lyon: IARC Press, 2001:177.

Gladish GW, Sabloff BM, Munden RF, et al. Primary thoracic sarcomas. *Radiographics* 2002;22:621–637.

Go C, Schwartz MR, Donovan DT. Molecular transformation of recurrent respiratory papillomatosis: viral typing and p53 overexpression. *Ann Otol Rhinol Laryngol* 2003;112:298–302.

Guillou L, Fletcher JA, Fletcher CDM, Mandahl N. Extrapleural solitary fibrous tumour and haemangiopericytoma. In: Fletcher DM, Unni KK, Mertens F, eds. *World Health Organization Classification of Tumours. Pathology and Genetics of Tumours of Soft Tissue and Bone.* Lyon: IARC Press, 2002:86–90.

Hammar SP. Lung and Pleural Neuroplasms. In: Dabbs DJ, ed. *Diagnostic Immunohistochemistry.* New York: Churchill-Livingstone, 2002:267–285.

Haque AK, Myers JL, Hudnall SD, et al. Pulmonary lymphomatoid granulomatosis in acquired immunodeficiency syndrome: lesions with Epstein-Barr virus infection. *Med Pathol* 1998:347–356.

Isaacson PG, Muller-Hermelink HK, Piris MA, et al. Extranodal marginal zone B-cell lymphoma of mucosa-associated lymphoid tissue (MALT lymphoma). In: Jaffee ES, Harris NL, Stein H, Vardiman JW eds. *Pathology and Genetics of Tumours of Haematopoietic and Lymphoid Tissues.* Lyon: IARC Press, 2001:185, 198–199.

Jaffe ES, Harris NL, Stein H, Vardiman JW, eds. *Pathology and Genetics of Tumours of Haematopoietic and Lymphoid Tissues.* Lyon: IARC Press, 2001.

James PL. Fine needle aspiration of soft tissue and bone. In: Atkinson BF, ed. *Atlas of Diagnostic Cytopathology.* Philadelphia: WB Saunders, 1992:602–618.

Jamovec J, Knuutila S. Kaposi sarcoma. In: Fletcher DM, Unni KK, Mertens F, eds. *World Health Organization Classification of Tumours. Pathology and Genetics of Tumours of Soft Tissue and Bone.* Lyon: IARC press, 2002:170–172.

Kaufmann O, Georgi T, Dietel M. Utility of 123C3 monoclonal antibody against CD56 (NCAM) for the diagnosis of small cell carcinomas on paraffin sections. *Hum Pathol* 1997;28(12):1373–1378.

Kerr DM. Pulmonary preinvasive neoplasia. *J Clin Pathol* 2001;54:257–271.

Kinsley BL, Mastery LA, Mergo PJ, et al. Pulmonary mucosa-associated lymphoid tissue lymphoma: CT and pathologic findings. *AJR Am J Roentgenol* 1999;172:1321–1326.

Kitamura H, Kameda Y, Ito T, et al. Cytodifferentiations of atypical adenomatous hyperplasia and bronchioloalveolar lung carcinoma: analysis by morphometry and the expressions of p53 and carcinoembryonic antigen. *Am J Surg Pathol* 1996;20:553–562.

Kovalski R, Hansen-Flaschen J, Lodato RF, et al. Localized leukemic pulmonary infiltrates: diagnosis by bronchoscopy and resolution with therapy. *Chest* 1990;97:674–678.

Laucirica R, Schultenover SJ. Body cavity fluids. In: Ramzy I, ed. *Clinical Cytopathology and Aspiration Biopsy. Fundamental Principles and Practice,* 2nd ed. New York: McGraw-Hill, 2001:205–223.

Leube RE, Rustad TJ. Squamous cell metaplasia in the human lung: molecular characteristics of epithelial stratification. *Virchows Arch B Cell Pathol Incl Mol Pathol* 1991;61:227–253.

Lin BT, Colby T, Gown AM, et al. Malignant vascular tumors of the serous membranes mimicking mesothelioma: a report of 14 cases. *Am J Surg Pathol* 1996;20:1431–1439.

Lukeman JM. Malignant neoplasms of the respiratory tract. In: Ramzy I, ed. *Clinical Cytopathology and Aspiration Biopsy,* 2nd ed. New York: McGraw-Hill, 2001:183–186.

Marick EL, Nascimento AG, et al. Desmoplastic small round cell tumor: a clinicopathologic, immunohistochemical, and molecular study of 32 tumors. *Am J Surg Pathol* 2002;26(7):823–835.

McMullan DM, Wood DE. Pulmonary carcinoid tumors. *Semin Thorac Cardiovasc Surg* 2003;15(3):289–300.

Miyoshi T, Yukitoshi S, Sakae O, et al. Early-stage adenocarcinomas with a micropapillary pattern, a distinct pathologic marker for a significantly poor prognosis. *Am J Surg Pathol* 2003;27(1):101–109.

Moran CA, Suster S, Fishback N, Koss MN. Primary intrapulmonary thymoma: a clinicopathologic and immunohistochemical study of eight cases. *Am J Surg Pathol* 1995;19:304–312.

Moran CA, Travis WD, Rosado-de-Christenson M, et al. Thymomas presenting as pleural tumors. *Am J Surg Pathol* 1992;16:138–144.

Mori M, Rao SK, Popper HH, et al. Atypical adenomatous hyperplasia of the lung: a probable forerunner in the development of adenocarcinoma of the lung. *Mod Pathol* 2001;14:72–84.

Nicholson SA, Beasley MB, Brambilla E, et al. Small cell lung carcinoma (SCLC): a clinicopathologic study of 100 cases with surgical specimens. *Am J Surg Pathol* 2002;26(9):1184–1197.

Ohori NP. Uncommon endobronchial neoplasms. In: Cagle PT, ed. *Diagnostic Pulmonary Pathology.* New York: Marcel Dekker, 2000:685–718.

Ordonez N, Ladanyi M. Alveolar soft part sarcoma. In: Fletcher DM, Unni KK, Mertens F, eds. *World Health Organization Classification of Tumours. Pathology and Genetics of Tumours of Soft Tissue and Bone.* Lyon: IARC Press, 2002:208–210.

Ordonez NG. The immunohistochemical diagnosis of mesothelioma: a comparative study of epithelioid mesothelioma and lung adenocarcinoma. *Am J Surg Pathol* 2003;27:1031–1051.

Patel AM, Ryu JH. Angiosarcoma in the lung. *Chest* 1993;103:1531–1535.

Politiek MJ, et al. A 49-year-old woman with well-differentiated fetal adenocarcinoma. *Neth J Med* 2001;58:177–180.

Potenza L, Luppi M, Morselli M, et al. Leukaemic pulmonary infiltrates in adult acute myeloid leukemia: a high-resolution computerized tomography study. *Br J Haematol* 2003;120:1058–1061.

Ralfkiaer E, Jaffe ES. Mycosis fungoides and Sezary syndrome. In: Jaffe ES, Harris NL, Stein H, Vardimann JW eds. *Pathology and Genetics of Tumours of Haematopoietic and Lymphoid Tissues.* Lyon: IARC Press, 2001:211, 216–220, 223.

Rao SK, Fraire AE. Alveolar cell hyperplasia in association with adenocarcinoma of lung: an immunohistochemical profile. *Mod Pathol* 1995;8:165–169.

Raymond AK, Ayala AG, Knuutila S. Conventional osteosarcoma. In: Fletcher DM, Unni KK, Mertens F, eds. *World Health Organization Classification of Tumours. Pathology and Genetics of Tumours of Soft Tissue and Bone.* Lyon: IARC Press, 2002:264–270.

Roggli VL, Cagle PT. Pleura, pericardium, and peritoneum. In: Silverberg SG, ed. *Principles and Practice of Surgical Pathology,* 4th ed. Hoboken: Wiley Medical, 2004 *(in press).*

Rossi G, Cavazza A, Brambilla E, et al. Pulmonary carcinomas with pleomorphic, sarcomatoid, or sarcomatous elements: a clinicopathologic and immunohistochemical study of 75 cases. *Am J Surg Pathol* 2003;27:311–324.

Sheehan KM, Curran J, Kay EW, et al. Well-differentiated fetal adenocarcinoma of the lung in a 29–year-old woman. *J Clin Pathol* 2003;56:478–479.

Shimosato Y, Mukai K. Tumors of the mediastinum. In: *Atlas of tumor pathology,* 3rd ed. Washington, DC. Armed Forces Institute of Pathology, 1997.

Stein H, Delsol G, Pileri S, et al. Classical Hodgkin lymphoma. In: Jaffe ES, Harris NL, Stein H, Vardiman JW eds. *Pathology and Genetics of Tumours of Haematopoietic and Lymphoid Tissues.* Lyon: IARC Press, 2001:172–261.

Sterner D, Roggli V, Mori M, et al. Prevalence of pulmonary atypical alveolar cell hyperplasia in an autopsy population: a study of 100 cases. *Mod Pathol* 1997;10:469–473.

Suster S, Moran C. Tumors of the lung and pleura. In: Fletcher C, ed. *Diagnostic Histopathology of Tumors,* 2nd ed. London: Churchill-Livingstone, 2000.

Syed S, Haque AK, Cowan DF, et al. Desmoplastic small round cell tumor of the lung. *Arch Pathol Lab Med* 2002;126:1226–1228.

Travis WD, Colby TV, Corin B, et al. Epithelial tumors. In: *WHO International Histological Classification of Tumours,* 3rd ed. Heidelberg: Springer, 1999:25–46.

Travis WD, Colby TV, Corin B, et al. Histological typing of lung and pleural tumours. New York: Springer-Verlag, 1999.

Travis WD. Pathology of lung cancer. *Clin Chest Med* 2002;23(1):65–81.

Travis WD, Brambilla E, Harris CC. Tumours of the lung. In: *World Health Organization Classification of Tumours. Pathology and Genetics of Tumours of the Lung, Pleura, Thymus, and Heart.* Lyon: IARC press, 2004 *(in press).*

Ullman R, Petzmann S, Klemen H, et al. The position of pulmonary carcinoids within the spectrum of neuroendocrine tumors of the lung and other tissues. *Genes Chromosomes Cancer* 2002;34(1):78–85.

Ullmann R, Bongiovanni M, Halbdwedl I, et al. Is high-grade adenomatous hyperplasia an early bronchioalveolar adenocarcinoma? *J Pathol* 2003;201(3):371–376.

Vadasz P, Egervary M. Mucoepidermoid bronchial tumors: a review of 34 operated cases. *Eur J Cardiothoracic Surg* 2000;17:566–569.

Van Ruth S, Van Coevorden F, Peterse JL, et al. Alveolar soft part sarcoma: a report of 15 cases. *Eur J Cancer* 2002;38:1324–1328.

Weiss SW, Bridge JA. Epithelioid haemangioendothelioma. In: Fletcher DM, Unni KK, Mertens F, eds. *World Health Organization Classification of Tumours. Pathology and Genetics of Tumours of Soft Tissue and Bone.* Lyon: IARC Press, 2002:173–174.

Yamzaki K. Pulmonary well-differentiated fetal adenocarcinoma expressing lineage-specific transcription factors (TTF-1 and GATA-6) to respiratory epithelial differentiation: an immunohistochemical and ultrastructural study. *Virchows Arch* 2003;442(4):393–399.

Yousem SA, Colby TV. Pulmonary lymphomas and lymphoid hyperplasias. In: Knowles DM, ed. *Neoplastic Hematopathology.* Baltimore: Williams & Wilkins, 1992:985–986.

Zaer FS, Braylan RC, Zander DS, et al. Multiparametric flow cytometry in the diagnosis and characterization of low-grade pulmonary mucosa-associated lymphoid tissue lymphomas. *Mod Pathol* 1998;11:525–532.

Zander DS, Iturraspe JA, Everett ET, et al. Flow cytometry: in vitro assessment of its potential application for diagnosis and classification of lymphoid processes in cytologic preparations from fine needle aspirates. *Am J Clin Pathol* 1994;101:577–586.

Zhang PJH, Livolsi VA, Brooks JJ. Malignant epithelioid vascular tumors of the pleura: report of a series and literature review. *Hum Pathol* 2000;31:29–34.

Section 4: Benign Neoplasms

Batori M, Lazaro M, Lonardo MT, et al. A rare case of pulmonary neurofibroma: clinical and diagnostic evaluation and surgical treatment. *Eur Rev Med Pharmacol Sci* 1999;3(4):155–157.

Cagle PT. Tumors of the lung (excluding lymphoid tumors). In: Thurlbeck WM, Churg AM, eds. *Pathology of the Lung,* 2nd ed. New York: Thieme, 1995:437–552.

Carney JA. The triad of gastric epithelioid leiomyosarcoma, functioning extra-adrenal paraganglioma, and pulmonary chondroma. *Cancer* 1979;43:374–382.

Cesario A, Galetta D, Margaritora S, et al. Unsuspected primary pulmonary meningioma. *Eur J Cardiothorac Surg* 2002;21(3):553–555.

Churg A. Localized pleural tumors. In: Cagle PT, ed. *Diagnostic Pulmonary Pathology.* New York: Marcel Dekker, 2000:719–734.

Clayton AC, Saloma DR, Keeney GL, et al. Solitary fibrous tumor: a study of cytologic features of six cases diagnosed by fine-needle aspiration. *Diagn Cytopathol* 2001;25:172–176.

Colby TV, Koss MN, Travis WD. Carcinoid and other neuroendocrine tumors. In: *Tumors of the Lower Respiratory Tract.* Washington, DC: Armed Forces Institute of Pathology, 1994:294–307.

Colby TV, Koss MN, Travis WD. Miscellaneous benign epithelial tumors. In: *Tumors of the Lower Respiratory Tract.* Washington, DC: Armed Forces Institute of Pathology, 1994:57.

Colby TV, Koss MN, Travis WD. Tumors of salivary gland type. In: *Tumors of the Lower Respiratory Tract.* Washington, DC: Armed Forces Institute of Pathology, 1994:64.

Colby TV, Koss MN, Travis WD. Miscellaneous tumors and tumors of uncertain histogenesis. In: *Tumors of the Lower Respiratory Tract.* Washington, DC: Armed Forces Institute of Pathology, 1994:85.

Comin CE, Caldarella A, Novelli A, et al. Primary pulmonary meningioma: report of a case and review of the literature. *Tumori* 2003;89:102–105.

Dail D. Uncommon tumors. In: Dail DH, Hammar SP, eds. *Pulmonary Pathology,* 2nd ed. New York: Springer-Verlag, 1994:1279–1462.

Faul JL, Berry GJ, Colby TV, et al. Thoracic lymphangiomas, lymphangiectasis, lymphangiomatosis, and lymphatic dysplasia syndrome. *Am J Respir Crit Care Med* 2000;161:1037–1046.

Gaffe MJ, Mills SE, Askin FB. Minute pulmonary meningothelial-like nodules: a clinicopathologic study of so-called minute pulmonary chemodectoma. *Am J Surg Pathol* 1988;12(3):167–175.

Govender D, Sabaratnam RM, Essa AS. Clear cell "sugar" tumor of the breast: another extrapulmonary site and review of the literature. *Am J Surg Pathol* 2002;26(5):670–675.

Hayashi T, Fleming MV, Stetler-Stevenson WG, et al. Immunohistochemical study of matrix metalloproteinases (MMPs) and their tissue inhibitors (TIMPs) in pulmonary lymphangioleiomyomatosis (LAM). *Hum Pathol* 1997;28:1071–1078.

Hsu HS, Wang CY, Li WY, et al. Endotracheobronchial neurofibromas. *Ann Thorac Surg* 2002; 74(5):1704–1706.

Kiryu T, Kawaguchi S, Matsui E, et al. Multiple chondromatous hamartomas of the lung: a case report and review of the literature with special reference to Carney Syndrome. *Cancer* 1999;85:2557–2561.

Kuroda M, Oka T, Horuichi H, et al. Giant cell tumor of the lung: an autopsy case report with immunohistochemical observations. *Pathol Int* 1994;44(2):158–163.

Langston C, Askin FB. Pulmonary disorders in the neonate, infant, and child. In: Thurlbeck WM, Churg AM, eds. *Pathology of the Lung,* 2nd ed. New York: Thieme, 1995:151–194.

Markaki S, Edwards C. Intrapulmonary ganglioneuroma. A case report. *Arch Anat Cytol Pathol* 1987;35(3):183–184.

Maruyama H, Seyama K, Sobajma J, et al. Multifocal micronodular pneumocyte hyperplasia and lymphangioleiomyomatosis in tuberous sclerosis with a TSC2 gene. *Mod Pathol* 2001;14(6):609–614.

Mendes W, Ayoub A, Chapchap P, et al. Association of gastrointestinal stromal tumor (leiomyosarcoma), pulmonary chondroma, and nonfunctional retroperitoneal paraganglioma. *Med Pediatr Oncol* 1998;31:537–540.

Muir TE, Leslie KO, Popper H, et al. Micronodular pneumocyte hyperplasia. *Am J Surg Pathol* 1998; 22(4):465–472.

Murer B. Fibrohistiocytic tumours of the lung and pleura. EU-Project on Rare Pulmonary Diseases. ESP Congress, Ljubliana, 2003.

Niho, S, Yokose, T, Nishiwaki, Y, et al. Immunohistochemical and clonal analysis of minute pulmonary meningothelial-like nodules. *Hum Pathol* 1999;30(4):425–429.

Ohori NP. Uncommon endobronchial neoplasms. In: Cagle PT, ed. *Diagnostic Pulmonary Pathology.* New York: Marcel Dekker, 2000:685–718.

Orosz Z, Toth E, Viski A. Osteoclastoma-like giant cell tumor of the lung. *Pathol Oncol Res* 1996; 2(1–2):84–88.

Pinkard NB. Enlarged airspaces. In: Cagle PT, ed. *Diagnostic Pulmonary Pathology.* New York: Marcel Dekker, 2000:349–358.

Popper HH, Juettner-Smolle FM, et al. Micronodular hyperplasia of type II pneumocytes: a new lung lesion associated with tuberous sclerosis. *Histopathology* 1991;18(4):347–354.

Prasad AR, Tazelaar HD, Cagle PT, et al. Primary giant cell tumors of the lung. *Mod Pathol* 2001;14(1):225A.

Spinelli M, Claren R, Colombi R, Sironi M. Primary pulmonary meningioma may arise from meningothelial-like nodules. *Adv Clin Pathol* 2000;4:35–39.

Stocker JT, Dehner LP. Acquired neonatal and pediatric diseases. In: Dail DH, Hammar SP, eds. *Pulmonary Pathology,* 2nd ed. New York: Springer-Verlag, 1994:191–254.

Tazelaar HD, Kerr D, Yousem SA, et al. Diffuse pulmonary lymphangiomatosis. *Hum Pathol* 1993;24:1313–1322.

Travis WD, Colby TV, Corrin B, et al. *WHO Histological Typing of the Lung and Pleural Tumors,* 3rd ed. Berlin: Springer-Verlag, 1999.

Travis WD, Brambilla E, Harris CC. Tumours of the lung. In: *World Health Organization Classification of Tumours. Pathology and Genetics, Tumours of the Lung, Thymus, and Heart.* Lyon: WHO, 2004 *(in press).*

Wilson RW, Gallateau-Salle F, Moran C. Desmoid tumors of the pleura: a clinicopathologic mimic of localized fibrous tumour. *Mod Pathol* 1999;12:9–14.

Wojcik EM, Sneige, N, Lawrence DD, et al. Fine-needle aspiration cytology of sclerosing hemangioma of the lung: case report with immunohistochemical study. *Diagn Cytopathol* 1993;9:304–309.

Yana S. Exacerbation of pulmonary lymphangioleiomyomatosis by exogenous estrogen used for infertility treatment. *Thorax* 2002;57:1085–1086.

Yilmaz A, Bayramgurler B, Aksoy F, et al. Pulmonary glomus tumor: a case initially diagnosed as carcinoid tumor. *Respirology* 2002;7:369–371.

Yousem SA. Benign epithelial neoplasms of the distal lobular unit of the lung. In: Cagle PT, ed. *Diagnostic Pulmonary Pathology.* New York: Marcel Dekker, 2000:627–648.

Section 5: Histiocytosis

Arico M, Girschikofsky M, Genereau T, et al. Langerhans cell histiocytosis in adults: report from the International Registry of the Histiocyte Society. *Eur J Cancer* 2003;39:2341–2348.

Cousar JB, Casey TT, Macon WR, et al. Lymph nodes. In: Sternberg SS, ed. *Diagnostic Surgical Pathology,* 3rd ed. Philadelphia: Lippincott Williams & Wilkins, 1999:151–155.

Desai SR, Ryan SM, Colby TV. Smoking-related interstitial lung diseases: histopathological and imaging perspectives. *Clin Radiol* 2003;58:259–268.

Egan AJM, Boardman LA, Tazelaar HD, et al. Erdheim-Chester disease: clinical, radiologic, and histopathologic findings in five patients with interstitial lung disease. *Am J Surg Pathol* 1999;23(1):17–26.

Foucar E, Rosai J, Dorfman R. Sinus histiocytosis with massive lymphadenopathy (Rosai-Dorfman disease): review of the entity. *Semin Diagn Pathol* 1990;7:19–73.

Mahar AM, Sporn TA, Roggli VL. Pulmonary extranodal Rosai-Dorfman disease: an unusual mimic of pulmonary carcinoma. Third Biennial Summer Symposium, Pulmonary Pathology Society, Snowmass Village, CO, July 30, 2003.

Rush WL, Andrido JAW, Galateau-Salle F, et al. Pulmonary pathology of Erdheim-Chester disease. *Mod Pathol* 2000;13(6):747–754.

Zander DS, Mergo PJ, Foster RA, et al. Pulmonary parenchymal sinus histiocytosis with massive lymphadenopathy (Rosai-Dorfman disease): report of a case with immunohistochemical studies. *Mod Pathol* 1997;10:174A.

Section 6: Benign and Borderline Lymphoid Proliferations

Abbondanzo SL, Rush W, Bijwaard KE, et al. Nodular lymphoid hyperplasia of the lung: a clinicopathologic study of 14 cases. *Am J Surg Pathol* 2000;24:587–597.

ATS/ERS international multidisciplinary consensus classification of the idiopathic interstitial pneumonias. *Am J Respir Crit Care Med* 2002;165:277–304.

Kradin RL, Mark EJ. Benign lymphoid disorders of the lung, with a theory regarding their development. *Hum Pathol* 1983;14:857–867.

Travis WD, Colby TV, Koss MN, et al. *Non-neoplastic Disorders Of The Lower Respiratory Tract.* Washington, DC: Armed Forces Institute of Pathology and American Registry of Pathology, 2001.

Section 7: Focal Lesions and Pseudotumors

Chapman SJ, Cookson WO, Musk AW, et al. Benign asbestos pleural diseases. *Curr Opin Pulm Med* 2003;4:266–271.

Colby TV, Koss MN, Travis WD. Tumor-like conditions. In: *Tumors of the Lower Respiratory Tract.* Washington, DC: Armed Forces Institute of Pathology, 1994:857–863, 870.

Colby TV, Yousem SA. Lungs. In: Sternberg SS, ed. *Histology for Pathologists,* 2nd ed. Philadelphia: Lippincott Williams & Wilkins, 1997:433–460.

Fletcher CDM. *Diagnostic Histopathology of Tumors.* London: Churchill Livingstone, 2000.

Griffin CA, Hawkins AL, Dvorak C, et al. Recurrent involvement of 2p23 in inflammatory myofibroblastic tumors. *Cancer Res* 1999;59:2776–2780.

Joines RW, Roggli VL. Dendriform pulmonary ossification: report of two cases with unique findings. *Am J Clin Pathol* 1989;91:398–402.

Lawrence B, Perez-Atayde A, Hibbard MK, et al. TPM3-ALK and TPM4-ALK oncogenes in inflammatory myofibroblastic tumors. *Am J Pathol* 2000;157:377–384.

Miyake HY, Kawagoe T, Hori Y, et al. Intrapulmonary lymph nodes: CT and pathological features. *Clin Radiol* 1999;54:640–643.

Muller KM, Friemann J, Stichnoth E. Dendriform pulmonary ossification. *Pathol Res Pract* 1980;168:163–172.

Ndimbie OK, Williams CR, Lee MW. Dendriform pulmonary ossification. *Arch Pathol Lab Med* 1987;111:1062–1064.

Roggli VL, Oury T. Interstitial fibrosis, predominantly mature. In: Cagle PT, ed. *Diagnostic Pulmonary Pathology.* New York: Marcel Dekker, 2000:77–102.

Travis WD, Colby TV, Corrin B, et al. Histological typing of tumors of lung and pleura, 3rd ed. New York: Springer-Verlag, 1999:61–66.

Travis WD, Colby TV, Koss MN, et al. Miscellaneous diseases of uncertain etiology. In: King DW, ed. *Non-neoplastic Disorders of the Lower Respiratory Tract.* Washington, DC: American Registry of Pathology and the Armed Forces Institute of Pathology, 2002:857–900.

Yousem SA. Pulmonary apical cap: a distinctive but poorly recognized lesion in pulmonary surgical pathology. *Am J Surg Pathol* 2001;25:679–683.

Section 8: Granulomatous Diseases

Azumi N. Immunohistochemistry and in situ hybridization techniques in the detection of infectious organisms. In: Connor DH, ed. *Pathology of Infectious Diseases.* Stamford, CT: Appleton and Lange, 1997:35–44.

Bynum LJ, Pierce AK. Pulmonary aspiration of gastric contents. *Am Rev Respir Dis* 1976;114: 1129–1136.

Cagle PT. Tumors of the lung (excluding lymphoid tumors). In: Thurlbeck WM, Churg AM, eds. *Pathology of the Lung,* 2nd ed. New York: Thieme, 1995:437–552.

Chandler FW. Approaches to the pathologic diagnosis of infectious diseases. In: Connor DH, ed. *Pathology of Infectious Diseases.* Stamford, CT: Appleton and Lange, 1997:3–9.

Chandler FW, Watts JC. Fungal infections. In: Dail DH, Hammar SP, eds. *Pulmonary Pathology,* 2nd ed. New York: Springer-Verlag, 1994:351–428.

Churg A, Carrington CB, Gupta R. Necrotizing sarcoid granulomatosis. *Chest* 1979;76:406–413.

Colby TV, Carrington CB. Interstitial lung disease. In: Thurlbeck WM, Churg AM, eds. *Pathology of the Lung,* 2nd ed. New York: Thieme, 1995:589–738.

Didolkar MS, Gamarra MC, Hartmann RA, Takita H. Lipoid granuloma of the lung: clinicopathologic observations. *J Thorac Cardiovasc Surg* 1973;66:122–126.

Elliott CG, Colby TV, Kelly TM, Hicks HG. Charcoal lung: bronchiolitis obliterans after aspiration of activated charcoal. *Chest* 1989;96:672–674.

Hakala M, Paako P, Huhi E, et al. Open lung biopsy of patients with rheumatoid arthritis. *Clin Rheumatol* 1990;9:452–460.

Haque AK. The pathology and pathophysiology of mycobacterial infections. *J Thorac Imaging* 1990;5:8–16.

Hruban RH, Hutchins GM. Mycobacterial infections. In: Dail DH, Hammar SP, eds. *Pulmonary Pathology,* 2nd ed. New York: Springer-Verlag, 1994:331–350.

James DG, Jones WW. *Sarcoidosis and Other Granulomatous Disorders.* Philadelphia: WB Saunders, 1985.

Kashiwabara K, Toyonaga M, Yamaguchi Y, et al. Sarcoid reaction in primary tumor of bronchogenic large cell carcinoma accompanied with massive necrosis. *Intern Med* 2001;40(2):127–130.

Kin T, Shimano Y, Shinomiya Y, et al. Double cancers of the lung and esophagus associated with a sarcoid-like reaction in their regional lymph nodes: report of a case. *Jpn J Surg* 1999;29:260–263.

Koss MN, Hochholzer L, Feinegen DS, et al. Necrotizing sarcoid-like granulomatosis: clinical, pathologic and immunopathologic findings. *Hum Pathol* 1980;2[Suppl]:510–519.

Kriebel D, Brain JD, Sprince NL, Kazemi H. The pulmonary toxicity of beryllium. *Am Rev Respir Dis* 1988;137:464–473.

Kwon KY, Colby TV. Rhodococcus equi pneumonia and pulmonary malakoplakia in acquired immunodeficiency syndrome. *Arch Pathol Lab Med* 1994;118:744–748.

Marty AM, Neafie RC. Protozoal and helminthic diseases. In: Saldana MJ, ed. *Pathology of Pulmonary Disease.* Philadelphia: JB Lippincott, 1994:489–502.

Newman LS, Kreiss K, King TE, et al. Pathologic and immunologic alterations in early stages of beryllium disease: re-examination of disease definition and natural history. *Am Rev Respir Dis* 1989;139:1479–1486.

Pinckard JK, Rosenbluth DB, Patel K, et al. Pulmonary hyalinizing granuloma associated with Aspergillus infection. *Int J Surg Pathol* 2003;11(1):39–42.

Popper HH, Klemen H, Colby TV, et al. Necrotizing sarcoid granulomatosis: is it different from nodular sarcoidosis? *Pneumologie* 2003;57(5):268–271.

Popper HH. Granulomas and granulomatous inflammation. In: Cagle PT, ed. *Diagnostic Pulmonary Pathology.* New York: Marcel-Dekker, 2000:287–330.

Rosen Y, Amorosa JK, Moon S, et al. Occurrence of lung granulomas in patients with stage I sarcoidosis. *AJR Am J Roentgenol* 1977;129:1083–1085.

Russell AFR, Suggit RIC, Kazzi JC. Pulmonary hyalinizing granuloma: a case report and literature review. *Pathology* 2000;32:290–293.

Schmidt RA. Iatrogenic injury: radiation and drug effects. In: Dail DH, Hammar SP, eds. *Pulmonary pathology,* 2nd ed. New York: Springer-Verlag, 1994:779–806.

Sharma OP. Sarcoidosis. *Dis Mon* 1990;36:469–535.

Siegal H. Human pulmonary pathology associated with narcotic and other addictive drugs. *Hum Pathol* 1972;3:55–66.

Tomashefski JR, Hirsch CS. The pulmonary vascular lesions of intravenous drug abuse. *Hum Pathol* 1980;11:133–146.

Travis WD, Colby TV, Koss MN, et al. Lung infections. In: King DW, ed. *Non-neoplastic Disorders of the Lower Respiratory Tract.* Bethesda, MD: American Registry of Pathology and AFIP, 2002:539–728.

Travis WD, Colby TV, Koss MN, et al. Bronchial disorders. In: King DW, ed. *Non-neoplastic Disorders of the Lower Respiratory Tract.* Bethesda, MD: American Registry of Pathology and AFIP, 2002:381–434.

Wright JL. Consequences of aspiration and bronchial obstruction. In: Thurlbeck WM, Churg AM, eds. *Pathology of the Lung,* 2nd ed. New York: Theime, 1995:1111–1128.

Youh G, Hove MGM, Wen J, et al. Pulmonary malakoplakia in acquired immunodeficiency syndrome: an ultrastructural study of morphogenesis of Michaelis-Gutmann bodies. *Mod Pathol* 1996;9:476–483.

Yousem SA, Colby TV, Carrington CB. Lung biopsy in rheumatoid arthritis. *Am Rev Respir Dis* 1985;131:770–777.

Section 9: Diffuse Pulmonary Hemorrhage

Bonsib SM. Goodpasture syndrome and the diffuse alveolar hemorrhage syndrome. In: Saldana MJ, ed. *Pathology of Pulmonary Disease.* Philadelphia: JB Lippincott, 1994:723–731.

Burns AP, Fisher M, Li P, et al. Molecular analysis of HLA class II genes in Goodpasture's disease. *QJM* 1995;88:93–100.

Churg A. Recent advances in the diagnosis of Churg-Strauss syndrome. *Mod Pathol* 2001;14: 1284–1293.

Corrin B. *Pathology of the Lungs.* London: Churchill Livingstone, 2000.

DeRemee RA, Anton RC, Cagle PT. Pulmonary angiitis and granulomatosis. In: James DG, Zumla A, ed. *The Granulomatous Disorders.* Port Chester, NY: Cambridge University Press, 1999:127–137.

Hay JG. Clinical diagnosis of pulmonary hemorrhage. In: Cagle PT, ed. *Diagnostic Pulmonary Pathology.* New York: Marcel Dekker, 2000:271–283.

Hirohata S, Kikuchi H. Behçet's disease. *Arthritis Res Ther* 2003;5:139–146.

Jennette JC, Falk RJ. Small-vessel vasculitis. *N Engl J Med* 1997;337:1512–1523.

Katzenstein A-LA. *Katzenstein and Askin's Surgical Pathology of Non-neoplastic Lung Disease,* 3rd ed. Philadelphia: WB Saunders Company, 1997.

Khoor A, Tazelaar HD. Pulmonary hemorrhage. In: Cagle PT, ed. *Diagnostic Pulmonary Pathology.* New York: Marcel Dekker, 2000:251–270.

Magro CM, Morrison C, Pope-Harman A, et al. Direct and indirect immunofluorescence as a diagnostic adjunct in the interpretation of nonneoplastic medical lung disease. *Am J Clin Pathol* 2003;119:279–289.

Masi AT, Hunder GG, Lie JT, et al. The American College of Rheumatology 1990 criteria for the classification of Churg-Strauss syndrome (allergic granulomatosis and angiitis). *Arthritis Rheum* 1990;33:1094–1100.

Milman N, Pedersen FM. Idiopathic pulmonary haemosiderosis: epidemiology, pathogenic aspects and diagnosis. *Respir Med* 1998;92:902–907.

Noth I, Strek ME, Leff AR. Churg-Strauss syndrome. *Lancet* 2003;361:587–594.

Rossi SE, Erasmus JJ, McAdams HP, et al. Pulmonary drug toxicity: radiologic and pathologic manifestations. *Radiographics* 2000;20:1245–1259.

Travis WD, Colby TV, Koss MN, et al. Diffuse parenchymal lung diseases. In: King DW, ed. *Non-neoplastic Disorders of the Lower Respiratory Tract.* Washington, DC: Armed Forces Institute of Pathology and American Registry of Pathology, 2001:49–50.

Travis WD, Koss MN. Vasculitis. In: Dail DH, Hammar SP, eds. *Pulmonary Pathology,* 2nd ed. New York: Springer-Verlag, 1994:1027–1096.

Wagenvoort CA, Mooi WJ. Vascular diseases. In: Dail DH, Hammar SP, eds. *Pulmonary pathology,* 2nd ed. New York: Springer-Verlag, 1994:985–1026.

Section 10: Pulmonary Hemorrhage with Vasculitis

Abrahams C, Catachatourian R. Bone fragment emboli in the lungs of patients undergoing bone marrow transplantation. *Am J Clin Pathol* 1983;79:360.

Almagro P, Julia J, Sanjaume M, et al. Pulmonary capillary hemangiomatosis associated with primary pulmonary hypertension: a report of 2 new cases and review of 35 cases from the literature. *Medicine (Baltimore)* 2002;81:417–424.

Bjornsson J, Edwards WD. Primary pulmonary hypertension: a histopathologic study of 80 cases. *Mayo Clin Proc* 1985;60:16–25.

Bloor CM. Acute pulmonary thromboembolism and other forms of pulmonary embolization. In: Saldana MJ, ed. *Pathology of Pulmonary Disease.* Philadelphia: JB Lippincott, 1994:171–178.

Burke AP, Farb A, Virmani R. The pathology of primary pulmonary hypertension. *Mod Pathol* 1991;4:269–282.

Carrington CB, Liebow AA. Pulmonary veno-occlusive disease. *Hum Pathol* 1970;1:22–324.

Cotran RS, Kumar V, Collins T. *Robbins Pathologic Basis of Disease,* 6th ed. Philadelphia: WB Saunders Company, 1999.

English JC. Pulmonary vascular lesions. In: Cagle PT, ed. *Diagnostic Pulmonary Pathology.* New York: Marcel Dekker, 2000:359–412.

Gagnadoux F, Capron F, Lebeau B. Pulmonary veno-occlusive disease after neoadjuvant mitomycin chemotherapy and surgery for lung carcinoma. *Lung Cancer* 2002;36:213–215.

Garcia-Palmier M. Cor pulmonale due to Schistosoma mansoni. *Am Heart J* 1964;68:714.

Gonzales-Vitale JC, Garcia-Bunuel R. Pulmonary tumor emboli and cor pulmonale in primary carcinoma of the lung. *Cancer* 1976;38:2105.

Hardin L, Fox LS, O'Quinn AG. Amniotic fluid embolism. *South Med J* 1991;84:1046.

Haque AK, Gokhale S, Rampy BA, et al. Pulmonary hypertension in sickle cell hemoglobinopathy: a clinicopathologic study of 20 cases. *Hum Pathol* 2002;33:1037–1043.

Hoffman JI, Abraham RM, Heymann MA. Pulmonary vascular disease with congenital heart lesions: pathologic features and causes. *Circulation* 1981;64:873.

Katsumura Y, Ohtsubo K. Incidence of pulmonary thromboembolism, infarction and haemorrhage in disseminated intravascular coagulation: a necroscopic analysis. *Thorax* 1995;50:160–164.

Lammers RJ, Bloor CM. Edema, emboli, and vascular anomalies. In: Dail DH, Hammar SP, eds. *Pulmonary Pathology.* New York: Springer-Verlag, 1988:986–988.

Mattox KL, Beall AC, Ennix CL, et al. Intravascular migratory bullets. *Am J Surg* 1979;137:192–195.

Pietra GG, Edwards WD, Kay JM, et al. Histopathology of primary pulmonary hypertension: a qualitative and quantitative study of pulmonary blood vessels from 58 patients in the National Heart, Lung, and Blood Institute, Primary Pulmonary Hypertension Registry. *Circulation* 1989;80:1207–1221.

Primary Pulmonary Hypertension. Executive Summary from the World Symposium–Primary Pulmonary Hypertension 1998. Evian, France: World Health Organization, 1999.

Rich S, Levitsky S, Brundage BH. Pulmonary hypertension from chronic pulmonary thromboembolism. *Ann Intern Med* 1988;108:425.

Shannon JJ, Vo NM, Stanton PE Jr, et al. Peripheral arterial missile embolization: a case report and 22-year literature review. *J Vasc Surg* 1987;5:773–778.

Spencer H. *Pathology of the Lung,* 4th ed. Oxford: Pergamon Press, 1985.

Tron V, Magee F, Wright JL, et al. Pulmonary capillary hemangiomatosis. *Hum Pathol* 1986;17:1144.

Virmani R, Roberts WC. Pulmonary arteries in congenital heart disease: a structure function analysis. In: Roberts WC, ed. *Adult Congenital Heart Disease.* Philadelphia: FA Davis, 1987:79–80.

Wagenvoort CA, Wagenvoort N. Primary pulmonary hypertension: a pathologic study of the lung vessels in 156 clinically diagnosed cases. *Circulation* 1970;42:1163.

Wagenvoort CA, Wagenvoort N. The pathology of pulmonary veno-occlusive disease. *Virchows Arch [A]* 1974;364:69–79.

Wagenvoort CA. Capillary hemangiomatosis of the lung. *Histopathology* 1978;2:401.

Section 11: Large Airways

Busse WW, Lemanske LF. Advances in immunology: asthma. *N Engl J Med* 2001;344:350–362.

Dail DH. Eosinophilic infiltrates. In: Dail DH, Hammar SP, eds. *Pulmonary Pathology,* 2nd ed. New York: Springer-Verlag, 1994:537–566.

Flint JDA. Vasculitis. In: Cagle PT, ed. *Diagnostic Pulmonary Pathology.* New York: Marcel-Dekker, 2000:413–428.

Guinee DG. Pulmonary eosinophilia. In: Cagle PT, ed. *Diagnostic Pulmonary Pathology.* New York: Marcel Dekker, 2000:195–218.

Jenkins HA, Cool C, Szefler SJ, et al. Histopathology of severe childhood asthma: a case series. *Chest* 2003;124:32–41.

Kobzik, L. The lung. In: Cotran RS, Jumar V, Collin T, eds. *Robbins' Pathologic Basis of Disease,* 6th ed. Philadelphia: WB Saunders, 1999:697–755.

Kwon KY, Myers JL, Swensen SJ, et al. Middle lobe syndrome: a clinicopathological study of 21 patients. *Hum Pathol* 1995;26:302–307.

Reich JM, Johnson RE. Mycobacterium avium complex pulmonary disease presenting as an isolated lingular or middle lobe pattern: the Lady Windermere syndrome. *Chest* 1992;101:1605–1609.

Sobonya RE. Fungal diseases, including allergic bronchopulmonary aspergillosis. In: Thurlbeck WM, Churg AM, eds. *Pathology of the Lung,* 2nd ed. New York: Thieme, 1995:303–332.

Thurlbeck WM. Chronic airflow obstruction. In: Thurlbeck WM, Churg AM, eds. *Pathology of the Lung,* 2nd ed. New York: Thieme, 1995:739–826.

Section 12: Small Airways

Popper HH. Bronchiolitis obliterans: organizing pneumonia. *Verh Dtsch Ges Pathol* 2002;86:101–106.

Schlesinger C, Vheeraraghavan S, Koss MN. Constrictive (obliterative) bronchiolitis. *Curr Opin Pulm Med* 1998;4:288–293.

Travis WD, Colby TV, Koss MN, et al. Idiopathic interstitial pneumonia and other diffuse parenchymal lung diseases. In: King DW, ed. *Non-neoplastic Disorders of the Lower Respiratory Tract.* Washington, DC: American Registry of Pathology and the Armed Forces Institute of Pathology, 2002:49–232.

Wright JL, Cagle PT, Churg A, et al. Diseases of the small airways. *Am Rev Respir Dis* 1992;146(1): 240–262.

Section 13: Alveolar Infiltrate

Allen JN, Pacht ER, Gadek JE, et al. Acute eosinophilic pneumonia as a reversible cause of noninfectious respiratory failure. *N Engl J Med* 1989;321:569–574.

Beasley MB, Franks T, Galvin J, et al. Acute fibrinous and organizing pneumonia: a histologic pattern of lung injury and possible variant of diffuse alveolar damage. *Arch Pathol Lab Med* 2002;126:1064–1070.

Bedrossian CW, Kuhn C, Luna MA, et al. Desquamative interstitial pneumonia-like reaction accompanying pulmonary lesions. *Chest* 1977;72:166–169.

Dail DH. Metabolic and other diseases. In: Dail DH, Hammar SP, eds. *Pulmonary Pathology,* 2nd ed. New York: Springer Verlag, 1994:707–777.

Epler GR, Colby TV, McLoud TC, et al. Bronchiolitis obliterans organizing pneumonia. *N Engl J Med* 1985;312:152–158.

Hogg JC. Pulmonary edema. In: Thurlbeck WM, Churg A, eds. *Pathology of the Lung,* 2nd ed. New York: Thieme Medical Publishers, 1995:375–383.

Ikehara K, Suzuki M, Tsubarai T, Ishigatsubo W. Lipoid pneumonia. *Lancet* 2002;359:1300.

Katzenstein A. Acute lung injury patterns: diffuse alveolar damage and bronchiolitis obliterans-organizing pneumonia. In: Katzenstein A-LA, ed. *Katzenstein and Askin's Surgical Pathology of Non-neoplastic Lung Disease.* Philadelphia: WB Saunders, 1997:15–32, 33–40.

Keller Ca, Frost A, Cagle PT, Abraham JL. Pulmonary alveolar proteinosis in a painter with elevated pulmonary concentrations of titanium. *Chest* 1995;108:277–280.

Morrissey WL, Gaensler EA, Carrington CB, et al. Chronic eosinophilic pneumonia. *Respiration* 1975;32:453–468.

Nicholson AG. Classification of idiopathic interstitial pneumonias: making sense of the alphabet soup. *Histopathology* 2002;41(5):381–391.

Simon HB. Pulmonary infections. In: Dale DC, ed. *Scientific American Medicine.* 2003 WebMD.

Tazelaar HD, Linz LJ, Colby TV, et al. Acute eosinophilic pneumonia: histopathologic findings in nine patients. *Am J Respir Crit Care Med* 1997;155:296–302.

Tomashefski JF Jr. Pulmonary pathology of the adult respiratory distress syndrome. *Clin Chest Med* 1990;11:593–619.

Travis WD, King TE Jr, Bateman ED, et al. ATS/ERS international multidisciplinary consensus classification of idiopathic interstitial pneumonias. Unpublished material.

Travis WD, Colby TV, Koss MN, et al. Bronchiolar disorders. In: King DW, ed. *Non-neoplastic Disorders of the Lower Respiratory Tract.* Bethesda, MD: American Registry of Pathology and AFIP, 2002:353–360.

Travis WM, Colby TV, Koss MN, et al. Diffuse parenchymal lung diseases. In: King DW, ed. *Non-neoplastic Disorders of the Lower Respiratory Tract.* Bethesda, MD: American Registry of Pathology and AFIP, 2002:89–102.

Wagenvoort CA, Mooi WJ. Vascular disorders. In: Dail DH, Hammar SP, eds. *Pulmonary Pathology,* 2nd ed. New York: Springer-Verlag, 1994:986–988.

Wright, JL. Adult respiratory distress syndrome. In: Thurlbeck WM, Churg A, eds. *Pathology of the Lung.* New York: Thieme Medical Publishers, 1995:387–397.

Section 14: Tobacco-Related Diseases

Cosio Piqueras MG, Cosio MG. Disease of the airways in chronic obstructive pulmonary disease. *Eur Respir J Suppl* 2001;34:41s–49s.

Demedts M, Costabel U. ATS/ERS international multidisciplinary consensus classification of the idiopathic interstitial pneumonias. *Eur Respir J* 2002;19:794–796.

Desai SR, Ryan SM, Colby TV. Smoking-related interstitial lung diseases: histopathological and imaging perspectives. *Clin Radiol* 2003;58(4):259–268.

Park JS, Brown KK, Tuder RM, et al. Respiratory bronchiolitis-associated interstitial lung disease: radiologic features with clinical and pathologic correlation. *J Comput Assist Tomogr* 2002;26(1):13–20.

Travis WD, Colby TV, Koss MN. Diffuse parenchymal lung diseases. In: King, DW, ed. *Non-neoplastic Disorders of the Lower Respiratory Tract.* Washington, DC: American Registry of Pathology and the Armed Forces Institute of Pathology, 2002:169–176.

Yousem SA, Colby TV, Gaensler EA. Respiratory bronchiolitis-associated interstitial lung disease and its relationship to desquamative interstitial pneumonia. *Mayo Clin Proc* 1989;64(11):1373–1380.

Section 15: Diffuse Interstitial Lung Diseases

Barrios R. Hypersensitivity pneumonitis. In: Saldana M, ed. *Pathology of Pulmonary Disease.* Philadelphia: Lippincott Williams and Wilkins, 1994:755–765.

Boag AH, Colby TV, Fraire AE, et al. The pathology of interstitial lung disease in nylon flock workers. *Am J Surg Pathol* 1999;23(12):1539–1545.

Cagle PT. Chronic interstitial pneumonia with specific histologic features. In: Saldana M, ed. *Pathology of Pulmonary Disease.* Philadelphia: JB Lippincott, 1994:341–355.

Cagle PT. Non-specific ("usual") interstitial pneumonia, interstitial fibrosis and the honeycomb lung. In: Saldana M, ed. *Pathology of Pulmonary Disease.* Philadelphia: JB Lippincott, 1994:341–355.

Cappeluti E, Fraire AE, Schaefer OP. A case of "hot tub lung" due to Mycobacterium avium complex in an immunocompetent host. *Arch Intern Med* 2003;163:845–848.

Casey MB, Tazelaar, Myers JL, et al. Noninfectious lung pathology in patients with Crohn's disease. *Am J Surg Pathol* 2003;27(2):213–219.

Cheung OY, Muhm JR, Helmers RA, et al. Surgical pathology of granulomatous interstitial pneumonia. *Ann Diagn Pathol* 2003;7(2):127–138.

Churg A. Nonneoplastic disease caused by asbestos. In: Churg A, Green FHY, eds. *Pathology of Occupational Lung Disease.* Baltimore: Williams & Wilkins, 1998:277–338.

Churg A, Colby TV. Diseases caused by metals and related compounds. In: Churg A, Green FHY, eds. *Pathology of Occupational Lung Disease.* Baltimore: Williams & Wilkins, 1998:77–128.

Colby TV, Carrington CB. Interstitial lung disease. In: Thurlbeck WM, Churg AM, eds. *Pathology of the Lung,* 2nd ed. New York: Thieme, 1995:589–738.

Corrin B. Occupational lung disease. In: Corrin B, ed. *Pathology of the Lungs.* London: Churchill Livingstone, 2000:279–320.

Dail DH. Metabolic and other diseases. In: Dail DH, Hammar SP, eds. *Pulmonary Pathology,* 2nd ed. New York: Springer-Verlag, 1994:707–778.

Frost AE, Keller CA, Brown RW, et al. Giant cell interstitial pneumonitis: disease recurrence in the transplanted lung. *Am Rev Respir Dis* 1993;148:1401– 1404.

Gibbs AR, Wagner JC. Diseases due to silica. In: Churg A, Green FHY, eds. *Pathology of Occupational Lung Disease.* Baltimore: Williams & Wilkins, 1998:209–234.

Green FHY, Churg A. Pathologic features of occupational lung disease. In: Churg A, Green FHY, eds. *Pathology of Occupational Lung Disease.* Baltimore: Williams & Wilkins, 1998:21–44.

Green FHY, Churg A. Diseases due to nonasbestos silicates. In: Churg A, Green FHY, eds. *Pathology of Occupational Lung Disease.* Baltimore: Williams & Wilkins, 1998:235–276.

Green FHY, Vallyathan V. Coal workers' pneumoconiosis and pneumoconiosis due to other carbonaceous dusts. In: Churg A, Green FHY, eds. *Pathology of Occupational Lung Disease.* Baltimore: Williams & Wilkins, 1998:129–208.

Kern DG, Kuhn C, Ely EW, et al. Flock worker's lung: broadening the spectrum of clinicopathology, narrowing the spectrum of suspected etiologies. *Chest* 2000;117(1):251–259.

Khoor A, Leslie KO, Tazelaar HD, et al. Diffuse pulmonary disease caused by nontuberculous Mycobacteria in immunocompetent people (hot tub lung). *Am J Clin Pathol* 2001;115(5): 755–762.

Myers JL, Colby TV, Yousem SA. Common pathways and patterns of lung injury. In: Dail DH, Hammar SP, eds. *Pulmonary Pathology,* 2nd ed. New York: Springer-Verlag, 1994:57–78.

Pardo A, Barrios R, Gaxiola M, et al. Increase of lung neutrophils in hypersensitivity pneumonitis is associated with lung fibrosis. *Am J Respir Crit Care Med* 2000;161(5):1698–1704.

Selman M. Hypersensitivity pneumonitis. In: Schwarz MI, King TE Jr, eds. *Interstitial Lung Disease,* 3rd ed. Hamilton: BC Decker, 1998:393–422.

Thurlbeck WM. Chronic airflow obstruction. In: Thurlbeck WM, Churg AM, eds. *Pathology of the Lung,* 2nd ed. New York: Thieme, 1995:739–826.

Travis WD, Colby TV, Koss MN, et al. Diffuse parenchymal lung diseases. In: King DW, ed. *Non-neoplastic Disorders of the Lower Respiratory Tract.* Bethesda, MD: American Registry of Pathology and AFIP, 2002:115–122.

Travis WD, Colby TV, Koss MN, et al. Lung infections. In: King DW, ed. *Non-neoplastic Disorders of the Lower Respiratory Tract.* Bethesda, MD: American Registry of Pathology and AFIP, 2002:638–660.

Travis WD, Colby TV, Koss MN, et al. Idiopathic interstitial pneumonia and other diffuse parenchymal lung diseases. In: King DW, ed. *Non-neoplastic Disorders of the Lower Respiratory Tract.* Washington DC: American Registry of Pathology and The Armed Forces Institute of Pathology, 2002:49–232.

Travis WD, Colby TV, Koss MN, et al. Connective tissue and inflammatory bowel diseases. In: King DW, ed. *Non-neoplastic Disorders of the Lower Respiratory Tract.* Bethesda, MD: American Registry of Pathology and AFIP, 2002:310–313.

Wright JL. Adult Respiratory Distress Syndrome. In: Thurlbeck WM, Churg A, eds. *Pathology of the Lung,* 2nd ed. New York: Thieme, 1995:387–397.

Section 16: Idiopathic Interstitial Pneumonias

Cagle PT. Usual or nonspecific interstitial pneumonia, interstitial fibrosis and the honeycomb lung. In: Saldana M, ed. *Pathology of Pulmonary Disease.* Philadelphia: JB Lipincott, 1994:325–339.

Cagle PT. Chronic interstitial pneumonias with specific histologic features. In: Saldana M, ed. *Pathology of Pulmonary Disease.* Philadelphia: JB Lipincott, 1994:341–355.

Dail DH. Intraalveolar exudates/infiltrates. In: Cagle PT, ed. *Diagnostic Pulmonary Pathology.* New York: Marcel Dekker, 2000:155–178.

Demedts M, Costabel U. ATS/ERS international multidisciplinary consensus classification of the idiopathic interstitial pneumonias. *Eur Respir J* 2002;19:794–796.

Flaherty KR, Colby TV, Travis WD, et al. Fibroblastic foci in usual interstitial pneumonia: Idiopathic versus collagen vascular disease. *Am J Respir Crit Care Med* 2003;167(10):1410–1415.

Katzenstein AL, Zisman D, Litzky LA, et al. Usual interstitial pneumonia: histologic study of biopsy and explant specimens. *Am J Surg Pathol* 2002;26(12):1567–1577.

Katzenstein AL, Myers JL, Mazur MT. Acute interstitial pneumonia: a clinicopathologic, ultrastructural, and cell kinetic study. *Am J Surg Pathol* 1986;10:256–267.

Olson J, Colby TV, Elliott CG. Hamman-Rich syndrome revisited. *Mayo Clin Proc* 1990;65: 1538–1548.

Roggli VL, Oury T. Interstitial fibrosis, predominantly mature. In: Cagle PT, ed. *Diagnostic Pulmonary Pathology.* New York: Marcel Dekker, 2000:77–100.

Sharma A. Interstitial lymphocytic infiltrates. In: Cagle PT, ed. *Diagnostic Pulmonary Pathology.* New York: Marcel Dekker, 2000:49–73.

Talamadge KE. Clinical diagnosis of interstitial infiltrates. In: Cagle PT, ed. *Diagnostic Pulmonary Pathology.* New York: Marcel Dekker, 2000:103–140.

Travis WD, Colby TV, Koss MN, et al. Idiopathic interstitial pneumonia and other diffuse parenchymal lung diseases. In: King DW, ed. *Non-neoplastic Disorders OF THE Lower Respiratory Tract.* Washington, DC: American Registry of Pathology and The Armed Forces Institute of Pathology, 2002:49–232.

Vourlekis JS, Brown KK, Cool CD, et al. Acute interstitial pneumonitis: case series and review of the literature. *Medicine (Baltimore)* 2000;79:369–378.

Vourlekis JS, Schwarz MI, Cool CD, et al. Nonspecific interstitial pneumonitis as the sole histologic expression of hypersensitivity pneumonitis. *Am J Med* 2002;112:490–493.

Yi, ES. Interstitial and intraalveolar fibrosis, predominantly immature. In: Cagle PT, ed. *Diagnostic Pulmonary Pathology.* New York: Marcel Dekker, 2000:141–154.

Zander DS. Idiopathic Interstitial pneumonias and the concept of the trump card. [Editorial] *Chest* 2004;125:359–360.

Section 17: Specific Infectious Agents

Abromova FA, Grinberg LM, Yampolskaya OV, Walker DH. Pathology of inhalation anthrax in 42 cases from the Sverdlovsk outbreak of 1979. *Proc Natl Acad Sci USA* 1993;90:2291–2294.

Arbustini E, Grasso M, Diegoli M, et al. Histopathologic and molecular profile of human cytomegalovirus infection in patients with heart transplants. *Am J Clin Pathol* 1992;98:205–213.

Arean VM. The pathologic anatomy and pathogenesis of fatal human leptospirosis (Weil's disease). *Am J Pathol* 1962;40:393–423.

Baird JK, Neafie RC, Marty AM. Parasitic Infections. In: Dail DH, Hammar SP, eds. *Pulmonary Pathology,* 2nd ed. New York: Springer Verlag, 1994:491–536.

Bausch DG, Ksiazek TG. Viral hemorrhagic fevers including hantavirus pulmonary syndrome in the Americas. *Clin Lab Med* 2002;22:981–1020, viii.

Becroft DM. Histopathology of fatal adenovirus infection of the respiratory tract in young children. *J Clin Pathol* 1967;20:561–569.

Becroft DM, Osborne DR. The lungs in fatal measles infection in childhood: pathological, radiological and immunological correlations. *Histopathology* 1980;4:401–412.

Bertoli F, Espino M, Arosemena JR, et al. A spectrum in the pathology of toxoplasmosis in patients with AIDS. *Arch Pathol Lab Med* 1995;119:214–224.

Bigio EH, Haque AK. Disseminated cytomegalovirus infection presenting with acalculous cholecystitis and acute pancreatitis. *Arch Pathol Lab Med* 1989;113:1287–1289.

Bogucki S, Weir S. Pulmonary manifestations of intentionally released chemical and biological agents. *Clin Chest Med* 2002;23(4):777–794.

Bosken CH, Myers JL, Greenberger PA, Katzenstein ALA. Pathologic features of allergic bronchopulmonary aspergillosis. *Am J Surg Pathol* 1988;12:216–222.

Catterall JR, Hofflin JM, Remington JS. Pulmonary toxoplasmosis. *Am Rev Respir Dis* 1986;133:704–705.

Chandler FW, Connor DH. Actinomycosis. In: Connor DH, Chandler FW, eds. *Pathology of Infectious Diseases.* Stamford, CT: Appleton & Lange, 1997:391–396.

Chandler FW. Nocardiosis. In: Connors DH, Chandler FW, eds. *Pathology of Infectious Diseases.* Stamford, CT: Appleton & Lange, 1997:701–708.

Chandler FW. Blastomycosis. In: Connor DH, Chandler FW, eds. *Pathology of Infectious Diseases.* Stamford, CT: Appleton and Lange, 1997:943–1615.

Chandler FW, Watts JC. Cryptococcosis. In: Connor DH, Chandler FW, eds. *Pathology of Infectious Diseases.* Stamford, CT: Appleton and Lange, 1997:989–997, 1617.

Chandler FW, Watts JC. Fungal infections. In: Dail DH, Hammar SP, eds. *Pulmonary Pathology,* 2nd ed. New York: Springer-Verlag, 1994:351–411.

Chandler FW, Watts JC. Histoplasmosis capsulate. In: Connor DH, Chandler FW, eds. *Pathology of Infectious Diseases.* Connecticut: Appleton and Lange, 1997:857–868.

Charrel RN, de Lamballerie X. Arenaviruses other than Lassa virus. *Antiviral Res* 2003;57:89–100.

Clark BM, Greenwood BM. Pulmonary lesions in African histoplasmosis. *J Trop Med Hygiene* 1968;71:4–10.

Cohen PR, Beltrani VP, Grossman ME. Disseminated herpes zoster in patients with human immunodeficiency virus infection. *Am J Med* 1988;84:1076–1080.

Connor DH, Lack EE. Tuberculosis. In: Connor DH, Chandler FW, eds. *Pathology of Infectious Diseases.* Stamford, CT: Appleton and Lange, 1997.

Crnich CJ, Gordon B, Andes D. Hot tub-associated necrotizing pneumonia due to Pseudomonas aeruginosa. *Clin Infect Dis* 2003;36:e55.

Cupples JB, Blackie SP, Road JD. Granulomatous Pneumocystis carinii pneumonia mimicking tuberculosis. *Arch Pathol Lab Med* 1989;113:1281–1284.

DeBrito T, Bohm GM, Yasuda PH. Vascular damage in acute experimental leptospirosis of the guinea pig. *J Pathol* 1979;128:177–182.

De Mazione N, Salsa RA, Paredes H, et al. Venezuelan hemorrhagic fever: clinical and epidemiological studies of 165 cases. *Clin Infect Dis* 1998;26(2):308–313.

Ding Y, Wang H, Shen H, Li Z, et al. The clinical pathology of severe acute respiratory syndrome (SARS): a report from China. *J Pathol* 2003;200:282–289.

Donisi A, Suardi MG, Casari S, et al. Rhodococcus equi infection in HIV-infected patients. *AIDS* 1996;10:359.

England DM, Hochholzer L. Primary pulmonary sporotrichosis: report of eight cases with clinicopathologic review. *Am J Surg Pathol* 1985;9:193–204.

Feldman S. Varicella-zoster virus pneumonitis. *Chest* 1994;106[1 Suppl]:22S–27S.

FloresBM, Garcia CA, Stamm WE, Torian BE. Differentiation of Naegleria fowleri from Acanthamoeba species by using monoclonal antibodies and flow cytometry. *J Clin Microbiol* 1990;28:1999–2005.

Fish DG, Ampel NM, Galgiani JN, et al. Coccidiomycosis during human immunodeficiency virus infection: a review of 77 patients. *Medicine* 1990;69:384–391.

Fraire AE, Libraty D, Dizon JR, et al. Immunopathology of early stage severe acute respiratory syndrome (SARS). *Mod Pathol* 2004;17[Suppl 1]:336A.

Franks T, Chong PY, Chui P, et al. Lung pathology of severe acute respiratory syndrome (SARS): a study of 8 autopsy cases from Singapore. *Hum Pathol* 2003;34:743–748.

Fraser RS. Protozoal and helminthic pulmonary infections. In: Thurlbeck WM, Churg AM, eds. *Pathology of the Lung,* 2nd ed. New York: Thieme, 1995:333–348.

Fraser DW, Tsai TR, Orenstein W, et al. Legionnaires' disease: description of an epidemic of pneumonia. *N Engl J Med* 1977;297:1189.

Friedland LR, Raphael SA, Deutsch ES, et al. Disseminated Acanthamoeba infection in a child with symptomatic human immunodeficiency virus infection. *Pediatr Infect Dis J* 1992;11:404–407.

Feldman PS, Cohan MA, Hierholzer WJJ. Fatal Hong Kong influenza: a clinical, microbiological and pathological analysis of nine cases. *Yale J Biol Med* 1972;45:49–63.

Gal AA, Koss MN, Striegle S, et al. Pneumocystis carinii Infection in the acquired immunodeficiency syndrome. *Semin Diagn Pathol* 1989;6:287–299.

Genta RM, Haque AK. Strongyloidiasis. In: Connor DH, Chandler FW, eds. *Pathology of Infectious Diseases.* Stamford, CT: Appleton and Lange, 1997:1567–1576.

Godwin JH, Stopeck A, Chang VT et al. Mycobacteremia in acquired immunodeficiency syndrome. *Am J Clin Pathol* 1991;95:369–375.

Graham BS, Snell JD Jr. Herpes simplex virus infection of the adult lower respiratory tract. *Medicine (Baltimore)* 1983;62(6):384–393.

Green WR, Williams AW. Neonatal adenovirus pneumonia. *Arch Pathol Lab Med* 1989;113:190–191.

Greenfield RA, Brown BR, Hutchins JB, et al. Microbiological, biological, and chemical weapons of warfare and terrorism. *Am J Med Sci* 2002;323(6):326–340.

Gremilion DH, Crawford GE. Measles pneumonia in young adults: an analysis of 106 cases. *Am J Med* 1981;71:539–542.

Gullett J, Mills J, Hadley K, et al. Disseminated granulomatous Acanthamoeba infection presenting as an unusual skin lesion. *Am J Med* 1979;67:891–895.

Hans CS, Miller W, Haake R, Weisdorf D. Varicella zoster infection after bone marrow transplantation: incidence, risk factors, and complications. *Bone Marrow Transplant* 1994;13:277–283.

Haque AK. Pathology of common pulmonary fungal infections. *J Thorac Imaging* 1992;7(4):1–11.

Haque AK. The pathology and pathophysiology of mycobacterial infections. *J Thorac Imaging* 1990;5:8–16.

Haque AK, Schnadig V, Rubin SA, et al. Pathogenesis of human strongyloidiasis: autopsy and quantitative parasitological analysis. *Mod Pathol* 1994;7:276–288

Harding CV. Blastomycosis and opportunistic infections in patients with acquired immunodeficiency syndrome. An autopsy study. *Arch Pathol Lab Med* 1991;115:1133–1136.

Javaly K, Horowitz HW, Wormser GP. Nocardiosis in patients with human immunodeficiency virus infection: report of 2 cases and review of the literature. *Medicine* 1992;71:128.

Jaax NK, Fritz DL. Anthrax. In: Connor DH, Chandler FW, eds. *Pathology of infectious diseases.* Stamford, CT: Appleton and Lange, 1997:397–406.

Jortani SA, Snyder JW, Valdes R. The role of the clinical laboratory in managing chemical or biological terrorism. *Clin Chem* 2000;46(12):1883–1893.

Kawamoto F. Rapid diagnosis of malaria by fluorescence microscopy with light microscope and interference. *Lancet* 1991;337:200–202.

Kazandjian D, Chiew R, Gilbert GL. Rapid diagnosis of Legionella pneumophila serogroup1 infection with the Binax enzyme immunoassay urinary antigen test. *J Clin Microbiol* 1997;35:954.

Khalifa MA, Lack EE. Herpes simplex virus infection. In: Connor DH, ed. *Pathology of Infectious Diseases.* Stamford, CT: Appleton and Lange, 1997:147–152.

Kim EA, Lee KS, Primack SL, et al. Viral pneumonias in adults: radiologic and pathologic findings. *Radiographics* 2002;Spec No:S137–S149.

Kissane JM. Staphylococcal Infections. In: Connors DH, Chandler FW, eds. *Pathology of Infectious Diseases.* Stamford, CT: Appleton & Lange, 1997:805–816.

Klatt EC, Shibata D. Cytomegalovirus infection in the acquired immunodeficiency syndrome: clinical and autopsy findings. *Arch Pathol Lab Med* 1988;112:540–544.

Kocher AS. Human pulmonary dirofilariasis: report of three cases and brief review of the literature. *Am J Clin Pathol* 1985;84:19–23.

Kuhn, C. III. Bacterial infections. In: Thurlbeck WM, Churg AM, eds. *Pathology of the Lung,* 2nd ed. New York: Thieme, 1995:267–302.

Kwon KY, Colby TV. Rhodococcus equi pneumonia and pulmonary malakoplakia in acquired immunodeficiency syndrome. *Arch Pathol Lab Med* 1994;118:744.

Lazarus AA, Deveraux A. Potential agents of chemical warfare. *Postgrad Med* 2002;112(5):133–140.

Lee SH, Barnes WG, Schaetzel WP. Pulmonary aspergillosis and the importance of oxalate crystal recognition in cytology specimens. *Arch Pathol Lab Med* 1986;110:1176–1179.

Levine SJ, White DA, Fels AOS. The incidence and significance of Staphylococcus aureus in respiratory cultures from patients infected with the human immunodeficiency virus. *Am Rev Respir Dis* 1990;141:89.

Lieberman D, Porath A, Schlaeffer F, et al. Legionella species community-acquired pneumonia: a review of 56 hospitalized adult patients. *Chest* 1996;109:1243.

Little BW, Tihen WS, Dickerman JD, Craighead JE. Giant cell pneumonia associated with parainfluenza virus type 3 infection. *Hum Pathol* 1981;12:478–481.

Ma P, Visvesvara GS, Martinez AJ, et al. Naegleria and Acanthamoeba infections: review. *Rev Infect Dis* 1990;12:490–513.

Marchevsky AM, Bottone EJ, Geller SA, et al. The changing spectrum of disease, etiology, and diagnosis of mucormycosis. *Hum Pathol* 1980;11:457–464.

Martinez AJ, Markowitz SM, Duma RJ. Experimental pneumonitis and encephalitis caused by acanthamoeba in mice: pathogenesis and ultrastructural features. *J Infect Dis* 1975;131(6):692–699.

Miller RR. Viral infections of the respiratory tract. In: Thurlbeck WM, Churg AM, eds. *Pathology of the Lung,* 2nd ed. New York: Theime, 1995:195–222.

Miller RR. Mycoplasma, chlamydia, and coxiella infections of the respiratory tract. In: Thurlbeck WM, Churg AM, eds. *Pathology of the Lung,* 2nd ed. New York: Thieme, 1995:223–228.

Mitchell TG, Perfect JR. Cryptococcosis in the era of AIDS: 100 years after the discovery of Cryptococcus neoformans. *Clin Microbiol Rev* 1995;8:515–548.

Monath TP, Barrett AD. Pathogenesis and pathophysiology of yellow fever. *Adv Virus Res* 2003;60:343–395.

Nahass GT, Goldstein BA, Zhu WY, et al. Comparison of Tzanck smear, viral culture, and DNA diagnostic methods in detection of herpes simplex and varicella-zoster infection. *JAMA* 1992;268:2541–2544.

Naib ZM, Stewart JA, Dowdle WR, et al. Cytologic features of viral respiratory tract infections. *Acta Cytol* 1968;12:162–171.

Nash G, Kerschma RL, Herndier B, Dubey JP. The pathological manifestations of pulmonary toxoplasmosis in the acquired immunodeficiency syndrome. *Hum Pathol* 1994;25:652–658.

Neilson KA, Yunis EJ. Demonstration of respiratory syncytial virus in an autopsy series. *Pediatr Pathol* 1990;10:491–502.

Nicholls JM, Poon LLM, Lee KC, et al. Lung pathology of fatal severe acute respiratory syndrome. *Lancet* 2003;361:1773–1778.

Nicodemo AC, Duarte MIS, Alves VAF, et al. Lung lesions in human leptospirosis: microscopic, immunohistochemical, and ultrastructural features related to thrombocytopenia. *Am J Trop Med Hygiene* 1997;56:181–187.

Nolte KB, Feddersen RM, Foucar K et al. Hantavirus pulmonary syndrome in the United States: pathologic description of a disease caused by a new agent. *Hum Pathol* 1995;26:110–120.

Olano JP, Walker DH. Human ehrlichioses. *Med Clin North Am* 2002;86(2):375–392.

Pappagianis D, Chandler FW. Coccidiomycosis. In: Connor DH, Chandler FW, eds. *Pathology of Infectious Diseases.* Stamford, CT: Appleton and Lange, 1997:977–1617.

Phillips RE, Warrell DA. The pathophysiology of severe falciparum malaria. *Parasitol Today* 1986;2:271–282.

Portnoy LG. Dirofilariasis. In: Connor DH, Chandler FW, eds. *Pathology of Infectious Diseases.* Stamford, CT: Appleton and Lange, 1997:1391–1396.

Radoycich GE, Zuppan CW, Weeks DA, et al. Patterns of measles pneumonitis. *Ped Pathol* 1992;12: 773–786.

Rinaldi MG. Invasive aspergillosis. *Rev Infect Dis* 1983;5:1061–1077.

Rosenbloom M, Leikin JB, Vogel SN, et al. Biological and chemical agents: a brief synopsis. *Am J Ther* 2002;9(1):5–15.

Rotterdam H. Mycobacterium avium complex (MAC) infection. In: Connor DH, Chandler FW, eds. *Pathology of Infectious Diseases.* Stamford, CT: Appleton and Lange, 1997:657–669.

Sarinas PS, Chitkara RK. Ascariasis and hookworm. *Semin Respir Infect* 1997;12(2):130–137.

Schwartz E. Pulmonary schistosomiasis. *Clin Chest Med* 2002;23(2):433–443.

Schwartz DA, Geyer SJ. Klebsiella and rhinoscleroma. In: Connors DH, Chandler FW, eds. *Pathology of Infectious Diseases.* Stamford, CT: Appleton & Lange, 1997: 589–596.

Schwartz TF, Zaki SR, Morzunov S, et al. Detection and sequence confirmation of Sin Nombre virus RNA in paraffin-embedded human tissues using one-step RT-PCR. *J Virol Methods* 1995;51:349–356.

Sepkowitz KA, Brown AE, Telzak EE, et al. Pneumocystis carinii pneumonia among patients without AIDS at a cancer hospital. *JAMA* 1992;267:832–837.

Shields AF, Hackman RC, Fife KH, et al. Adenovirus infections in patients undergoing bone-marrow transplantation. *N Engl J Med* 1985;312:529–533.

Slavin MA, Meyers JD, Remington JS, Hackman RC. Toxoplasma gondii infection in marrow transplant recipients: a 20 year experience. *Bone Marrow Transplant* 1994;13:549–557.

Srinivasan A, Wolfenden LL, Song X, et al. An outbreak of Pseudomonas aeruginosa infections associated with flexible bronchoscopes. *N Engl J Med* 2003;348:221.

Stocker JT, Conran RM, Fishback N. Respiratory syncytial virus. In: Connor DH, ed. *Pathology of Infectious Diseases.* Stamford, CT: Appleton and Lange, 1997:287–295.

Stout JE, Yu VL. Legionellosis. *N Engl J Med* 1997;337:682.

Sugar AM. Mucormycosis. *Clin Infect Dis* 1992;14:S126–S129.

Tappero JW, Ashford DA, Perkins BA. Leptospira species (Leptospirosis). In: Mandell GL, Bennett JE, Dolin R, eds. *Principles and Practice of Infectious Diseases.* Philadelphia: Churchill Livingstone, 2000.

Tesh RB. Viral hemorrhagic fevers of South America. *Biomedica* 2002;22:287–295.

Travis WD, Colby TV, Koss MN, et al. Lung infections. In: King DW, ed. *Non-neoplastic Disorders of the Lower Respiratory Tract.* Bethesda, MD: American Registry of Pathology and AFIP, 2002:539–728.

Travis WD, Colby TV, Koss MN, et al. Bronchial disorders. In: King DW, ed. *Non-neoplastic Disorders of the Lower Respiratory Tract.* Bethesda, MD: American Registry of Pathology and AFIP, 2002:381–434.

Urbanetti JS. Toxic inhalation injury. In: Zajtchuk R, Bellamy RF, eds. *Medical Aspects of Chemical and Biological Warfare. Textbook of Military Medicine.* Washington, DC: Office of the Surgeon General, Department of the Army, 1997:47–70.

Wachowski O, Demirakca S, Muller KM, Sheurlen W. Mycoplasma pneumoniae associated organizing pneumonia in a 10 year old boy. *Arch Dis Child* 2003;88(3):270–272.

Walker DH, Crawford CG, Cain BG. Rickettsial infection of the pulmonary microcirculation: the basis for interstitial pneumonitis in Rocky Mountain spotted fever. *Hum Pathol* 1980;11:263–272.

Walker DH, Dumler SJ. Rickettsial infections. In: Connor DH, Chandler FW, Manz HJ, et al, eds. *Pathology of Infectious Diseases.* Stamford, CT: Appleton & Lange, 1997:789–799.

Walker DH, Valbuena GA, Olano JP. Pathogenic mechanisms of diseases caused by Rickettsia. *Ann NY Acad Sci* 2003;990:1–11.

Watts JC, Chandler FW. Aspergillosis. In: Connor DH, Chandler FW, eds. *Pathology of Infectious Diseases.* Stamford, CT: Appleton and Lange, 1997:933–1117.

Watts JC, Chandler FW. Pneumocystosis. In: Connor DH, Chandler FW, eds. *Pathology of Infectious Diseases.* Stamford, CT: Appleton and Lange, 1997:1241–1251.

Winn WC JR, Chandler FW. Bacterial infections. In: Dail DH, Hammar SP, eds. *Pulmonary Pathology,* 2nd ed. New York: Springer-Verlag, 1994:255–330.

Winn WC, Walker DH. Viral infections. In: Dail DH, Hammar SP, eds. *Pulmonary Pathology,* 2nd ed. New York: Springer-Verlag, 1994:429–464.

World Health Organization. Severe and complicated malaria. *Trans Roy Soc Trop Med Hygiene* 1990;84[Suppl 2]:1–65.

Yuoh G, Hove MGM, Wen, J, Haque AK. Pulmonary malakoplakia in acquired immunodeficiency syndrome: an ultrastructural study of morphogenesis of Michaelis-Gutmann bodies. *Mod Pathol* 1996;9(5):476.

Zaki SR, Greer PW, Coffield LM, et al. Hantavirus pulmonary syndrome: pathogenesis of an emerging infectious disease. *Am J Pathol* 1995;146:552–579.

Zaki SR. Hantavirus-associated diseases. In: Connor DH, ed. *Pathology of infectious diseases.* Stamford, CT: Appleton and Lange, 1997:125–136.

Zander DS, Cicale MJ, Mergo P. Durable cure of mucormycosis involving allograft and native lungs. *J Heart Lung Transplant* 2000;19:615–618.

Section 18: Transplant-Specific Pathology

Bando K, Paradis IL, Similo S, et al. Obliterative bronchiolitis after lung and heart-lung transplantation: an analysis of risk factors and management. *J Thorac Cardiovasc Surg* 1995;110:4–13.

Baz MA, Layish DT, Govert JA, et al. Diagnostic yield of bronchoscopies after isolated lung transplantation. *Chest* 1996;110:84–88.

Cagle PT. Lung transplant pathology. In: Churg AM, ed. *Pathology of the Lung,* 3rd ed. New York: Thieme Medical Publishers, 2004 *(in press).*

Cagle PT, Brown RW, Frost A, et al. Diagnosis of chronic lung transplant rejection by transbronchial biopsy. *Mod Pathol* 1995;8:137–142.

Collins J, Muller NL, Leung AN, et al. Epstein-Barr-virus-associated lymphoproliferative disease of the lung: CT and histologic findings. *Radiology* 1998;208:749–759.

Cooper JD, Billingham M, Egan T, et al. A working formulation for the standardization of nomenclature and for clinical staging of chronic dysfunction in lung allografts. International Society for Heart and Lung Transplantation. *J Heart Lung Transplant* 1993;12:713–716.

Dail DH, Hammar SP, eds. *Pulmonary Pathology,* 2nd ed. New York: Springer-Verlag, 1994.

DePerrot M, Liu M, Waddell TK, et al. Ischemia-reperfusion-induced lung injury. *Am J Respir Crit Care Med* 2003;167:490–511.

Frost AE, Jammal CT, Cagle PT. Hyperacute rejection following lung transplantation. *Chest* 1996;110:559–562.

Griffith BP, Magee MJ, Gonzalez IF, et al. Anastomotic pitfalls in lung transplantation. *J Thorac Cardiovasc Surg* 1994;107:743–753.

Harris NL, Ferry JA, Swerdlow SH. Posttransplant lymphoproliferative disorders: summary of Society for Hematopathology Workshop. *Semin Diagn Pathol* 1997;14:8–14.

Hosenpud JD, Bennett LE, Keck BM, et al. The Registry of the International Society for Heart and Lung Transplantation: eighteenth official report—2001. *J Heart Lung Transplant* 2001;20:805–815.

Keller CA, Cagle PT, Brown RW, et al. Bronchiolitis obliterans in recipients of single, double and heart-lung transplantation. *Chest* 1995;108:277–280.

Knowles DM. Immunodeficiency-associated lymphoproliferative disorders. *Mod Pathol* 1999;12: 200–217.

Knowles DM, Cesarman E, Chadburn A, et al. Correlative morphologic and molecular genetic analysis demonstrates three distinct categories of posttransplantation lymphoproliferative disorders. *Blood* 1995;85:552–565.

Kshettry VR, Kroshus TJ, Hertz MI, et al. Early and late airway complications after lung transplantation: incidence and management. *Ann Thorac Surg* 1997;63:1576–1583.

Nalesnik MA. Clinicopathologic characteristics of post-transplant lymphoproliferative disorders. *Recent Results Cancer Res* 2002;159:9–18.

Nalesnik MA. The diverse pathology of post-transplant lymphoproliferative disorders: the importance of a standardized approach. *Transplant Infect Dis* 2001;3:88–96.

Saldana MJ, ed. *Pathology of Pulmonary Disease.* Philadelphia: JB Lippincott, 1994.

Scornik JC, Zander DS, Baz MA, et al. Susceptibility of lung transplants to preformed donor-specific HLA antibodies as detected by flow cytometry. *Transplantation* 1999;68:1542–1546.

Siddiqui MT, Garrity ER, Husain AN. Bronchiolitis obliterans organizing pneumonia-like reactions: a nonspecific response or an atypical form of rejection or infection in lung allograft recipients? *Hum Pathol* 1996;27:714–719.

Urbanski SJ, Kossakowska AE, Curtis J, et al. Idiopathic small airways pathology in patients with graft-versus-host disease following allogeneic bone marrow transplantation. *Am J Surg Pathol* 1987;11:965–971.

Wolff D, Reichenberger F, Steiner B, et al. Progressive interstitial fibrosis of the lung in sclerodermoid chronic graft-versus-host disease. *Bone Marrow Transplant* 2002;29:357–360.

Yousem SA. Alveolar lipoproteinosis in lung allograft recipients. *Hum Pathol* 1997;28:1383–1386.

Yousem SA. The histological spectrum of pulmonary graft-versus host disease in bone marrow transplant recipients. *Hum Pathol* 1995;26:668–675.

Yousem SA, Berry GJ, Cagle PT, et al. Revision of the 1990 working formulation for the classification of pulmonary allograft rejection: lung rejection study group. *J Heart Lung Transplant* 1996;15:1–15.

Yousem SA, Duncan SR, Griffith BP. Interstitial and airspace granulation tissue reactions in lung transplant recipients. *Am J Surg Pathol* 1992;16:877–884.

Yousem SA, Randhawa P, Locker J, et al. Posttransplant lymphoproliferative disorders in heart-lung transplant recipients: primary presentation in the allograft. *Hum Pathol* 1989;20:361–369.

Zander DS. Transplant-related pathology. In: Cagle PT, ed. *Diagnostic Pulmonary Pathology.* New York: Marcel Dekker, 2000:461–484.

Zander DS, Baz MA, Visner GA, et al. Analysis of early deaths after isolated lung transplantation. *Chest* 2001;120(1):225–232.

Section 19: Lung Pathology in Collagen Vascular Disease

Katzenstein A-LA, ed. *Katzenstein and Askin's Surgical Pathology of Non-neoplastic Lung Disease,* 3rd ed. Philadelphia: W.B. Saunders, 1997.

Travis WD, Colby TV, Koss MN, et al. *Non-neoplastic Disorders of the Lower Respiratory Tract.* Washington, DC: Armed Forces Institute of Pathology and American Registry of Pathology, 2001.

Section 20: Therapeutic Drug Reactions and Radiation Effects

Casey MB, Tazelaar HD, Myers JL, et al. Noninfectious lung pathology in patients with Crohn's disease. *Am J Surg Pathol* 2003;27:213–219.

Colby TV, Carrington CB. Interstitial lung disease. In: Thurlbeck WM, Churg AM, eds. *Pathology of the Lung,* 2nd ed. New York: Thieme Medical Publishers, 1995:589–738.

Donaldson L, Grant IS, Naysmith MR, Thomas JS. Acute amiodarone-induced lung toxicity. *Int Care Med* 1998;24:626–630.

Foster RA, Zander DS, Mergo PJ, et al. Mesalamine-related lung disease: clinical, radiographic, and pathologic manifestations. *Inflamm Bowel Dis* 2003;9(5):308–315.

Fraire AE, Guntupalli KK, Greenberg SD, et al. Amiodarone pulmonary toxicity: a multidisciplinary review of current status. *South Med J* 1993;86(1): 67–77.

Imokawa S, Colby, TV, Leslie KO, et al. Methotrexate pneumonitis: review of the literature and histopathological findings in nine patients. *Eur Respir J* 2000;15:373–381.

Kaushik S, Hussain A, Clarke P, Lazar HL. Acute pulmonary toxicity after low-dose amiodarone therapy. *Ann Thorac Surg* 2001;72:1760–1761.

Martin WJ, Rosenow EC. Amiodarone pulmonary toxicity: recognition and pathogenesis. *Chest* 1988;93:1067–1075.

Ramzy I. Effects of radiation, chemotherapy, and other therapeutic modalities. In: Ramzy I, ed. *Clinical Cytopathology and Aspiration Biopsy.* New York: McGraw-Hill, 2001:135–143.

Rosiello RA, Merrill WW. Radiation-induced lung injury. *Clin Chest Med* 1990;11(1):65–71.

Rothman RB, Ayestas MA, Dersch CM, et al. Aminorex, fenfluramine, and chlorphentermine are serotonin transporter substrates: implications for primary pulmonary hypertension. *Circulation* 1999;100:869–875.

Tomita T, Zhao Q. Autopsy findings of heart and lungs in a patient with primary pulmonary hypertension associated with use of fenfluramine and phentermine. *Chest* 2002;121:649–652.

Travis WD, Colby TV, Koss MN, et al. Drug and radiation reactions. In: King DW, ed. *Non-neoplastic Disorders of the Lower Respiratory Tract.* Bethesda, MD: American Registry of Pathology and AFIP, 2002:321–347.

Section 21: Forensic Pathology

Bailey ME, Fraire AE, Greenberg SD, et al. Pulmonary histopathology in cocaine abusers. *Hum Pathol* 1994;25(2):203–207.

Ganesan S, Felo J, Tomashefski JR, et al. Embolized crospovidone (poly [N-vinyl-2–pyrrolidone] in the lungs of intravenous drug users. *Mod Pathol* 2003;16(4):286–292.

Herndon DN, Langner F, Thompson P, et al. Pulmonary injury in burned patients. *Surg Clin North Am* 1987;67:31–46.

Karch SB. Pathology of the lung in near-drowning. *Am J Emerg Med* 1986;4:4–9.

Kay JM. Vascular disease. In: Thurlbeck WM, Churg AM, eds. *Pathology of the Lung,* 2nd ed. New York: Thieme, 1995:931–1066.

Roggli VL, Shelburne JD. Pneumoconioses, mineral and vegetable. In: Dail DH, Hammar SP, eds. *Pulmonary Pathology,* 2nd ed. New York: Springer-Verlag, 1994:867–900.

Spitz WU, Fisher RS. *Medicolegal Investigation of Death: Guidelines for the Application of Pathology to Crime Investigation,* 2nd ed. Springfield IL: Charles C. Thomas, 1980.

Thompson PB, Herndon DN, Trabor DL, et al. Effect on mortality of inhalation injury. *J Trauma* 1986;26:163–165.

Toor AH, Tomashefski JF Jr, Kleinerman J. Respiratory tract pathology in patients with severe burns. *Hum Pathol* 1990;21:1212–1220.

Wagner RB, Jameson PM. Pulmonary contusion: evaluation and classification by computed tomography. *Surg Clin North Am* 1989;69:31–40.

Section 22: Metabolic Disorders/Storage Diseases

Cagle PT, Ferry GD, Beaudet AL, Hawkins EP. Clinicopathologic conference: pulmonary hypertension in an 18-year-old girl with cholesteryl ester storage disease (CESD). *Am J Med Genet* 1986;24:711–722.

Colby TV, Carrington CB. Interstitial lung disease. In: Thurlbeck WM, Churg A, eds. *Pathology of the Lung,* 2nd ed. New York: Thieme Medical Publishers, 1995:690–696.

Dail DH. Metabolic and other diseases. In: Dail DH, Hammar SP, eds. *Pulmonary Pathology,* 2nd ed. New York: Springer-Verlag, 1994:728–736.

Lauta VM. Pulmonary alveolar microlithiasis: an overview of clinical and pathological features together with possible therapies. *Respir Med* 2003;97(10):1081–1085.

Moran CA, Hochholzer L, Hasleton PS, et al. Pulmonary alveolar microlithiasis. A clinicopathologic and chemical analysis of seven cases. *Arch Pathol Lab Med* 1997;121(6):607–611.

Nicholson AG, Wells AU, Hooper J, et al. Successful treatment of endogenous lipoid pneumonia due to Niemann-Pick type B disease with whole-lung lavage. *Am J Respir Crit Care Med* 2002; 165(1):128–131.

Travis WD, Colby TV, Koss MN, et al. *Non-neoplastic Disorders of the Lower Respiratory Tract.* Bethesda, MD: American Registry of Pathology and AFIP, 2002:890–892.

Section 23: Nonneoplastic Lesions of the Pleura

Bowman RR, Rosenblatt R, Myers LG. Pleural endometriosis. *BUMC Proc* 1999;12:193–197.

Cagle PT. Pleural histology. In: Light RW, Lee YC, eds. *Textbook of Pleural Diseases.* London: Arnold, 2003:249–255.

Churg A. Diseases of the pleura. In: Thurlbeck WM, Churg AM, eds. *Pathology of the Lung,* 2nd ed. New York: Thieme, 1995:1067–1110.

Churg A, Colby TV, Cagle PT, et al. US-Canadian Mesothelioma Reference Panel. The separation of benign and malignant mesothelial proliferations. *Am J Surg Pathol* 2000;24:1183–1200.

Corrin B. Pleura and chest wall. In: Corrin B, ed. *Pathology of the Lungs.* London: Churchill Livingstone, 2000:607–642.

Dail DH. Uncommon tumors. In: Dail DH, Hammar SP, eds. *Pulmonary Pathology,* 2nd ed. New York: Springer-Verlag, 1994:1279–1462.

Galateau-Salle F, Cagle PT. Nonmalignant versus malignant proliferations on pleural biopsy. In: Cagle PT, ed. *Diagnostic Pulmonary Pathology.* New York: Marcel Dekker, 2000:555–570.

Guinee DG. Pulmonary eosinophilia. In: Cagle PT, ed. *Diagnostic Pulmonary Pathology.* New York: Marcel Dekker, 2000:195–218.

Light RW. Pleural effusions due to obstetric and gynecological conditions. In: Light RW, Lee YC, eds. *Textbook of Pleural Diseases.* London: Arnold, 2003:419–427.

Madjar S, Weissberg D. Thoracic splenosis. *Thorax* 1994;49(10):1020–1022.

Roggli VL, Cagle PT. Pleura, pericardium, and peritoneum. In: Silverberg SG, ed. *Principles and Practice of Surgical Pathology,* 4th ed. Wiley Medical, 2004 *(in press).*

Sarda R, Sproat I, Kurtycz DF, et al. Pulmonary parenchymal splenosis. *Diagn Cytopathol* 2001;24(5):352–355.

Syed S, Zaharopoulos P. Thoracic splenosis diagnosed by fine-needle aspiration cytology: a case report. *Diagn Cytopathol* 2001;25(5):321–324.

Section 24: Pediatric Pulmonary Pathology

Armin A, Castelli M. Congenital adrenal tissue in the lung with adrenal cytomegaly: case report and review of the literature. *Am J Clin Pathol* 1984;82(2):225–228.

Boggs S, Harris MC, Hoffman DJ, et al. Misalignment of pulmonary veins with alveolar capillary dysplasia: affected siblings and variable phenotypic expression. *J Pediatr* 1994;124:125–128.

Bonikos DS, Bensch KG, Northway WH, et al. Bronchopulmonary dysplasia: the pulmonary pathologic sequel of necrotizing bronchiolitis and pulmonary fibrosis. *Hum Pathol* 1976;7:643–666.

Chambers HM. Congenital acinar aplasia: an extreme form of pulmonary maldevelopment. *Pathology* 1991;23:69–71.

Cohen MC, Kaschula ROC. Primary pulmonary tumors in childhood: a review of 31 years experience and the literature. *Pediatr Pulmonol* 1992;14:222–232.

Cole FS, Hamvas A, Nogee LM. Genetic disorders of neonatal respiratory function. *Pediatr Res* 2001;50:157–162.

Dehner LP, Watterson J, Priest JR, et al. Pleuropulmonary blastoma: a unique intrathoracic pulmonary neoplasm of childhood. *Perspect Pediatr Pathol* 1995;18:214–226.

DeMello DE, Nogee LM, Heymans S, et al. Molecular and phenotypic variability in the congenital alveolar proteinosis syndrome associated with inherited surfactant protein B deficiency. *J Pediatr* 1994;124:43–50.

Deterding RR, Fan L, Morton R, et al. Persistent tachypnea of infancy (PTI): a new entity. *Pediatr Pulmonol* 2001;Suppl 23:72–73.

Deterding RR, Pye C, Fan LL, et al. Neuroendocrine cell hyperplasia of infancy. *(submitted).*

Faul JL, Berry GJ, Colby TV, et al. Thoracic lymphangiomas, lymphangiectasis, lymphangiomatosis, and lymphatic dysplasia syndrome. *Am J Respir Crit Care Med* 2000;161:1037–1046.

Fisher M, Roggli V, Merten D, et al. Coexisting endogenous lipoid pneumonia, cholesterol granulomas, and pulmonary alveolar proteinosis in a pediatric population. *Pediatr Pathol* 1992;12:365–383.

Janney CG, Askin FB, Kuhn C. Congenital alveolar capillary dysplasia: an unusual cause or respiratory distress in the newborn. *Am J Clin Pathol* 1981;76:722–727.

Jensen HB, Leach CT, McClain KL, et al. Benign and malignant smooth muscle tumors containing Epstein-Barr virus in children with AIDS. *Leuk Lymphoma* 1997;27:303–314.

Katzenstein A-LA, Gordon LP, Oliphant M, et al. Chronic pneumonitis of infancy. *Am J Surg Pathol* 1995;19:439–447.

Kershisnik MM, Kaplan C, Craven CM, et al. Intrapulmonary neuroglial heterotopia. *Arch Pathol Lab Med* 1992;116(10):1043–1046.

Langston C. New concepts in pathology of congenital lung malformations. *Semin Pediatr Surg* 2003;12(1):17–37.

Langston C. Misalignment of pulmonary veins and alveolar capillary dysplasia. *Pediatr Pathol* 1991;11:163–170.

Langston C, Askin FB. Pulmonary disorders in the neonate, infant, and child. In: Thurlbeck WM, Churg AM, eds. *Pathology of the Lung,* 2nd ed. New York: Thieme, 1995:151–194.

Lee ES, Locker J, Nalesnik M, et al. The association of Epstein-Barr virus with smooth-muscle tumors occurring after organ transplantation. *N Engl J Med* 1995;332:19–25.

Marchevsky AM. Lung tumors derived from ectopic tissues. *Semin Diagn Pathol* 1995;12(2):172–184.

Nogee LM, deMello DE, Dehner LP, et al. Pulmonary surfactant protein B deficiency in congenital pulmonary alveolar proteinosis. *N Engl J Med* 1993;328:406–410.

Nogee LM, Dunbar AE, Wert SE, et al. A mutation in the surfactant protein C gene associated with familial interstitial lung disease. *N Engl J Med* 2001;344(8):573–579.

O'Brodovich HM, Mellins RB. Bronchopulmonary dysplasia: unresolved neonatal acute lung injury. *Am Rev Respir Dis* 1985;132:694–709.

Oppenheimer EH, Esterly JR. Pathology of cystic fibrosis: review of the literature and comparison with 146 autopsied cases. In: Rosenberg HS, Bolande RP, eds. *Perspectives in Pediatric Pathology, vol. 2.* Chicago: Year Book, 1975.

Orenstein DM, Winnie GB, Altman H. Cystic fibrosis: a 2002 update. *J Pediatr* 2002;140:156–164.

Priest JR, Watterson J, Strong L, et al. Pleuropulmonary blastoma: a marker for familial disease. *J Pediatr* 1996;128:220–224.

Rabah R, Poulik JM. Congenital alveolar capillary dysplasia with misalignment of pulmonary veins associated with hypoplastic left heart syndrome. *Pediatr Dev Pathol* 2001;4:167–174.

Reyes C, Abuzaitoun O, DeJong A, et al. Epstein-Barr virus associated smooth muscle tumors in ataxia-telangiectasia: a case report and review. *Hum Pathol* 2002;133:133–136.

Rutledge JC, Jensen P. Acinar dysplasia: a new form of pulmonary maldevelopment. *Hum Pathol* 1986;17:1290–1293.

Stocker JT. The respiratory tract. In: Stocker JT, Dehner LP, eds. *Pediatric Pathology,* 2nd ed. Philadelphia: Lippincott Williams & Wilkins, 2001:445–517.

Stocker JT, Drake RM, Madewell. Congenital cystic adenomatoid malformation of the lung. Classification and morphologic spectrum. *Hum Pathol* 1977;8:155–171.

Stocker JT, Madewell JE. Persistent interstitial pulmonary emphysema: another complication of the respiratory distress syndrome. *Pediatrics* 1977;59:847–857.

Tazelaar HD, Kerr D, Yousem SA, et al. Diffuse pulmonary lymphangiomatosis. *Hum Pathol* 1993;24:1313–1322.

Tomashefski JF Jr, Dahms B, Abramowsky CA. The pathology of cystic fibrosis. In: Davis PB, ed. *Cystic Fibrosis.* New York: Marcel Dekker, 1994:435–489.

Vargas SO, Nose V, Fletcher JA, et al. Gains of chromosomes 8 are confined to mesenchymal components in pleuropulmonary blastoma. *Pediatr Dev Pathol* 2001;5:221–222.

Wright JR. Pleuropulmonary blastoma: a case report documenting transition from type I (cystic) to type III (solid). *Cancer* 2000;88:2853–2858.

Zimmerman JJ, Farrell PM. Advances and issues in bronchopulmonary dysplasia. *Curr Prob Pediatr* 1995;24:159–170.

Index

D

I

N

O

P